A Practice Manual for Community Nursing in Australia

Dedication

This manual is dedicated to the many Australians who have needed the care of community nurses. We also dedicate this manual to Australia's community nurses who are fulfilling one of the most challenging roles in health care and are devoted to the well-being of Australian people needing their care.

A Practice Manual for Community Nursing in Australia

Edited by

Debbie Kralik
RN, PhD
Director of Research
Royal District Nursing Service
South Australia

Katherine Trowbridge
RN (Mstr Nsg Science – Nrs Prac)
Research Associate
Royal District Nursing Service
South Australia

Judy Smith
RN (Mstr Nsg), BApplSc (Nsg), DipApplSc (Nsg)
Executive Director of Nursing and Client Services
Royal District Nursing Service
South Australia

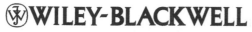
WILEY-BLACKWELL

A John Wiley & Sons, Ltd., Publication

This edition first published 2008
© 2008 Blackwell Publishing Ltd

Blackwell Publishing was acquired by John Wiley & Sons in February 2007. Blackwell's publishing programme has been merged with Wiley's global Scientific, Technical, and Medical business to form Wiley-Blackwell.

Registered office
John Wiley & Sons Ltd, The Atrium, Southern Gate, Chichester, West Sussex, PO19 8SQ, United Kingdom

Editorial offices
9600 Garsington Road, Oxford, OX4 2DQ, United Kingdom
350 Main Street, Malden, MA 02148-5020, USA

For details of our global editorial offices, for customer services and for information about how to apply for permission to reuse the copyright material in this book please see our website at www.wiley.com/wiley-blackwell.

Library of Congress Cataloging-in-Publication Data
A practice manual for community nursing in Australia / edited by Debbie Kralik, Katherine Trowbridge, Judy Smith.
       p.   ;   cm.
   Includes bibliographical references and index.
   ISBN 978-1-4051-5964-7 (pbk. : alk. paper)   1. Community health nursing—
Australia—Handbooks, manuals, etc.   I. Kralik, Debbie.   II. Trowbridge, Katherine.
III. Smith, Judy, 1949–
   [DNLM: 1. Community Health Nursing—Australia. WY 106 P8955 2008]
   RT98.P74 2008
   610.73′43–dc22
                                              2008017517

A catalogue record for this book is available from the British Library.

Set in 9.5/11.5 pt Sabon by Aptara Inc., New Delhi, India

1   2008

Contents

List of contributors

Paul Arbon, RN, PhD
Professor of Nursing (Population Health), School of Nursing and Midwifery, Flinders University, Adelaide, South Australia

Cathy Bennett, BA, Grad Dip Hlth Counselling
Clincial Nurse Consultant in Palliative Care, Royal District Nursing Service (RDNS) of SA Inc, Adelaide, South Australia

Norah Bostock, RN, MRCNA, Grad Cert Health (Continence), TAA Cert IV
Continence Nurse Advisor, Royal District Nursing Service (RDNS) of SA Inc, Adelaide, South Australia

Moya Conrick, RN, RM, Dip App Sc, BN, MClEd, PhD
Lecturer, Griffith University, Nathan, Queensland, Australia

Elizabeth Crock, RN, Cert Infectious Diseases Nursing, BSc, Grad Dip Ed (Women's Studies), PhD
Clinical Nurse Consultant HIV/AIDS, Royal District Nursing Service (RDNS), Melbourne, Victoria, Australia

Janette Curtis, RN, BA, Dip Public Health, PhD, FRCNA, MACMHN
HBS Faculty International Advisor and Director of Mental Health Nursing, School of Nursing, Midwifery and Indigenous Health, The University of Wollongong, New South Wales, Australia

Gay Edgecombe, RN, RM, CHN, BachApplSc (Nsg), MS, PhD
Professor, Community Child Health Nursing, Division of Nursing and Midwifery, RMIT University, Victoria, Australia

Irene Ellis, FRCNA, MEd (Monash), BEd Studies, GradDipNurs (Child & Family Health), RN, Midwife
Coordinator, Child & Family Health Nursing, School of Health Sciences, Division of Nursing & Midwifery, RMIT University, Victoria, Australia

Carmen George, RN, Dip Appl Sc (Nsg), Grad Dip Adult Edn, STN (Credentialled)
Previous Director, Clinical Nursing Specialist Services, Adelaide, South Australia

Jane Giles, MN, BEd, Grad Cert (Diab Ed), RN, CDE
Clinical Nurse Manager, Diabetes Outreach (SA DoH Programme), The Queen Elizabeth Hospital, Woodville, South Australia

Stephen Harding, MMHN, CrMHN, RN, FRCNA, FACMHN, FAAG
Clinical Nurse Consultant, Mental Health/Dementia, Royal District Nursing Service (RDNS) of SA Inc, Adelaide, South Australia, and Visiting Fellow, School of Nursing, Queensland University of Technology, Queensland, Australia

Jennifer Harland, RN, Grad Cert (ICU), Grad Cert (Mental Health), MA (Applied Ethics)
Lecturer/Manger Clinical Education, School of Nursing, Midwifery and Indigenous Health, The University of Wollongong, New South Wales, Australia

Belinda Henderson, MAdv Health Practice (Infection Control), BNursSC (Nursing)
Clinical Nurse Consultant, Infection Control, Infection Management Services, Princess Alexandra Hospital, Brisbane, Queensland, Australia

Pauline Hill, MEd(St), BN(Ed), DipAppSc (Nsg), RN, PhD Candidate
Flinders University of South Australia, Senior Lecturer, School of Nursing & Midwifery, University of South Australia, Adelaide, South Australia

Scott King, RN, BN, MRCNA, Dip Bus, Cert IV TAA
Clinical Nurse Consultant, Disabilities Division, Royal District Nursing Service (RDNS) of SA Inc, Adelaide, South Australia

Debbie Kralik, RN, PhD
Director of Research, Royal District Nursing Service (RDNS) of SA Inc, Adelaide, South Australia

Anne Maddock, RN, RM, BN, MSc (Primary Health Care)
Manager of Clinical Governance, St Vincent's Health, Melbourne, Victoria, Australia

Creina Mitchell, DipAppSci (Ng), BAppdSci (Ad Ng), GradDipComp, MPH, RN, Midwife, MCHN
Lecturer, Maternal and Child Health, Division of Nursing and Midwifery, La Trobe University, Victoria, Australia

Rhonda Nay, RN, BA, M Litt, PhD
Professor of Gerontic Nursing, and Director of the Australian Centre for Evidence-Based Aged Care, La Trobe University, Melbourne, Victoria, Australia

Megan O'Donnell, Bachelor of Social Sciences (Psychology)
Research Officer, Australian Centre for Evidence-Based Aged Care, La Trobe University, Melbourne, Victoria, Australia

Carolyn Roe, RN, BN, Grad Dip Soc Science Counselling, Dip NSc, Cert IV, WPAT
Occupational Nurse, Tenneco Pty Ltd, South Australia

Dianne Roughton, RN, RPN, Grad Cert in Health (Palliative Care)
Clinical Nurse Consultant in Palliative Care, Royal District Nursing Service (RDNS) of SA Inc, Adelaide, South Australia

Ramon Shaban, RN, EMT-P, BSc, BN, DipAppSc (Amb), PGDipPH&TM, GCertInfCon, MCHealthPrac (Hons), MEd, PhD Candidate
Clinical Research Fellow – Infection Control, Princess Alexandra Hospital, Brisbane, Queensland, Australia, and Postgraduate Convenor – Infection Control and

Prevention, School of Nursing and Midwifery, Research Centre for Clinical and Community Practice Innovation, Griffith University, Brisbane, Queensland, Australia

Julianne Siggins, RN, RM, RPN, BBus (Hmn Res Mgt), MBA
Divisional Director, Southern Public Programs, Royal District Nursing Service (RDNS) of SA Inc, Adelaide, South Australia

Colleen Smith, RN, DipT (Ned), BEd, MEd, PhD
Senior Lecturer, School of Nursing and Midwifery, University of South Australia, Adelaide, South Australia

Sue Templeton, RN, BN, MnSc (NursPrac)
CNC Advanced Wound Specialist, Royal District Nursing Service (RDNS) of SA Inc, Adelaide, South Australia

Deryn Thompson, RN, BNg, PC Allergy Nursing
Assoc Member & Nat Rep ASCIA, Allergy Nurse Professional, Allergy SA, Adelaide, South Australia, and Lecturer in Allergy Nursing, University of South Australia, Adelaide, South Australia

Elaine Tooke, RMDN, RN, BN, Dip Appl Sci (Developmental Disability), Grad Cert Stomal Therapy, Cert IV TAA
Clinical Nurse Consultant, Disabilities Division, Royal District Nursing Service (RDNS) of SA Inc, Adelaide, South Australia

Katherine Trowbridge, RN, BN (Mstr Nsg Science – Nrs Prac)
Research Associate, Royal District Nursing Service (RDNS) Inc, Adelaide, South Australia

Lisa Turner, RN, MNurs (Clin Edn), BNurs, Cert IV in WPAT, MRCNA
Clinical Education Consultant, Royal District Nursing Service (RDNS) of SA Inc, Adelaide, South Australia

Antonia van Loon, RN, DipAppSc (CHN), BN, MN (Research), PhD
Senior Researcher, Royal District Nursing Service (RDNS) of SA Inc, Adelaide, South Australia, and Adjunct Senior Lecturer, Flinders University, Adelaide, South Australia

Kate Visentin, MN, Grad Cert (Diab Ed), DipAppSc (Nsg), RN
Research Associate, Royal District Nursing Service (RDNS) of SA Inc, Adelaide, South Australia

Yvonne White, RN, RM, BN, MN (Hons)
Lecturer, The University of Wollongong, New South Wales, Australia

Margaret Winbolt, RN, GradDip Adv Nurs (Gerontic Nursing), PhD Candidate
Research Officer, Australian Centre for Evidence-Based Aged Care, La Trobe University, Melbourne, Victoria, Australia

Preface

This manual has been developed to support Australian community nurses in their work. It is a 'practical' companion text for the book *Community Nursing in Australia* also published with Wiley-Blackwell. Chapter authors are nurses who are central figures and experts in their fields and in Australian community nursing, who work across diverse specialties, with people from diverse cultural backgrounds and in areas that are often uniquely Australian.

It was our intention to develop a resource that would provide guidance to the novice community nurse, be utilised by student nurses as they grapple with the complexities of community nursing and be a resource for experienced community nurses as they reflect on and confirm their practice. For administrators establishing or expanding their community nursing services or moving traditional hospital-based services into the community or closer to people's homes, this text will assist in the development of community services.

Community nursing is an expanding horizon of careers, opportunities and innovation. The contents of this *Community Nursing Practice Manual* will be a revelation for those who currently do not comprehend the breadth of community nursing practice, and for practising community nurses, it will be a confirmation of the ever-growing, comprehensive and empowering role they play within the community and the pivotal role they play in the health of the Australian population. For example Chapter 1 describes approaches to care, bridging theory and practice and examining community nursing roles and the changing boundaries to practice.

Community nurses work in the uncontrolled environments of people's homes, community centres, parklands, schools and rural and remote communities. They connect with people who are lonely and isolated. Their tools of trade are their motor vehicles, their mobile phones and, in some cases, their backpacks. Their tools can also include computers, syringe drivers, vacutexs and intravenous pumps. The broad and varied nature of the chapters of this manual provide testament to the ever-changing and diverse environments in which these skilled nurses practise.

Community nurses often practise as sole practitioners and yet are an integral part of a team working with the client's general practitioner, the client's carer and of course most importantly, the client. They fill many and varied roles. Community nurses are found in roles such as diabetes educators and practice nurses; they nurse within homeless programmes, palliative care programmes and hospital in the home programmes; they are community mental health nurses, district nurses, midwives, immunisation nurses, rural and remote nurses, Royal Flying Doctor Service nurses, continence nurse advisors, wound management nurses, nurses providing disability services, school nurses, nurses working in the areas of correctional services and nurse practitioners. Technology to support aspects of practice becomes important when working across such diverse roles, geographical locations and clinical specialties. Chapter 23 details some of the technology required to support community nursing and predicts future trends. Common to community nurses in whatever role they are working is that quality care is being provided. Chapter 2 discusses the principles of clinical governance and application in community nursing across the spectrum.

Chapter 3 discusses issues surrounding informed consent, which is pertinent to practice as community nursing clients range from the very young (Chapter 14) to the oldest (Chapter 17). They can be homeless (Chapter 10), have either an acute or chronic health condition (Chapter 8), or both. The care these nurses provide for their clients extends to support for their families and carers. In many cases these nurses almost become part of the extended family of the client. It is the knowledge and skills of community-based palliative care nurses that support and empower palliative care clients to die at home. These nurses not only support the client and the family in the final time of life, but also provide bereavement care and often attend the client's funeral. Chapter 18 is devoted to community-based palliative care.

Community nurses do not have the immediate backup of their peers. Backup and support are, in the first instance, by phone. They cannot call a 'code' of any colour; they have to be self-reliant. Their emergency support comes by way of an ambulance and their crisis support is frequently the police. Chapter 5 examines issues of mandatory reporting and incident management, while Chapter 7 identifies the importance of planning and nursing response in disaster management. Fundamental to the capacity of a community nurse to respond effectively in any situation are the skills of assessment, which have been discussed in Chapter 4.

Community nursing is not for everyone. Community nurses tend to be humble, often refraining from boasting about what they do and the differences they make in the lives of the people they work with. They do not boast about how they put their arms around the shoulders of a dying man's wife and tell her she is doing a great job looking after him. They do not talk about how the face of the older woman lights up every day when they visit and they do not boast about how, after many long months of wound care, the older man's leg ulcer has finally healed. Chapter 21 details the skill and knowledge required to promote wound healing when working with community-based clients.

So what is it that makes community nurses such special people – people who are able to work in this ever-changing environment and provide a vast array of care to their community and the community as a whole? They bring to their role a diverse skill set. This skill set is evidenced by discussions and guidelines provided in many chapters, focusing on the varied clinical aspects of community nursing care where nurses make a profound difference to people they are working with, who are facing adverse health situations, including people needing help with mental health, addiction, medications, continence, stoma care, diabetes, nutrition and personal care.

Skimming over the chapter headings of this book will confirm for the reader the traits that these nurses bring to their role:

Resourcefulness + Hardiness + Compassion + Knowledge + Skill + Competence + Empathy + Confidence + Self-reliance + Integrity = Community nurses

We anticipate that reading this manual will provide insight into the work of community nurses and enable nurses themselves to effectively meet the changing needs of people in our communities who are challenged by adverse health situations.

Debbie Kralik
Katherine Trowbridge
Judy Smith

Acknowledgements

Many people contributed to the development of this manual. Firstly, we acknowledge the authors of the chapters, experts in their fields whose knowledge and experiences we have depended on. We thank our colleagues at the Royal District Nursing Service in South Australia who were always interested and provided support and feedback throughout the writing and editing process. In particular, we thank Natalie Howard and Lois Dennes for being the point of liaison, for providing expert administrative support and for always keeping us 'on track'. We also thank Fiona Johnstone and Dr Antonia van Loon for their support and editing skills.

Chapter 1

Approaches to community nursing care

Antonia van Loon

Introduction

Australian community nurses practise using research-based knowledge and skills that are underpinned by a philosophy of primary health care. A variety of factors impact the community nurse's chosen approach to care and these are discussed in this chapter. Some examples of these factors are:

- The nurse's personal philosophy for practice, including the beliefs, values and attitudes that form their personal philosophy for practice
- The community nursing role and the legislation and organisational influences
- The person receiving the care and their sociocultural situation and personal beliefs, values, attitudes and communication styles
- The care context and the realities of working within uncontrolled environments, such as the care recipient's home
- The specific needs and challenges of working with diverse populations within Australian society, such as Indigenous Australians; those living in rural and remote areas; and those living in the community with disabilities, chronic conditions, substance misuse, poverty, mental illness, family violence and homelessness
- Future trends, such as the move towards self-management models, the provision of research-based clinical pathways and the pressures of competitive funding

Background

Legal and professional factors influencing approaches to care

Choosing an approach to care must always be guided by the legal and professional parameters of practice within which a community nurse works, whether that position is salaried or voluntary. All care provided by community nurses must accord with the national standards developed by the Australian Nursing and Midwifery Council (ANMC), which provide the framework for professional nursing practice in Australia. These include the ANMC National Competency Standards for Registered and Enrolled

Nurses [1, 2], the Code of Ethics for Nurses in Australia [3] and the Code of Professional Conduct for Nurses in Australia [4]. Additionally, each nurse is obliged to be aware of and comply with the common law and the legislative requirements of the relevant state/territory legislation that governs health care and nursing practice within the jurisdiction in which the nurse is employed. This can be challenging when one's community nursing practice moves across jurisdictions, as is the case with national call centres and some rural and remote nursing practices.

Additional parameters of practice are determined by employing organisations which have their own policies, protocols, pathways and procedures to govern their service. The community nurse must know, adhere to and be accountable to those directives. Each nurse must always practise within their own professional scope of practice, adhering to the standards and boundaries delineated by specific professional, educational and organisational requirements, to which the nurse is accountable.

Principles of primary health care influencing approaches to care

Primary health care (PHC) is a World Health Organization (WHO) endorsed philosophy of health care formulated in 1978 to redress global health inequities and assert as fundamental the human right to health [5–7]. PHC is defined as:

> ...essential care based upon practical, scientifically sound and socially acceptable methods and technology made universally accessible to individuals and families in the community through their full participation and at a cost that the community and country can afford to maintain at every stage of their development in the spirit of self-reliance and self-determination [8, p. 3].

Definitions are open to interpretation and debate continues as to how such a concept can simultaneously be a guiding philosophy, a set of activities, a level of care and a strategy for care delivery. The PHC vision was 'health for all by the year 2000'. The strategy was aimed at reorganising health services to promote sustainable global and local health outcomes by recognising that well-being depended on a broad range of social, political, economic and environmental factors [8, 9]. It was followed by a paradigm shift that challenged the Western world's prevailing health care focus on disease treatment and cure at any cost, to shift attention to disease prevention and heath promotion. This was done to make health care more available, affordable, acceptable, accessible and sustainable to all the world's people [10].

The Declaration of Alma-Ata [11] refers to eight fundamental activities that must occur to improve global health. These are:

- Education concerning prevailing health problems and the methods of preventing and controlling them
- Promotion of food supply and proper nutrition
- Provision of an adequate supply of safe water and basic sanitation
- Provision of maternal and child health care, including family planning
- Immunisation against the major infectious diseases
- Appropriate control of locally endemic diseases
- Appropriate treatment of common diseases and injuries
- Provision of essential drugs [8, p. 6]

PHC principles advocate a health care approach that is promotive, preventative, curative and rehabilitative and includes 'all activities that contribute to health at the interface between the community and the health system' [11, p. 4]. Therefore, as a strategy, PHC reflects care that transitions health system boundaries and focuses attention on community needs, which it contends should be self-determined rather than imposed by outsiders.

We can reflect on these idealistic notions 30 years later to see that in Australia today, local groups may have some input into government activities, but the direction of spending remains the province of state/territory and federal policy makers who are often far removed from local situations. The failure of health policy and expenditure to resolve the ailing health of Indigenous Australians is a case in point. The life expectancy of Australians at birth has risen to be one of the highest in the world. For females it is 83.0 years, which is third behind Japan and France, and for males 78.1 years, which is second only to Japan [12, p. 2]. However, life expectancy for Indigenous Australians during the same period (2002–2004) is 59.4 years for males and 64.8 years for females, indicating the imperative for genuine community engagement of Indigenous people in policy, planning and delivery of health care so that such inequity can be redressed.

In 1986 the Ottawa Charter challenged governments to be responsible and accountable for five action areas that would promote health:

- Advocacy, enabling and mediation to build healthy public policies
- Creating supportive environments
- Strengthening community action
- Developing personal skills
- Reorienting health services [7, 13]

The Ottawa Charter underscored the importance of intersectoral and multidisciplinary partnerships that considered more than the medical aspect of disease and health and kept in mind the context of the person's life [14].

PHC reinforces the concept that health is entrenched in the social frameworks that enable people to contribute in a meaningful way to their society, both relationally and economically [10, 15, 16]. The PHC framework includes social determinants that impact health, such as the social gradient, stress, early life, social exclusion, work, unemployment, social support, addiction, food and transport [17]. Thus, choosing an approach to care grounded by PHC principles requires attention to social determinants as much as to population profiling and disease management determinants.

Community nurses can develop ways to work in partnership with clients to help them make informed health choices. The community nurse using PHC principles to guide practice will seek to promote self-management in individuals and communities as part of an approach to care. Such an approach necessarily involves inclusion and mutual respect as essential aspects in building a healthy approach to care [18].

Approaches focused on PHC principles are under threat, as the emphasis of the current health system is biomedical, and focused on disease/condition management in the community. Community nurses see this as a barrier that prohibits health-promoting approaches to care [19]. It is difficult to promote health only in the context of a specific disease. It is important that nurses understand PHC principles if they are to provide health-promoting approaches to practice. This involves broadening one's education regarding personal and community strategies to conduct health promotion activities. It also relies on organisations valuing such care and enabling it via appropriate resource allocation.

The nurse's personal approach to care

Community nurses value what they are doing as worthwhile work that is making a difference in people's lives. Their motivation comes from the capacity to help people and influence quality health outcomes for clients [20]. Factors that enable such values are esteemed and those that constrain them are perceived as barriers that may frustrate nurses and lead to job dissatisfaction. How each nurse's values conflict and conform to organisational, professional, community and client values will impact their approach to care. Understanding these values, beliefs and attitudes is central to the community nurse's professional role and integral to quality client outcomes.

Personal beliefs, attitudes and values and a philosophy for practice

Each person brings their own value system to the nurse/client interaction. Values emerge from a confluence of factors such as the person's culture, race, ethnicity, religion and associated beliefs, attitudes, rituals and understandings. How a community nurse approaches care will depend on their perspectives of the person, community, health, disease, illness, wellness and their role in the nurse/client interaction. Value clashes may occur between individuals holding different beliefs. It is therefore important that the community nurse is aware of their values and open to assessing and sensitively considering the client's value systems when choosing an approach to care. Value clashes are known to occur between generations and can lead to miscommunication between nurses, health team workers, family and clients. In multicultural and Indigenous Australia, there are a plethora of beliefs around health and illness and it is important that the approach selected by the community nurse is underpinned by tolerance, respect, sensitivity and integrity.

The community nurse's education and experience

Sound knowledge is the foundation for needs assessment and caregiving in community nursing practice. It is built on an amalgam of theoretical (knowing that) and practice-based (knowing how) knowledge [21]. Contemporary community nurses must be accomplished knowledge workers. Community nurses have expanding and evolving knowledge and skill sets and increasingly need to apply acute interventions within home settings. Consequently, educational and theoretical models for community nursing should be embedded in the community context rather than adapted from acute care, because this is the context in which the knowledge will be used and applied. Community nurses work independently and so they need to be able to translate theory, public policy and research knowledge into practice with effect [22, 23].

Nurses advocate for clients in the initiation and coordination of other services and may have to broker client care. Thus, the approach to care they choose should be based on research evidence because the client is reliant on the knowledge that the community nurse holds. The community nurse needs to be well educated. She/he is expected to know why they are doing activities; how to do the activity and perform it with proficiency; and how to problem-solve any unanticipated issues along the way. The nurse needs excellent decision-making skills and needs to know how to adjust plans of care when they monitor and evaluate the outcomes of nursing activities [24]. They must know how, when and where to access more assistance if needed [20]. Each nurse must have sufficient self-awareness to realise when they do not know, so they can ask for help in a timely manner. As such, the nurse's personal educational preparation and professional experience will influence the approach to care that they choose.

The community nursing role

The shifting focus of community nursing impacts approaches to care

Australian community nurses have traditionally had two key foci: the provision of PHC with its health education, disease prevention and health promotion focus, and the provision of community-based clinical care [25]. In recent years the community nurse's role has begun to shift, directing more attention to the provision of disease recovery nursing care for transitioning clients as they move out of the hospital environment and into the community context. Additionally, the community nurse's role has become more focused on the provision of early intervention measures to prevent exacerbations or complications for clients with chronic illness/conditions or to prevent unnecessary hospital (re)admission.

Nurses are using cutting-edge technology to provide increasingly complex primary nursing and health care across the lifespan. The changing social demographic in Australia will require care to be provided to many older people with higher acuity and complex comorbid health needs within their homes. Currently, over 560 000 older Australians have a profound or severe limitation. This means that 22% of the population is affected by some pre-existing disability [26, 27]. The number of older people with profound disability impacting their capacity to self-care is projected to increase rapidly. These people often require resource-intensive approaches to care, and nurses may have to advocate and argue for such expenditure, as the resources are unlikely to be freely available to sustain individualised approaches to care. Community nurses need to know how to collect pertinent data, interpret it and articulate it in order to make a case for funding clinical care management decisions so that community services can shift resources and remain responsive. Arguing the case for a particular approach to care in a competitive funding environment will require the provision of accurate research evidence and knowledge, and accompanying efficient and fluid structures, policies, processes and guidelines.

Person-centred approaches to care

Currently, community nurses increasingly assist clients and their carers/families to self-manage their health situation within their home environment. This help now includes locating and liaising with appropriate support services, advocating for clients and increasingly brokering health information and services to help clients attain the skills they require to maximise the self-management of their illness/disorder. Such nursing roles require person-centred approaches to care.

Nurses find reward and gain motivation in person-centred care [20, 28]. Community nurses are touched by the varying clients with whom they work and the diverse environments in which they work. They are welcomed into the privacy of their client's home and share personal space with their family. A large study of effective and ineffective cancer care, taken from the perspective of people with cancer, revealed the importance of human connection, of being known in a meaningful way, as a component of quality nursing care [29]. The home setting provides a unique person-centred understanding of what it is to be ill. It facilitates a close therapeutic relationship that enables a shared understanding of the illness experience so that nurses can alleviate the suffering and loneliness that often accompany illness [30]. Community nurses who have such personal access into the homes and lives of the ill person are well situated to interpret the person's expressions of their experience and this shared understanding forms the basis of a relationship that can be intimate and therapeutic.

While nurses can and do experience a degree of powerlessness working within the home care context, that power imbalance is quickly redressed by their educational and occupational status, which continues to be a source of power for nurses within the client/nurse relationship. Power moves towards balance when clients are able to control their own life and care decisions [31].

It is in such a person-centred approach to care that community nurses use 'ways of doing' with/for the client that involve the nursing process of planning, implementing, monitoring and evaluating care. These 'ways of doing' may include purposeful additions to the normal daily tasks and routines that take place within the ordinary nurse/client relationship. Here nurses use themselves therapeutically via their 'ways of being', which include dialoguing with the client, provision of compassionate presence and various forms of connecting and communicating with the client [32]. Dialogue with the client involves informing, sharing, paraphrasing, questioning, confronting, reassuring, mediating, joking and planning. The nurse is available, listening attentively, sitting with the client, anticipating the client's needs and being there for the duration of the experience.

Gerrish says that nurses employ six principles as they conceptualise and practise person-centred approaches to care: respecting individuality, providing holistic care, focusing on nursing needs, promoting independence, partnership and negotiation of care and also equity and fairness [33]. Community nurses using PHC principles prioritise client involvement in decision making as part of their everyday clinical practice. It is easy to assume that because care is occurring in the context of a client's home, the person is involved in care and treatment decisions. This assumption is false. Community nurses must devote time to relationship building in their practice to garner client participation [34]. Luker *et al.* interviewed district nursing teams to determine the factors that contributed or detracted from quality palliative care [35]. Factors enabling the formation of a positive relationship with the client were esteemed and strategies used to achieve such a relationship included establishing early contact with the client and their family, ensuring continuity of care, spending time with the client and providing more than the physical aspects of care. They verified that knowing the client and their family was an essential antecedent to the provision of high-quality palliative care. The nurse/client relationship was the vehicle through which this person-centred approach to care was delivered.

Continuity of care is the basis for firm nurse/client relationships [36]. Research demonstrates that regular contact with a community nurse is associated with a strong sense of security for home-based cancer patients and their primary carers. This security is a significant component of client's and carer's physical and psychosocial well-being – a point that should not be forgotten by community health services when the temptation to employ agency staff arises [36]. Another study by Richardson found that psychological well-being of clients was enhanced by less restricted personal interaction with nurses [37]. In many cases, health professional's interaction focused on the person's disease and physical problems, but the client's perception of 'feeling better' was most often focused on enhancement of psychological health and well-being, which was genuinely sustained by consistent therapeutic interactions that centred on the whole person. Needless to say, there is evidence that a person-centred approach to care provides quality outcomes for the client and their family while providing job satisfaction for nurses [20].

The person receiving care

Changing population demographic influences the approach to care

Along with many other developed countries, Australia has vastly improving life expectancies for men which are predicted to increase to 92.2 years and for women to 95.0 years by the year 2050–2051 [38]. Australian mortality rates continue to drop, and as the post–Second World War 'baby boomers' approach retirement age, the demand for health and community services will escalate. At the same time Australia's birth rates are dropping, so children will make up a smaller part of Australia's population, while those over 65 years increase [38]. This demographic shift will impact economic, social and health policy, as older people require alternative housing options, income support, provision of health services, disability services and community care [39].

It cannot be presumed that every older person will have health care needs, but research shows that the age-specific prevalence of profound disability (that requiring supportive care) increases from about 5% at age 70 years to 50% at age 90 years [40]. Many older Australians do not have access to an extended family due to geographic distance, divorce, couples having fewer or no children, changing attitudes to caring for the elderly within the family and the growth of two-income families that may not have the time or inclination to provide intensive and extended supportive care to their elders. Thus the future client base of community nursing is likely to include an increased number of frail older people with increasingly complex care needs and multiple comorbid conditions.

Approaches to care in multicultural Australia

Australia is a multicultural country with people born overseas making up 33% of the older Australian population in 2004 [38]. Of that group, 61% come from culturally and linguistically diverse (CALD) backgrounds [38]. It may be assumed that the support for older people is higher in these communities, but this is not the case [41]. As a group, migrants tend to be quite healthy and use fewer resources than the rest of the population [38]. This may be due to their resilience developed through their life experiences of migration, or it may be due to their lifestyle. Whatever the case, the diversity of Australia's population poses culturally specific issues for community nurses. Not the least of these is that older migrants may revert to their language of origin. There may also be additional cultural challenges within the family as the second generation adopt Australian norms and decline to provide extended support, accommodation or care to their ageing parents and grandparents. We live in a time where people are increasingly mobile and this reduced access to support may leave people from CALD backgrounds feeling isolated and rejected in their time of need.

The need is apparent for culturally competent community nurses who seek to understand the client's cultural influences and preferences and meet their language and communication needs. Core personal differences relating to family, education, finances, religion, sexuality, community and ethics are some of the areas that are influenced by varying cultural perspectives. In a study conducted in the UK, district nurses demonstrated a lack of confidence regarding ethnicity and cultural difference. They had a limited understanding of culturally appropriate care and the practices they were using could have been considered discriminatory and inequitable [42]. Clearly, nurses need to be willing to recognise that expertise exists within other cultural groups. The client's skills, knowledge and healthy ways of coping need to be acknowledged and sustained, while those practices that challenge health must be confronted with sensitivity. It does take time to establish rapport and acceptance before a nurse can assess client needs accurately, influence their health choices, provide care that is culturally appropriate, utilise designated CALD resources and advocate for such culturally appropriate services.

Nurses need to use many styles of communication and seek to understand the finer nuances of body language that are peculiar to particular cultures. They should check for culturally sensitive ways of assessing client needs, check their own ethnocentrism and ensure health information is provided in accessible language that promotes transcultural health literacy. The nurse needs to be aware of culturally mediated perceptions regarding health and illness. For example Indigenous Australians view health as integral to people, country and the other things that are happening in their life, so their presentation of mental illness such as depression can be different from a Caucasian English-speaking client's presentation [43]. Benson suggests that when assessing Indigenous people and those from other cultural backgrounds, broad assessment questions will yield productive answers [43, pp. 19–20]. She suggests the following questions as a starting point for community nurses:

1. What is the main problem you would like me to help you with today?
2. How is this problem affecting you?
3. Why do you think it started when it did?
4. What do you most fear about this problem?
5. What solutions have you tried or have you thought of?
6. What were you hoping that I would do for you today?
7. How can your family and community help you with your problem?
8. How will we know when you are well again?
9. When would you like to come back?

The care context

The home is a central defining concept of community for most district and home nurses, with notions surrounding the nature of the relationships that exist within that setting influencing the approach to care [44]. Other branches of community nursing, such as those nurses working in drug and alcohol services or among homeless people, view their community context differently, where 'home' is seen as an environmental context of care. On the other hand, faith community nurses perceive community as the cultural or geographic group that their faith community serves [45, 46]. Similarly, community nurses working in rural and remote areas understand community as the people that they service within a geographic boundary. Suffice to say, the community care context has a relational focus or a population focus and the perspective the nurse holds will influence their approach to care.

The client's home environment as the care context

The redesign of health and community care is ongoing, as client and community needs and economic demands dictate which approaches to care are to be preferred and funded. The future is likely to see the expansion of the scope of community nursing practice. This will necessitate application of generalist and specific knowledge and skill sets unique to acute care being employed in the community context, which will pose challenges. Obviously, the principles of infection control are the same whether one is dressing a wound in a hospital or in the home setting. However, application of universal precautions presents a challenge in the home environment where water may be scarce or the environment itself may be crowded and unhygienic. The nurse does not control the community setting; it is managed by clients and carers, so care needs to be negotiated. Consequently, innovation and improvisation may be necessary to get even simple tasks done with effect.

Similarly, the issue of personal safety within the client's home will influence the approach to care. All community nurses face the unpredictable when moving into the personal space of clients. They face different risks, such as clutter, spillage, poor hygiene, obstacles, pets (especially protective dogs) and slippery surfaces. Services have protocols for managing such risks in the community. However, there are other hidden risks in family homes which include the presence of weapons, violent behaviour, drug and alcohol misuse, domestic squalor, neglect and abuse and criminal activity, all of which pose danger and require nurses to think and react quickly and carefully. Community nurses need excellent assessment, communication and interpersonal skills to defuse tense situations, de-escalate conflict, and/or consider their self-preservation and extricate themselves from a dangerous situation quickly and safely. It is important to anticipate health and safety risks and prepare plans in advance where possible. Strategies such as backup support, telephone numbers pre-programmed into the mobile phone, negotiation of meetings in public places can promote safety. The nurse should exercise their right to decline to provide care if they believe their safety may be compromised.

The client's relationships in the family/home as the care context

Community nurses are quick to point out that family relationships influence their approach to care. Some families are a resource, both practically and emotionally, to the client, and when open communication flows, a valued care partnership ensues [20, 47]. However, families that are suffering can impact care if they are demanding, unresponsive or obstructive. When the client's family is suffering, the community nursing role extends to supporting and sustaining them as well as the client [47].

The employing organisation's focus on the care context

The Australian government has specific guidelines for community organisations that care for clients of the Department of Veterans' Affairs [48]. These guidelines clearly detail quality assurance processes that include auditing of the organisation's compliance with the prescribed guidelines, accreditation processes and clinical pathways. Organisations must adhere to the guidelines to obtain funding and this will influence the approaches to care that are available to nurses.

Organisational values influence the context for care

A recent study of district nurses in South Australia found that the nurses valued excellence as a practice and organisational norm [20]. Organisational structures that provide accountability frameworks and engender organisational trust are esteemed. Collegiality is unanimously viewed as a value to be embraced. Nurses enjoy working relationships that are mutual and reciprocal and in which constructive feedback and information is shared. The organisation that provides participation and development for its team members and enables them to work autonomously within their scope of professional practice raises satisfaction for nurses. These district nurses are not interested in competition; rather they want to work in teams that display a refined sense of loyalty to an agreed purpose and that provide mutual stimulation, which motivates staff to work towards achieving agreed goals. In such an environment, healthy debate is encouraged, facilitated and moderated, and because the context is safe, transparent and open, innovation is encouraged and valued. It is true that when an organisation's values align with the employed nurse's values, the potential for creative synergy is enhanced and this affects quality care, improves morale and provides intrinsic motivation among the nurses while increasing the likelihood of quality client outcomes [20].

Issues and concepts

Working in multidisciplinary teams

The work of the community nurse is changing in response to health system demands and altering population demographics. The community nurse role has traditionally had a PHC focus on health promotion, disease prevention, early identification and intervention. But this is now pressured by systemic changes which are forcing early discharge from acute care, hospital avoidance programmes, introduction of intermediate care services, ageing in place policies and deinstitutionalisation of mental health and disability services. Such policy changes are shaping the community nurse's focus and workload. For example district nurses are seeing more adult clients who receive shorter, intensive, clinically focused services and are then discharged from care, rather than receiving a lower intensity service over a longer period of time [25]. It is noted that this expanded acute care role is impacting workload, but staffing numbers are not increasing commensurate with client acuity and intensity and this is resulting in less time for holistic PHC [25]. This is necessitating the development of partnerships with community organisations to advocate for clients and broker aspects of client care. Community-based nurses are the professionals most frequently visiting older people in their homes and as such they must adopt strategic approaches that ensure clients receive the services to which they are entitled [49].

We can learn from the studies conducted in the UK where partnership has become central to public health and social care policy. The literature is largely sceptical about the feasibility of effective partnerships between health professionals, even to the point of saying that interprofessional relationships are the Achilles' heel of partnerships between health and social care [50]. The power struggles that occur between health professionals pose challenges to the nurse's chosen approach to care. For example general practitioners in the UK exercise increasing authority over district nurses and practice nurses in their employ and this has required the nurses to develop assertive communication skills and become more business-like in tightly controlling their working relationships [51]. The demands of such partnerships require different skill sets, such as business acumen, negotiation skills and emotional intelligence, to meet the needs of direct patient care and cooperative consultation within a multidisciplinary team [52].

The needs of vulnerable community groups

There are many vulnerable groups in Australian society that require a careful approach to care. They include people with mental illness, addictions and disabilities; survivors of trauma and abuse; the homeless; and the frail aged. Policies of reintegration and de-institutionalisation have increased the opportunity for integration into the community for such people. Such policies have amplified the number of challenging environments that community nurses enter and the types of testing behaviour with which they must deal [53]. The demands of mental health nursing, in particular, extend beyond the established skills of providing care to skills in emotional intelligence and resilience as nurses are called on to role-model, educate and support clients on how to live and function in the community [54]. Many of these vulnerable people struggle to access health care and to navigate the complexities of self-management. They often have compounding comorbid disease and lack the skills, the finances or the desire to adequately feed and care for themselves. These people experience difficulty accessing the specialised assessment, care and treatment that they require within mainstream health services. This is particularly true for clients with mental illness and addiction to drugs and alcohol, who have complex health and social care needs. They often encounter a discourse of prejudice by mainstream acute and community health services. It is not unusual for service providers to shape their approach to care by a discourse of risk, constructing themselves as vulnerable and at risk in the client care context [55]. This is partly due to the workers' knowledge deficit and lack of experience in how to work with such client groups.

A report on the experiences of Indigenous Australians using mainstream health services highlights their experience of prejudice and ignorance [56]. This is also a key theme in Goold and Liddle's book on Indigenous nurses' accounts of their nursing care and work in Australian health services [57]. Few aspects of mainstream health services were perceived as helpful but it was viewed as positive that some mainstream health workers were recognising Aboriginal and Torres Strait Islander people as a special needs group. There was appreciation for the increased awareness of Aboriginal history and the desire to learn culturally appropriate methods of dealing with Indigenous Australians. At the very least it was suggested that community nurses should realise the importance of understanding life circumstances and family and kinship relationships to work effectively with this population [58].

The addition of diagnostic labels may exacerbate prejudicial discrimination which militates against quality health outcomes for clients. For example the label of 'personality disorder' is one that may set in motion a stereotypical response by health professionals, namely, 'Oh well, there is nothing we can do for them'. This and other diagnostic labels have profound impact on the care received by Indigenous clients with mental illness and clients who have experienced the trauma of sexual abuse in childhood [56, 59, 60].

The first step in addressing such care deficits is to raise awareness of how prejudice and ignorance impact on the nurse's approach to care. This awareness must be followed up with education regarding the nuances of care management for groups with special needs. It underscores the importance of community nursing services providing continuing education for staff.

Future trends in approaches to care

Australian community nurses need to choose viable, helpful and practical approaches to care. To meet the changing demands on community services and the variable needs of special groups, community nursing services may have to redesign service options so that continuity of care is improved, service duplication is avoided and clients can be assisted in self-managing their illness/condition. Even with the best intentions regarding quality health and community care, it is likely that cost rationalisation will occur. Decision making regarding approaches to care will be affected by economic imperatives and the viability of meeting service demands within budget constraints. This will require community nurses to be able to argue their case for their chosen approach to care for particular clients, client groups and indeed whole services. To do this they will need to be able to provide an evidence/research base for their practice and a sound clinical rationale for their choices.

Providing the research/evidence base for practice

When providing any clinical nursing activity, the community nurse should be able to undertake a full and thorough assessment. When providing care, she/he should know how to provide that care to a quality standard. This includes understanding the anticipated effect of the activity, the contraindications for its use, being aware of any possible side effects and how to avoid or mitigate these. All nursing requires a thorough understanding of how to monitor the activities, which includes problem solving and evaluating outcomes, and how to alter care as required, referring on to other health professionals as necessary.

The important outcome of locating an evidence base for practice is to have a standardised approach among community health care providers. The approach used to develop and inform evidence-based guidelines is largely one of systematic reviews of predominantly quantitative research studies. It is noted by Smith and MacDonald that such research foci often ignore minority groups [61]. This reduces the capacity to respond to individual patient's needs, using a PHC approach which aims to provide a holistic, preventive, empowering method to work with and in communities [61].

It is likely that uniform clinical pathways and accompanying tools will be developed. Funding and audit requirements will be linked to these pathways. Community nurses will have to ensure that they are able to provide meaningful research input into the development of the protocols, guidelines and tools that will accompany clinical pathways. It is imperative that community nursing organisations have quality research centres to support their practice. Suffice to say, the approach to care chosen by individuals and organisations will be influenced by their development and understanding of the research base for their practice. Disseminating research can assist monitoring and help entrench best practice by linking clinical pathways to health outcomes which achieve an agreed standard across multiple providers in various jurisdictions. Research findings need to be communicated and disseminated via the published literature so that they become part of the evidence base for community nursing practice. Additionally, representatives from community nursing organisations need to be present in policy-making ventures so that they have a voice in the directions community nursing takes. Developing the research base requires resources and infrastructure and, in a competitive funding environment, it is tempting for organisations to think that someone else can provide that research.

Approaches to care that promote self-management by clients

There are many assumptions made about the benefits of self-management, but recent research indicates that some clients lack knowledge about their condition and its treatment. They are confused about different nursing roles and about whom they should enlist in their care partnership [62]. As discussed, community nurses who underpin their practice with PHC principles will want to educate and empower clients towards self-care. Community nurses need to use refined skills in client education and knowledge translation and transfer, to promote self-management. Much has been written on this subject, indicating that this approach to care is appreciated by most clients and their carers, and produces effective health outcomes once the client is supported in gaining the skills they need to manage their care [63–70].

The future impact of market forces on approaches to care

Nursing care is being opened to market forces because organisations need to tender for government contracts. Organisations are expected to provide cost-effective care that produces quality outcomes while being responsive to growing consumer demand.

Governments cannot carry the financial burden of the ageing population's health requirements. For example nurses know that providing care to the dying requires 24-h palliative care; yet cost constraints prohibit organisations providing 24-h hospice-at-home community palliative care services. Addressing these issues requires pragmatic approaches to care that consider partnerships, where some services are provided by carers and trained volunteers who are able to access a network of specialists with broader knowledge and skills. Perhaps outcomes will be improved by approaches that employ professional nurse case managers or nurse practitioners who manage the care and broker high-quality, cost-effective and value-for-money client services. Nurses will need to interface with allied health services and volunteer community support structures. However, such care managers must have designated responsibilities and the accompanying authority to make clinical decisions and delegate care when appropriate or such approaches to care will fail.

The capacity for services to move with the client across the continuum of health care will be helpful, but raises the issue of professional boundaries and role delineation. It is increasingly difficult to define what professional knowledge is particular and unique to which professional and who should be responsible for what aspects of client care in the community. Such questions raise issues about credentialing and supervising carers in a climate of increased litigation. Is the risk worth the money saved? Very large studies (19 000 nurses) in the USA clearly indicate that maintaining a professional credentialed workforce does save money, improve client outcomes and decrease adverse events while increasing client and nurse satisfaction [71–73].

It is well documented that many adverse medical events can be avoided if appropriate and timely referral occurs [74, 75]. A major cause of adverse events is the failure of communication between caregivers, because the authority gradient hinders communication and teamwork [76]. Such system failures need to be addressed by having fluid communication policies and protocols that promote the movement of client data across the continuum of care. The future community nurse will need excellent assessment skills that are grounded in a sound knowledge base and an outstanding capacity to communicate that knowledge across the health care continuum. This again highlights the need for developing the research and knowledge base of community nursing practice and promoting fluid and efficient methods for knowledge to transfer into practice via policies, processes and guidelines.

Summary

Australian community nurses face a variety of issues which impact their chosen approach to care and some of these have been discussed in this chapter. Non-negotiable factors include the legal and professional standards that prescribe nursing care. The nurse will also hold their own personal approach to care based on their beliefs, attitudes and values and their philosophy for practice. This will be shaped by their education and experience. However, external influences on the community nursing role are shifting the focus of community nursing from person-centred approaches to care to disease management and this is impacting the approaches to care nurses can employ. The client or the person receiving care is changing as the population demographic alters and the number of older Australians grows. The multicultural configuration of

Australia and the needs of vulnerable community groups require sensitive and flexible approaches to care.

The care context in which community nurses operate is often the client's home, but sometimes it is the client's relationships within the family or extended community, as in the case of Indigenous Australians, where kinship and relationship to country underpin the care context. The employing organisation's values and service structures will influence the approaches to care available to the community nurse. Approaches that promote client self-management are embraced by clients, caregivers and funders as the new way forward. However, the confluence of care needs of clients with multiple co-morbid conditions clearly requires partnership and multidisciplinary team approaches to care. Designing approaches that meet these changing requirements will remain a future challenge. Community nurses are uniquely placed to influence this future by developing and using a research/evidence base to inform their practice. This will enable them to select approaches to care that are proved to provide quality client outcomes.

Useful resources

Guidelines for accreditation of community nursing organisations:

The Australian Council on Health Care Standards (ACHS) – ACHS EquIP Standards at http://www.achs.gov.au/

Quality Improvement Council (QIC) accreditation programme delivered by Australian Health and Community Services Standards (AHCSS) at http://www.latrobe.edu. au/qic

SAI Global Assurance Services, a subsidiary of Standards Australia – ISO 9001 Certification at http://www.sai-global.com/

Department of Veterans' Affairs Clinical Pathways for the planning and delivery of best practice standards of care at http://www.dva.gov.au/health/provider/community_ nursing/cnindex.htm

References

1. Australian Nursing and Midwifery Council (ANMC) (2006) *National Competency Standards for Registered and Enrolled Nurses.* Australian Nursing and Midwifery Council, Dickson, ACT.
2. ANMC (2006) *National Competency Standards for Registered and Enrolled Nurses.* Australian Nursing Council, Dickson, ACT.
3. ANMC (2002) *The Code of Ethics for Nurses in Australia.* Australian Nursing and Midwifery Council, Dickson, ACT.
4. ANMC (2003) *The Code of Professional Conduct for Nurses in Australia.* Australian Nursing and Midwifery Council, Dickson, ACT.
5. Banerji, D. (2003) Reflections on the twenty-fifth anniversary of the Alma-Ata declaration. *International Journal of Health Services,* 33(4), 813–18.
6. Grootjans, J. and Townsend, M. (2005) Grounding co-ordinating contexts for sustainability and health, in J. Brown, J. Grootjans, J. Ritchie, M. Townsend and G. Verrinder (eds) *Sustainability and Health.* Allen & Unwin, Crows Nest, NSW, pp. 83–130.
7. McMurray, A. (2003) *Community Health and Wellness: A Socio-Ecological Approach,* 2nd edition. Mosby, Sydney.
8. Tablot, L. and Verrinder, G. (2005) *Promoting Health: The Primary Health Care Approach,* 3rd edition. Elsevier, Sydney.

9. Vaughan, C. (2004) Determinants of health: Case studies from Asia and the Pacific, in H. Keleher and B. Murphy (eds) *Understanding Health – A Determinants Approach*. Oxford University Press, South Melbourne, pp. 97–112.

10. Baum, F. (2002) *The New Public Health: An Australian Perspective*. Oxford University Press, South Melbourne.

11. World Health Organization (1978) *Primary Health Care: Report on the International Conference on Primary Health Care*, Alma-Ata, USSR, 6–12 September 1978. Health for All Series No. 1. World Health Organization, Geneva, pp. 2–79.

12. Australian Institute of Health and Welfare (AIHW). (2006) *Australia's Health 2006*. Australia's health no. 10. Australian Institute of Health and Welfare, Canberra.

13. Catford, J. (2004) Health promotion: Origins, obstacles and opportunities, in H. Keleher and B. Murphy (eds) *Understanding Health – A Determinants Approach*. Oxford University Press, South Melbourne pp. 134–51.

14. Macdonald, J. (2004) Primary health care: A global overview. *Primary Health Care Research and Development*, 5(4), 284–8.

15. Keleher, H. (2004) Public and population health: Strategic responses, in H. Keleher and B. Murphy (eds) *Understanding Health – A Determinants Approach*. Oxford University Press, South Melbourne pp. 97–112.

16. Pender, N., Murdaugh, C. and Parsons, M. (2006) *Health Promotion in Nursing Practice*, 5th edition. Pearson/Prentice Hall, Upper Saddle River.

17. Wilkinson, R. and Marmot, M. (2003) *Social Determinants of Health: The Solid Facts*, 2nd edition. World Health Organization, Denmark.

18. Lumby, J. (2001) *Who Cares? The Changing Health Care System*. Allen & Unwin, Crows Nest.

19. Dympna, C. (2007) Nurses' perceptions, understanding and experiences of health promotion. *Journal of Clinical Nursing*, 16(6), 1039–49.

20. Van Loon, A.M. and Kralik, D. (2006) *Clinical Leadership in the Context of Community Nursing*. Royal District Nursing Service Foundation of SA, Adelaide, South Australia.

21. Kennedy, C. (2004) A typology of knowledge for district nursing assessment practice. *Journal of Advanced Nursing*, 45(4), 401–9.

22. Daghfous, A. (2004) Knowledge management as an organisational innovation: An absorptive capacity perspective and a case study. *International Journal of Innovation and Learning*, 1(4), 409.

23. Breu, K., Hemingway, C.J., Strathern, M. and Bridger, D. (2001) Workforce agility: The new employee strategy for the knowledge economy. *Journal of Information Technology*, 17, 21–31.

24. Bryans, A. and McIntosh, J. (1996) Decision making in community nursing: An analysis of the stages of decision making as they relate to community nursing assessment practice. *Journal of Advanced Nursing*, 24(1), 24–30.

25. Kemp, L.A., Harris, E. and Comino, E. (2005) Changes in community nursing in Australia: 1995–2000. *Journal of Advanced Nursing*, 49(3), 307–14.

26. Australian Bureau of Statistics (ABS) (1999) *1998 Disability, Ageing and Carers: Disability and Long Term Health Conditions*. Australian Bureau of Statistics, Canberra.

27. AIHW (2004) Carers in Australia: Assisting frail older people and people with a disability, in Department of Health and Ageing (ed.). *Ageing*. Aged care series no. 8. AIHW and the Australian Government, Canberra, p. 108.

28. Dunne, K., Sullivan, K. and Kernohan, G. (2005) Palliative care for patients with cancer: District nurses' experiences. *Journal of Advanced Nursing*, 50(4), 372–80.

29. Thorne, S., Kuo, M., Armstrong, E., McPherson, G., Harris, S. and Hislop, G. (2005) 'Being known': Patients' perspectives of the dynamics of human connection in cancer care. *Psychooncology*, 14(10), 887.

30. Öhman, M. and Söderberg, S. (2004) District nursing – sharing an understanding by being present. Experiences of encounters with people with serious chronic illness and their close relatives in their homes. *Journal of Clinical Nursing*, 13(7), 858–66.

31. Oudshoorn, A., Ward-Griffin, C. and McWilliam, C. (2007) Client–nurse relationships in home-based palliative care: A critical analysis of power relations. *Journal of Clinical Nursing*, 16(8), 1435–43.

32. Van Loon, A. (2001) Assessing the spiritual needs of older persons, in S.K. Garrett and S. Koch (eds) *Assessing Older People – A Work Book*. MacLennan & Petty, Melbourne, pp. 51–73.

33. Gerrish, K. (2000) Individualized care: Its conceptualization and practice within a multi-ethnic society. *Journal of Advanced Nursing*, 32(1), 91–9.

34. Millard, L., Hallett, C. and Luker, K. (2006) Nurse–patient interaction and decision-making in care: Patient involvement in community nursing. *Journal of Advanced Nursing*, 55(2), 142–50.

35. Luker, K., Austin, L., Caress, A. and Hallett, C. (2000) The importance of 'knowing the patient': Community nurses' constructions of quality in providing palliative care. *Journal of Advanced Nursing*, 31(4), 775–82.

36. McKenzie, H., Boughton, M., Hayes, L, Forsyth, S., Davies, M., Underwood, E. and McVey, P. A sense of security for cancer patients at home: The role of community nurses. *Health and Social Care Community*, 15(4), 352–9.

37. Richardson, J. (2002) Health promotion in palliative care: The patients' perception of therapeutic interaction with the palliative nurse in the primary care setting. *Journal of Advanced Nursing*, 40(4), 432–40.

38. ABS (2004) *Australian Social Trends, 2004. 4102.0.* Australian Bureau of Statistics, Canberra.

39. Rowland, D. (2003) An ageing population: Emergence of a new stage of life? in S. Khoo and P. McDonald (eds) *The Transformation of Australia's Population: 1970–2030.* UNSW Press, Sydney pp. 239–65.

40. Giles, L.C., Cameron, I.D. and Crotty, M. (2003) Disability in older Australians: Projections for 2006–2031. *Medical Journal of Australia*, 179, 130–33.

41. Ward, B., Anderson, K. and Sheldon, M. (2005) Patterns of home and community care service delivery to culturally and linguistically diverse residents of rural Victoria. *Australian Journal of Rural Health*, 13(6), 348–52.

42. Peckover, S. and Chidlaw, R. (2007) The (un)-certainties of district nurses in the context of cultural diversity. *Journal of Advanced Nursing*, 58(4), 377–85.

43. Benson, J. (2007) A culturally sensitive consultation model. *Synergy*, 1, 5–7, 18–19.

44. McGarry, J. (2003) The essence of 'community' within community nursing: A district nursing perspective. *Health and Social Care Community*, 11(5), 423–30.

45. Van Loon, A.M. (1998) The development of faith community nursing programs as a response to changing Australian health policy. *Health Education and Behavior*, 25(6), 790–99.

46. Van Loon, A.M. (2001) The challenges and opportunities of faith community (parish) nursing in an ageing society, in E. MacKinlay, J.W.P. Ellor and S.K. Pickard (eds) *Aging, Spirituality and Pastoral Care: A Multi-National Perspective.* Haworth Press, New York, pp. 167–80.

47. Benzein, E., Johansson, B. and Saveman, B. (2004) Families in home care – a resource or a burden? District nurses' beliefs. *Journal of Clinical Nursing*, 13(7), 867–75.

48. Department of Veterans' Affairs (2001) *The Guidelines for the Provision of Community Nursing Care.* Australian Government Department of Veterans' Affairs, Canberra.

49. Goodman, C., Robb, N., Drennan, V. and Woolley, R. (2005) Partnership working by default: District nurses and care home staff providing care for older people. *Health and Social Care Community*, 13(6), 553–62.

50. Hudson, B. (2002) Interprofessionality in health and social care: The Achilles' heel of partnership? *Journal of Interprofessional Care*, 16(1), 7–17.
51. Speed, S. and Luker, K. (2006) Getting a visit: How district nurses and general practitioners 'organise' each other in primary care. *Sociology of Health & Illness*, 28(7), 883–902.
52. McQueen, A. (2004) Emotional intelligence in nursing work. *Journal Advanced Nursing*, 47(1), 101–8.
53. Mueser, K., Bond, G., Drake, R. and Resnick, S. (1998) Models of community care for severe mental illness: A review of research on case management. *Schizophrenia Bulletin*, 24(1), 37–74.
54. Warelow, P. and Edward, K. (2007) Caring as a resilient practice in mental health nursing. *International Journal of Mental Health Nursing*, 16(2), 132–5.
55. Peckover, S. and Chidlaw, R. (2007) Too frightened to care? Accounts by district nurses working with clients who misuse substances. *Health and Social Care Community*, 15(3), 238–45.
56. Department of Health and Ageing (1995) *Ways Forward: National Aboriginal and Torres Strait Islander Mental Health Policy National Consultancy Report*. Commonwealth of Australia, Canberra.
57. Goold, S. and Liddle, K. (2005) *In Our Own Right: Black Australian Nurses' Stories*. eContent Management, Sydney.
58. De Crespigny, C., King, M., Van Loon, A.M. and Groenkeer, M. (2004) *Clinical Management of Aboriginal People with Co-Existing Diabetes and Alcohol Related Health Problems – A Review*. Flinders University School of Nursing and Midwifery, Adelaide.
59. Van Loon, A.M. and Kralik, D. (2005) *Reclaiming Myself after Child Sexual Abuse*. Royal District Nursing Service Foundation Research Unit, Catherine House Inc, Centacare, Adelaide.
60. Van Loon, A., Koch, T. and Kralik, D. (2004) Care for female survivors of child sexual abuse in emergency departments. *Accident and Emergency Nursing*, 12, 208–14.
61. Smith, J. and MacDonald, J. (2001) Evidence-based health care and community nursing: Issues and challenges. *Australian Health Review*, 24(3), 133–40.
62. Luker, K., Wilson, K., Pateman, B. and Beaver, K. (2003) The role of district nursing: Perspectives of cancer patients and their carers before and after hospital discharge. *European Journal of Cancer Care*, 12(4), 308–16.
63. Department of Health (2000) The expert patient: A new approach to chronic disease management for the 21st century. *United Kingdom National Health Service*. London: Department of Health.
64. Lorig, K., Seleznick, M., Lubeck, D., Ung, E., Chastain, R.L. and Holman, H.R. (1989) The beneficial outcomes of the arthritis self-management course are not adequately explained by behavior change. *Arthritis and Rheumatism*, 32(1), 91–5.
65. Kennedy, A. and Rogers, A. (2001) Improving self-management skills: A whole systems approach. *British Journal of Nursing*, 10(11), 734–7.
66. Buetow, S., Goodyear-Smith, F. and Coster, G. (2001) Coping strategies in the self-management of chronic heart failure. *Family Practice*, 18(2), 117–22.
67. Clark, N.M., Gong, M. and Kaciroti, N. (2001) A model of self-regulation for control of chronic disease. *Health Education and Behavior*, 28(6), 769–82.
68. Willems, D. (2000) Managing one's body using self-management techniques: Practicing autonomy. *Theoretical Medicine and Bioethics*, 21(1), 23–38.
69. Eastwood, S., Kralik, D. and Koch, T. (2002) Compromising and containing: Self-management strategies used by men and women who live with multiple sclerosis and urinary incontinence. *Australian Journal of Holistic Nursing*, 9(1), 33–43.
70. Kralik, D., Koch, T., Price, K. and Howard, N. (2004) Chronic illness self-management: Taking action to create order. *Journal of Clinical Nursing*, 13(2), 259–67.

71. McGillis Hall, L., Doran, D., Baker Ross, G., Pink, G.H., Sidani, S., O'Brien-Pallas, L. and Donner, G.J. (September 2003) Medical care. *Nurse Staffing Models As Predictors of Patient Outcomes*, 41(9), 1096–109.

72. Aiken, L.H. (2002) Superior outcomes for magnet hospitals: the evidence base, in M.L. McClure and A.S. Hinshaw (eds), *Magnet Hospitals Revisited: Attraction and Retention of Professional Nurses*. American Nurses Publishing, Washington, DC, pp. 61–81.

73. Needleman, J., Buerhaus, P., Mattke, S., Stewart, M. and Zelevinsky, K. (2002) Nurse-staffing levels and the quality of care in hospitals. *New England Journal of Medicine*, 346(22), 1715–22.

74. Wilson, R., Runciman, W., Gibberd, R., Harrison, B., Newby, L. and Hamilton, J. (1995) The quality in Australian health care study. *Medical Journal of Australia*, 163(9), 458–71.

75. Wilson, R., Harrison, B., Gibberd, R. and Hamilton, J. (1999) An analysis of the causes of adverse events from the Quality in Australian Health Care Study. *Medical Journal of Australia*, 170, 411–15.

76. Leape, L. (2005) Questions and answers with Dr Lucian Leape. *4th Australasian Conference on Safety and Quality in Health Care*, Melbourne, Australia.

Chapter 2

Clinical governance

Anne Maddock

Introduction

This chapter discusses the role of the community nurse in the provision of safe and quality care and strategies to enact their accountability and responsibility in clinical governance.

> The contemporary view of quality and safety incorporates clinical governance where all staff in an organisation share responsibility and accountability so that risks are minimised and opportunities for clinical excellence are enhanced through continuous monitoring and improvement of services [1].

Clinical governance is defined as 'the system by which the governing body, managers and clinicians share responsibility and are held accountable for patient care, minimising risks to consumers, and for continuously monitoring and improving the quality of clinical care' [2, p. 4]. This chapter incorporates primary health care principles within a clinical governance approach for community nursing. Specific areas covered in this chapter are:

- The realities of community care delivery.
- Clinical governance frameworks and accountability.
- Clinical excellence and key tools.
- Managing change and change strategies.

The context of community care

The factors impacting on the context of community care include:

- The changing and diverse complexity of illness and disease comorbidities that people experience as they live longer.
- The increasing number of people who want to be cared for in their homes.
- Health care delivery that is becoming more complex with multiple services that require multidisciplinary team approaches to care provision and complex policy and strategic guidance to ensure quality and safe outcomes.

These factors give rise to a range of clinical safety and quality challenges that community nurses face on a daily basis. Some examples include:

- Assisting clients with their management of chronic conditions can involve complex care coordination and liaison with other health services and various professionals. It is important to foster the client's self-management and consider the ways they have been managing their chronic disease over many years, acknowledging that they are the experts of their own health and daily living activities [3].
- Coordinating medication management and providing assistance with comorbid chronic condition management because these clients are often on multiple medications that compound the complexity of their illness experience that requires community nurses to work across interfaces to ensure that the management of medications is current, safe and effective [4]. For example a study undertaken in 2005 identified that a key cause of adverse medication events was the transfer of people from primary to secondary care [5].
- As the population ages the prevalence of falls is increasing and many frail elderly struggle with bodily function; inadequate access to, and consumption of, a nutritious diet requires community nurses to be aware of safety measures within people's homes. Community nurses need to advise clients about safe and effective environments to prevent harm from falls [4].
- The prevention of pressure ulcers is another challenge for community nurses. One expert witness in several court cases and inquests has noted that 'nurses are increasingly being held account for pressure ulcers that have been the cause of death in their patients' [6]. Therefore community nurses need to employ strategies to minimise the incidence of pressure ulcers, utilising evidence-based pressure ulcer prevention and management strategies.
- The uncontrolled and variable hygiene of the home care context can confront community nurses with infection control management issues and so nurses need to adopt 'an infection control system that supports safe practice and a safe environment for consumers/patients and health care workers' [4, p. 104].
- The number of people experiencing leg ulcers is projected to double over the next 25 years. 'An Australian study found that only 19% of patients who should have been receiving compression therapy were in fact doing so' [7, p. 45], making evidence-based chronic leg ulcer management a key role for community nurses. This role can be complicated by the potential for ineffective treatment when the client is between nursing visits and providing self-care if they cannot apply the bandages as required.
- There is an increasing need to manage challenging client and community behaviours, such as aggression, which requires the community nurses to implement safe management systems that ensure their own safety and the safety and well-being of clients, staff, visitors and contractors [4].

Consequently, the community context and its accompanying challenges require community nurses to adopt a clinical governance approach to effect change to their practice. Such an approach:

- Employs strategies that access, implement, monitor, support and disseminate research findings for clinical excellence in practice, in particular the provision of safe and quality outcomes.

- Employs strategies that reduce inappropriate variation in care and minimise the risk that care may not be beneficial.
- Adopts strategies that encourage learning from past mistakes rather than blaming, to produce practice standards for high-quality services.
- Participates in strategies that lead to the sharing of effective practice with colleagues and that address failures in performance across the care interfaces.
- Employs effective strategies of self-agency to facilitate the delivery of high-quality and safe care between visits and on discharge from the service [3, 8].

Clinical governance frameworks and accountability

A product of the evolution of clinical governance across the world is the artificial distinctions that have occurred between clinical and non-clinical governance and risk management, with the introduction and implementation of clinical governance frameworks [9]. This has been necessary to bring clinical safety and quality to the fore of policy and decision makers' minds. Integrated governance recognises the dynamic tension of competing governance elements whilst breaking down these distinctions. When community nurses put the client and their safety and the quality of the services that they receive at the centre of their decision making, they can make decisions about safety and quality as close as possible to the point of care.

Clinical governance provides the structure in which everyone in the organisation demonstrates accountability 'for continuously improving the quality of their services and safeguarding high standards of care by creating an environment in which excellence in clinical care can flourish' [10, p. 65].

There is a need for organisations to have a clinical governance framework in place to provide a frame of reference to:

- 'Assess to what extent there are systems, processes and appropriate levels of resources in place to improve the safety and quality of client care' [1].
- 'Continue to improve the safety and quality of client care' [1].
- Create 'change through a common understanding of what clinical governance is, the interrelationship between structure and processes and lines of responsibility and accountability' [1].

The key elements of a clinical governance framework for each organisation appear to be more a product of time and evolution of clinical governance in that organisation, as opposed to one being more right than the other.

From the author's experience there are six key elements commonly identified in clinical governance frameworks:

- Organisational structure.
- Patient consumer involvement.
- Human resource management.
- Infrastructure support functions.
- Measurement and evaluation in the dimension of quality areas.
- Exploration across the whole care continuum.

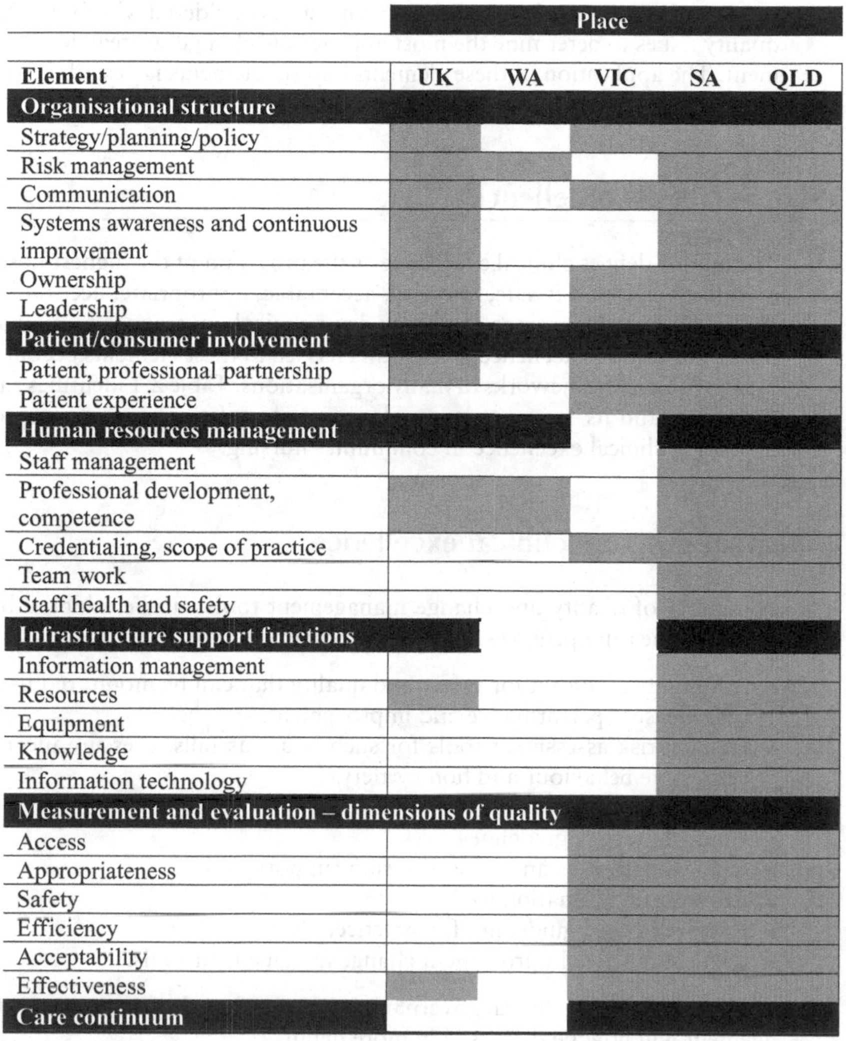
Place
Element
UK
WA
VIC
SA
QLD
Organisational structure
Strategy/planning/policy
Risk management
Communication
Systems awareness and continuous improvement
Ownership
Leadership
Patient/consumer involvement
Patient, professional partnership
Patient experience
Human resources management
Staff management
Professional development, competence
Credentialing, scope of practice
Team work
Staff health and safety
Infrastructure support functions
Information management
Resources
Equipment
Knowledge
Information technology
Measurement and evaluation – dimensions of quality
Access
Appropriateness
Safety
Efficiency
Acceptability
Effectiveness
Care continuum

Figure 2.1 Clinical governance elements – an evolution.

All of these elements, either individually or collectively, can impact on the safety and quality of health care. The frameworks and the corresponding key elements and subelements of clinical governance are noted in Figure 2.1. These elements are included in clinical governance frameworks due to their impact on safety and quality health care as it evolved in the United Kingdom (UK), Western Australia (WA), Victoria (VIC), South Australia (SA) and Queensland (QLD) [11–15]. The examples depicted in Figure 2.1 demonstrate an increase in the scope of clinical governance from the National Health Service in the UK in 1999 to frameworks developed in QLD in 2006 and all comply with the most recent version of the Australian Council on Healthcare Standards of quality for health care service provision [4]. The organisational structure and process subelements listed in Figure 2.1 are foundational to the operation of safety and quality service provision and must be considered when reviewing safety and quality issues to determine the most appropriate change strategy for quality improvement. The application of these elements and subelements is described in the following section.

What is clinical excellence?

The author defines clinical excellence as the provision of the highest possible standard of clinical care that is safe, effective, acceptable, appropriate, accessible and efficient [15]. These six dimensions of quality drive clinical governance frameworks [13]. The pursuit of clinical excellence in Australia has led to these elements becoming embedded into the quality frameworks of many organisations. Table 2.1 identifies each dimension of quality and its scope and provides examples of the key areas to consider when managing clinical excellence in community nursing.

Tools that promote clinical excellence

A number of quality and change management tools can be adopted by community nurses to measure progress towards clinical excellence, including:

- A minimum data set for safety and quality that can be monitored using scorecards that measure performance and improvement.
- Clinical risk assessment tools for such issues as falls, pressure ulcers, violent and aggressive behaviour and home safety.
- Clinical audit tools.
- Clinical practice guidelines.
- Clinical pathways and other decision support tools.
- Review and evaluation tools.
- Research-based guidelines for practice.
- Clinical practice improvement change management tools.

The link between clinical governance, safety and quality outcomes and change management will now be discussed in more detail.

Managing change and change strategies

Features of effective change management

The unpredictable, dynamic and multifaceted nature of change is a learning process that is neither linear nor sequential, but a continuous process of transition that involves adjusting goals, tackling unanticipated events and managing disruptions [16, p. 156].

Change management strategies impact on health care processes in order to create sustainable change. 'Change will not work unless it is owned and led by clinical teams' and that change 'has to be manageable, testing incremental improvements' [17, p. 56]. Questions have been raised in relation to policy being a useful driver of change without

Table 2.1 Measurement and monitoring of clinical excellence [1].

Dimension and scope	Management of excellence in community nursing
Safety of health care: • Safe progress through all parts of the system • Risk minimised in care delivery processes	• Reducing medication error, falls rates, infection or pressure ulcers and workplace violence • Accurate client identification • Safe use of blood products • Effective clinical handover
Effectiveness of health care: • Treatment received will produce measurable benefit • Treatment, intervention or service achieves the desired outcome	• Monitoring client outcomes • The treatment produced the desired outcome, such as compression therapy, readmission rates for the same problem • The adoption of clinical pathways and variance tracking • Communication with other service providers
Appropriateness of care: • The intervention will produce the desired outcome • Expected health benefit exceeds the expected negative consequences Evidence is used to do the right thing to the right patient, at the right time, avoiding and under utilisation	• Peer review and monitoring of the appropriateness of treatment regimes • Client involvement in decision making • The availability of best practice guidelines for treatment and interventions
Acceptability of care: • Opportunities for health consumers to participate collaboratively • Degree to which a service meets or exceeds the expectations of informed consumers	• Monitoring of client satisfaction with the service provided • Client awareness of their rights and responsibilities • Involvement of consumers in the review and development of care regimes
Access to services: • Equitable access to health services • Availability of services, physical and information access	• Monitoring client access to services and care regimes • Hospital avoidance capacity • The provision of the right service
Efficiency of service provision: • Resources are utilised to achieve value for money • Allocation of resources to provide the greatest benefit to consumers • Allocative efficiency • Technical efficiency: reducing costs and minimisation of waste	• Monitoring the cost of different care regimes compared to the client outcomes • The activity of the community nurse service • Length of stay

clinician support, as 'policies are enacted largely if clinicians decide to do so, and they determine the circumstances of implementation' [18, p. 11]. Consequently, enlisting the support of clinicians is essential to effectively implementing change.

Several facilitators for sustainable change have been identified by Sibthorpe *et al.* [19]. These include:

- Political sustainability – having individual champions and good linkages.
- Institutional sustainability – having good relationships, structures and processes.
- Financial sustainability – including the availability of necessary funds.
- Economic sustainability – referring to income advantage and workload.
- Client sustainability – including the resilience of the client base, the right setting, acceptance of the provider and the service being embedded in its patient community.
- Workforce sustainability – having the right staffing, skills and motivation factors [19].

It is important to foster the social relationships, networks and champions that will affect the political, financial and societal forces that create the context within which change happens. Specifically the need for a solid policy footing, ongoing funding and enduring client demand and workers that are both able to adapt innovation and adapt to innovation are required for sustainable change. Flexibility and factors that influence workers such as '... perceived client need, the adequacy of staffing levels and mix, staff training and skills, workload, compatibility of new with existing roles and tasks, institutional support, patient and community receptivity and support, perceived effectiveness, economic viability, and feed back of information' [19, p. S77] all impact clinicians' capacity to excel in a changing clinical care environment. These themes reflect the core elements of clinical governance frameworks described earlier in this chapter.

How can community nurses adopt the clinical governance framework?

It is important that community nurses adopt the guiding principles of their organisation's clinical governance framework in their daily practice. For example: .

- Apply the *structural elements* through the implementation of effective processes and procedures that comply with the organisation's risk and continuous improvement strategies.
- Consider the criticality of the *health care interface* and *multidisciplinary team* and *patient partnerships* in their decision making to effect safe and quality outcomes.
- Seek out and apply *research-based knowledge* sources for *evidence-based practice* to ensure the appropriateness and effectiveness of treatments and interventions.
- Seek out and utilise appropriate *technology* for point-of-care decision making.
- Seek to influence the *infrastructure support* requirements needed to provide safe and quality outcomes.
- Ensure there is appropriate *human resource support* with adequate knowledge, competence, skills and staffing numbers [4, 14, 20].

Applying a clinical governance framework for continuous improvement

So how can community nurses apply a clinical governance framework to their practice? Let us look at three high-risk clinical care situations that community nurses are confronted with each day, namely medication management, falls prevention and pressure ulcer prevention.

Medication management

Structural elements – Community nurses need to demonstrate leadership in the application of risk and continuous improvement management strategies to reduce medication errors. Community nurses need to be aware of the relevant Australian State or legislation and standards, and they need to facilitate a patient-safety culture.

Health care interface and the multidisciplinary team – Community nurses need to facilitate teamwork and appropriate and effective medication management through the use of regular medication review. Community nurses should be alert to the potential of medication error across the interface and respond appropriately, making decisions that are inclusive of the total client journey by establishing timely and effective communication processes with appropriate health services and providers.

Patient partnerships – Community nurses need to ensure that there are acceptable levels of consumer involvement in care and enhance or maintain self-management. Wherever possible, they should help the client understand the rationale for their medication, its rationale for use and the appropriate use, administration and storage of the medications in the home. They can assist with provision of dose administration aids and help clients maintain and monitor accurate medication lists.

Knowledge resources and evidence-based practice – Community nurses need to ensure they have access to evidence-based knowledge and information resources to provide safe, appropriate and effective treatment regimes and interventions. Community nurses need to ensure safe, appropriate and secure storage of medicines and facilitate the appropriate disposal of medicines. Community nurses need to employ safe documentation and communication of medication orders and administration.

Technology – Community nurses need to use technology accurately and understand the rationale for its use. They should provide input into the development and ongoing sustainability of the necessary technology for the provision of safe and quality medication management within a community context.

Infrastructure support – Community nurses need to provide input into the accessibility and effectiveness of the infrastructure support required to ensure excellence in safe and quality medication outcomes. For example are there adequate knowledge sources such as MIMS On-line and available clinical experts that they can access when they have pharmacological enquiries?

Human resource support – Community nurses need to communicate with their manager on human resource requirements for the provision of safe and quality medication management, such as workforce design and flow, training, development and credentialing requirements, scope of practice required for medication administration, safe staffing and feedback that will be important for workforce planning [7, 20].

Falls prevention

Structural elements – Community nurses need to demonstrate leadership in the application of risk and continuous improvement management strategies to reduce client falls and the extent of injury associated with falls. Community nurses need to be aware of relevant policy in the areas of restraints (minimisation in use), management of the confused client and manual handling, which are essential for falls management. Community nurses need to facilitate a client-safety culture and be aware of referral sources within the community in which they are working.

Health care interface – Community nurses need to facilitate teamwork with community partners, regarding safety in the home environment and the use of best-practice preventative strategies that effect minimisation of risk for falls.

Client partnerships – Community nurses need to ensure that there are acceptable levels of consumer involvement in their care, enhancing or maintaining self-management as long as possible.

Knowledge resources and evidence-based practice – Community nurses need to utilise risk-screening and -assessment processes as early as possible after the admission of the client and employ the required falls minimisation strategies in use in their organisation using a documented risk reduction plan. They should be aware of best practice in this area-effect strategies such as the 'implementation of simple, safe and effective measures such as vitamin D and calcium supplements could prevent many fractures' and therefore serious injuries as a result of falls [7, p. 42].

Infrastructure support – Community nurses need to facilitate access to the necessary equipment required for falls prevention and provide feedback to their managers on the accessibility, appropriateness and effectiveness of the equipment provided. Community nurses should ensure that there are effective maintenance programmes in place for any equipment they use/loan.

Human resource support – Community nurses need to ensure they access education on evidence-based falls prevention [21].

Pressure ulcer prevention

Structural elements – Community nurses need to demonstrate leadership in the application of risk and continuous improvement management strategies to reduce pressure ulcer prevalence and harm associated with pressure ulcers. Monitoring pressure ulcer prevalence and external-service-acquired pressure ulcers is important. Community nurses need to be aware of relevant organisation policy and standards and facilitate a client-safety culture.

Health care interface – Community nurses need to facilitate teamwork and appropriate and effective reduction of pressure ulcer prevalence by employing a partnership approach to improvement. This may require liaison with general practitioners regarding medical management of the ulcers. It may include preventative strategies that assist with mobility and movement using community volunteers, carers and other allied health professionals.

Multidisciplinary team – Community nurses should ensure that there are mechanisms in place to provide feedback to service providers on the prevalence of external-service-acquired pressure ulcers and strategies to reduce their occurrence.

Client partnerships – Community nurses need to ensure that there are acceptable levels of consumer involvement in their care, enhancing or maintaining self-management as long as possible. This can be challenging when clients struggle to apply pressure bandages on their own and so it may involve enlisting other people to partner with the client to effect care.

Knowledge resources and evidence-based practice – Community nurses need to utilise risk-screening and -assessment processes and employ evidenced-based pressure ulcer prevention strategies through a documented risk reduction plan in line with best practice. They should be contributing to the advancement of professional knowledge in this area and its application to the community context.

Infrastructure support – Community nurses need to facilitate access to the necessary equipment required for pressure ulcer prevention and provide feedback to their manager on the accessibility, appropriateness and effectiveness of equipment provision. Community nurses should ensure that there are effective maintenance programmes in place for all equipment.

Human resource support – Community nurses need to provide feedback to their manager on the availability of staff, with adequate evidence-based knowledge of pressure ulcer prevention and safe staffing requirements to provide a high-quality and safe service [22].

Applying a clinical governance framework to practice as described above requires the selection of the most appropriate change management strategy to ensure improvement and sustainability of safe and quality outcomes. The following section will provide a range of strategies from which community nurses can choose, depending on the issue at hand.

Choosing the most appropriate approach to clinical practice improvement

Previous authors have highlighted 'the need for formal methods of improving practice' [23, p. 460]. In order to enact their role in clinical governance, community nurses need to be aware of, and employ, appropriate clinical practice improvement approach that sustains change. The organisation's capacity to learn and change as an outcome of information and knowledge transfer is a critical activity and is foundational to efforts to secure improvements in the quality and safety of care and services [14].

A sound change management approach is essential. 'Change in complex organisations such as community health services is unlikely to be a straightforward process and is likely to require more than one approach' [16, p. 156]. Therefore, the change management approach of telling people the 'correct thing to do, rarely leads to systemic change' [24, p. 156]. Furthermore, 'changing deep seated culture and embedded practices may be more generational in scope than many think' [25, p. 12]. Clinical service provision can be analysed from a number of different approaches.

> Prospective analyses of systems are increasingly being explored in health care on the reasonable argument that it is better to examine safety proactively and to prevent incidents before they happen [25, p. 242].

Community nurses need to be involved in fostering a learning culture to advance clinical practice improvement [1].

A guide to improvement

The challenge for the community nurse is to choose the right change management strategy, depending on the issue at hand. In some cases there may need to be a blend of strategies; however, this needs to be put into the context of understanding that 85% of workplace problems can be attributed to 'the capability of the system in which (people) work (not) the performance of individual people' [26, p. 9]. Key elements of a successful improvement strategy have been highlighted as:

- Understanding what needs to improve or utilising processes that secure that understanding.
- Engaging the key stakeholders in the improvement.
- Utilisation of a fluid and flexible plan.
- Having executive support.
- Reflecting on successes at key milestones.
- Communication.
- An evaluation strategy.
- Sharing the results through an effective communication strategy [22].

Summary

This chapter provides an overview for community nurses to implement a clinical governance approach for sustainable improvement in safety and quality health care outcomes. The chapter covers areas that are essential for a community nurse to grasp to facilitate the achievement of their role and responsibility in clinical governance. These include:

- The context of community care delivery.
- Clinical governance frameworks and the community nurse's accountability for their application in the work environment.
- Expectations in the pursuit of clinical excellence and key tools for use.
- How to manage options for sustainable change management.

Clinical governance may be viewed as complex and ethereal to clinicians at the client interface, but it is imperative that community nurses understand that they are pivotal to quality health outcomes and the pursuit of clinical excellence for their clients.

Useful resources

Community nurses need to keep abreast of advances in improvement strategies in health care. This can be facilitated by visiting the following websites:

The Joint Commission at www.jcaho.org
National Patient Safety Association at www.npsa.nhs.uk
Nation al Health Service Modernisation Agency at www.wise.nhs.uk
National Institute of Clinical Studies at www.nics.com.au
Institute of Healthcare Improvement at www.ihi.org
Agency for Healthcare Research and Quality at www.ahrq.gov

References

1. Maddock, A. (2008) Quality and safety in community health care, in D. Kralik and A. van Loon (eds) *Community Nursing in Australia*. Blackwell Publishing, Oxford, UK.
2. Australian Council on Health Care Standards (ACHS) (2004) *ACHS News*, 12, 4.
3. Koch, T., Jenkin, P. and Kralik D. (2005) Chronic illness self management: Locating the 'self'. *Journal of Advanced Nursing*, 48(5), 484–92.
4. ACHS (2006) *The ACHS EQuIP 4 Guide. Part 1: Accreditation, Standards, Guidelines*. Australian Council on Healthcare, Zetland, NSW.
5. Midlov, P., Bergkvist, A., Bondesson, A., Eriksson, T. and Hoglund, P. (2005) Medication errors when transferring elderly patients between primary health care and hospital. *Pharmacy World and Science*, 27(2), 116–20.
6. Hampton, S. (2005) Death by pressure ulcer: Being held account when ulcers develop. *Journal of Community Nursing*, 19(7), 26. Available at www.jcn.co.uk (viewed 26 March 2007).
7. National Institute of Clinical Studies (NICS) (2005) *Evidence-Practice Gaps Report*, Vol. 2. National Institute of Clinical Studies, Australia.
8. Zeh, P. (2002) Clinical governance and the district nurse. *Journal of Community Nursing* [serial online], 16(4), 1–11. Available at www.jcn.co.uk (viewed 16 June 2003).
9. Cauchi, S. (2005) Integrated governance: Is this the future? *Professional Nurse*, 20(7), 53–5.
10. Scally, G. and Donaldson, L.J. (1998) Clinical governance and the drive for quality improvement in the new NHS in England. *BMJ*, 317, 65.
11. NHS Clinical Governance Support Team (1999) *Seven Pillars of Clinical Governance*. Available at http://www.cgsupport.nhs.uk/downloads/Seven_Pillars.doc (viewed March 2007).
12. Department of Health, Western Australia (2005) *Clinical Governance Framework*. Office of Safety and Quality in Health Care, Western Australia. Available at www.safetyandquality.health.wa.gov.au (viewed March 2007).
13. Victorian Quality Council (2005) *Evaluation of Victorian Quality Council Better Quality, Better Health Care: A Safety and Quality Improvement Framework for Victorian Health Services*. Department of Human Services, The Victorian Quality Council, Victoria.
14. Balding, C. and Maddock, A. (2006) *South Australian Safety and Quality Framework & Strategy 2006–2009: Project Report and Resource Documents*. Department of Health, Government of South Australia, South Australia. Available at www.safetyandquality.sa.gov.au (viewed 1 March 2007).
15. Maddock, A. and Smith, J. (2007) *Risk Assessment and Management Framework Development Project for the Maternity Services Steering Committee, Queensland*. Available from secretariatmssc@health.qld.gov.au.
16. Telford, T., Maddock, A., Isam, C. and Kralik, D. (2006) Managing change in the context of a community health organisation. *Australian Journal of Primary Health*, 12(2), 156–66.
17. Lock, L. (2003) Healthcare redesign: Meaning, origins and application. *Journal of Quality and Safety in Healthcare*, 12, 56.
18. Braithwaite, J., Black, D. and Westbrook, J.I. (2003) Policy effects on clinical work: Less change than envisaged? *Clinical Governance Bulletin*, 3(6), 11.
19. Sibthorpe, M., Glasgow, N.J. and Wells, R.W. (2005) Emergent themes in the sustainability of primary health care innovation. *Medical Journal of Australia*, 183(10), S77–80.
20. Australian Pharmaceutical Council (2006). *Guiding Principles for Medication Management in the Community*. Commonwealth of Australia, Australian Capital Territory.
21. Victorian Quality Council (2006) *Evaluation of the Effectiveness of the 'Minimising Risk of Falls and Fall-Related Injuries: Guidelines for Acute, Subacute and Residential Settings' Final Report*. Department of Human Services, The Victorian Quality Council, Victoria.
22. Victorian Quality Council (2006) *Successfully Implementing Change*. Department of Human Services, The Victorian Quality Council, Victoria.

23. Wilson, R.M. and Harrison, B.T. (2002) What is clinical practice improvement? *International Medical Journal*, 32, 460.

24. Maddock, A. (2008) 'Risky business' – risk management in community nursing, in D. Kralik and A. van Loon (eds) *Community Nursing in Australia*. Blackwell Publishing, Oxford, UK.

25. Vincent, C.A. (2004) Analysis of clinical incidents: A window on the system not a search for root causes. *Quality and Safety in Health Care*, 13, 242.

26. Australian Quality Council (AQC) (1996) Principles of quality management and improving organisations: Systems thinking and organisational learning, in AQC (ed.) *Certificate IV. Quality Management Assessment Participant Guide*, pp. 9–34, 40. Australian Quality Council, Australia.

Chapter 3

Informed consent

Elizabeth Crock

Introduction

This chapter examines the issue of informed consent in community nursing contexts. The historical origins of the doctrine of informed consent are explored, followed by identification of the important elements of informed consent, competence to consent, assessment of decision-making capacity, surrogate decision making and children and consent. The aim of this chapter is to enhance nurses' understanding of the legal and moral frameworks related to consent processes which serve to protect and promote people's rights and welfare within health care, including those of children and of people with disabilities. Cases from the law are described and the literature is drawn on to discuss nurses' ethical responsibilities in relation to consent processes and protecting the vulnerable from harm in health care delivery.

Defining the terms

'Informed consent' within health care refers to a person's autonomous authorisation of a specific medical intervention or participation in research [1, 2]. The doctrine of informed consent is most often discussed in relation to procedures or treatments prescribed by doctors; however, there has been little discussion in the nursing literature about the ethical requirement for informed consent to nursing care [3, 4]. Even so, it is recognised within the nursing profession that nurses are obliged to obtain clients' consent prior to performing nursing procedures [4]. This obligation is equally applicable to all nurses regardless of work settings. Moreover, the right to informed consent is in accordance with the principles of primary health care, in particular their focus on full participation, self-determination and a rights-based approach to health care [5]. Ethical, lawful consent processes and practices are also integral to clinical governance, in the interests of quality client care, and the minimization and management of risk in clinical care [6].

The right of people to provide informed consent to care and treatment within health care is acknowledged in a range of Australian and international nursing guidelines and documents. For example in the Australian Code of Ethics for Nurses [7, p. 3], it is stated that 'nurses accept the rights of individuals to make informed choices in relation to their care'. The code goes on to explain:

1. Individuals have the right to make decisions related to their own health care on the basis of accurate and complete information given by health care providers. Nurses must be satisfied that they have the person's consent for any care or treatment they are providing. If individuals are not able to provide consent for themselves, nurses have a role in ensuring that valid consent is obtained from the appropriate substitute decision maker.
2. Nurses have a responsibility to inform people about the nursing care that is available to them, and people are entitled morally to accept or reject such care. Nurses have a responsibility to respect the decisions made by each individual.
3. Illness and/or other factors may compromise a person's capacity for self-determination. Where able, nurses should ensure that such persons continue to have adequate and relevant information to enable them to make informed choices about their care and treatment and to maintain an optimum degree of self-direction and self-determination [7, p. 3].

Similarly, the Australian Code of Professional Conduct for Nurses [8, p. 2] stipulates that nurses must support 'the informed decision-making of an individual'. In addition, it is expected that nurses 'must also ensure that the person is represented by an appropriate advocate if unable to speak or decide independently'. These statements serve as both guidelines for nurses' conduct and standards to which nurses are expected to adhere.

The requirement for nurses to obtain informed consent is also recognised internationally. For example the International Council of Nurses' Code of Ethics stipulates that practising nurses/managers ought to provide 'sufficient information to permit informed consent and the right to choose or refuse treatment' [9, p. 5]. Nurse educators and researchers ought to provide 'teaching/learning opportunities related to informed consent', and National Nurses' Associations ought to provide 'guidelines, position statements and continuing education related to informed consent' [9, p. 5].

These statements make it clear that nursing as a profession acknowledges its independent responsibility and accountability in relation to the doctrine of informed consent. Informed consent obligations have both moral (ethical) and legal implications. It is important for community nurses to understand the legal and ethical rationale behind the principles of informed consent so that the principles are applied appropriately in their work context [4].

Historical perspective on consent

Consent has been formally recognised as a prerequisite to medical intervention and human experimentation only recently in the history of Western health care. Human experimentation was the first area which became subject to the ethical and legal requirement of informed consent. Significantly, Grodin [10] suggests that all ethical codes related to human experimentation appear to have been developed in response to specific abuses and that, in all cases, violations have continued after the promulgation of the codes.

The requirement that physicians gain the consent of patients prior to surgery has been traced to the year 1767 and the case of Slater v. Baker & Stapleton in the USA. Early American decisions held such cases to be founded in the law of battery. A North American physician, William Beaumont, devised a code in 1833 dealing with human experimentation, in which 'voluntary consent' was deemed a necessary condition of experimentation [11]. In Germany in 1891, a Prussian minister issued a directive to prisons that tuberculin for the treatment of tuberculosis ought not to be used 'against the patient's will' [12, p. 1445]. But the first known, detailed European regulations relating to consent to human experimentation was a Prussian directive issued by the minister of religious, educational and medical affairs in Germany in 1900, which stipulated that such experimentation was 'absolutely prohibited' if 'the person concerned has not declared unequivocally that he [*sic*] consents to the intervention' [10, p. 127]. Interestingly, this directive was issued following public debate about experiments conducted by venereologist Albert Neisser, who inoculated several children and three prostitutes with syphilis serum without their consent, resulting in their contracting the disease [10]. Nevertheless, medical interventions for the purposes of treatment, diagnosis or immunisation remained exempt from the requirements of the directive [10].

The doctrine of voluntary informed consent for experimentation on prisoners was confirmed as an essential element of ethical medical practice, following the Nuremberg trials of the Nazi doctors in Germany in 1945, although the term 'informed consent' did not appear until 10 years following the trials [1]. Those doctors, with the collaboration of nurses in many cases, had conducted injurious, agonising and often fatal experiments on prisoners throughout the Second World War [13]. The emphasis on people's rights to refuse or accept to take part in medical research stems directly from these atrocities. These rights were codified in the Nuremberg Code of 1948 and, later, in the Declaration of Helsinki of 1964 [14].

Informed consent is now a central ethical and legal principle in the provision of health care, including nursing care; its requirement is not limited to circumstances of human experimentation, but is applicable to all health care interventions, with certain well-defined exceptions (such as in life-threatening situations) [1]. Whilst in the USA and Canada, the requirement for informed consent uses a 'reasonable patient' standard model of consent (which stresses that a practitioner can be found to have committed 'trespass or battery' if performing a procedure without consent), the Australian and New Zealand legal model has traditionally used a 'reasonable practitioner' standard, which emphasises negligence and malpractice [3]. Recently, this has been changing however, and it now appears that Australian courts have begun applying a tougher standard for the information that doctors should provide to patients – that is, what the 'reasonable patient' might expect, rather than what a reasonable body of practitioners might think [15] (see Box 3.1).

Justification for and elements of informed consent

Historically, there have been two main ethical justifications for informed consent. The avoidance of harm, unfairness and exploitation has been the primary justification for the doctrine [1]. More recently, however, the emphasis has been placed

---

Box 3.1   Duty to disclose

In an Australian case known as Rogers v Whitaker (1992) [16], an ophthalmologist failed to mention the possibility of sympathetic ophthalmia, a serious though rare complication of eye surgery which can result in blindness, even though the patient concerned had asked about possible harm to her intact eye. The patient became almost completely blind when this complication occurred. The court judged that it was the doctor's duty to disclose 'material' risks – that is, a risk that 'in the circumstances of the particular case, a reasonable person ..., if warned of the risk, would be likely to attach significance to it or if the medical practitioner is, or should reasonably be aware that the particular patient, if warned of the risk, would be likely to attach significance to it' [15, p. 39, 16].

---

on the requirement to protect a person's autonomous choice or self-determination [1, 3].

Consent is both an ethical requirement and a legal doctrine [3]. The legal approach focuses on the health practitioner's duty to disclose relevant information, whereas the moral or ethical approach focuses on the principle of respect for persons and their right to make autonomous decisions about their care [3,11]. Functions of informed consent processes include the protection of patients, avoiding fraud and duress, encouraging self-scrutiny by health professionals and promoting 'rational' and systematic ethical decision making [3, p. 136].

Faden and Beauchamp [11, p. 274] identify the following five elements as critical to informed consent: disclosure, comprehension, voluntariness, competence and consent. Expanding on these, Beauchamp and Childress [1] note that:

- Disclosure must include all the relevant information – that is, both risks and possible benefits of the procedure or service, as well as the risks or benefits of not having it provided.
- The person must be competent to make a decision (both rational and prudent).
- The person must comprehend both the information being given and the implications of consent.

Finally, consent must be freely given (see also [1, 3, pp. 141–7]). A person must feel and *be* free to refuse to undergo the procedure, without prejudice. In this regard, a person's freedom to choose can be impaired or enhanced by cultural, religious and psychological forces, as it can by external factors such as legal requirements or by their location (such as a nursing home, prison or immigration detention centre) [17]. Consequently, there would need to be a compelling reason to support the performance of any nursing or medical procedure on a person without voluntary informed consent. Consent is not required, however, in an emergency when delaying treatment would jeopardise a person's life or well-being [1, 18]. The required elements of informed consent are relevant to all settings and professions [2] (see Box 3.2).

> **Box 3.2   Essential elements of informed consent**
>
> - Disclosure
> - Comprehension
> - Voluntariness
> - Competence
> - Consent

How much and what type of information must be given?

Information should be presented in a form that is clear and comprehensible at a level the person can understand – this may be written, may need to be in the client's own language or given with an interpreter present. Information should be presented in a way that maximises a client's understanding as well as the possible impacts of their decision on the basis of the standard of what a 'reasonable' individual in the client's position would be able to understand and make a reasonably informed decision about [2, p. 106]. Ideally, the nurse ought to be sure that the form of the information (written or oral) is comprehensible to the client, the language is one in which the client is literate, jargon is avoided and the timing of the giving of information takes into account the client's mental state, fatigue and level of distractibility [2]. Questions may be asked by the nurse to elicit comprehension.

Restricted disclosure or withholding of all information is sometimes justified, for example when the practitioner judges that disclosure might cause such distress that it would hinder or complicate treatment or even pose psychological damage to the client [2]. In such cases courts have allowed restricted disclosure, under the name of 'therapeutic privilege'. Some authors have criticised 'therapeutic privilege', pointing out that there is little evidence to support the notion that disclosure of relevant medical information prior to a treatment decision would harm patients [3, 19].

The specific content, manner and timing of presentation of information or data (for example written or oral) may vary as a function of legal requirements, agency policies, client characteristics and/or the setting in which services are provided [2]. As mentioned earlier, for a person to be able to provide informed consent, they must be competent to make the decision. The issue of competence warrants further discussion.

Consent as a process

Some authors describe consent as a process rather than as a single or static event [24, 25]. Davis [24] states that experienced nurses view consent as a process that occurs over time. Usher and Arthur [25] view consent as an 'ongoing consensual process that involves the nurse and patient in mutual decision-making and ensures that the patient is kept informed at all stages of the treatment process' [25, p. 692]. In community nursing contexts, consent as a process seems to be most apt, as the nurse is actively engaged in the establishment and ongoing processes of consent. Consent 'must be constantly re-evaluated' to check whether the original consent still holds true for the client [3, p. 146]. In this way, the client remains involved in decision making throughout the care episode, and is kept informed about and involved in negotiating their treatment options and goals [25].

Benefits of informed consent

Alongside the obvious benefits to clients of upholding their rights to self-determination (autonomy) and respecting their wishes and decisions, the use of proper informed consent procedures has been reported to decrease clients' anxiety, improve clients' compliance with medical treatments and contribute to more rapid recovery. In some contexts, clients may be more favourably disposed towards practitioners who take the time and effort to provide information for informed consent [26]. Basic requirements of the process of gaining informed consent are identified in the example given in Box 3.4.

Competence

Competence, or the capacity for autonomous choice, refers to a person's ability to make decisions for her- or himself [1]. For a person to be considered competent, she or he must have the cognitive capacity to make a competent decision concerning a proposed therapeutic relationship or procedure to be contemplated [2]. It should be noted that there is a presumption of competence for adults aged over 18 years in Australia and that competent adults have the legal and moral right to make 'bad' or 'risky' decisions that others may see as being against their best interests [20]. Specifically, people are judged competent to make a decision if they are:

- Informed of the facts and probabilities.
- Able to understand the facts and probabilities.
- Able to make a voluntary choice (not coerced).
- Able to make a reasoned choice.
- Able to communicate that choice [21, pp. 199–200].

Judgements of capacity can be distinguished from judgements of competence – it is the health professional who assesses capacity and incapacity, whereas it is the legal system that determines competence [1]. Thus, competency is a legal construct. The burden of proof regarding competence lies with the practitioner. If the client is not competent, another person must be appointed to consent on the client's behalf (see the section on 'Surrogate decision makers and consent', below).

The legal system relies on the expert advice of clinicians regarding the client's disability and the effect of the disability on decision-making capacity. The terms 'competence' and 'incompetence' are nevertheless frequently used by health professionals whose judgements may lead them to override a person's decisions, to advocate for others to make the decisions (family members or other surrogates), to request that a guardian be appointed or to seek involuntary institutionalisation on a person's behalf [1].

The importance of clients having access to properly trained interpreters in obtaining informed consent cannot be overstated (see Box 3.3). Implications of a lack of provision of adequate information and subsequent informed consent to treatment can include poor adherence to medication and treatment regimens, poorer follow-up and attendance at medical appointments, lower rates of preventative or health promotion strategies being offered and taken up (such as breast self-examination and Pap smear testing) and much poorer satisfaction with health services overall. Bischoff [23] describes how minority and migrant patients are likely to be treated less aggressively for a range of cancers, receive less specialist cardiac care, receive less antiretrovirals for HIV infection, receive fewer paediatric prescriptions and those with mental illness are more likely to be misdiagnosed and to receive inadequate treatment. All these outcomes can be related to failures in information giving and adequate informed consent processes being followed for people who do not speak or understand the dominant language.

Surrogate decision makers and consent

Where a person lacks the capacity to provide informed consent, 'surrogate' (substitute) consent may be obtained. Guardianship and Administration Boards, sometimes referred to as Adult Guardianship Boards, have developed as a means of facilitating medical treatment (and other decisions) for people over 18 years with a disability, who are unable to give their own consent to dental, medical or special procedures, because they are incapable of understanding the nature and effect of the

---

Box 3.3 Failures of informed consent and the importance of access to qualified interpreters

1. Some health professionals in Australian hospitals use the term 'veterinary medicine', meaning treating patients 'as if they are unconscious' in emergency departments with poor access to interpreter services: 'One time, someone from the emergency department . . . said, "Well you need to get an interpreter" . . . and then they said, "If we can't get an interpreter, we will just treat them as if they are unconscious" ' (in effect, this means relying on a possibly unnecessary barrage of diagnostic investigations rather than diagnostic questioning of the patient) [22, p. 152].

2. 'One night I (interpreter) was called urgently to the hospital because somebody was about to suffer a ruptured appendix and would not give his consent to an operation – he just refused to. I found out why he refused to. They had asked a cleaner to come and interpret for him orally, to look at the consent form and give it to him in his language. God bless her, she did not have enough language skills and she said, 'They want to cut something from your tummy', and he said, 'I am not going to have anything cut from my tummy or anywhere else', and he was very, very ill. But he was also a gentleman who had a lot of personal strength to refuse to sign the consent form . . . . He could have died. In fact, the moment he had signed, the trolley was waiting to take him to the operating theatre' [22, p. 147].

Box 3.4   Consenting to become a client of a nursing service

It is common practice for clients to be required to sign a consent form when becoming clients of a service. This is an example of informed consent.
The following provides an outline of basic requirements of the process:

1. Explain the nature and orientation of your role and, where relevant, the perspective you come from (for example health promotion, feminist midwife or Gestalt-trained mental health nurse) and the relevant aspects and boundaries of your role. State your credentials (registered nurse, midwife or other specialist qualifications).
2. Any costs of the service should be disclosed, along with options for clients who are unable to pay.
3. Explain how records are kept within your agency and how the client can access the files. Explain that records are kept for the client's benefit and for communication between health care workers. As a general rule, clients should have access to their files as long as information contained therein is not misleading or detrimental to the client. Explain the essential elements of the Privacy Act and any limits to confidentiality.
4. If providing a service/treatment, explain the likely treatment benefits, risks and alternatives.
5. Disclose any consultation or supervision requirements of your agency and the possible impact of such a relationship on the current nurse/client relationship.
6. Disclose the client's rights and responsibilities, including how complaints can be made [2].
7. Obtain the client's verbal or written consent.

---

proposed treatment or they are incapable of communicating their consent. Prior to any applications for guardianship where a decision is made regarding competency, preventive measures should first be explored [20]. These measures could include documents such as wills, enduring powers of attorney, advance directives and 'elder care contracts'.

The Australian Guardianship and Administration Committee is the peak body of the Australian organisations responsible for guardianship and financial administration for people who are unable to make their own decisions. Each state and territory has its own organisation(s) which performs these roles, usually referred to as the Office of the Public Advocate or Guardianship Tribunals, as well as state trustees or financial administrators. In addition, each state/territory has its own Guardianship and Administration Act or Adult Guardian Act, which governs the agencies concerned. (These acts are all available online, and community nurses should be familiar with the relevant act for their jurisdiction.)

In general, within the Guardianship Acts, medical treatment includes any surgical or medical procedures or examinations and any preventative, palliative or rehabilitative care normally carried out or under the supervision of a registered medical practitioner. There are three types of substitute consent:

- Consent by the person responsible – guardian, spouse including same-sex spouse (in some jurisdictions though not all), close personal friend, sibling.
- Consent deemed by law.
- Consent given by the Guardianship and Administration Board.

There will be some situations where it is mandatory to obtain consent for a specific procedure through the board. Whilst the specific procedures vary a little between states, such treatments include any treatment that is likely to lead to infertility, termination of pregnancy, removal of tissue for transplant, administration of drug of addiction, psychosurgery and any treatment involving an aversive stimulus [27]. Substitute or surrogate consent need not be obtained for emergency care or first aid, administration of prescribed medications within recommended dosages or visual examination of mouth, throat, nasal cavity, eyes or ears. If care is considered 'necessary', consent by a substitute is not required as long as the patient does not object. As a general rule, community nursing, including district nursing care, would be deemed 'necessary'. If 'necessary' care has been carried out, or supervised, without consent of a substitute but in good faith that the requirements of the act have been complied with, the practitioner would not be guilty of assault or battery or professional misconduct.

In order to appoint a substitute or surrogate decision maker, the following conditions need to be met:

- The person has a disability, as a result of which there is an impairment of decision-making capacity.
- There is a 'need'.
- An immediate decision is required.
- There is substantial risk of harm to the person or others.
- Less restrictive options have been unsuccessful [20].

'Disability' could include a wide range of issues, such as mental illness, intellectual impairment, dementia and acquired brain injuries; however, the person must also have impaired decision-making capacity. Thus, just because a person has a specific diagnosis does not mean that they are incapable of making decisions. For example as Bennett and Hallen [28, p. 487] comment, 'It is not the presence or absence of dementia *per se* that potentially compromises capacity but the presence of specific cognitive deficits which may selectively impact upon different aspects of the person's decision-making ability'.

Importantly, assessing decision-making capacity is about ensuring the freedom of competent individuals while protecting those who lack competence from possible harm. In any event, assessments of decision-making capacity and the appointment of substitute decision makers deserve due consideration and are generally not undertaken unless genuine need is evident. Even where decision-making capacity is doubtful, less restrictive alternatives should be attempted first. Examples may include the appointment of case managers, increased services and supports, counselling, trials and education [20]. The appointment of case managers, however, should be subject to informed consent processes and potentially can have significant implications for client autonomy and privacy. If there is genuine concern about decision-making capacity, the imposition of case management itself can entail rights violations. Cognitive capacity assessment at this stage can provide an opportunity to identify people's strengths as well as their weaknesses that might jeopardise their decision-making abilities. Ideally, a person's strengths can be used to compensate for weaknesses, and targeted training or education might help individual clients to remain independent [20]. Even in cases where a surrogate decision maker has been appointed, the person may still be able to participate in decision making. In addition, guardians and administrators are legally obliged to include the person in decision making wherever possible.

Problems with competency assessments

The use of the word 'competency' as a blanket term can lead to the mistaken notion that a person is either completely 'competent' or completely 'incompetent'. In fact, a person's decision-making capacity is assessed in regard to a specific decision, at a specific point in time, under specific circumstances [20]. Furthermore, people who lack decision-making capacity can continue to make their own decisions as long as they are not at substantial risk of harm. Issues can also arise concerning how 'harm' is defined, what is meant by a substantial risk and who should properly decide these things [3, p. 152].

There can be considerable disagreement between professionals around competency assessments and a lack of convergence in the clinical findings [3, 20]. Some clients may receive 'borderline' results, which do not give a clear indication of their decision-making capacity, so there is a need for a flexible and individualised approach. (For a detailed overview of the legal context in Australia regarding competency, see Bennett and Hallen [28].)

Informed refusal – challenging 'informed consent'

As discussed earlier, protection of clients' rights to autonomy, or to exercise self-determination, is considered to be the essential principle underlying the doctrine of informed consent. Therefore, and as a corollary, it is implied that clients have the right to refuse consent. As Schweitzer and Puig-Vergès [29, p. 776] comment, 'The freedom to oppose must be accepted for every person facing a medical intervention: for the respect of individual liberty requires it'. Autonomy is a Western ideal, and within Western health care systems, even if a client refuses to undergo a recommended medical procedure on the basis of information received about risks, it is still the case that any competent person is entitled to do this, regardless of what others might think of their refusal [3, 11]. Johnstone [3, p. 144] asserts that 'at best, all attending health professionals can morally do is persuade patients non-coercively about the known benefits of undergoing a given medical procedure; but they are not entitled to interfere with the patient's choice if such persuasion fails'.

As Johnstone [3] and other authors have pointed out, issues about competency rarely arise when patients agree with and consent to a doctor's recommended or prescribed treatments. The question of a client's competency tends to arise mostly when they refuse treatment and that refusal is considered by health workers to be irrational. Others disagree with this focus on autonomy and see it as a cultural bias. For example Glick [30] describes a case in which a district judge in Israel ordered the force-feeding of a group of political prisoners engaged in a hunger strike after prison doctors judged their

---

Box 3.5   Informed refusal of nursing care by a competent person

M. was a 50-year-old morbidly obese woman with a long medical history. As a result she had developed large areas of skin breakdown and ulceration resulting in unrelieved pain. Five people were needed to turn her and wash her. She adamantly refused to be turned or to have wound care done. Nursing staff involved became very distressed and an ethics consultation was held.

Discussing this case, Dudzinski and Shannon [31] point out that if staff are assured that M's decision-making capacity is intact, her refusal is informed, she is aware of the possible benefits of the nursing care proposed and risks, benefits and the consequences of refusal, and her refusal is not coerced in any way, a response based solely on respect for her autonomy would allow her to remain in 'an ever increasing swamp of faeces and urine', supporting her 'right to die buried in human waste' [31, p. 612]. This approach is consistent with legal and ethical standards that allow competent patients to refuse treatment.

The authors proposed a 'negotiated reliance' approach in an effort to compromise, which treads lightly on the patient's autonomy while minimising the distress caused to others – care providers can ask for only a minimum of hygiene while agreeing to provide aggressive pain management [31, p. 608].

After ethics consultation, and in view of M's ongoing refusal of turning and management of bowel incontinence, the nursing staff negotiated turning M once per day and shifted the plan to palliative care goals. The authors later believed that M should have received 'conscious sedation' for turning and for hygiene and should have been turned only to manage her bowel incontinence, not according to any set daily routine [31].

---

lives to be in danger. The judge in this case stated that 'when there is a conflict between life and dignity, the preservation of life takes precedence' and thus the prisoners' autonomy was overridden [30, p. 954].

Even those authors who agree in theory with the focus on autonomy appear to be more reluctant to accept a client's decision to refuse treatment or care than to accept their agreement. Nurses regularly encounter refusal of nursing care by clients, and many find such situations extremely challenging and sometimes morally distressing, although this has not been discussed in depth in the literature. Dudzinski and Shannon [31] describe one such case of a woman who refused pressure area care and incontinence management, as outlined in Box 3.5.

Despite the focus on autonomy and rhetoric about respecting clients' informed refusal, and its perceived Western cultural bias, there continue to be notable cases where competent adults are denied the right to refuse treatment or care. In recent years, there have been cases in the UK where court-ordered caesareans for mentally competent women have been performed against their autonomous wishes – even after it was determined that such operations were unlawful [32, 33]. Similar cases have occurred in the USA, denying women the rights generally accorded to other competent people [34].

Implied or tacit consent

Consent can be written, oral or given by implication. Some argue that for consent to be valid, written consent is neither sufficient nor necessary [4]. Nurses in particular have argued that clients express consent to nursing procedures 'by implication'. Implied consent may be given by, for example, rolling up a sleeve prior to an injection or putting out an arm prior to a blood pressure reading. Implied consent is recognised in ethics and law, but it must also comprise the elements of informed consent; it merely lacks verbal or written affirmation. Practitioners are still expected to respect a person's refusal of any specific examinations or treatments [35].

Aveyard [36] has described how nurses proceed with providing care without formally seeking consent, as long as the patients do not object. Aveyard raises the concern that in many such cases, the patient can be said to have acquiesced or complied, but 'cannot be said to have given implied consent' [36, p. 204]. Others have questioned the use of 'tacit' or 'implied' consent. For example mass immunisations without explicit consent are given in some nursing homes in Holland, in order to maximise immunisation rates which can increase protection for all residents by fostering 'herd immunity'. Verweij and van den Hoven [37] argue that this deviation from standard informed consent processes is not ethically justified, because nursing homes that do request informed consent also have high vaccination rates that may be sufficient to promote herd immunity. Second, tacit consent is valid only if everyone knows they have a choice to refuse. Particularly in institutional settings, patients have been found to comply, to fit in with nurses' routines, to 'toe the line' rather than participate in decision making. Aveyard [36, p. 206] cautions nurses that implied consent can often be indistinguishable from compliance and to assume that this constitutes implied consent is to 'risk administering care without consent'. Coerced consent is also legally invalid. In any case it is recommended that nurses document when they have explained the procedure and the client has consented to it, whether the consent was implied or explicit [18]. In the community nursing context, nurses who are involved in group immunisation-giving or other procedures must be aware of their responsibilities in gaining informed consent from each client, whether or not consent is 'implied'.

Children and consent

All Australian jurisdictions assert that minors do not have the 'capacity' to provide informed consent. Legal incapacity is intended to protect minors, as consent expressed by minors is considered 'insufficiently free and enlightened' [29, p. 777], because minors are assumed to be unable to defend their own interests. Consent for minors is systematically delegated to parents or a legal guardian. There may be exceptions in the case of 'emancipated minors' who are living independently and supporting themselves. In some circumstances, the common law recognises that minors can seek specific advice and support, for example on pregnancy counselling, sexually transmissible infections and substance use, without the consent of a legal guardian or parents [38]. The principles in such circumstances include that the child needs to understand the advice given, that the doctor cannot persuade the child to inform her or his parents/guardian and that the treatment is in the child's best interests [38].

There is specific legislation in some states (New South Wales and Victoria) relating to the medical treatment of minors. In any case, it is considered good therapeutic practice for nurses to provide appropriate information to children to encourage their voluntary participation in recommended therapies.

Challenges and controversies in consenting on behalf of children and the disabled

There remain numerous contemporary examples where parents or legal guardians have made decisions on behalf of their children which the children later disagree with, regret and challenge or which violate the child's right to bodily integrity and, in the opinion of some legal commentators, can also constitute assault and child abuse [39]. Foremost amongst these are parental decisions to have genital surgery performed on children born with intersex conditions. (An intersex person is a person who, because of a genetic condition, was born with reproductive organs or sex chromosomes that are not exclusively male or female. (Legislation Act 2001, Republication no. 55, 10 November 2007. Commonwealth of Australia, Canberra, p. 128.)) These cases are disturbing, as the children do later attain competence and then would have the capacity to make their own decisions. Similarly, decisions have been made to sterilise or perform hysterectomies on young girls with intellectual or physical disabilities. Most often these children have intellectual disabilities and may never be able to attain 'competence'.

Some medical procedures proposed for children (up to 18 years of age) require approval of the Family Court – these include non-therapeutic sterilisation, hysterectomy, gender reassignment and organ donation (see Box 3.6). In New South Wales, permission is required from the Guardianship Board for the prescription of long-term injectable contraceptives and other 'special medical treatment' [38]. Even so, hundreds (and possibly over a thousand) of unauthorised sterilisations on young girls with disabilities are reported to have been performed in Australia since the legal determination known as Marion's case in 1992 [40–42]. In relation to this, Nicholson [39] encourages a more proactive stance by health care workers who might find themselves in the position of whistleblowers if they are witness to such cases, as well as registration boards who he suggests ought to impose sanctions. Thus, community nurses involved

---

Box 3.6   Marion's case

In the early 1990s, the Australian Family Court had been presented with an application for the sterilisation of a 14-year-old girl with a severe disability and incapacity to provide consent, with the aim of preventing pregnancy and menstruation. The matter went to the Australian High Court, which made the landmark decision that court or tribunal authority is needed before any child can be lawfully sterilised (unless the sterilisation occurs as a result of surgery to treat some other disease or malfunction). Authorisation is allowed only if sterilisation is determined to be in the child's best interests after alternative and less invasive procedures have failed or if it is certain that no other procedure or treatment will work. It should be a procedure of 'last resort'. Thus, parental consent is ineffective where a proposed intervention is 'invasive, permanent and irreversible and not for the purpose of curing a malfunction or disease' [39, p. 1].

in the care of such children ought not to turn a blind eye when such procedures are proposed and indeed may have a moral (and legal) duty to act – for example to conscientiously object to participate and to report the situation to relevant authorities, cognizant of the personal and professional sensitivities and risks this might entail. Nicholson [39, p. 3] adds that health care workers should heed advice as to 'the criminal and civil liability that may attach to direct and also indirect involvement in an unauthorised procedure; and the statutory consequences of not fulfilling mandatory reporting requirements in respect of "abuse".'

The fact that such unlawful procedures are still performed and receive little attention in the media or in the nursing literature reflects the critical importance for nurses of understanding the legal framework governing consent and substitute consent, which is intended to protect the vulnerable from harm. If nurses are uncertain about their legal obligations involving the consent of a child or adolescent to medical treatment or nursing care, advice should be sought from their employing body and/or professional and industrial organisation.

Future trends

Advance directives

Advance directives (sometimes referred to as 'living wills') are written or oral statements that people make when they are mentally competent in order to influence treatment decisions which may arise when they are no longer competent to make them. The directives come into force only if and when the person becomes 'incompetent' [21] (see Box 3.7). For example a person may make a decision to refuse artificial hydration

---

Box 3.7   Ulysses contracts – advance directives and mental health care

Ulysses was the character in Greek mythology who asked his sailors to bind him to the mast of his ship, and to plug their own ears with wax, to avoid being seduced to their death by the Sirens of Cyrene. Advance directives for psychiatric care [43] ('Ulysses contracts') have been proposed for people with a mental illness who are 'in remission' and are competent to give prior authorisation for treatment in the future when they may be incompetent, refusing treatment and non-compliant [43]. At times of mental health crisis, people may lack insight into their condition and possible harm that may arise. It has been suggested that this type of advance directive can help prevent relapses and sustain good mental health [44]. Ethical and legal concerns however are raised about Ulysses contracts. For example some say that they undermine the legal right to refuse treatment or that levels of competence in psychiatric patients can shift from day to day and thus it can be difficult to determine when to intervene. However, if safeguards and processes (such as opportunities to revoke consent and ongoing communication about treatment options) are in place to ensure protection of people's significant moral interests, welfare and well-being, such advance directives may have a role in enhancing mental health care (see also Johnstone [3]).

and nutrition if in a vegetative state, to decline renal dialysis or to decline hospital admission. Generally, basic care or palliative care cannot be refused. Advance directives can direct another person to make decisions on one's behalf and/or instruct health care workers about one's values and treatment preferences, or both of these [3]. A written document ('Enduring power of attorney') may be completed or the directive may be informal and verbal. Some guidelines stipulate that people should not be able to refuse basic care in advance or instruct others to refuse it on their behalf (where 'basic care' means medical and nursing care measures essential to provide comfort and alleviate pain and distress). This includes the provision of warmth, shelter, hygiene measures and management of distressing symptoms, such as pain and breathlessness, and provision of oral food and fluids, but not artificial feeding. Emergency care should not be withheld while seeking the advance directive or interpreting it [21].

Consent to health promotion

Consent to medical treatments and research has been the focus of most of the bioethics literature regarding consent [3, 45]. Little has been written, however, about consent processes in relation to health promotion interventions [45]. This might include information people require prior to participating in health screening, such as for breast cancer, cervical cancer or prostate cancer. Pfeffer argues that 'there is no good reason why informed consent' should not be sought for health promotion interventions, which are neither neutral nor harmless, and that 'blind compliance or non-compliance fails to respect human rights' [45, p. 230]. Community nurses are frequently at the forefront of health promotion activities and interventions, and this may well be an area in which they have much to contribute in terms of developing improved informed consent and informed refusal processes and practices.

Consent and research nurses

Nurses are increasingly involved in medical as well as nursing research in all settings in which they work, and as mentioned earlier in this chapter, they can be held independently accountable for ensuring that informed consent has been obtained and for the legal implications of violations of people's right to informed consent. Several historic and current examples have been given of dubious or unethical practices in research and treatment, in some of which nurses have been implicated. Karigan [46] describes a scenario in which a client is to receive an investigational drug, but there is no evidence of a signed consent form and the physician concerned cannot produce it when asked. Should the nurse proceed with the treatment or demand to see the consent form or consult with the nurse manager, colleagues or the hospital ethics committee first? Karigan [46] concludes that simply assuming the protocol is being followed is not acceptable and that the nurse has responsibility to the client first, as well as to the research team.

In one study, clinical research nurses were surveyed to determine their attitudes, perceptions and behaviours regarding the informed consent process [47]. The study recognised that nurses are well qualified to survey the informed consent process. The researchers found that 41% of the nurses reported that they had assisted on a research protocol where the participant did not understand the consent document, but was nevertheless enrolled; 27% of the nurses said they assisted in research where participants did not understand that the intervention was for research and not treatment purposes; and 11% assisted in research where they felt subjects had been coerced into participating. In many cases, these nurses had acted to try to rectify problems with the consent process and some had refused to administer a study intervention; however, 10% also said that they never or only rarely contacted a study investigator if they perceived a problem with the consent process. Davis [24] also found that nurses assumed the roles of 'watchdog' to monitor the informed consent process, 'advocate' to mediate on behalf of clients, 'resource person' to provide information on alternatives, 'coordinator' to preserve an open, friendly atmosphere for discussion and 'facilitator' to clarify differences between involved parties. Studies such as these indicate the important quality improvement role nurses can have in ensuring that consent processes are properly addressed.

Involvement in clinical research trials can offer nurses additional career opportunities whilst offering patients new and improved treatments [46]. Nurses in community settings are also being asked with increasing frequency, by other professionals and by hospital staff, to perform tasks related to research projects, sometimes as part of fee-for-service arrangements. In this environment, it is critical that participating agencies and individual nurses are confident that appropriate ethics approval and informed consent processes have been followed and, where nurses believe they have not, that they have the right and the opportunity not to participate in such research. Ideally, participating nurses should have the opportunity to contribute to the research process and not be simply utilised as data collectors. Nurses themselves ought to decide what will be their role and their level of involvement in medical research, or they risk taking on more responsibility and accountability without the corresponding authority and acknowledgement of their roles.

Summary

This chapter has examined the issue of consent in nursing contexts with a focus on community nursing. The history and theoretical underpinnings of the doctrine of informed consent have been explored and its essential elements explained. Although the specific application of the elements of informed consent have not been widely discussed in the nursing literature [4, p. 202], these elements are equally relevant to nurses as they are for other health professionals. Along with explicit consent, the issues of tacit or implied consent, clients' rights to informed refusal of care and the challenges these can pose for nurses have been discussed.

Competence, assessment of decision-making capacity, surrogate decision making and children and consent have been examined, with a view to enhancing nurses' understanding of the legal and moral frameworks which serve to protect and promote people's rights within health care, including children and people with disabilities. Cases from the law and cases described in the literature have been drawn on to promote debate and critical thinking amongst nurses regarding their roles and their ethical responsibilities in relation to consent processes and protecting the vulnerable from harm within health care.

The issue of advance directives outlining treatment and care decisions in general as well as in mental health care has been examined in the light of emerging and future approaches to consent. Other emerging issues such as consent in health promotion and research have been briefly canvassed.

Parsons [2] notes that informed consent is more than an ethical or legal mandate – the promotion of informed consent is a reflection of the nature of the helping relationship that is respectful of people's autonomy and values their full participation. This type of relationship according to Parsons is 'the hallmark of the ethical practitioner' [2, p. 114]. Community nurses have a role in helping to develop and promote responsive, accountable and carefully considered consent practices in all work settings, and can thereby help promote the human rights, dignity, well-being and interests of all people for whom they care.

References

1. Beauchamp, T. and Childress, J. (2001) *Principles of Biomedical Ethics*, 5th edition. Oxford University Press, Oxford, UK.
2. Parsons, R.D. (2001) *The Ethics of Professional Practice*. Allyn and Bacon, Boston, pp. 101–18.
3. Johnstone, M.J. (2004) *Bioethics: A Nursing Perspective*, 4th edition. Harcourt Australia, Sydney.
4. Aveyard, H. (2002) The requirement for informed consent prior to nursing care procedures. *Journal of Advanced Nursing*, 37(3), 243–9.
5. World Health Organization (WHO) (1978) *The Alma Ata Declaration*. World Health Organization, Geneva.
6. Australian Commission on Safety and Quality in Health Care (2006) *Measurement for Improvement Toolkit (Part B)*. Commonwealth of Australia, Canberra.
7. Australian Nursing and Midwifery Council Inc (ANMC Inc) (2002) *Code of Ethics for Nurses in Australia*. Australian Nursing and Midwifery Council Inc, Canberra.
8. ANMC Inc (2003). *Code of Professional Conduct for Nurses in Australia*. Australian Nursing and Midwifery Council Inc, Canberra.
9. International Council of Nurses (2005) *The ICN Code of Ethics for Nurses*. International Council of Nurses, Geneva.
10. Grodin, M.A. (1992) Historical origins of the Nuremberg code, in G.J. Annas and M.A. Grodin (eds) *The Nazi Doctors and the Nuremberg Code: Human Rights in Human Experimentation*. Oxford University Press, New York, pp. 121–44.
11. Faden, R. and Beauchamp, T. (1986) *A History and Theory of Informed Consent*. Oxford University Press, New York.
12. Vollmann, J. and Winau, R. (1996) Informed consent in human experimentation before the Nuremberg code. *British Medical Journal*, 313(7070), 1445–9.
13. Annas, G.J. and Grodin, M.A. (eds) (1992) *The Nazi Doctors and the Nuremberg Code: Human Rights in Human Experimentation*. Oxford University Press, New York.
14. Ijsselmuiden, C. and Faden, R. (1999) Research and informed consent in Africa – another look, in J. Mann, S. Gruskin, M. Grodin and G. Annas (eds) *Health and Human Rights*. Routledge, New York, pp. 363–72.
15. Skene, L. and Smallwood, R. (5 January 2002) Informed consent: Lessons from Australia. *British Medical Journal*, 324, 39–41.
16. Rogers v Whitaker (1993) *Australian Law Journal*, 67(1), 47–55.
17. Bloch, S. and Salzburg, M. (2003) Informed consent in psychiatric research. *Current Opinion in Psychiatry*, 16(6), 679–84.

18. Brent, N. (July 1993) How informed are you about consents? *Nurses' Service Organization Risk Advisor Newsletter*, 1–2.
19. Buchanan, A. (1978) Medical paternalism. *Philosophical Public Affairs Summer*, 7(4), 371–90.
20. Mullaly, E. (2006) *Psychologists, the Elderly and the Law*. Paper presented at Caulfield General Medical Centre, Melbourne.
21. Randall, F. and Downie, R.S. (1999) *Palliative Care Ethics: A Companion for All Specialties*, 2nd edition. Oxford University Press, Oxford, UK.
22. Johnstone, M.J. and Kanitsaki, O. (2005) *Cultural Safety and Cultural Competence in Health Care and Nursing: An Australian Study*. RMIT University, Division of Nursing and Midwifery, Melbourne.
23. Bischoff, A. (2003) *Caring for Migrant and Minority Patients in European Hospitals: A Review of Effective Interventions*. A Study commissioned by the Ludwig Boltzmann Institute for the Sociology of Health and Medicine. Neuchatel and Basel, Vienna.
24. Davis, A.J. (1988) The clinical nurse's role in informed consent. *Journal of Professional Nursing*, 4(2), 88–91.
25. Usher, K. and Arthur, D. (1998) Process consent: A model for enhancing informed consent in mental health nursing. *Journal of Advanced Nursing*, 27(4), 692–7.
26. Sullivan, T., Martin, W. and Handelsman, M. (1993) Practical benefits of an informed consent procedure. *Professional Psychology Research and Practice*, 24(2), 160–63.
27. Tasmanian Guardianship Board (2006) *Guardianship Fact Sheet 2*. Guardianship and Administration Board, Hobart.
28. Bennett, H. and Hallen, P. (2005) Guardianship and financial management legislation: What doctors in aged care need to know. *International Medical Journal*, 35(8), 482–7.
29. Schweitzer, M.G. and Puig-Vergès, N. (1996) The child and its health, in E. Verhellen (ed.) *Monitoring Children's Rights*. Martinus Nijhoff Publishers, The Hague, pp. 775–83.
30. Glick, S.M. (1997) Unlimited human autonomy: A cultural bias? *New England Journal of Medicine*, 336(13), 954–6.
31. Dudzinski, D.M. and Shannon, S.E. (2006) Competent patients' refusal of nursing care. *Nursing Ethics*, 13(6), 608–21.
32. Cahill, H. (1999 An Orwellian scenario: Court ordered caesarean and women's autonomy. *Nursing Ethics*, 6(6), 494–505.
33. Kitzinger, S. (1998) Court ordered caesareans in the UK. *Birth: Issues in Perinatal Care*, 25(3), 202–3.
34. Lindgren, K. (October 1996) Maternal–fetal conflict: Court ordered caesarean section. *Journal of Obstetric, Gynecologic and Neonatal Nursing*, 25(8), 653–6.
35. Syse, A. (14 October 2000) Norway: Valid (as opposed to informed) consent. *Lancet*, 356(9238), 1347–8.
36. Aveyard, H. (2002) Implied consent prior to nursing procedures. *Journal of Advanced Nursing*, 39(2), 201–7.
37. Verweij, M. and van den Hoven, M. (9 February 2002) Influenza vaccination rates and informed consent in Dutch nursing homes: Survey of nursing home physicians. *British Medical Journal*, 324, 328.
38. Bird, S. (2007) Children and adolescents: Who can give consent? *Australian Family Physician*, 30(3), 165.
39. Nicholson, A. (19 October 1999) *Medical Abuse: An Extract From the Keynote Address Presented at the 7th Australasian Conference on Child Abuse and Neglect*. Defence for Children International, Perth, Australia.
40. Brady, S. and Grover, S. (1997) *The Sterilisation of Girls and Young Women in Australia: A Legal, Medical and Social Context*. A Report commissioned by the Disability Discrimination Commissioner. Human Rights and Equal Opportunity Commission, Canberra.

41. Brady, S., Britton, J. and Grover, S. (2001) *The Sterilisation of Girls and Young Women in Australia: Issues and Progress.* A report commissioned jointly by the Sex Discrimination Commissioner and the Disability Discrimination Commissioner at the Human Rights and Equal Opportunity Commission. HREOC, Canberra.

42. Joint Standing Committee on Treaties (1998). *Executive Summary: United Nations Convention on the Rights of the Child (17th report).* Parliament of the Commonwealth of Australia, Canberra, p. 286.

43. Widdershoven, G. and Berghmans, R. (2001) Advance directives in psychiatric care: A narrative approach. *Journal of Medical Ethics,* 27, 92–7.

44. Puran, N. (2005) Ulysses contracts: Bound to treatment or free to choose? *The York Scholar,* 2, 42–51.

45. Pfeffer, N. (2004) 'If you think you've got a lump, they'll screen you.' Informed consent, health promotion, and breast cancer. *Journal of Medical Ethics,* 30, 227–30.

46. Karigan, M. (2001) Ethics in clinical research: The nursing perspective. *American Journal of Nursing,* 101(9), 26–30.

47. Murff, H., Pichert, J., Byrne, D., Hedstron, C., Black, M., Churchill, L., *et al.* (July–August 2006) General Clinical Research Center Staff Nurse Perceptions. *IRB: Ethics and Human Research The Hastings Center,* 28(4), 8–12.

Further readings

Bennett, H. and Hallen, P. (2005) Guardianship and financial management legislation: What doctors in aged care need to know. *International Medical Journal,* 35(8), 482–7.

Dalinis, P. (2005) Informed consent and decisional capacity. *Journal of Hospice and Palliative Nursing,* 7(1), 52–7.

Johnstone, M. (2004) *Bioethics: A Nursing Perspective,* 4th edition. Churchill Livingstone, Sydney.

Ladd, R., Pasquerella, L. and Smith, S. (2002) *Ethical Issues in Home Health Care.* Charles C. Thomas Publisher Limited, Springfield.

Chapter 4

Assessment

Lisa Turner, Julianne Siggins and Stephen Harding

Introduction

This chapter examines the factors most likely to influence the community client's ability to remain in the community and the role that the community nurse has to play in facilitating this outcome – that is, for the person to be supported to remain at home or, when required, to transition smoothly to an alternative care facility. Community nurses require a specific body of knowledge to work effectively in the community regardless of their clinical focus or location. Exploration and an understanding of how to develop this specific knowledge and incorporate this information into the community nursing assessment process will be the focus of this chapter.

Community nurses come into contact with clients who have complex health care needs every day in the community practice setting. Community nurses practise in diverse settings such as clinics, the client's home, or mobile services across urban, rural and remote locations. 'Care for people with chronic diseases usually involves multiple health care providers in multiple settings' [1]. A large proportion of community clients are living with a chronic disease [2] and require nursing assistance to enable them to remain in their homes, thus avoiding hospital admissions or placement in a residential aged care facility [1]. To be effective in the role of a community nurse, an understanding of the many factors that impact on a client living in the community is paramount. Positive health outcomes are reliant not only on addressing the disease process but also on understanding the 'whole' client. Psychosocial and environmental factors, social support systems, functional deficits, resilience and life experience all impact on the ability of an individual to remain living in the community.

Assessment

Some older adults or people living with a disability or debilitating chronic conditions perceive that living alone in the community with no or minimal supports is a significant means of maintaining independence and self-worth, which, in turn, enables them to maintain choice and control. However, this belief may place the person at risk of self-neglect, as functional and cognitive deterioration can go undetected and frequently result in the occurrence of a major crisis, such as sustaining an injury in a fall.

Independence is an actual or perceived state in which people maintain, adjust, access or exchange physical, cognitive and social support, spiritual, housing and financial resources within social, cultural, political and economic environments in order to maximise self-care and ability and control over the course of daily life [3].

Maintaining independence safely and effectively is determined by [4]:

- *Physical function* – the person's ability to function at home, i.e. successfully undertake personal and domestic activities of daily living.
- *Social ability* – the person's involvement in social activities, i.e. their ability to maintain contact with others, or frequency of visits away from the home environment.
- *Physical health* – which is the state of physical well-being, i.e. the number of visits to their general practitioner (GP), the number of days spent in bed and the number of medications taken.

Causative factors which influence a person's capacity for independence include their level of cognitive function, functional status, level of physical activity, presence of comorbidities, level of resilience, the presence of a depressive illness or symptoms, fear of safety in the community, polypharmacy (multiple medications), financial status and income, attentional demands (see definition in Carer's assessment section), nutritional health, oral health, fear of falling and their social supports [3]. The changing health care environment in Australia has resulted in acutely ill people, with degenerative conditions being cared for at home [5]. As a consequence, community nurses are being required to focus their care delivery towards more technical and specialised services [6]. However, it is imperative for community nurses to ensure that nursing assessment of clients occurs at each visit to enable the identification of any causative factors that may impact on the client's physical, emotional and social well-being.

The community nurse is required to gather information that informs practice which ultimately leads to positive client outcomes [7]. Information gathering is fundamental to enabling the community nurse to undertake assessment of the client's health needs and should culminate in the formation of a health care plan. An understanding of the principles of primary health care assists the community nurse to be effective in this role. Primary health care can be defined as:

> socially appropriate, universally accessible, scientifically sound first level care provided by a suitably trained workforce supported by integrated referral systems and in a way that gives priority to those in most need, maximises community and individual self-reliance and participation and involves collaboration with other sectors [1].

Primary health care includes the following [1]:

- Health promotion.
- Illness prevention/early intervention.
- Care of the sick.
- Advocacy.
- Community development.

The community nurse may play an integral role in the client remaining at home, acting as the conduit for communication between health care providers and the client (see Figure 4.1). Assessment is a fundamental role in community nursing because it

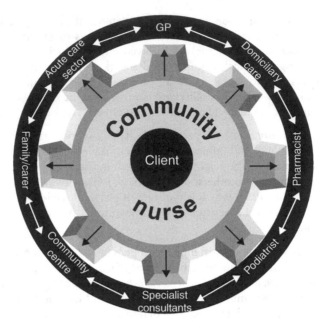

Figure 4.1 The community nurse as a conduit for communication between the client and other health care providers.

sets the scene and the approach to an episode of care and the working relationship that follows [8]. The process of assessment with a client creates the opportunity to learn more about the individual and their circumstances, experiences, perspectives, hopes and plans for the future [9].

The role of the community nurse in assessment of the community client

Patient or client assessment by community nurses is central to the provision of high-quality care [10]. Assessment in the home setting can be a complex process, requiring the community nurse to possess a wide range of knowledge and skills. There are several approaches to the assessment of the community client. These approaches include formal, structured questionnaire-based assessment and informal, conversation-based assessment, both of which draw on nursing concepts (e.g. the nursing process) and theories (e.g. primary health care approaches). However, what can be lacking in the assessment process is the client's perspective. The importance of this inclusion and its contribution to care planning and improved client outcomes cannot be overstated. This process is likely to lead to holistic care and, to be effective, it requires negotiation of care within a relationship that develops throughout the episode of care or duration of care.

The development of a therapeutic relationship between the client and the community nurse is often the foundation for successful and desirable client outcomes [11]. The community nurse, in some cases, must advocate for the client and facilitate the coordination of care when the client is unable to do so independently. For example the younger person living with cerebral palsy in a supported community house with care undertaken by unlicensed careworkers may require a community nurse to advocate on behalf of the client for appropriate care provision. The careworker may also require support in delivery of care through appropriate education and training undertaken by the community nurse. Ultimately, the assessment process should be based on sound primary health care principles and be person centred in its approach.

What should the approach to assessment include?

The assessment process culminates in care planning and since the client is central to the health care team, the community nurse must continually incorporate the client's experiences, ideas, goals and needs into care planning. This plan helps to identify how the client's various wishes will be met and by whom. It also facilitates reassessment when changes in the client's functioning or family supports occur, through provision of baseline assessment data, thus enabling recognition of changes when they occur. The process is 'needs' based [8], with the needs of the client being the focus, not the availability of services.

> The process of assessment can be seen as ongoing (never static), where needs are identified by the older person and the person carrying out the assessment as part of the care planning process [12].

The assessed needs of clients are not always able to be met by the services. This presents a complex dilemma for community nurses; however, utilising a need-based approach ensures that the needs of the client are incorporated into the care plan, with strategies put in place to explore how unmet needs may be met. The community nurse provides information about available services (including that of the community nursing service) and facilitates the process of addressing the care needs gap. The client remains the focus of care and intervention by the nurse working collaboratively with them to identify their needs. This is what 'person-centred' care is all about.

Assessment of one area such as care for a wound should have clear links to additional assessment in the future as the wound heals, rather than be considered in isolation. Assessment takes place at different levels. For example a community client may have a need for a wound care assessment, a nutritional assessment, and an assessment of pain and their risk of developing pressure ulcers. Unidentified health issues may also be uncovered during the assessment process. For example if unexplained delay in wound healing occurs, despite all factors for this being addressed, it may be that comorbidities, such as diabetes, are identified. This emphasises the importance of a comprehensive client-centred assessment methodology for all community clients.

Ensuring that the concerns and issues for the client are at the centre of their care can be achieved if the community nurse seeks to understand and incorporate the client's perspectives and uses a collaborative approach to care. Through experience, the author has come to know a person-centred approach to assessment which requires the community nurse to undertake key activities. These include but are not restricted to:

- Creation of an appropriate environment for the assessment process to take place.
- Establishment of a therapeutic relationship that is based on mutual respect and openness about the purpose of the assessment.
- Acknowledgement of the client's abilities, strengths and resources.
- Being an active listener.
- Being non-judgemental.
- Setting of mutually agreed goals for care.
- Ensuring that the outcomes of the assessment are clarified with the client and the health care goals for the future are realistic and achievable.

The key activities listed above require the assessor to value and understand the information that the client has shared, recognising that this information may come both verbally and non-verbally. Also, often overlooked in the process of assessment are the perspectives of informal carers or family members. The risk of excluding the perspectives of significant others from the assessment process is the development of an incomplete or a less effective plan of care.

Time constraints and environmental assessment

Person-centred assessment takes time – a resource not always freely available in the authors' experience. Recognition of the limits lack of time may place on the community nurse in undertaking a comprehensive person-centred assessment requires a 'balance' to be achieved between the traditional approach (formal interview) to assessment as opposed to observation of the client and their environment. This requires the community nurse to devise innovative methods for undertaking assessment, such as commencing assessment while providing nursing care. In the author's opinion, the 'flow' of information is richer when incorporating key questions designed to explore health issues and concerns from the client's perspective whilst undertaking a technical nursing task, such as changing a wound dressing. Observation of the client's home environment can identify unmet needs. One such example of this is as follows:

> Upon entering the home of a community client the nurse noted that there were unpaid bills on the kitchen table, lack of fresh food in the fridge and numerous bags of rubbish on the floor. During the assessment process the client invited the nurse into her bedroom and when asked what medication she was taking the client instructed the nurse to open her bedside drawer. The nurse noted a large number of 'untaken' tablets in the bottom of the drawer as well as a medication dose administration aid.

It would be reasonable to conclude from the above scenario the need to explore further the client's ability to independently manage medication, financial affairs, grocery shopping and home maintenance. It is however essential not to make assumptions that the client wants to change their situation or that they have a choice about how they are living. All of the above were discovered through observation rather than direct questioning of the client. A formal questionnaire approach to assessment undertaken in just one room of the house would not have revealed what was discovered through the approach described in the scenario.

A useful strategy employed by the author when visiting a client at home is to ask permission to see the bathroom and other rooms where the care is to be undertaken. This provides valuable insight into the client's realm and often 'fills in the gaps' for the nurse's assessment. When time constraints are not recognised as barriers to effective assessment, the community nurse may approach assessment by prioritising the technical nursing needs or tasks. This may result in the loss of 'client centredness', with the community nurse adhering to rigid or unbending frameworks for assessment. The challenge for the community nurse is to develop approaches to assessment that allow for the client-centred approach to be upheld whilst simultaneously meeting the demand for community nursing services. The context of practice can thus influence the outcomes of the assessment approach in that it imposes real-life constraints, such as limited time and resources, on the community nurse.

Assessment structure

The community nursing assessment should include assessment of the client's:

- Functional capacity (disability/ability).
- Attentional demands.
- Cognitive function.
- Nutritional health.
- Environment.

The structure of the assessment process is challenging and highly dependent on the community client's presentation at the time of assessment. The community nurse often 'flies blind' and may not have the advantage of prior information before the client is met for the first home visit. Unknown issues may include home and environmental factors, cultural background, language issues, cognitive function and the client's willingness to accept assistance, and these may impact on the community nurse's ability to remain 'client centred' in approach.

What is the purpose of assessment?

'Health promotion and empowerment are central to health visiting practice and should be reflected in the way the needs are assessed' [13]. The central purpose of the community nursing assessment is to *promote* health with the focus on *prevention* (of development of other health problems) and *support*, making a difference, rather than fostering a dependent relationship between the community nurse and the client. The author believes that in order for the assessment process to achieve its purpose it is important to 'set the scene' from the first contact. This ensures that the client is aware that a 'partnership' is to be embarked on with mutually agreed goals identified and set. This is achieved via the utilisation of the community nurse's expertise and knowledge and contribution from the client. This encourages the client to engage with the community nurse and a rapport to develop.

Primary screening

Screening the client (involving asking a series of questions via the telephone and undertaken by a referral officer) prior to the first visit serves the following purposes:

- Identification of potential and actual risks for the visiting nurse (e.g. aggressive animals, visitors, environmental hazards like broken floor boards, unstable steps and slippery floors).
- Confirmation of correct address details.
- An opportunity to commence information gathering with demographic data collection, such as the client's age, marital status, health insurance status (thus meeting the needs of various funding bodies).
- An opportunity to gather information from the client's perspective (invaluable when matched with the 'real' observations made when visiting the client in their home).
- An opportunity to gather information for referral to other services.
- Confirmation that the client is aware of the referral.
- Confirmation of the need for a community nursing service.
- Inappropriate referrals can be screened and diverted to appropriate services.

The initial assessment

Once primary screening has occurred and the need for the service is confirmed, the community nurse then visits the client's home to undertake the initial assessment. Even before the house is entered much can be learnt about the client. The state of repair of the house, the condition of the garden and even the health of the family pet can contribute to an understanding of the client's ability to manage at home. However, it is at this point that it is essential that conclusions are not drawn about the client's ability to self-care and to remember that the client has a choice about the way they live. All of the observed environmental factors are utilised as a foundation to work from, with integration of these observations into the creation of an overall 'picture' of the client's health care status and way of life.

Establishing a relationship of empowerment and support

A community nurse brings to the assessment process their ability to:

- Get to know the client.
- Get to know the carers.
- Work with the client to identify what actions to take to assist the client to meet unmet needs.
- Know/recognise knowledge deficits in nurse, client and carers.
- Know community resources and services [14].

This knowledge and the information gathered form the framework for establishing a rapport with the client, which assists in the identification of the client's needs. If a relationship based on trust, mutual respect and honesty is established at the outset of assessment, the client remains the focus and is more likely to feel supported throughout the episode of care [15]. The community nurse builds on this relationship as the client becomes more comfortable and begins to share frustrations and challenges, which can be incorporated into a plan of care to assist with the achievement of the long-term goals of care.

Functional capacity assessment

In the author's opinion a relationship built on trust and mutual respect allows the formal aspects of the assessment to commence. Before a plan of care can be developed the client's functional capacity should be understood. Reduced functional capacity can be a major adverse outcome of age-related chronic and/or debilitating conditions. This includes conditions such as osteoarthritis, cerebrovascular disease and cardiovascular disease, which may result in the client having difficulty effectively performing routine activities of daily living, such as mobilising or showering [16].

A potential consequence of reduced functional capacity is the fear of falling. This fear is associated with frailty in older people and contributes to significant psychological and physical conditions, such as depression, anxiety, social isolation and loneliness, culminating in further functional decline and ultimately falls [17].

Physical limitations may impact on the client's ability to be fully involved in meeting their unmet health care needs. For example a client with rheumatoid arthritis may have a reduced capacity to be active with dexterous tasks (e.g. self-medicating via a dose administration aid), and for this reason functional capacity needs to be assessed prior to planning the care. Functional capacity includes factors such as:

- The client's ability to transfer independently, with assistance, or not be able to transfer at all.
- The client's ability to walk short distances or longer distances on uneven surfaces, or climb stairs.
- The client's ability to manage activities of daily living:
  - Showering
  - Mouth care
  - Grooming
  - Dressing
  - Toileting
- The client's ability to manage domestic work, cleaning, gardening, shopping and house maintenance.
- The client's visual and hearing impairments.
- The client's cognitive status.

Gaps in functional capacity can be identified and solutions explored with the client. Often, there are other community services available which the client may be unaware of. The community nurse draws on their knowledge of the local resources and services available to facilitate the client to contact the appropriate agency. However, it is important that the client, rather than the community nurse, makes this contact when able. Experience tells the author that this engenders a partnership approach to the client's health plan. It has the added benefit of empowering the client to be active in their health choices and does not create a reliance on the community nurse to advocate for the client when the client has the capacity and ability to do so themselves.

Attentional demands

Our daily lives comprise activities which constantly demand our attention, e.g. catching a bus, driving a car or crossing a road. Due to the extra-mental effort required to cope with these demands, our ability to function can be impacted upon. Attentional demands in everyday living can cause fatigue in the neural mechanisms of the brain which are responsible for cognitive processes, particularly concentration [18]. The cognitive impairment resulting from such fatigue renders routine daily activities, such as decision making and remembering information, more difficult.

Ageing and other chronic conditions can result in loss and change in motor, sensory, physiological and cognitive functioning abilities, including vision and hearing impairment, physical discomfort, anxiety and mild cognitive impairment [16]. For example picking up the newspaper from the front lawn can be a mentally taxing exercise, which requires numerous attentional demands. Strategies for reducing attentional demands include:

Physical – The reduction of the glare from polished floors; the provision of readily visible cues to locate specific rooms in a complex house design; increasing the colour contrasts between floors, walls and stairs; reducing clutter and potential hazards, e.g. floor mats and rugs in the home. Referral to a community-based occupational therapist will enable a home-safety assessment to be undertaken with suggested environmental alterations being discussed with the client.

Informational – The community nurse should avoid using medical jargon in conversation and ensure that medical terminology and procedures are explained simply and succinctly. Written material provided by the community nurse should adhere to the aforementioned principles and be accompanied by a verbal explanation on presentation to the client.

Behavioural – Appropriate referral by the community nurse to community-based organisations will ensure the availability of assistive devices such as a wheelie walker with an attached tray table that will improve the client's independence and level of control.

Affective – The identification of significant issues such as social isolation, absence of family supports, loneliness and grief due to the loss of a partner or someone significant in the client's life requires attention. Referral to a community-based grief counsellor or bereavement service can provide support and assistance to the grieving client. The exploration of community social interaction groups, through community health care centres and local councils, will provide access to social engagement activities. These may range from telephone link-up morning tea groups to involvement in various interest groups which meet at a central location. Community buses or volunteer transport is frequently available to assist with transportation.

Cognitive screening and older people

Through working with older people, particularly those 70 years and older and those who are physically ill, the author has observed a higher incidence of cognitive impairment. This is important as an Australian study of admissions to a tertiary teaching hospital of people aged over 75 years found rates of cognitive disorder of about 26% [19]. This cognitive impairment was largely due to delirium and dementia.

Cognitive impairment is difficult to identify in general conversation and so screening is important, particularly as some causes (e.g. depression and delirium) are more common in older people and are treatable. Also, medical disorders and treatments may contribute to, or mimic, mental/cognitive disorders, making older people susceptible to missed or misdiagnosis. Early identification of impairment from any cause allows for appropriate therapeutic intervention and facilitation of health and community support services. The burden of untreated mental illness on the client, caregivers and services is high and the routine use of screening instruments in health services may assist in the objective identification of cognitive impairment and assist in establishing the cause. The identification of cognitive impairment is important for health service provision because at little cost to the health service, it assists in our understanding of people's capacity to engage in treatment and care, supports our clinical management and supports post-service planning.

Why screen?

The presence of cognitive impairment means that the likelihood of a diagnosis of dementia is high [20]. Cognitive impairment can however more commonly arise with delirium and depression – as well as dementia. Mental and/or cognitive disorder may also be the first sign of *physical* disorder [20]. Older people may not present with the classic picture of a disease, and advancing age is more likely to bring multiple physical disorders. Equally, the increasing number of physical illnesses associated with ageing will likely bring an increase in the number of drugs prescribed to treat them, and multiple medications increase the risk of adverse effects – e.g. delirium [21, 22]. Impaired orientation and a presenting problem of confusion are strongly associated with falls [23]. Short-term confusional states associated with acute illness and particularly with being in unfamiliar environments, such as hospital wards, pose a high risk of falls for older people.

Cognitive screening in the assessment process

Cognitive screening can be an element of the initial contact with a client so that the baseline occurs at the time the initial history is collected. The history, including a list of current medications from all sources, such as those prescribed, over-the-counter, herbal and illegal substances, and other pertinent information, such as alcohol intake, with corroboration from carers, can be an important part of cognitive screening. Screening as part of the initial assessment will ensure a baseline against which to identify any change in function and will provide information relating to the progression of symptoms (including effect on memory, behaviour and speech) and function (including activities of daily living, ADLs) as well as offer an impression of usual cognitive function. This information could be drawn from relevant information on recent eating habits, ability to manage medications and other aspects of daily life.

Benefits of screening

The formal cognitive screening process is important, as there is no indication that cognitive function can be accurately determined through conversation, particularly if the client's impairment is mild [24] or primarily affects executive functions. In fact, the evidence points to a need for formal screening to determine impairment, particularly in mild and moderate impairment groups [25]. There is evidence that cognitive screening should be routine at admission assessment in health services because it identifies impairment, regardless of cause [26]. This position is supported by the 'best practice approaches to minimise functional decline in the older person across the acute, sub-acute and residential aged care settings' [27] and the 'Clinical Practice Guidelines for the Management for Delirium in Older People', which recommend a structured screening process for the most common cognitive disorder, delirium [27].

Cognitive screening (using a validated tool as part of a detailed history) at the point of entry to a service supports or enhances assessment processes [28]. It provides a baseline against which any cognitive change can be measured and identifies those at risk of further cognitive impairment [29]. Early identification of cognitive impairment assists in diagnostic and management plans and permits anticipation by health professionals of problems in care or the patient's comprehension of or adherence to treatment regimens [30]. Given the predictive relationship of cognitive impairment and deficits in instrumental activities of daily living, it may also facilitate planning future care needs [31]. Screening as part of assessment should not be dismissed on the grounds that patients will be adversely affected because few people experience the process as intrusive or distressing [32]. Nor should it be avoided because of issues of time, as there are a number of tools appropriate for screening that require little time to administer.

Documenting medical history

The biggest challenge in documenting health history with a client is ensuring that the client remains focused on the most relevant aspects. It is here the client or the carer/guardian often shares their 'life history', and innovative 'redirection' by the community nurse is required if the client or carer drifts off on a tangent. However, a balance between redirection and open conversation must be found, as too much direction provided during this process can result in valuable information being missed.

Connecting the discovered comorbidities (e.g. diabetes and its relationship to delayed wound healing, poor nutritional status and falls prevalence, and constipation and urinary incontinence) to the presenting nursing need and the impact these may have on a client's life assists in maintaining the focus and automatically involves the client in the planning phase that occurs later. If there is a cognitive deficit then the carer or family often becomes the conduit for sharing this information. Again the community nurse needs to be 'inventive' in facilitating this situation as the client can quickly become the 'subject' of the conversation rather than remaining at the 'centre' of the care. Deliberate involvement of the client by the community nurse helps assist the confused or disorientated client to remain involved at a level that does not cause distress. For example often the parents of a child with Type I diabetes are the ones to 'take control' rather than involve the child. The nurse has an important role in ensuring that the child remains the focus of care through involvement of the child (if possible) right from the start – another example of 'scene setting'.

Addressing the presenting referral request or nursing need

The focus of care for the client is often on the presenting need, e.g. wound management for a chronic leg ulcer, support and education for a new diagnosis of diabetes, or continence issues requiring further investigation. Whilst this is a good starting point, the presenting need (often seen as the 'nursing' task by the client and the referrer) can be a symptom of a much larger problem. It is easy for the community nurse to assume that the presenting clinical issue is also the need with the highest priority for the client. It is here that 'client-centred care' must become the focus. The community nurse must ensure that the client perspective is gained by asking questions that are open ended, enquiring and non-judgemental. Questions could include the following:

- What is your understanding of why we (community nursing service) have been asked to come and provide assistance?
- What areas of your life are affected by your presenting need?
- Are there other health issues impacting on your quality of life?
- Who do you see as your main support at home?
- What would you like to gain from my (the community nurse's) involvement in your care?

Thus, addressing the presenting issue is an opportunity for the community nurse to get his or her 'leg in the door', but should not remain the only priority for care.

The client's perspective

Gaining the client's perspective and assessing how this may affect health care outcomes requires an understanding or insight into living with a chronic disease. Most community clients are living with a chronic disease [1]. In 2001, 78% of respondents in the National Health Survey [33] said that they had one or more long-term health condition (one that has lasted or is expected to last for 6 months or more). Among those aged 15 years and over, this prevalence was 87%. The corresponding levels in 1995 were 76 and 83%. Understanding the associated risk factors for chronic disease helps the community nurse to promote health. Those risk factors include:

- Inadequate diet and nutrition.
- Physical inactivity.
- Tobacco smoking.
- Alcohol misuse.
- High blood pressure.
- High blood cholesterol.
- Excess weight and body mass index [33].

Special note. The community nurse should not miss the opportunity to provide information to clients on reducing or quitting smoking, improving exercise levels, consideration of weight loss/nutritional programmes so that they can make informed decisions about their own health care outcomes. This continues to reinforce the need for the client to remain involved in their health care plan and thus be responsible for their health care outcomes.

Nutritional health

The nutritional health of older people living in the community is one of the most significant indicators of health and influences the older person's ability to live independently

[34]. Nutritional health is affected by numerous factors including depression, functional disability, poor oral health and financial difficulties.

Community nurses have regular, ongoing contact with older clients and therefore have an opportunity and obligation to conduct a nutritional risk assessment of these clients to predict and/or identify the potential for undernutrition or malnutrition. The community nurse should also weigh the client weekly or fortnightly to monitor the client's progress.

The nutritional risk assessment may identify *undernutrition* due to an unbalanced diet. Referral to a community-based dietitian will provide the opportunity for education and the formulation of a balanced meal plan for the client and carer.

Malnutrition due to an absence of food in the home may be the result of financial hardship. The community nurse should immediately access community agencies that provide interim food packages, with prompt referral to a community social worker for assistance with ongoing financial resources.

Once an older client is identified as being at risk, the community nurse should work with the client to eliminate or control the risk. For example oral or dental conditions require referral to a dental clinic for management. Poor nutritional health often results in significant weight loss, which will produce ill-fitting, uncomfortable dentures. New dentures or modification of existing dentures can be obtained through referral to a dental hospital; however, it is important to engage the general practitioner's assistance in obtaining a priority appointment to enable the hasty procurement of new dentures, thus reducing further deterioration of the client's nutritional status.

In the event the nutritional risk assessment suggests the presence of depressive symptoms (loss of appetite or energy to prepare meals), the community nurse will need to facilitate the need for the client to be assessed by a geriatrician or psychogeriatrician.

Overcoming nutritional health risks resulting from physical disability can be achieved through several options ranging from the implementation of in-home meal delivery, e.g. Meals on Wheels, to the acquisition of equipment and home modifications as a result of a home assessment conducted by an occupational therapist.

Pressure ulcer prevention and prediction

The Australian Wound Management Association (AWMA) [35] states that a risk assessment for potential to develop pressure ulcers should be performed on any individual on admission to a health care facility or home care facility. Despite general consensus that pressure ulcers are preventable, they remain an expensive consequence in any health care setting. The social cost is also an important consideration. Pain, loss of independence and decreased mobility impact on the client's ability to remain at home, thus avoiding a hospital admission.

In order to prevent and predict pressure ulcers, the community nurse should:

- Undertake a risk assessment on admission to any health care facility or home care service, following a change of health status and at appropriate intervals throughout the continuum of care.
- Document the 'at-risk status' and risk factors following a change in the individual's condition.

- Identify the 'at-risk' client and plan interventions which will prevent pressure ulcer formation; skin integrity inspection is fundamental in this process.
- Facilitate the use of the most effective pressure-relieving devices.
- Educate both the client and the carer in the area of pressure area care.

This process, combined with a commitment to ongoing review and re-evaluation of the effectiveness of interventions and the risk for development of pressure ulcers in the future, is paramount in the prevention of pressure ulcer formation [35].

Planning care

Once the assessment process is completed, the community nurse through identification of health care deficits formulates a plan of care. The client must be involved in identifying goals of care with the guidance of the community nurse. The long-term goals must be reviewed on a regular basis through short-term objectives or expected milestones. The short-term objectives allow both the community nurse and the client the opportunity to measure the effectiveness of the plan of care against expected outcomes. For example if the community nurse identifies poor nutritional status as an underlying reason for delayed wound healing, they should set a short-term objective that focuses on achieving better nutrition [35]. Implementing client education, adjustment of medications and lifestyle changes along with monitoring the long-term goal of care against the short-term goals provides both the client and the nurse with a yardstick – or a method for remaining on track towards the long-term goal. Planning of care should be directly linked to the outcomes of the assessment process. When this occurs, in the author's experience the client remains the focus of care and takes on the responsibility for health care outcomes. This is due in part to the formation of a partnership that begins with the initial assessment and continues to develop and strengthen throughout the planning process.

Discharge planning from the community nursing service should also begin at this point. This continues to 'set the scene' from the community nurse's perspective and reinforces a partnership approach to the client's care. The client remains involved in the planning of all aspects of their care and continues to remain jointly responsible for their health care outcomes.

Prioritisation of health care needs

One of the challenges for the community nurse is prioritising the client's health care needs. This is particularly important when multiple health care needs are identified at the completion of the initial assessment. A suggested strategy to facilitate this process is to continue to include the client in the decisions that are made during the prioritisation phase. Asking the client what health problem impacts most on their quality of life is a good place to start. Often, it is easy for the community nurse to be seen as 'taking over' and assuming that what they (nurses) identify as the key goal for care is the same as what is important for the client. A tool that supports this process is the Client-Generated Index (CGI) [36]. Through a series of discussion points this tool allows the client to identify how the presenting nursing need and all their other health care problems impact on their quality of life. The most important aspect in this assessment process is what can be learnt about the client and their perspective on their health care status. A good example of how this process is effective can be learnt from the following scenario:

A 92-year-old woman is referred to a community nursing organisation for management of skin tears sustained via a traumatic injury to the left lower leg. The client is blind, cognitively intact and quite withdrawn during the initial admission visit. The wounds are relatively minor and the client seems happy for the community nurse to manage as she sees fit. The community nurse asks the client how the wounds on her leg are affecting her quality of life. The client replies, 'They are the least of my worries. I just wish that you could get my interfering daughter out of my life! She is what makes my life awful.' Following further discussion it is discovered that the client's daughter has restricted many activities that the client had previously enjoyed: hearing her grand daughter play the piano, going to the theatre and having other family members visit her at home. The daughter has full control of her mother's money and is not allowing her mother to make any decisions for herself. Following further discussion via the CGI, it is discovered that her daughter has at times when the client had asked for money become verbally abusive, stating that she needed all her pension to make up for her loss of income, due to her having to take care of her mother.

It can be seen that if the community nurse in the above scenario had not taken the time to explore things from the client's perspective, the above 'elder abuse' would not have been discovered. 'Elder abuse is a single or repeated act, occurring within any relationship where there is an expectation of trust, which causes harm or distress to an older person' [37]. The community nurse has a moral obligation to report any suspected or confirmed acts of elder abuse. The use of a client advocate is one possible strategy to use in the case of elder abuse. The National Aged Care Advocacy Programme is one such example [38].

Nursing documentation

Nurses routinely spend 15–25% of their workday documenting client care [39]. Professional documentation is an integral part of community nursing. It is an important communication tool between all the health service providers. Nursing documentation has multiple uses such as forming the basis for evidence of care, research, legal analysis and determining allocation of resources.

Documentation can be defined as 'any written or electronically generated information about a client that describes the care or services provided to that client' [34]. Reasons for documentation can broadly speaking be described under the following headings:

- Facilitation of communication.
- Promotion of good nursing care.
- Meet professional and legal standards.

Requirements for documentation and the sharing, storage and disposal of this information are directed by statutory regulation (e.g. Nurses act 1999 and Privacy Act 1988), Standards of Practice (e.g. NBSA Guiding Principles for Documentation and the

Australian Nursing and Midwifery Council Competencies (ANMC)) [40, 41], agency policy and procedure, and legal principles.

Documentation includes, but is not limited to, the following:

- An assessment of the client's health care status.
- Nursing interventions carried out and the effectiveness of these interventions.
- A care plan reflecting the needs and goals of care.
- Changed care needs.
- Information reported to other health care providers and, if appropriate, their responses.
- Client and carer education.
- Evidence of client advocacy undertaken by the nurse [40].

The challenge for all nurses is the increasing need for documentation. The subsequent impact that this demand has on availability of resources to undertake documentation is often foremost in the nurse's mind. It is however not an acceptable excuse for poor or absence of documentation.

The community nursing setting requires documentation to be clear, concise, timely and contemporaneous [40]. Good documentation assists in the smooth transition of the client from one health service provider to the next. For the documentation to be effective it should be systematic in its approach [39], and regardless of whether it uses a 'focus charting' [39], 'narrative' or 'SOAP/SOAPIER', the outcome remains the same; i.e. it is 'up to' scrutiny should (in the worst case) it end up before a court of law. In today's information technologically advanced world, electronically held data are becoming more commonplace [39, 40]. If technology is used, the principles of access, storage, retrieval and transmittal of information remain the same [34, 36]. If electronically held documentation is the approach used by the agency then it is imperative that it is supported by sound documentation policies. Equally important is that 'precautions must be taken to ensure that nurses and midwives are fully informed of appropriate, safe and secure use of electronic information systems' [40].

Specialist assessments (diabetes, continence, mental health and wound management)

During the assessment process, the community nurse often identifies the need for additional specialist nursing assessments. It is rare that a client living with a chronic disease has only one nursing problem. A difficulty with self-administration of medication can be due to underlying cognitive deficit, dementia, depression or poor dexterity due to severe rheumatoid arthritis. Delayed wound healing can be due to unidentified diabetes or poorly controlled blood glucose levels if diabetes is already known [42]. The community nurse plays a vital role in identifying and assessing comorbidities because through a comprehensive assessment process they develop an understanding of the client and all of the components (pieces) that make the client the unique individual that they are.

Without having an understanding of how all of the pieces of the puzzle fit together (see Figure 4.2) and their relationship to each other, the clients' health care needs cannot be met. It would be pointless setting a goal of healing the wound if the issues of poor

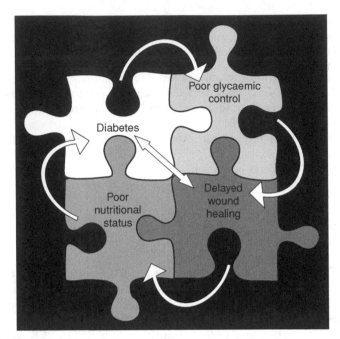

Figure 4.2 Identifying likely comorbidities.

nutritional status and poor glycaemic control were not addressed. Incorporated into this approach is the recognition of the need to make a referral onto a specialist nurse. This does not negate the need for the community nurse to have a sound knowledge base in many areas related to chronic disease processes but to also possess the ability to identify when the client's needs are beyond the scope of practice of the community nurse.

Evaluation of care

Inherent in successfully achieving planned client outcomes is the continual reassessment of the care being delivered. The reassessment process allows the community nurse to evaluate the care, set new goals of care (if required) and continue to build the relationship that has developed between the client and the community nurse. In the author's opinion, this maintains the 'client-centred' approach to the care delivered and ensures that the client remains involved in the planning of care.

Community integration

The author believes the community nurse has an important role in fostering a relationship which engenders in the client a desire to return to independence. For this outcome to be achieved, the client needs to be successfully 'integrated' back into the community (Figure 4.3). Through experience the author has come to understand community

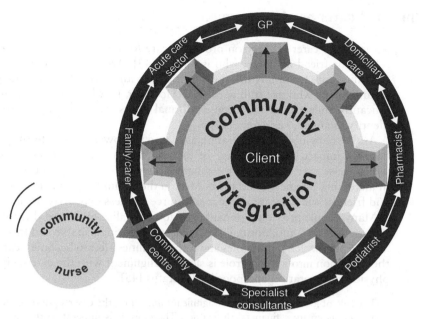

Figure 4.3 Community integration.

integration as the ability of the client and the nurse to work together to either initiate or re-initiate contact with other health care services, who may be providing ongoing support to the client and the carer. A good example of this process is described below:

Following the successful treatment of a venous leg ulcer with the outcome being a healed wound, the community nurse discussed with the client their impending discharge from the community nursing service. This discussion included strategies such as:

- Ensuring the client was able to verbalise how to access the community nursing service should it be required again.
- Discussing with the client what ongoing services were being provided and ensuring that contact was made with the key people from these services (e.g. domiciliary nursing care, home maintenance, home meal delivery service, regular podiatry and specialist medical appointments etc.).
- Identifying or reiterating with the client their long-term health care goals.
- Notifying the GP of the completion of the community nursing service and the outcomes of the service.
- Including the client's carer/family member in all of the above.
- Discussions, if appropriate.

Once the strategies have been explored 'jointly' with the community nurse and client, a smooth transition from a partnership approach to the client's care and a return to client independence is more likely to be achieved.

Informal carer needs assessment

An informal carer is a person providing care for a disabled, vulnerable, frail or sick relative or friend at home, who is unpaid [43]. Around 2.3 million Australians are providing care for family members or friends with a disability, mental illness, chronic conditions or who are frail aged [42]. However, it is believed that this figure is significantly underestimated, because informal carers are frequently 'hidden' and do not identify themselves as carers [44].

As the 'baby-boomer' generation ages, and the lower rates of fertility and mortality have an impact, the percentage of the population aged over 65 years will double, whilst those over 80 years are estimated to treble. This ageing population will result in increasing care needs and the burden on the community, which is usually on family and friends, will increase as the main source and less expensive form of care [16].

Many people providing unpaid care do not realise or regard themselves as carers. 'Informal caring' and 'normal' family life are indistinguishable and there is no identifiable point at which family roles and responsibilities alter to become a carer. Frequently, the transition into a caring role is slow, in alignment with the care recipient's gradual physical deterioration and poor health status [45].

> The role of a carer, however, has significant impact on the carer's physical and mental health as well as creating financial difficulties. Therefore it is imperative that an assessment and identification of the carer's needs be undertaken whilst also ensuring that access to support services is easy [46].

Caregiving encompasses an enormous range of responsibilities and levels of commitment from occasional assistance with transport or shopping through to 24 h a day care. Jarvis and Worth [43] identified that carers provide care in a variety of ways. Many carers provide assistance with instrumental activities of daily living, including meal preparation, managing money, shopping, doing housework and using a telephone. Others also provide assistance with routine activities of daily living, such as showering, dressing, toileting, grooming and feeding [47].

There are significant restrictions imposed on carers by the necessity to ensure day-to-day and frequent moment-to-moment care delivery in an effort to maintain the well-being of the care recipient. The stress of these demands is far more taxing than most physical tasks. Carers, especially full-time or primary carers, describe the role as all-encompassing, consuming every day and every waking hour of their day [48].

Carers frequently experience anxiety and anguish about the impact on their life created by the provision of care to the care recipient whilst grappling with the sense of responsibility for ensuring the well-being of the care recipient. As a result, carers discover that decisions about their own lives are restricted by concern for the care recipient [49].

The National Carers Coalition Report suggests that one of the most significant issues identified by carers is their isolation, which therefore increases the carer's risk of developing depression and its associated physical effects. Carers frequently relinquish a career, financial independence, freedom and a social life to undertake a caregiver role [50].

Consequently, carers are themselves likely to become disabled due to the stress of caring and the physical demands, for example, of lifting and continual sleep deprivation. Caregiver stress not only affects the caregiver's health and quality of life, but has a negative effect on the care recipient's outcomes [51]. Part-time or secondary carers who are still working believe that going to work is a break from caring and reduces isolation. It provides them with a sense of self, support and social interaction.

In addition to their roles as hands-on care providers and care managers, family caregivers are also trusted companions, surrogate decision makers and client advocates. Many caregivers meet the demands of caring for a relative or friend in the midst of their own deteriorating health. Family caregivers are far less likely to observe or participate in preventative health behaviours due to stress and exhaustion and may even have a high risk of mortality [45].

Composition of an informal carer needs assessment

The purpose of an informal carer needs assessment is to evaluate the needs of the carer in an effort to provide tailored support based on their needs. The assessment should be holistic, and needs to identify the types of assistance provided by the carer, including:

- Cooking.
- Medication administration.
- Financial situation.
- Hygiene assistance.
- Emotional support.

The assessment should also examine:

- The effect on the carer's life as a result of being a carer.
- The problems being experienced in the role.
- Any assistance currently provided to assist with the execution of the role [50].

One assumption commonly held by health professionals is that the carer is planning to continue to provide all of the required care to the care recipient, e.g. personal hygiene and continence management. However, this may be in complete contrast to the informal carer's desire or need, who may be physically exhausted by this activity which may also have resulted in significantly eroding their 'normal' relationship with the care recipient. The carer may still be happy to continue aspects of the care delivery whilst attempting to regain their former relationship with the care recipient.

Therefore, it is imperative that the needs of the informal carer are considered rather than an assumption being made that the carer will be able to continue to provide the same level of care, e.g. the informal carer meeting the needs of a young person with significant intellectual and physical disability. Often adult services may not be tailored or may not even be in place to meet the needs of such a young person. Thus, this places an increasing burden on the informal carer to continue to meet the needs of the young person due to the 'gap' in available services.

Community nurses should consider the 'informal carer' as a client of their service and should be sensitive to verbal and non-verbal cues which highlight their need for assistance. The duration of a visit to a client may prohibit the ability of the community nurse to spend time talking to the informal carer. However, if the carer has indicated a need to talk, another visit should be scheduled to explore the issue(s), preferably without the care recipient being present [52].

Informal carers may feel isolated and have little access to interaction with others. Carers may also feel excluded from any interaction between the community nurse and the care recipient, usually because the nurse is engaged in a conversation with their back towards the carer. This clearly demonstrates that open communication is an important factor in the relationship between the community nurse and the informal carer [52].

Clearly, there are time and resource implications associated with the informal carer needs assessment conducted by the community nurse. These would include the need for education in assessment of carer needs and the development of protocols to guide the community nurse in the provision of appropriate referral to services which can assist in the achievement of these needs.

Significant areas of need for the carer are:

- *Respite* which is often deemed inadequate and inaccessible in times of crisis and may not accommodate the needs of the informal carer. The respite needs to be available in the home and available at short notice in the event of a crisis.
- *Provision of information* which is available in the carer's local region, language and available via telephone or pamphlet.
- *General support* achieved through attendance at support groups, with respite available to ensure that this occurs.
- *General support* in the form of practical assistance with activities which the carer has in limited time or is too exhausted to undertake, such as housework, gardening and assistance with financial issues.
- *Medical monitoring* of the informal carer that should occur on a regular basis, with respite organised to enable attendance at the appointment. Informal carers routinely neglect their health, as they have difficulty finding time and available carers to assist them.
- *Referral and coordination of services* is a critical element in ensuring that the carer has access to the services required to meet their needs. It is frequently too difficult for the informal carer to navigate the pathway to access appropriate services, due to its complexity and the informal carer's exhaustion.
- *Advocacy* which refers to the need for someone to represent the informal carer's needs to service providers.
- *Education and training* of the informal carer to ensure that they have the relevant skills to undertake the various aspects of their role, e.g. showering, dressing and dietary needs [50].

Due to their frequently long-term relationships with clients and their carers, community nurses are in a position to teach carers the skills required to undertake aspects of the carer role and to provide the informal carer with support which will sustain them. It is acknowledged, however, that this does not address the needs of the carer beyond upskilling them to deliver care [43].

Summary

The community nurse plays an important role in the maintenance of clients' well-being. Through the development of partnerships, effective assessment and planning of care with the client and evaluation of that care, the community nurse can help to integrate the client back into the community. Careful documentation underpins the community nurse's practice and assists in the facilitation of independence rather than foster dependence. Cultural sensitivity and developing a relationship built on mutual respect and trust also promotes improved client outcomes. Incorporating strong primary health care principles and approaches to care results in improved client health care outcomes and successful community integration. Strong communication skills, resilience and determination on the community nurse's behalf to explore with the client or the informal carer factors impacting on their quality of life all lead to successful integration of the client back into the community. This is the ultimate goal of the community nurse and, once achieved, sees the community nurse leave the client, comfortable in the thought that the client's health care outcomes have been improved through their involvement (Figure 4.3).

References

1. Australian Primary Health Care Research Institute (APHCRI) (2006) Available at http://www.anu.edu.au/aphcri/ (viewed 24 September 2007).
2. Iliffe, S. (2006) Case management of chronic diseases and long-term conditions: Make haste slowly. *Primary Health Care Research and Development*, 7, 185–7.
3. Aminzadeh, F., Dalziel, W., Wilson, M., Deane, N. and Papahariss-Wright, S. (2005) Effectiveness of outpatient geriatric assessment programs. *Journal of Gerontological Nursing*, 31, 19–25.
4. Australian and New Zealand Health Policy (2006) Institute APHC, APHCRI. Available at http://www.anzhealthpolicy.com/content/pdf/1743-8462-4-16.pdf (viewed 24 September 2007 and 1 December 2007).
5. Jeong, S.-S. and Stein, I. (13 September 2003) Ageing in place. *Geriaction*, 21, 2.
6. Anderson, B. (2006) Relatives in end-of-life care – Part 1: A systematic review of the literature the five last years, January 1999–February 2004. *Journal of Clinical Nursing*, 15, 1158–69.
7. McCormack, B. (2006) *Development of a Framework for Person-Centred Nursing*. Blackwell Publishing Pvt Ltd, Oxford, p. 477.
8. Dewing, J. and Pritchard, E. (2004) *Nursing Assessment with Older People: A Person-Centred Approach*. Royal College of Nursing, London.
9. Heath, H. (2000) *Nursing Assessment and Older People*. Royal College of Nursing, London.
10. Caffrey, R.A. (July 2005) Community care gerontological nursing: The independent nurse's role. *Journal of Gerontological Nursing: Health and Medical Complete*, 31(7), 21.
11. Williams, C. and Tappen, R. (March 1999) Can we create a therapeutic relationship with nursing home residents in the later stages of Alzheimers? *Journal of Psychosocial Nursing Mental Health Services*, 37(3), 29.
12. Webster, J. (2004) Person-centred assessment with older people. *Nursing Older People*, 16(3), 22–6.
13. Cowley, H. (2002) An empowerment approach to needs assessment in health visiting practice. *Journal of Clinical Nursing*, 11, 640–50.
14. Kennedy, C. (2002) The decision making process in a district nursing assessment. *British Journal of Community Nursing*, 7(10), 505–13.
15. Yamashito, M., Forchuk, C. and Mound, B. (April–June 2005) Nurse case management: Negotiating care together with a developing relationship. *Perspectives in Psychiatric Care: Health & Medical Complete*, 41(2), 62.

16. Austin, J. (2004) *Carers – Who's Going to Care?* Carers Australia, Deakin, p. 31.
17. Australian Bureau of Statistics (1998) *Disability, Ageing and Carers: Summary Tables.* Australian Bureau of Statistics, Canberra.
18. Australian Institute of Health and Welfare (1999) *Australia's Welfare 1999 Services and Assistance.* Australian Institute of Health and Welfare, Canberra.
19. Ames, D. and Tuckwell, V. (1994) Psychiatric disorders among elderly patients in a general hospital. *Medical Journal of Australia,* 160(11), 671–5.
20. Meagher, D. and Trzepacz, P. (1998) Delirium phenomenology illuminates pathophysiology, management and course. *Journal of Geriatric Psychiatry and Neurology,* 11(3), 150–56.
21. Hollister, L. (1986) Drug-induced psychiatric disorders and their management. *Medical Toxicology,* 1, 428–48.
22. Patten, S. and Hope, E. (1994) Neuropsychiatric adverse drug reactions: Passive reports to Health and Welfare Canada's adverse drug reaction database (1965–present). *International Journal of Psychiatry in Medicine,* 24(1), 45–62.
23. Salgado, R., Lord, S., Ehrlich, F., Janji, N. and Rahman, A. (2004) Predictors of falling in elderly hospital patients. *Archives of Gerontology and Geriatrics,* 38, 213–19.
24. Bowers, J., Jorm, A., Henderson, S. and Harris, P. (1990) General practitioners' detection of depression and dementia in elderly patients. *Medical Journal of Australia,* 153, 192–6.
25. Callahan, C., Hendrie, H. and Tierney, W. (1995) Documentation and evaluation of cognitive impairment in elderly primary care patients. *Annals of Internal Medicine,* 122, 422–9.
26. US Preventable Services Task Force (2003) *Guide to Clinical Preventive Services.* US Preventable Services Task Force, Office of Disease Prevention and Health Promotion, Washington, DC.
27. Department of Human Services, Victoria (2006) *Clinical Practice Guidelines for the Management for Delirium in Older People.* Australian Health Ministers Advisory Council.
28. Flicker, L., Logiudice, D., Carlin, J. and Ames D. (1997) The predictive value of dementia screening instruments in clinical populations. *International Journal of Geriatric Psychiatry,* 12, 203–9.
29. Laurila, J., Pitkala, K., Strandberg, T. and Tilvis, R. (2004) Detection and documentation of dementia and delirium in acute geriatric wards. *General Hospital Psychiatry,* 26(1), 31–5.
30. Iliffe, S., Manthorpe, J. and Eden, A. (2003) Sooner or later? Issues in the early diagnosis of dementia in general practice: A qualitative study. *Family Practice,* 20, 376–81.
31. Kiosses, D. and Alexopoulos, G. (2005) IADL functions, cognitive deficits and severity of depression: A preliminary study. *American Journal of Geriatric Psychiatry,* 13(3), 244–9.
32. Jorm, A., Henderson, A., Scott, R., Mackinnon, A., Korten, A. and Christensen, H. (1994) Do mental health surveys disturb? Further evidence. *Psychological Medicine,* 24(1), 233–7.
33. Australian Institute of Health and Welfare (2007) *National Health Survey.* Available at http://www.aihw.gov.au/cdarf/data_pages/incidence_prevalence/index.cfm (viewed 11 September 2007).
34. Nursing Documentation (2007) *CRNBC Practice Support.* College of Registered Nurses of British Columbia, British Columbia.
35. Australian Wound Management Association (2001) *Clinical Practice Guidelines for the Prediction and Prevention of Pressure Ulcers.* Available at http://www.awma.com.au/publications/publications.php (viewed 14 October 2007).
36. Author? *Personal Privacy Protection in Health Care Information Systems.* Australian Standard; AS 4400-1995.
37. Aged Care, Australia (2007) *Prevention of Elder Abuse.* Available at http://www.agedcareaustralia.gov.au/internet/agedcare/publishing.nsf/Content/Prevention+of+elder+abuse?Open&etID=WCMEXT05-WCME-79JBAR (viewed 1 December 2007).
38. The National Aged Care Advocacy Program (2007) Available at http://www.health.gov.au/internet/wcms/publishing.nsf/Content/ageing-advocacy.htm (viewed 1 December 2007).

39. Guguerty, B., Maranda, M., Beachley, M., Navarro, V., Newbold, S., Hawk, W., *et al.* (May 2007) Challenges and opportunities in documentation of the nursing care of patients. *A Report of the Maryland Nursing Workforce Commission, Documentation Work Group.* Available at http://www.mbon.org/commossion2/documentation_challenges.pdf (viewed 16 June 2008).

40. Nurses Board of South Australia (2006) *Standards of Documentation.* Nurses Board of South Australia, Kensington, South Australia.

41. Australian Nursing and Midwifery Council (2006) *RN Competency Standards.* Available at http://www.anmc.org.au/professional_standards/index.php (viewed 1 December 2007).

42. Lilley, S. and Levine, G. (1998) Management of hospitalized patients with type 2 diabetes mellitus. *Practical Therapeutics.* Available at http://www.aafp.org/afp/980301ap/lilley.html (viewed 9 December 2007).

43. Navaie-Waliser, M., Feldman, P., Gould, D., Levine, C., Kuerbis, A. and Donelan, K. (2002) When the caregiver needs care: The plight of vulnerable caregivers. *American Journal of Public Health*, 92(3), 409–13.

44. Carers Australia (2006) Available at http://www.carersaustralia.com.au (viewed 9 December 2007).

45. Kilmer, D. (1996) *A Model Carer Assessment Tool for Health and Community Services Agencies in South Australia – Modified Version.* Carers Association of South Australia, Adelaide, p. 10.

46. Maddock, A., Isam, C. and Kilner, D. (1998) *Carers' Needs Assessment Trial: Who Are the Carers and What Are Their Needs?* Royal District Nursing Society of SA, Adelaide.

47. Jarvis, A. and Worth, A. (2005) Meeting carers information needs. *Community Practitioner*, 78(9), 322–6.

48. Carers Coalition Submission to The Council of Australian Governments (COAG) (1999) Canberra, Australia.

49. SANE Australia (July 2007) *More Than Half of All Family Carers Report Decline in Health and Wellbeing.* Media Release. SANE Australia, Victoria.

50. Twigg, J., Atkin, K. and Perring, C. (1990) *Carers and Services: A Review of Literature.* HMSO, London.

51. Simon, C., Kumar, S. and Kendrick, T. (2002) Who cares for the carers? A district nurse perspective. *Family Practice*, 19, 29–35.

52. Gregory, N., Collins-Atkins, C., Macpherson, R., Ford, S.A. and Palmer, A. (2006) Identifying the needs of carers in mental health services. *Nursing Times*, 103(17), 33.

Chapter 5

Incident management and mandatory reporting

Anne Maddock and Katherine Trowbridge

Introduction

Community nurses have a pivotal role to play in the reduction of risk. This chapter examines the role of the community nurse in the provision of safe and quality care through the implementation of strategies to enact their accountability and responsibility in incident management and mandatory reporting. The intention is to build on nurses' knowledge of primary health care (PHC) principles within a risk management approach in community nursing. Specific areas covered in this chapter include:

- Incident definitions and contemporary requirements in incident reporting and management.
- Safety challenges for community nurses and community nursing organisations, including:
  – Community nurses' injury prevention and management.
  – The management and prevention of infectious diseases to minimise safety implications for community nurses, clients, their families and significant others.
- Mandatory reporting in the areas of child abuse and the reporting of elder abuse and firearms.
- Management of the death of a client in a community setting.

The contemporary view of incident management and mandatory reporting requires that all staff in an organisation share responsibility and accountability so that risks are minimised. Safe and quality service provision protects community nurses, clients, their families and significant others.

Incident reporting

Key definitions

Incident reporting includes some common terms that the community nurse should be familiar with. These are as follows:

An incident

An incident is 'an event or circumstance that could have, or did lead to unintended and/or unnecessary harm to a person, and/or complaint, loss or damage' [1, p. 31]. Incidents that gain a lot of national and international attention include medication, pressure ulcers, falls and infection control.

Clinical incident

A clinical incident is 'an event or circumstance that could have, or did lead to unintended and/or unnecessary harm' [1, p. 31] to a client, family member or significant other, and/or complaint, loss or damage in the process of delivering care or health service provision.

Error

An error includes 'all those occasions in which a planned sequence of mental or physical activities fails to achieve its intended outcome, and when these failures cannot be attributed to the intervention of some chance agency' [1, p. 31].

Near miss

A near miss is 'an incident that did not cause harm' [1, p. 31].

Sentinel event

A sentinel event is

> an unexpected occurrence involving death or serious physical or psychological injury, or the risk thereof. Serious injury specifically includes loss of limb or function. The phrase, 'or risk thereof' includes any process variation of which recurrence would carry a significant chance of a serious adverse outcome. Such events are called 'sentinel' because they signal the need for immediate investigation and response [1, p. 32].

Adverse event

An adverse event is 'an incident in which unintended harm resulted to a person receiving health care' [1, p. 30].

Incident reporting, monitoring and continuous improvement

Promoting the safety of clients, their families and significant others and staff through incident reporting is a key strategy used by organisations to identify and act on areas of improvement and to prevent such an occurrence from happening again. Community nurses have a responsibility to participate in incident reporting mechanisms. There is legislation in place to ensure all staff have a responsibility to report occupational, health and safety incidents. The same commitment should apply when it comes to the reporting of clinical incidents in relation to client, family and significant others' safety.

Many organisations, states and territories are promoting voluntary and anonymous clinical incident reporting mechanisms to facilitate accurate and no-blame and just approaches to incident reporting. Incidents can be reported and captured in a separate database due to the legislative or policy requirements set by different states or territories. Organisations may use computer-assisted incident reporting. Some of these computer-assisted programs are more rigorous and comprehensive than others. It is important that incident monitoring systems and processes have a no-blame philosophy in order to encourage reporting and to enable learning from incidents [2]. Organisations and community nurses need to adopt strategies to overcome disincentives for reporting incidents [3].

When incidents occur, investigation is required to identify opportunities for improvement so as to prevent a similar incident from recurring or the incident escalating to be more significant. If community nurses are diligent in incident reporting and investigation processes then factors contributing to the incident can be identified. A good reason for anonymous reporting is to force decision makers to truly identify the contributing factor and put in place strategies that will prevent it from recurring. Community nurses may need to advocate for a no-blame and just culture and processes in their organisation that allow for the identification of the contributing factors and/or root cause of incidents.

Incident management including open disclosure

It is important that organisations have in place a comprehensive, well-communicated incident management strategy. Incident management includes:

- Implementing immediate action to prevent escalation of the incident and treating the immediate problem.
- Reporting the incident to the appropriate staff members in the organisation, including lodging the incident report.
- Undertaking investigation as to why the incident occurred in the first place.
- Putting in place strategies to prevent the incident from recurring.
- Discussing the incident and subsequent management strategy (open disclosure) with the client, family member or significant other.

Open disclosure

The Australian Open Disclosure Standard [4] refers to open disclosure as open communication when things go wrong in health care. It is claimed that 'people will forgive medical errors when they are disclosed promptly, fully and compassionately' and, in fact, 'being open also decreases the trauma' felt by people following an incident [5, pp. 5, 7]. Open disclosure is about being open with clients, family and significant others following safety incidents [5]. The elements of open disclosure include:

- An expression of regret.
- A factual explanation of what happened and consequences of the event.
- Steps being taken to manage the event and prevent a recurrence.

Open disclosure is not an admission of liability but rather an expression of regret that the incident has occurred. The standard provides guidance on what to say and what not to say to patients and their families when implementing open disclosure. It also highlights the legal concerns with regard to freedom of information, privacy, defamation and qualified privilege [4]. Community nurses should locate their organisational policy on open disclosure or access the Australian Standard in full for additional information.

Mandatory incident reporting

There are requirements for mandatory reporting to health departments in most states and territories when a sentinel event occurs. The clinical risk manager of an organisation often holds responsibility for mandatory incident reporting. This approach is important because it has the capacity to:

- Provide state alerts on areas of significant risk.
- Provide aggregate data on significant incidents that occur infrequently in health services to identify trends and areas for improvement for statewide planning.
- Inform a national approach to these serious occurrences.

A root cause analysis investigation

A community organisation may put in place criteria to alert to early warnings of a significant or adverse event. This enables the organisation to investigate the root cause and respond appropriately in order to prevent escalation and put in place improvements so that a similar occurrence does not happen again. These types of incidents are normally best investigated utilising the root cause analysis methodology to ensure a thorough investigation is undertaken and the actual contributing factors are identified and acted on. A root cause analysis is 'a systematic process whereby the factors which contributed to an incident are identified' [4, p. 30]. This process involves significant resources and a high level of rigour. A root cause analysis aims to protect the anonymity of staff, clients and significant others who are involved. It should not be utilised when there is a clear indication of legal implications (e.g. breeach of duty of care and criminal acts). The following is an example of root cause analysis.

Telephone calls from clients to a community nursing organisation reveal that a nurse has 'missed' several visits that morning – several clients reported that they had not received their planned visit and as a result medications had been missed and wound care had not been attended to.

An immediate response by some managers may have been to 'blame' the nurse or hold the nurse accountable for those missed visits, *but* the root cause analysis revealed that:

- The visits had only been added to the nurse's list that morning.
- Although the staff member reallocating the visits thought that she had notified the nurse, she had in fact sent the message to the nurse's old phone because the organizational telephone list was out of date.
- The nurse never received the message alerting her to the additional client visits.

- The organisational system for updating telephone lists was where the real issue lay and the organisation needed to 'fix' that system.

When investigating incidents, using a root cause analysis approach more times than not organisations will find just as in this example that it is a system breakdown that led to the incident.

Some organisations have specific criteria in place to determine when a root cause analysis should be undertaken. For example the Royal District Nursing Service (RDNS) in South Australia will undertake a root cause analysis when:

- Incidents are of a determined high level of risk.
- There is an expression of serious concern about an outcome for a client.
- Legal action is explicitly communicated; however, it is important to note that in this case the organisation's lawyers should, in most instances, be responsible for the investigation due to protection under qualified privilege.
- There is an unexpected serious client outcome (death) and the apparent absence of any other contributing factors [6].

Responding to an incident

Example: a just culture where staff are held accountable for their actions

A community nursing organisation has a policy that directs staff not to carry client medications in their car. In fact the organisation has stickers on all of their cars, saying medications were not carried in cars. The organisation received a complaint from a client that a nurse was doing them a favour and had collected their medications from a pharmacy and left them in her car overnight and the car had been broken into and the medications, including narcotics, were stolen. In this instance, the nurse had to be counselled and held accountable for her actions. In practicing outside of recommended organisations policy, she had placed at risk herself (it could be alleged that she had stolen the medication) and the organisation; if the client had chosen to go to the press, the organisation would have been placed in a very difficult situation and the rest of her peers, and if the word got out on the streets 'that the community nurses were carrying narcotics', it would place all of her peers, the organisation and herself at an increased risk.

The incident reporting in community nursing practice should follow the principles outlined in Table 5.1 [8].

Safety challenges for community nurses and community nursing organisations

The organisation's chief executive officer, managers and supervisors and all staff work together in the provision of a healthy and safe workplace for all employees and aim to demonstrate measurable outcomes [9]. Specifically, the community nurse has a role in

Table 5.1 Principles in incident reporting.

Principle	Application – the community nurse ...
Apply *structural elements* through the implementation of effective processes in the organisation to avert risk and foster continuous systems improvement	• Needs to participate in the organisation's risk and incident monitoring programme • Is responsible for fostering a just culture in the organisation for open and honest incident reporting and management • Should participate in the continuous system improvement in medication management
Consider the criticality of the *health care interface* and *multidisciplinary team* and *client partnerships* in decision making required for safety and quality outcomes	• Should not be constrained in reporting by the thought that 'it is not our incident'. It is the decision-making responsibility of managers and executive on the system improvement processes required across the interface to achieve safety and quality in health care. The primary goal guiding system improvement should be the safety and quality of client care, regardless of who provided the care • Is required to be competent in medication management
Seek out and apply *knowledge resources and evidence-based practice* to ensure the appropriateness and effectiveness of service delivery	• Participates in the incident reporting, aggregated measurement, analysis and interpretation of incident reports to inform new knowledge in the organisation for system improvement opportunities
Seek out and utilise appropriate *technology* for point of decision making and subsequent incident reporting	• Should ensure that the OH&S technology priorities are communicated to management and executive. The community nurse has a duty of care to their client for safe and high-quality care, including accessing or advocating for the resources required • Have a duty of care to utilise technology available in accurate and timely incident reporting
Seek to influence the *infrastructure support* requirements needed to provide safe and quality outcomes	• Owe a duty to their clients to have ready access to the appropriate medical supplies and equipment such as portable resuscitation devices for OH&S and client quality and safety outcomes
Ensure there is appropriate *human resource support* – adequate knowledge, competence, skills and safe staffing	• Need to remain competent in incident reporting, investigation and management • Need to ensure they are competent in medication management in line with the latest evidence-based practice

For more detail of the application of these clinical governance principles, see Chapter 3 [7].

occupational health and safety (OH&S), according to their respective state or territory legislation, to adhere to the following responsibilities as an employee: (NB. Supervisors have additional responsibility – see relevant legislation.)

- Take care of their own and others' health and safety.
- Comply with policies, guidelines and directives and work instructions and reasonable directions.
- Use appropriate protective equipment.
- Not misuse items provided in the interest of OH&S.
- Not undertake work including driving if, through the consumption of alcohol or drugs, safety is impaired.
- Not undertake work that has an unacceptable level of risk of injury/illness.
- Report all hazards, risks, injuries and other incidents to their supervisor.
- Attend all compulsory training sessions provided.
- Participate in induction, graduated return to core duties programmes and functional assessment where a length of absence from core duties may have reduced their capability to work safely [9].

Safety challenges: injury reporting, management and prevention

A risk monitoring, assessment and management approach to injury prevention and management is important. It is also important that the community nurse assesses, communicates and manages potential and actual hazards in their workplace on a daily basis. This will maximise their safety and also the safety of their peers, clients, families and significant others. Community nurses often practice in uncontrolled environments, such as people's homes or industrial environments, and so an ongoing environmental assessment becomes a fundamental part of practice.

The key safety challenges for the community nurse include:

- *Safety hazards* – This may be as simple as the nurse not wanting to bother the client to rectify staff hazard issues. Examples may be suggesting that a rug be moved because it is a tripping hazard or requesting that the family pet be removed from the clinical care area when the nurse is present.
- *Personal security and safety* – This includes workplace violence, abuse or threats, manual handling injuries, or hazards related to access to appropriate equipment, compliance with no lift guidelines, the uncontrolled environment and lack of ready and timely access to additional staff support to meet the care requirements.
- *Rehabilitation* – The rehabilitation of injured employees back into the workplace.
- *Infection transmission* – This includes hand hygiene practices and the impact of infection prevention and control [10].

Hazard management

Hazard management incorporates a PHC focus on prevention, early intervention and rehabilitation. The community nurse is responsible for [11]:

- Undertaking hazard training and upgrade their knowledge on a regular basis.
- Applying the organisation's hazard identification and assessment guidelines to all areas of work on a regular basis.

- Reporting any issues identified through the hazard and incident reporting processes, and documenting in the client record.
- Reporting uncontrolled issues to their supervisor and OH&S representative.
- Speaking with the union worksite representative or organiser if the hazard is not adequately addressed.

For example RDNS in South Australia has a staff hazard identification and safety policy that pets are securely restrained when a nurse visits a client's home. This ensures that community nurses are safe at work from the risks of injury and ill health (e.g. bites or allergic reactions) caused by a client's pet, in a manner that does not adversely affect the client's well-being [11]. Exemptions may be applicable for guide dogs, hearing dogs and helper dogs where minimal risk is calculated.

Manual handling

Manual handling is 'any activity requiring the use of force exerted by a person to lift, lower, push, pull, carry or otherwise move, hold or restrain any person, animal, object or thing' [12]. Manual-handling-related activities for the community nurse may include activities such as transferring clients, squatting to provide wound care, carrying items to and from a vehicle or getting in and out of a vehicle.

Manual handling remains the single biggest threat to nurses' health and safety. The Australian Nursing Federation (ANF) adopted a 'Safer Manual Handling Policy' with the aim of addressing this threat. The policy seeks to eliminate manual handling of people in all but exceptional or life-threatening situations. Manual assistance may continue only if it does not involve lifting most or all of a client's weight. To implement the policy, the ANF developed 'No lift, No injury', a training programme to enable the implementation of the policy in the workplace [13]. Strategies to redesign operating procedures in the workplace to protect staff, wherever possible, should be considered [7]. It is however the community nurse's responsibility to:

- Use mechanical aids in accordance with the manufacturer's instructions.
- Use personal protective equipment (e.g. mask, gown and gloves).
- Use the appropriate numbers of staff required to do the task; otherwise delay completing the task until staff are available.
- Undertake appropriate education and training [12].

Elimination of manual handling has been successfully implemented in a wide range of health care services both in Australia and overseas. For nurses this has led to a significant reduction in the number and severity of back and other related injuries [13].

The rehabilitation of injured employees back into the workplace

The rehabilitation of injured employees back into the workplace is an integral part of the process of managing employee safety and rehabilitation. It is important to assist staff to achieve a best practicable level of recovery and return as quickly as possible to safe and suitable duties that are within documented medical directions and the employee's best interests [12]. The process to follow is usually associated with the relevant legislation and associated organisation policy, which may require the community nurse to:

- Immediately report the injury through the organisation's reporting processes.
- Undertake an immediate medical or allied health assessment of fitness to work.
- Be provided with the appropriate support processes in being rehabilitated back to work.
- Be provided with the appropriate support in returning to the most appropriate work tasks.

All organisations, depending on their state/territory requirements, will have specific requirements for supervisors and employees in the reporting of a work-related injury or illness. Community nurses need to comply with these requirements in a timely manner [14, 15].

The community nurse and the organisation in which they work should consider adopting the following clinical governance principles and strategies in the rehabilitation of injured employees back into the workplace:

- Comply with all policies, guidelines, directives and work instructions and all reasonable directions in terms of staff and client safety in the organisation. Community nurses should take reasonable care of their own and others' health and safety.
- Report any hazards that may compromise staff safety.
- Ensure that the latest evidence in maintaining staff safety is adopted, such as not undertaking work including driving if, through the consumption of alcohol or drugs, safety is impaired; not undertaking any work that has an unacceptable level of risk of injury/illness; and reporting all hazards, risks, injuries and other incidents to their supervisor.
- Ensure that the appropriate and required technological aids are available to foster sound OH&S.
- Use available equipment and supplies, use appropriate protective equipment and not misuse items provided in the interest of OH&S.
- Attend all compulsory training sessions such as orientation induction, graduated return to core duty programmes, return to work programmes and functional assessments [14].

Safety challenges: infection control, prevention and management

While it is not within the scope of this chapter to include the management and prevention of all possible infections and their cross infection, aspects of this topic do need to be emphasised (refer to Chapter 7 for more details). 'Infection control is the process of minimising the risks of developing infectious complications while providing health care' [16, p. 1]. The infection prevention and management challenges confronting community nurses are progressively changing as the world attempts to control infection progression that impacts on staff, clients, their families and significant others. Community nurses' responsibilities include provision of safe working conditions, use of personal protective equipment, adherence to polices and guidelines and maintenance of competency in infection control. As the community nurse works in such diverse locations, the need to be familiar with their organisational policy in this area and to be rigorous in its application is important.

Specifically, the community nurse has a role in preventing the spread of infection and in infection management by applying the following guidelines:

- Have knowledge of microbiology and modes of transmission of infection.
- Thoroughly handwash and use protective equipment provided.
- Keep any cuts and abrasions clean and covered.
- Avoid contact with other people's wounds or material contaminated by the wounds.
- Instruct people not to share razors, soap, ointments, balms, towels, washcloths, clothing and uniforms.
- Ensure single use of equipment or the appropriate reprocessing of instruments and equipment after use.
- Ensure immunisations are available.
- Follow appropriate waste management practices – handling, transport, storage and disposal.
- Participate in the organisation's infection screening, -surveillance and -control programmes.
- Have knowledge of when to adopt additional precautions, such as gloves, impermeable gowns, respirators or masks, goggles and face shields, and special handling equipment [16–20].

The reality of preparing for a pandemic

A pandemic is a virus that is capable of being transferred from human to human rapidly, because people have no natural immunity to the virus [21]. It is important for the community nurse to be aware of specific organisational plans and policies to manage any pandemic – such as SARS (severe acute respiratory syndrome virus) or influenza. Table 5.2 outlines the principles of risk reduction in relation to infection control.

Mandatory reporting

The community nurse has the same duty of care, ethics, conduct and reporting mandates as those working in other health care settings [22, 23]. A community nurse has a duty of care to the client to:

- Report all suspected incidences of child abuse and neglect (see Nurses' Act 1999 and Children's Protection Act 1993) [24].
- Report all suspected incidences of elder abuse.
- Report all cases of inappropriate use and storage of firearms (see Firearms Act 1977 [25] and Nurses' Act 1999 [Section 43]).
- Report all unexpected deaths as described in the Coroner's Act 2003 [26].

The community nurse is urged to seek the support of supervisors and organisational hierarchy in any situation where abuse is suspected.

Table 5.2 Reducing risk in infection control.

Principle	Application – the community nurse …
Apply *structural elements* through the implementation of effective processes in the organisation to avert infection risk	• Needs to take reasonable care of their own and others' health and safety by complying with all policies, guidelines work instructions and directives • Needs to take reasonable directions on reporting infection hazards and incidents • Should foster a culture of looking after the safety of all staff, clients and others
Consider the criticality of the *health care interface* and *multidisciplinary team* and *client partnerships* in decision making required for safety and quality outcomes	• Should ensure there are acceptable levels of consumer involvement in their care • Should enhance or maintain client awareness, empowerment and management through the use of effective education and change management strategies • Needs to ensure that all facilities in which they practise operate in terms of the reduction of infection risk. This may include the community nurse's role in reporting any hazards that may compromise staff, clients and others' safety

Seek out and apply *knowledge resources and evidence-based practice* to ensure the appropriateness and effectiveness of service delivery	• Has a responsibility to:
	  – Ensure they adopt latest evidence in maintaining infection control
	  – Participate in incident reporting, aggregated measurement, analysis and interpretation of incident reports to inform new knowledge in the organisation for system improvement opportunities

Seek out and utilise appropriate *technology* for point of decision making and subsequent incident reporting	• Should ensure:
	  – The technology priorities are communicated to management
	  – Executive and the appropriate and required technological aids are available to foster sound OH&S

Seek to influence the *infrastructure support* requirements needed to provide safe and quality outcomes	• Is required to always use appropriate protective equipment to reduce the threat of infection transmission
	• Owes their clients duty of care to readily access the appropriate medical supplies and equipment to:
	  – Reduce infection risk
	  – Provide the range of equipment and supplies that will reduce infection colonization and spread

Ensure there is appropriate *human resource support* – adequate knowledge, competence, skills and safe staffing	• Has a responsibility to remain competent in incident infection control, reporting, investigation and management

Defining mandatory reporting

Mandatory reporting is described in Australia as 'legislation which specifies who is required by law to report suspected cases of child abuse and neglect' [27, p. 1]. Mandatory reporting is considered by the Australian Institute of Family Studies to play a vital role in the early detection of child abuse and neglect. Its introduction aims to advance child protection.

Mandatory reporting requires that the community nurse overcome any reluctance to be involved in suspected cases of child abuse, by imposing a public duty to do so [27–29]. In Australia, child protection (involving child abuse and neglect) is a matter which falls within the constitutional powers of all states and territories (except Western Australia) and nurses are mandated and have a statutory duty to notify the Australian Government Child and Family Services Organisation in each state or territory of suspicion that a child has been abused or neglected [30]. In Australia, a child is considered any person up to the age of 18 years, except in NSW where the mandatory reporting obligation is up to the age of 16 years [30, 31].

Abuse and neglect can take many forms and may be prolonged or acute. For example the community nurse must be able to discern between bruises attributable to playtime and those that may signal abuse [32]. This can be difficult and the community nurse may need to seek guidance from Child and Family Services or a similar agency. Documenting all assessed physical or non-physical signs of abuse or neglect is a legal requirement of the community nurse and is proof of quality of care for the child [33].

The following definitions are applicable when reporting suspected abuse [34]:

- *Neglect* – inadequate supervision, non-provision of adequate nutrition, clothing, personal hygiene, failure to provide medical treatment, allowing chronic truancy.
- *Physical abuse* – hitting, shaking, burns, biting, pulling out hair, alcohol or ellicit drug administration.
- *Sexual abuse* – sexual suggestion, child prostitution, mutual masturbation, penile or other penetration of genital or anal region, exposing the child to pornographic material.
- *Emotional abuse* – devaluing, ignoring, rejecting, isolating, terrorising, chronic domestic violence in the child's presence [34].

The community nurse may experience the process of reporting suspected abuse or neglect as confronting and stressful. The community nurse must clearly document all forms of suspected abuse or neglect, including observed signs (e.g. bruising or cigarette burns), observed abuse situations or communication (e.g. a carer failing to provide nutritional food or fluids to an older person in their care) and communicate these concerns together with objective observations to the Australian Government Child and Family Services Organisation reporting officer in their state or territory. A reporting officer may organise counselling and/or advice for the reporting nurse and their expected role in the case. A risk assessment may be conducted to ascertain whether the person suspected of being abused needs to be removed from their home situation [34].

Elder abuse

Elder abuse is 'any act occurring within a relationship where there is an implication of trust, which results in harm to an older person. Abuse can include physical, sexual, financial, psychological and social abuse and/or neglect' [35, p. 2]. The reporting of suspected elder abuse is not a statutory duty for the community nurse, as at this time no Australian jurisdiction has supported mandatory reporting [35]. However, the nursing code of ethics and code of professional conduct offers broad guidelines supporting the community nurse to document and report any suspected ill treatment of a person in their care [22, 23]. A vulnerable adult can be defined as 'a person who is or may be in need of community care services by reason of mental or other disability, age or illness, and who is or may be unable to care for him or herself' [36, p. 43].

Types of elder abuse are described by Neno [36] as:

- *Physical* – hitting, slapping, burning, pushing, restraint, over dosage of medication.
- *Psychological* – shouting, swearing, frightening, blaming, ignoring, humiliating.
- *Financial* – unauthorised use of money, property or valuables.
- *Sexual* – forced sexual acts without consent.
- *Neglect* – deprivation of food, heat, comfort, clothing, essential medication and medical care.

Risk factors for elder abuse are:

- Social isolation.
- History of a poor-quality long-term relationship between the abused and the abuser.
- A pattern of family violence by the abuser.
- Dependence of the abused on the abuser.
- Mental health concerns (including depression) of the abused or the abuser.
- Poor control of chronic diseases of abused or the abuser [37].

There are a range of interventions available to the abused person, such as crisis care or similar agency, community support services, respite care, counselling, choices of treatment for the abuser, alternative accommodation or legal intervention [35]. The community nurse can contact one of these services on behalf of the client or the Australian Government Child and Family Services Organisation reporting officer in their state or territory who can provide advice on how to manage a suspected abuse situation. The community nurses employer may also be able to provide debriefing support to allow the nurse to talk about their experience in the abuse situation. Debriefing may occur via phone or two-way radio communication for those nurses who are working in remote communities [35].

Firearms reporting

Australian nurses are deemed to be 'prescribed persons' and therefore have reporting responsibilities/obligations to inform the firearms section of the state police department, or the local police authority for those nurses practising within rural or remote areas, when there is reasonable cause to believe that a person has a physical or mental illness, disability or deficiency that is likely to make the possession of a firearm by the person unsafe or that the person holds or intends applying for a firearms licence or possesses or has the intention of possessing a firearm [25].

Information which must be provided to the police is [25]:

- The person's name and address.
- The nature of their illness, disability or deficiency.
- The reason why, in the opinion of the prescribed person, it is or would be unsafe for the person to have possession of a firearm.

Death of a client in the community

Expected death in the home usually encompasses aspects of palliative care and is legislated by the Consent to Medical Treatment and Palliative Care Act (1995) and the Natural Death Act (1983). On the death of a client, the community nurse will need to notify the treating medical officer to request verification of the client's death and issue a certificate stating cause of death. In exceptional circumstances the funeral director can notify the treating medical officer [38]. The community nurse should be familiar with and respect the family's and the client's wishes, if known, in relation to death rituals, such as washing of the deceased's body, prayer and religious practices [39–41].

Unexpected death in the home or 'reportable death' requires the community nurse to immediately notify the treating medical officer of the circumstances surrounding the death and also to provide a statement to the police for the coroner. The community nurse may be the first person to find the deceased client or the last person to see the client alive. The Coroner's Act 2003 defines a reportable death as:

(a) Death of unexpected, unnatural, unusual, violent or unknown cause
(b) Death that occurs during, as a result of or within 24 h of:
    - The carrying out of a surgical or invasive procedure or investigation.
    - The administration of an anaesthetic.
    - Having been discharged from hospital as an inpatient or sought emergency treatment at the hospital.
    - Death of a baby in unusual circumstances.
    - Death of a person who resides in a supported residential facility.
    - Death in custody.
    - Death on an aircraft during a flight.
    - Death on a vessel during a voyage.
    - The death of a person protected under the Mental Health Act 1993, Guardianship and Administration Act 1993, Aged and Infirm Persons' Property Act 1940 or the Children's Protection Act 1993 [26].

The community nurse should be familiar with specific organisational directives related to death in the community, such as:

- Leaving in situ all tubing, needles and catheters from invasive procedures or transdermal patches untouched for the coroner's assessment (i.e. not disturbing the body or surroundings).
- Accurate documentation of the situation.

- Notification of the client's next of kin.
- Caring for the body of the deceased with dignity and respect.
- Respecting and advocating for the client's and family's religious, cultural and personal beliefs, reflecting cultural competence.
- Practising infection control procedures when handling the deceased person's body [42–47].

For the community nurse, managing the 'death of a client', including support for loved ones of the deceased, or involvement in a mandatory reporting situation such as child or elder abuse should be described as 'critical incident'. Involvement for the community nurse in an incident can be confronting and requires a need for debriefing to allow the nurse to verbalise their feelings, thoughts and concerns. Collegial support is also important. Community nursing organisations should have a staff support process in place for the community nurse in such events. This process of looking after yourself and colleagues will provide nurses with an avenue to debrief about the specific experience and articulate their reactions to the experience and acknowledge coping strategies.

Summary

This chapter has examined the fundamentals of incident management and mandatory reporting for community nurses in diverse community environments. The community nursing role is to promote health and disease prevention within the health care setting and also to communicate to clients and colleagues an understanding of how incidents and mandatory reporting should be managed. This management will be unique to each practice setting and be dependent on cultural, religious and belief systems for each individual client. Legislation and guidelines underpinning this management have been described. The community nurse in conjunction with their employing organisation needs to utilise a PHC approach to plan quality care for the client that is personalised, inclusive of the principles of clinical governance, and incorporates strategies to enact accountability and responsibility in the nursing role.

Useful resources

Australian Commission on Safety and Quality in Health Care (ACSQHC) (2006) *Measurement for Improvement Toolkit.* Commonwealth of Australia, Canberra.
World Health Organization (WHO) (2005) *World Alliance For Patient Safety: WHO Draft Guidelines for Adverse Event Reporting and Learning Systems – From Information to Action.* World Health Organization, Geneva.
Australian Government legislation at www.legislation.sa.gov.au
The Victorian Quality Council at http://www.health.vic.gov.au/qualitycouncil/ Institute of Healthcare Improvement at http://www.ihi.org/ihi
Department of Human Services Victoria Safety and Quality Branch at http://www.dhs.vic.gov.au/rrhacs/qualitybranch
The National Institute of Clinical Studies at http://www.nhmrc.gov.au/nics/asp/index.asp?
The Joint Commission at http://www.jointcommission.org/
The United Kingdom National Health Service at http://www.wise.nhs.uk

The United Kingdom National Health Service National Patient Safety Agency at http://www.npsa.nhs.uk

The World Health Organization Patient Safety website at http://www.who.int/patientsafety/en/

Department of Health South Australia Safety and Quality website and Department of Health Western Australia Safety and Quality websites http://www.health.sa.gov.au/safetyandquality/ and www.safetyandquality.health.wa. gov.au

Mental Health Services Australia at www.mental-health-services.com/

The Department of Families, Housing, Community Services and Indigenous Affairs (FaHCSIA) at www.facsia.gov.au/

Aged and Community Services Australia at www.agedcare.org.au/

World Health Organization (WHO) at www.who.int/violence_injury_prevention/

Department of Human Services (DHS) at www.humanservices.gov.au/

Firearms reporting at www.sapb.saboards.com.au/manreporting.htm

References

1. Australian Commission on Safety and Quality in Health Care (2006) *Measurement for Improvement Toolkit*. Australian Commission on Safety and Quality in Health Care, Sydney, Australia.
2. Burroughs, L. and Atkins, S. (2005) The Doncaster West approach to learning from significant events. *Clinical Governance Bulletin*, 6(2), 6–8.
3. Barach, P. and Small, S.D. (2000) Reporting and preventing medical mishaps: Lessons from non-medical near miss reporting systems. *BMJ*, 320(18), 759–63.
4. Australian Safety and Quality Council (2003) *Open Disclosure Standards: A National Standard for Open Communication in Public and Private Hospitals – Following an Adverse Event in Health Care*. Commonwealth of Australia, Australia.
5. Carthey, J. (2005) Being open with patients and their carers following patient safety incidents. *Clinical Governance Bulletin*, 5(5), 5–6.
6. Royal District Nursing Service (RDNS) (2005) *Adverse Events: In Analysis and Reporting Process*. Royal District Nursing Service, Adelaide, SA.
7. Maddock, A. (2008) Quality and safety in community health care, in D. Kralik and A. van Loon (eds) *Community Nursing in Australia*. Blackwell Publishing, Oxford, UK, pp. 84–97.
8. Australian Council on Healthcare Standards (2004) *News*. Australian Government Publishing, Sydney, New South Wales.
9. RDNS (2006) Employee safety and rehabilitation (ESR), in RDNS (ed.) *Manual – Safety and risk management*. Royal District Nursing Service, Adelaide, SA.
10. Storr, J. (2005) Preventing infection in hospital – should patient involvement be central to current hand hygiene strategies? *Clinical Governance Bulletin*, 5(5), 6–8.
11. RDNS (2006) Pets in client homes, in RDNS (ed.) *Manual – Safety and Risk Management*. Royal District Nursing Service, Adelaide, SA.
12. RDNS (2006) Manual handling guidelines, in RDNS (ed.) *Manual – Safety and Risk Management*. Royal District Nursing Service, Adelaide, SA.
13. Australian Nurses Foundation (2007) *Occupational Health and Safety and Manual Handling*. Australian Nurses Foundation. Available at www.anf.org.au/ (viewed May 2007).
14. RDNS (2007) *Injury Management Package*. Royal District Nursing Service, Adelaide, SA.
15. RDNS (2005) *Reporting a Work Related Injury/Illness*. Royal District Nursing Service, Adelaide, SA.
16. RDNS (2005) Infection control, in RDNS (ed.) *Manual – Community Care Services: Nursing*. Royal District Nursing Service, Adelaide, SA.

17. Therapeutic Goods Act (1989) Therapeutic Goods Act, as amended by the Therapeutic Goods Amendment (Medical Devices) Bill, 2002 and the Therapeutic Goods (Medical Devices) Regulations, Commonwealth of Australia, Canberra.

18. RDNS (2004) Infection control: Implementing standard and additional precautions – hand hygiene, in RDNS (ed.) *Community Care Services – Nursing*. Royal District Nursing Service, Adelaide, SA.

19. Yetman, L. (2006) A new 'superbug' leaves the hospital: Community-acquired methicillin-resistant *Staphylococcus aureus*. *Home Healthcare Nurse*, 24(4), 213–16.

20. Department of Health, Victoria (2005) *Rural Infection Prevention and Control Manual*. Rural Infection Control Practice Group, Victoria, Melbourne.

21. Department of Health and Ageing (2007) *Information on Influenza Pandemic*, Vol. 1. Commonwealth of Australia.

22. Australian Nursing and Midwifery Council (ANMC) (2005) *Code of Ethics for Nurses in Canberra, Australia*. Australian Nursing and Midwifery Council, pp. 1–6.

23. ANMC (2005) *Code of Professional Conduct for Nurses in Australia*. Australian Nursing and Midwifery Council, Canberra, Australia, pp. 1–4.

24. South Australian Government (1993) *Children's Protection Act 1993 – Notification of Abuse or Neglect*. Government of South Australia, Adelaide, SA, pp. 1–22.

25. South Australian Government (1977) *Firearms Act 1977 – Section 20*. SA Government, Adelaide, SA, pp. 1–12.

26. Federal Government of Australia (2003) *Coroner's Act 2003*. Government of Australia, Canberra.

27. Australian Institute of Family Studies (2005) *Mandatory Reporting of Child Abuse*. Resource sheet. Australian Government Institute of Family Studies, Canberra, Australia.

28. Tomison, A. (2002) Mandatory reporting: A question of theory versus practice. *Developing Practice: The Child Youth and Family Work Journal*, 4, 13–17.

29. Cashmore, J. (2002) Mandatory reporting: Is it the culprit? Where is the evidence? *Developing Practice: The Child Youth and Family Work Journal*, 4, 9–12.

30. Mathews, B.P., Walsh, K.M. and Fraser, J.A. (2006) Mandatory reporting by nurses of child abuse and neglect. *Journal of Law and Medicine*, 13(4), 505–17.

31. Ainsworth, F. (2002) Mandatory reporting of child abuse neglect: Does it really make a difference? *Child and Family Social Work*, 7(1), 57–63.

32. Harrison, S. (9–15 April 2003) Eyes wide shut. *Nursing Standard*, 15(30), 12.

33. Joint Commission on Accreditation of Healthcare Organisations (February 2006) Assessing risk in medical documentation. *Joint Commission Perspectives on Patient Safety*, 6(2), 3–4.

34. Government of South Australia, Department for Families and Communities (2007) *Child Safe Environments; Reporting Child Abuse and Neglect*. Guidelines for mandated notifiers. Department for Families and Communities, Adelaide, SA.

35. Sadler, P. (March 2006) *Elder Abuse: A Holistic Response*. Background paper. Aged and Community Services, Australia. Commonwealth Government Publishing Department, Canberra, pp. 1–13.

36. Neno, R. (2005) Identifying abuse in older people. *Nursing Standard*, 20(3), 43–7.

37. Rodriguez, M.W., Woolf, N. and Mangione, C. (2006) Mandatory reporting of elder abuse: Between a rock and a hard place. *Annals of Family Medicine*, 4(5), 403–9.

38. Ayris, W. (2002) Verification of expected death by district nurses. *British Journal of Nursing*, 7(7), 370–73.

39. Molzahn, A. (2004) Aboriginal beliefs about organ donation: Some Coast Salish viewpoints. *Canadian Journal of Nursing Research*, 36(4), 111–28.

40. Pitorak, E. (5 May 2005) Care at time of death. *Home Health Care Nursing*, 23, 318–27.

41. Joanna Briggs Institute (2006) *Evidence Summary – Last Officers*, 1(1), 1–4.

42. Kumari, K. (2006) Handling death and bereavement at work. *Therapy Today*, 17(4), 48.

43. Baldwin, D. (1999) Community-based experiences and cultural competence. *Journal of Nursing Education*, 38(5), 195–6.
44. Romeo, C. (2007) Caring for culturally diverse patients: One agency's journey toward cultural competence. *Home Health Nurse*, 25(3), 206–13.
45. Ivorine, B. (2006) Caring for patients of diverse religious traditions: Evangelical 'born again' Christians. *Home Health Care Nursing*, 24(10), 677–80.
46. Narayan, M. (2006) Caring for patients of diverse religious traditions: Catholicism. *Home Health Care Nursing*, 24(3), 183–6.
47. Ward, J. (2006) Caring for patients of diverse religious traditions: The Church of Jesus Christ of Latter-Day Saints. *Home Health Care Nursing*, 24(6), 396–8.

Chapter 6

Community infection control and prevention practice

Ramon Shaban and Belinda Henderson

Introduction

The aim of this chapter is to provide community nurses with practical guidelines for infection control and prevention in the Australian health care context. It is a resource for nurses practising in diverse community health contexts, such as district nursing, practice nursing, rural and remote nursing, domiciliary nursing, nursing within correctional services and school-based settings. This chapter:

- Reviews the contemporary infection control and prevention challenges for community nursing practice in the Australian context
- Describes contemporary infection control and prevention frameworks, standards, guidelines and practices for community nursing and health
- Examines standard precautions for infection control and prevention in community nursing settings
- Explores additional precautions for specific infections relevant to community nursing practice
- Identifies future challenges and contemporary strategies for infection control and prevention in community nursing and health

Reforms in community health care

Global reform of health care systems over the last 20 years has been driven by a renewed focus on community care. Treating disease and illness in community rather than hospital settings is the popular and preferred model [1]. Care for people who have mental illness, or who are older, disabled or intellectually impaired, is primarily undertaken in the community. The shift towards early discharge from hospital to home and increasing efforts to manage the care of older people, the disabled and chronically ill at home or in the community have been strategic initiatives [2]. 'Community' and 'primary health care' models for health service delivery are popular and prominent. Such models abandon biomedical models of health care for those with a greater emphasis on the social determinants of health, where individuals, families, groups and communities are placed at the centre of the systems of care. Community nursing is a specialty nursing practice at the centre of community care models.

These reforms and the focus towards community care have resulted in new demands on community nurses. Community nurses are adopting and adapting to new roles, extending their scope of practice, and consequently are more accountable for their clinical practice than ever before. The rapid changes in the health care environment continue to precipitate challenges for health professions, regarding the sufficiency of professional practice standards, education and training, and clinical policy and procedures that ensure quality, safety and accountability in health care. As health care provided in primary and community care settings becomes more complex, so too do the complexities and risks of infection [3].

Providing safe and quality health care is a complex business [4]. Preventing health care–acquired infections (HCAIs) is high on the agenda of quality and safety of health care. Public trust and confidence in our hospitals as clean and as safe places continues to be challenged by HCAIs [5]. Wherever health care is provided, HCAI is a risk. Infectious agents are present in almost all health care settings. Whether in community settings, hospitals, general practice, day surgery centres, respite and residential aged care facilities or elsewhere, there are variable risks for cross-infection. Those not associated with heath care delivery, such as ancillary and office workers and, of course, visitors and the general public, may also be at risk of infection when working or interacting with clients in health care settings. Some settings present greater risks and hazards than others. Although the level of risk may vary, hazards may remain or reoccur. In some cases, HCAIs are inconspicuous. In others, however, they are extremely serious, potentially life-threatening, and even fatal. For those who contract HCAI, the burden of infection is both economic and human, with dramatically increased length of service delivery, pain, suffering and at times death. Clearly, such burdens are unacceptable. For organisations and governments there are also significant financial and economic consequences.

Clinical governance and quality systems

Quality control measures that are based on risk identification and mitigation help minimise HCAIs. Infection control management plans (ICMPs) are formal and systematic clinical governance processes that enable institutions to meet their infection control and prevention obligations within the broader corporate mission and goal. They are designed to ensure that institutions and their people demonstrate accountability for quality in areas of infection control and prevention. ICMPs should risk-manage and reduce the incidence of preventable HCAIs within organisational frameworks and systems that ensure quality and safety in health care. Key elements of an infection control programme are outlined in Figure 6.1.

The infection control programme should inform the development of an ICMP. An ICMP also provides an opportunity to define the scope of an infection control programme within the boundaries of areas such as client demographics, epidemiology of infection and restricted resources. ICMPs should embrace, build and extend the organisational strategic plan. Additionally, the plan allows organisations to prioritise infection control activity in accordance with principles of risk management and develop

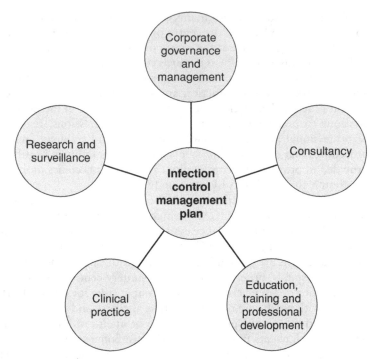

Figure 6.1 Standard elements of an infection control management programme.

appropriate professional and programme performance measures, thereby demonstrating professional and public accountability of the infection control programme in terms of cost-effectiveness and/or cost benefit [6]. Tools to assist the development of an ICMP are available from sources in the resources list at the end of this chapter.

The type of plan developed for the community context will depend on factors such as the requirements of the organisation, financial and human resources, and knowledge of infection control and management. Plans can be either long- or short-term. Long-term plans are often referred to as strategic plans, whereas short-term plans are called business or operational plans. These plans guide day-to-day and long-term activity. As such, the strategic intentions documented in the strategic plan or activities outlined in the operational plan should form the basis of the infection control committee's (ICC's) agenda, thereby assisting the ICC to steer activity in accordance with the ICMP [6].

Central to the success of an ICMP is its focus on infection control performance measures of both the organisation and its people. Good infection control outcomes rely on clinicians and service providers complying with infection control principles/standards and reporting various risk factors and/or situations that may lead to a risk of infection transmission. As such, leadership is required to obtain stakeholder buy-in at every level of the organisation. The input of stakeholders such as health workers – including nurses and doctors – and also consumers need to be sought when setting policies/guidelines, targets and performance measures. In most instances the performance being measured is that of the stakeholders. This fact needs to be clear for clinicians or service providers to be accountable for their action and outcomes [6].

Community infection control practice standards

Effective infection control guidelines and strategies for the control and prevention of HCAIs are required for all health contexts and settings, from large hospitals to community, home and practice settings [4]. Traditionally, guidelines and practice standards for infection control and prevention have focused on the acute care and hospital-based contexts. The general principles of infection control are, however, relevant to all health care settings, although specific settings may need their own requirements [1]. The success of these policies and procedures lies in ensuring they meet the demands and challenges of the specific settings and context in which they operate. Essentially, the basics of infection control and prevention apply.

In the Australian context, the standards for best-practice infection control and prevention are informed by a number of guidelines. The 'Infection Control Guidelines for the Prevention of Transmission of Infectious Diseases in the Health Care Setting' is the principal and authoritative standard on infection control and prevention across the range of health care establishments [1]. They are national infection control guidelines that encompass a variety of health care contexts and settings that are relevant to infection control and prevention, including community settings, and are designed to assist health care providers involved in direct client care to minimise the risk of infection [4]. They make specific reference to and recommendations for such settings that work alongside state or territory legislative requirements for work practices at the local level [4]. When using these guidelines, statutory requirements of the jurisdiction take precedence when difference exists [1]. Community nursing and health practice should be informed by policies and procedures established within clinical and corporate governance systems. On an individual level, policies and guidelines established for community nurses should reflect the diversity of their work. Such policies require tailoring to the specific practice environment – the community.

Managing the physical environment – multiple settings

Community nursing occurs in diverse settings, including people's homes, public events, rural and remote settings, community health centres and immunisation clinics. Nursing practice across diverse settings demands that community nurses develop expertise as specialist generalists, requiring them to develop and draw on knowledge and experiences of multiple contexts. Each of these settings is unique and often unpredictable and, more often than not, is resource-poor. Community nurses often work in uncontrolled environments and have time constraints. Care can be provided in less than ideal environmental conditions, which creates a challenge for compliance with basic infection control standards.

A key feature of community nursing practice is that it most often occurs in people's homes. Providing care in informal settings without the infrastructure or regulations of a hospital setting is the mainstay of community nursing practice; however, infection control standards applicable to the hospital context are not always readily transferable to community settings. In such settings, the client has control over the environment. Care is often provided by family, friends, volunteers, personal care attendants and home help, all of which are unregulated. The diversity of community practice brings with it many challenges for managing HCAIs.

Table 6.1 Checklist for planning care for patients with infection practices in community settings.

- Have detailed discharge summaries and client records been provided for this client?
- What is this client's medical history, particularly as it relates to infections and antibiotic treatment?
- Are there any particularly relevant conditions I should consider, such as MROs, immunocompromised states or chronic wounds?
- Was this client's most recent care provided in a setting where an infection surveillance system was in operation?
- Does the client have any epidemiologically significant infections?
- What care plans and pathways do I need to provide for this client, and what other staff/services were involved in the care process?
- What procedures need to be performed, and when?
- Where will procedures be carried out, and by whom?
- How can I and others decontaminate our hands and ensure good standards of hand hygiene?
- What types of clinical waste will be generated, and how will I need to dispose of it appropriately?
- What equipment is available to provide care safely and effectively?
- How do I go about acquiring the necessary equipment, such as sharps containers, for appropriate care?
- What support services will be required to provide care, such as allied health care professionals, and how will I contact them?
- Have I conducted a safety and risk assessment of the client and site I am required to visit?
- Have I established safety and emergency action plans for each of my site visits, which include access to mobile communication equipment?
- Have I ensured my personal development plan identifies areas for my professional development to meet the needs of contemporary community heath care practice relevant to infection control and prevention?
- What additional education, training or professional development, or resources, do I require to perform my role in a safe and effective manner?
- Have I identified colleagues with expertise in infection control, such as infection control practitioners, public health physicians and other mode experienced community nurses, whom I can contact for advice and assistance as required?

To meet these challenges, St John and Keleher argue that community nurses draw on 'public health, epidemiology, social science, communication, project management, case management, health promotion, research, combining with existing foundational general nursing knowledge and skills and specific specialty expertise' [1, p. 5].

The key to effective infection control practice in community care settings is planning and preparation [10]. Work practices at a local level should as much as possible be reflective of the diversity in social, cultural and environmental conditions community nurses are required to work in. Table 6.1 provides a checklist for community nurses in planning their work care practices.

The Basics – Standard Precautions

For the community nurse, the variety of physical environments where they work and provide care makes infection control and prevention challenging. ICMPs for community nurses require an assessment of the context-specific challenges of practice.

Table 6.2 Standard Precautions for community nursing practice [2].

Hand washing and hand hygiene

- Community nurses should wash their hands before and after contact with community-based clients. Where access to clean running water is difficult, clean water should be transported in canisters. Canisters may be fitted with a tap. If water is not accessible, single-use towelettes (with detergent) may be used before an alcoholic hand rub. Hands should then be washed with liquid handwash and running water at the first opportunity.
- Community nurses may use a clean, dry towel provided by the client or employer, provided a fresh area of the towel is used each time hands are dried. Paper towels can be used in cases where clients are unable to provide a clean, dry towel for nurses to use.

Personal protective equipment

- Employers are responsible for providing personal protective equipment, and community nurses should carry it in anticipation of exposure to blood and body substances. These basic requirements can be carried into the home in a work case and should include waterproof gown, gloves, masks and goggles.
- Care must be taken to wash hands before removing items from or returning clean items to the work case or bag. The work case or bag and other items carried in it (e.g. stethoscopes, sphygmomanometers and scales) should be cleaned regularly or if they become soiled.

Waste disposal

- Waste disposal must be carried out in accordance with local and state/territory regulations. The Australian and New Zealand standard for clinical and related wastes (AS/NZS 3816 Management of Clinical and Related Waste) does not cover general domestic waste. Attempts should be made to segregate wastes at point of generation.
- Hazards arise when handling, storing, transporting and disposing of waste. Blood and body fluids should be disposed of directly into the sewer system where possible. Heavily exudating wound dressings should be contained in a leak-proof bag and be double bagged before disposal. Care must be taken in the handling and disposal of sharps. Sharps and other clinical wastes must be disposed of according to state/territory guidelines.

Equipment and supplies

- Medical supplies and client equipment should be stored in a dry area out of reach of children and pets and away from the high-traffic areas of the home. All parts of any equipment should be dismantled, where possible, to allow physical removal of all particulate and biological matter. Equipment should be cleaned with detergent and water and dried thoroughly before it is transported into or out of the home.

---

[1] AS/NZS 3816 (1998) *Management of Clinical and Related Wastes.*

Table 6.2 outlines standard precautions that are a foundation for best-practice infection control and prevention in community care settings [4], including the most fundamental aspects of infection control and prevention – handwashing and hand hygiene.

Special issues for community contexts – Additional Precautions

Pandemic influenza

One of the oldest infectious diseases associated with significant morbidity and mortality to successfully escape eradication is influenza. Influenza and variants such as avian influenza and other respiratory infections have evolved over hundreds of years, survived the passing of time and the rise and fall of populations, and today are a significant global challenge [1]. Humans appear to be accidental hosts of avian influenza, which is spread through bird faeces and contaminated water or dust. Outbreaks of avian influenza have been recognised in poultry flocks in most countries of the world for many years, resulting in severe disease [7].

Outbreaks of pandemic influenza could have devastating economic and social consequences in Australia and around the world. The 'Australian Health Management Plan for Pandemic Influenza – Interim Infection Control Guidelines for Pandemic Influenza in Healthcare and Community Settings' [8] provides community nurses and other community-based health care professionals with the appropriate guidelines for the management of the outbreak of pandemic influenza. Essentially, it is suggested that infection control for influenza is probably better aimed at reducing community risk and household transmission [9]. Table 6.3 details the principles of infection control and prevention for pandemic influenza.

There are important work practices for community nurses to consider. Personal hygiene, such as covering the mouth during sneezes or coughs and hand decontamination, are likely to be more effective in deterring household infection transmission, particularly for airborne infections such as influenza. Table 6.4 outlines infection control and prevention work practices relevant to pandemic influenza.

Essentially, infection control and prevention of pandemic influenza in the community should focus on respiratory and hand hygiene. Avoiding direct contact with people with respiratory symptoms should be promoted when the pandemic is circulating in the community, which may be extended to keeping a distance of over 1 m between all people regardless of symptom status. The use of masks by persons with respiratory symptoms to limit aerosol spread is recommended. Although there is only limited evidence demonstrating the value of masks in community settings as a public health measure to decrease infections during a community outbreak, individuals may choose to wear a mask as part of individual protection strategies that include cough etiquette, hand hygiene and avoiding public gatherings [8]. People at high risk for complications of influenza, such as the immunocompromised and the elderly, should consider avoiding public gatherings when pandemic influenza is circulating in the community. The role of the community nurse in communicating these measures to individuals, families and communities is essential.

Gastrointestinal diseases and *Norovirus*

Many microorganisms are capable of producing symptoms of diarrhoeal disease. Gastrointestinal disease causes fluid loss and dehydration in people regardless of the cause. Outbreaks of infectious diseases can occur sporadically and there are organisms that cause infections seasonally in the community. Infections in health care may arise from staff, clients, visitors, air, food, water, sterile products, the environment and vermin. Most pathogens will enter the gastrointestinal tract via the faecal–oral route, from contaminated hands, food or fluids. Diarrhoea may be caused by many viral, bacterial and parasitic pathogens including, but not limited to, *Adenovirus, Rotavirus, Norovirus, Campylobacter* sp., *Clostridium difficile, Salmonella* sp., *Yersinia, Cryptosporidium* and *Giardia Lamblia* [10]. *Norovirus* (formerly known as Norwalk-like viruses) is a common cause of non-bacterial gastroenteritis. Outbreaks have been reported in the community, hospitals and aged care facilities [11]. *Norovirus* commonly occurs in winter months and is a syndrome of acute nausea, vomiting and explosive

Table 6.3 Principles of infection control and prevention for pandemic influenza [3].

Principles

Limit contact between infected and non-infected persons
a. Isolate infected persons (e.g. confine clients to a defined area as appropriate for the health care setting):
  - Limit contact to a small number of health care workers and close family and friends
  - Promote spatial separation in common areas (e.g. sit or stand as far away as possible, at least 1 m, from potentially infected persons) to limit contact between symptomatic and asymptomatic persons
b. Protect persons caring for influenza clients in health care and other special settings from contact with the pandemic influenza virus. Persons who must be in close client contact should wear appropriate personal protective equipment.
c. Contain infectious respiratory secretions:
  - Instruct clients who have 'flu-like' symptoms to use respiratory hygiene/cough etiquette (see below, 'Respiratory hygiene/cough etiquette')
  - Promote use of surgical masks by symptomatic persons in common areas (e.g. in waiting rooms) or when being transported (e.g. by ambulance)

Respiratory hygiene/cough etiquette
To contain respiratory secretions, all persons with signs and symptoms of a respiratory infection, regardless of presumed cause, should be instructed to:
  - Cover the nose/mouth when coughing or sneezing
  - Use tissues to contain respiratory secretions
  - Dispose of tissues in the nearest waste receptacle after use
  - Perform hand hygiene after contact with respiratory secretions and contaminated objects/materials
Health care facilities should ensure the availability of materials for adhering to respiratory hygiene/cough etiquette in waiting areas for clients and visitors:
  - Provide tissues and no-touch receptacles for used tissue disposal
  - Provide conveniently located dispensers of alcohol-based hand rub
  - Provide soap and disposable towels for handwashing where sinks are available

Surgical masks and separation of symptomatic persons
During periods of increased respiratory infection in the community, persons who are coughing should be offered a surgical mask to contain respiratory secretions. Coughing persons should be encouraged to sit as far away as possible (at least 1 m) from others in common waiting areas. Some facilities may wish to institute this recommendation year-round.

diarrhoea. Symptoms usually last between 24 and 48 h with an incubation period of the same; viral shedding continues for approximately 24 h after the symptoms cease [10]. The Norwalk-like viruses are small ribonucleic acid (RNA) viruses classified as caliciviruses. This virus is transmitted via the faecal–oral route. The literature suggests that active vomiting causes widespread aerosol dissemination of viral particles, causing environmental contamination and subsequent spread [12].

As stated previously, the general principles of infection prevention and control apply when providing care for clients in the community setting. Standard precautions involve strict hand hygiene after contact with people who have signs and symptoms of gastrointestinal disease. Health care providers should encourage clients to practise good hand hygiene and toilet hygiene. Health care providers themselves should not attend work when symptomatic of gastrointestinal disease of unknown or infectious origin.

Table 6.4 Work practices for infection control and prevention of pandemic influenza [3].

Work practices

Contact precautions
- When caring for clients with pandemic influenza, community nurses should be particularly vigilant to avoid touching their eyes, nose or mouth with contaminated hands (gloved or ungloved). Careful placement of personal protective equipment (PPE) before client contact will help avoid the risk of self-contamination whilst making PPE adjustments. Careful removal of PPE is also important.

Personal protective equipment
- PPE is used to protect the wearer from contact with the pandemic influenza virus. During the early phases of a pandemic when the transmission characteristics of the newly emergent virus are not fully understood, immunity to the virus is absent and a vaccine is not available. Adherence to appropriate PPE is recommended for all contacts with avian or pandemic influenza clients. In the later phases, recommendations will be updated in the light of increasing knowledge about the virus, availability of PPE and availability of antivirals and vaccines.
- Community nurses should wear a P2 (N95) mask, gown, gloves, eyewear and cap when in close client contact (1 m), when an aerosol-generating procedure is being performed or when in contact with contaminated client consumables.
- Gloves should never replace the need for hand hygiene. Gloves should be worn in accordance with standard precautions, i.e. when contact with respiratory secretions or other body fluids is anticipated (e.g. during provision of oral care, handling soiled tissues). They are not necessary when performing other tasks such as changing bed linen unless the linen is visibly soiled, provided hand hygiene is performed afterwards. Gloves should always be replaced between different client contacts. Always perform hand hygiene after glove removal.
- Gowns should be worn when attending to pandemic influenza clients. A disposable gown made of synthetic fibre or a washable cloth gown may be used. The gown should cover the wearer's clothing. Gowns are essential when soiling of clothes is anticipated (e.g. during invasive procedures or suctioning, nebulisation, bronchoscopy, chest physiotherapy or intubation). In such circumstances, a long-sleeved, cuffed and fluid repellent gown is recommended. Gowns should be worn only once and then disposed of in clinical waste bins appropriately.
- If a P2 (N95) mask is not available, a surgical mask should be worn. Change a mask when it becomes moist. The mask should never be reapplied after it has been removed. Do not leave them dangling around the neck. On touching or discarding a used mask, perform hand hygiene.

Hand hygiene
- Hand hygiene is a crucial practice to reduce the transmission of infectious agents in health care settings and is an essential element of standard precautions. The term 'hand hygiene' includes both handwashing with either plain or antimicrobial soap and water and use of alcohol-based products (gels, rinses, foams) containing an emollient that do not require the use of water.
- If hands are visibly soiled or contaminated with respiratory secretions, wash hands with soap (either plain or antimicrobial) and water. In the absence of visible soiling of hands, approved alcohol-based products for hand disinfection may be preferred over antimicrobial or plain soap and water because of their reduced drying of the skin and convenience. Always perform hand hygiene between client contacts and after removing PPE. Ensure that resources to facilitate handwashing (e.g. sinks with warm and cold running water, plain or antimicrobial soap, disposable paper towels) and hand disinfection (e.g. alcohol-based products) are readily accessible in areas in which client care is provided.
- In general, wearing goggles or a face shield for routine contact with clients with pandemic influenza is not necessary unless sprays or splatter of infectious material is likely, especially if the client is not wearing a surgical mask at the time.

Table 6.4 (*continued*)

Work practices

Disposal of solid waste
- Standard precautions are recommended for disposal of solid waste (clinical and non-clinical) that might be contaminated with a pandemic influenza virus. Contain and dispose of clinical waste in accordance with facility-specific and/or local or state/territory regulations for handling and disposal of medical waste, including used needles and other sharps. All other waste, including disposable gowns, gloves and masks and soiled tissues, should be disposed of in the general waste stream. Wear disposable gloves when handling contaminated waste. Perform hand hygiene after removal of gloves.

Linen and laundry
- Standard precautions are recommended for linen and laundry that might be contaminated with respiratory secretions from clients with pandemic influenza. If there is a linen service, place soiled linen directly into a laundry bag in the client's room. Contain linen in a manner that prevents the linen bag from opening or bursting during transport and while in the soiled linen holding area. Wear gloves and gown when directly handling visibly soiled linen and laundry (e.g. bedding, towels, personal clothing) as per standard precautions. Do not shake or otherwise handle soiled linen and laundry in a manner that might create an opportunity for disease transmission or contamination of the environment. Linen should be decanted directly from the bag into the washing machine without contact. It should be laundered on a normal hot cycle and then aired or tumble dried. Perform hand hygiene after removing gloves that have been in contact with soiled linen and laundry. Paper sheeting is a good alternative to standard linen sheets for use on client examination tables/couches and should be changed after each client.

Client care equipment
- Disposable equipment should be used wherever possible during the treatment and care of clients and should be disposed of appropriately in the general waste. If equipment is to be reused, then it should be disinfected in accordance with the manufacturer's instructions.
- Follow standard precautions for handling and reprocessing used client care equipment, including medical devices. Wear gloves when handling and transporting used client care equipment. Clean heavily soiled equipment with water and neutral detergent followed by a disinfectant solution (1) sodium hypochlorite (1000 parts per million of available chlorine, usually achieved by a 1 in 50 dilution of 5% liquid bleach), (2) granular chlorine (e.g. Det-Sol 5000 or Diver sol, to be diluted as per manufacturer's instructions), and (3) alcohol (e.g. isopropyl 70%, ethyl alcohol 60%). Follow current recommendations for cleaning and disinfection or sterilisation of reusable client care equipment. Decontaminate external surfaces of portable equipment that may be used on other clients. Combination detergent/disinfectant or alcohol wipes would be an acceptable method.

Environmental cleaning and disinfection
- Standard precautions recommended for cleaning and disinfection of environmental surfaces are important components of routine infection control in health care facilities
- Cleaning and disinfection of client-occupied rooms require appropriate PPE, including mask, gown and gloves. Keep areas around the client free of unnecessary supplies and equipment to facilitate daily cleaning. Give special attention to frequently touched surfaces (e.g. bedrails, bedside and overbed tables, TV controls, call buttons, telephones, lavatory surfaces including safety/pull-up bars, door knobs, commodes) in addition to floors and other horizontal surfaces.

Wound care

Wound care is a routine practice for community nurses. Wounds are often chronic and complex in nature, and community nurses often manage them in resource-poor environments. The environmental condition clients often live in compounds of the complexity of wound care, extending healing time, pain and suffering. Normal human skin is colonised with various types of microorganisms [13]. Bacteria are responsible for the majority of wound infections, including organisms such as coagulase-negative staphylococci and *Staphylococcus aureus*, with these organisms accounting for 14% and 20% of infected wounds respectively [14]. Because these and many other bacteria form part of the skin's normal flora, standard infection prevention and control principles including asepsis apply when managing wounds in the community.

Contamination of a wound or the presence of microorganisms does not necessarily mean that the wound is infected unless clinical signs and symptoms of infection are present, including fever, pain, swelling, induration, erythema, odour and warmth/heat [15]. The client, family and health care provider must be aware of these signs and symptoms of wound infection, and make referral to the principal health care provider when required. Treating wounds that are colonised or infected with epidemiologically significant organisms requires specialist skills obtained by adopting a multidisciplinary approach. In most instances, the aim is to promote wound healing rather than the removal of significant organisms. The successful treatment of such wounds requires community nurses to consult with other relevant experts, such as infection control practitioners, wound care nurses, stomal therapists and physicians. Community nurses should, in consultation with the multidisciplinary team, develop comprehensive wound management plans that incorporate principles of infection control and prevention, with a strong emphasis on standard precautions.

Multidrug-resistant organisms

The emergence and re-emergence of multidrug-resistant organisms (MROs) is an ongoing international health priority. Historically, *S. aureus* has been a major cause of HCAI. It is the leading cause of health care–acquired (HCA) pneumonia and surgical site infections, and the second leading cause of HCA bloodstream infections. It is also responsible for community-acquired infections such as osteomyelitis, septic arthritis, skin infections, endocarditis and meningitis [16]. Methicillin-resistant *S. aureus* (MRSA) continues to challenge the safety and quality of modern health care [17]. In some settings it is responsible for as many as 20% of all HCAIs. Endemic in most hospitals and epidemic in others, approximately 30% of all *S. aureus* infections present with some form of drug resistance [16].

Many other organisms show increased chemotherapeutic resistance. Vancomycin-resistant enterococci (VREs) were discovered in clinical settings around the world in the late 1980s and early 1990s. The emergence of *S. aureus* infection with intermediate resistance to vancomycin indicates that *S. aureus* strains are constantly evolving and may develop full resistance [16, 18]. Although MRSA, VRE and extended-spectrum β-lactamase and AmpC-producing Enterobacteriaceae have been the subject of much of this attention, the popular press is dominated by concerns about HCAIs by other MROs such as *Acinetobacter baumannii* [19]. Concern about carbapenem-resistant *A. baumannii* (CRAB) began when the first HCA outbreak occurred in the United States in 1991. Since then, CRAB infections and hospital-wide outbreaks have been reported in many other countries [19].

MROs are becoming increasingly relevant outside hospital settings. First reported in 1961, MRSA is internationally endemic and one of the most challenging bacterial pathogens affecting both patients in hospitals and clients in the community; however, its presentation and epidemiology continue to evolve. 'Community-acquired MRSA' (CA-MRSA), or MRSA occurring in otherwise healthy individuals with no risk factors for MRSA such as recent hospitalisation, surgical procedure or antibiotic administration, is emerging. In many parts of the world, infections cause a growing number of illnesses.

Efforts to control and prevent MROs have focused almost exclusively on reducing infections in hospital contexts. The main route of MRSA transfer is from one person to another, by direct or indirect contact [20]. Individuals transmit infection by failing to decontaminate their hands effectively before and after contact with individuals colonised or infected with MRSA. Hand hygiene before and after close contact with clients is the single most important measure for controlling and preventing the spread of infection [20]. Hand hygiene and decontamination practices for acute care nurses are the same for community nurses; in community contexts, hand hygiene is as important as it is in acute settings. The importance of hand hygiene has been highlighted in many health care settings with various campaigns to encourage frequent and thorough hand hygiene. New initiatives include the standard issue of alcohol hand gel at 'point of care' in all care settings [20].

Australian research has suggested that nurses rely on facilities provided by the client for hand hygiene and, in the main, nurses 'make do' when facilities, tools or time are inadequate [21]. Community nurses should decontaminate their hands, the universally acknowledged primary strategy for infection control and prevention. Convenience of equipment encourages compliance [20]. Controlling MROs is a contentious issue. Attempts to eliminate endemic MRSA in hospitals have proved difficult, costly and largely unsuccessful. Hand hygiene and standard precautions are the primary strategies for community nurses managing clients colonised and infected with MROs.

To participate fully in infection control and prevention strategies, community nurses require a comprehensive understanding of microbiology and how and why microorganisms develop resistance to antibiotics. This better prepares them for preventing the spread of MROs, including teaching clients and their families about infection control and antibiotic management. Continued reinvestment in integrated and comprehensive infection control programmes focusing on sound hand hygiene practice, surveillance and rational and justified use of antibiotics is often required. Ensuring infection control management programmes are inclusive and sensitive to the needs and context of community nursing and health practice is vital to reduce the morbidity and mortality arising from MRSA and other HCAIs [17]. Although there is much evidence that supports the position that wounds heal better at home or in community contexts where clients are not at risk of HCAIs [21, 22], community environments also present challenges to clients with respect to wound management and healing.

Responding to outbreaks

Managing outbreaks of infectious disease in community contexts is complex. There is general consensus that in the event of a national infectious disease emergency the Australian health system would 'work' [23]. Until recently, Australia's public health system response to pandemic outbreak was largely untested, and many of Australia's hospitals and facilities appeared underprepared. More recently, threats of emerging disease such as SARS (severe acute respiratory syndrome virus) and avian influenza have prompted countries around the world to examine their capacity to prevent, detect and respond to serious infectious diseases [23]. The threat of pandemic influenza has precipitated in Australia the development of outbreak management plans within governments, health service authorities and organisations nationally. 'Exercise Cumpston 2006' tested Australia's readiness for a potential pandemic influenza outbreak and also tested the Australian Health Management Plan for Pandemic Influenza [24]. A critical element of this exercise was the ability of hospitals to deal with a sudden influx of multiple casualties, often referred to as a 'surge capacity'. Most hospitals operate at or near capacity, so there is little flexibility to cope with an influx of people [23]. Consequently, there is little doubt that nationally Australian hospitals could not deal with such a crisis [23]. There is, however, little expectation that they should. In the event of national infectious disease outbreaks, it is entirely foreseeable that clients would remain and receive care in the community. With little capacity to admit people into hospital rapidly, hospital and district health services have developed disaster plans that anchor the care of those with infection in community settings. Community nurses must then be prepared with sound knowledge and skills regarding infection control and preparedness to expedite service procedures efficiently. Community nurses, therefore, have integral roles to play with the notification of suspected outbreaks of infectious disease and their ongoing community management.

State and territory governments have amended legislation to enable a more timely and effective response to the threat of epidemic or pandemic infectious diseases. These acts, such as the *Public Health Act 2005* (Queensland), provide improved measures for preventing, controlling and reducing risks to public health, particularly related to the identification of and response to notifiable conditions. They define important obligations for health care professionals such as community nurses and particular health care facilities involved in the provision of declared health services to minimise infection risks and provide a central legislative basis for responding to public health emergencies [25]. Community nurses must determine their obligations under the legislation within their own jurisdiction and establish collaborative links with officials from their respective public health units. Establishing these links and contacts is essential if the community nurse is to respond to the threat of an outbreak of a notifiable disease in their setting. In these instances, the community nurse forms an integral part of an outbreak investigation team, providing vital local information that is essential to the timely and appropriate response to public health emergencies.

Summary

HCAIs are no longer a problem solely for hospitals. Infection control and prevention must be a focus of all health care settings. Infectious diseases will continue to pose significant threats to the health, safety and well-being of the community. Emerging threats such pandemic influenza are clearly relevant to community nursing and health care. Improvements in technology and changing consumer demands are widening the range of services provided outside hospital settings. Expanding health care provision into community settings will increase the risks of HCAI. In a social and political environment where the demands on health care workers for safe and quality health care have never been so great, the ways in which community nurses manage infectious disease take on crucial importance [1]. Community infection control and prevention is an evolving specialist discipline informed by a body of specialist knowledge, evidence and experience in the community care context [1]. There will be a need for community infection control and prevention while there is continuing emphasis on community models of health care. Infection control and prevention is thus core business for the community nurse.

Useful resources

Australian Infection Control Association (AICA) at http://www.aica.org.au
Australian Society for Microbiology (ASM) at http://www.theasm.com.au
Centre for Healthcare Related Infection Surveillance and Prevention (CHRISP) at http://www.chrispqld.com
US Center for Disease Control and Prevention (CDC) at http://www.cdc.gov
Association for Professionals in Infection Control and Epidemiology (APIC) at http://www.apic.org

References

1. Shaban, R.Z. (2008) Infection control and prevention in community settings, in D. Kralik and A. van Loon (eds) *Community Nursing in Australia*. Blackwell Publishing, Oxford, pp. 184–97.
2. Wilson, J. (2003) Foreword, in J. Lawrence and D. May (eds) *Infection Control in the Community*. Churchill Livingstone, London.
3. National Institute for Health and Clinical Excellence (2003) *Infection Control, Prevention of Healthcare-Associated Infection in Primary and Community Care*. National Institute for Health and Clinical Excellence, London.
4. Department of Health and Ageing (2004) *Infection Control in the Health Care Setting: Guidelines for the Prevention and Transmission of Infectious Diseases*. Australian Government, Canberra.
5. Beasley, C. (2004) Editorial – healthcare associated infections prevention. *Nurse Manager*, 3(1), 2.
6. Griffith University (2007) *Contemporary Infection Control Practice*. School of Nursing and Midwifery, Griffith University, Brisbane.
7. Department of Health and Ageing (2006) *Avian Influenza*. Available at http://www.health.gov.au/internet/main/publishing.nsf/Content/health-avian_influenza-index.htm, (viewed 2007).
8. Department of Health and Aging (2006) *The Australian Health Management Plan for Pandemic Influenza – Interim Infection Control Guidelines for Pandemic Influenza in Healthcare and Community Settings*. Commonwealth of Australia, Canberra.
9. Weber, J.T. and Hughes, J.M. (2004) Beyond Semmelweis: Moving infection control into the community. *Annals of Internal Medicine*, 140(5). 397–8.
10. Farr, B.M. (2004) Nosocomial gastrointestinal tract infections, in C.G. Mayhall (ed.) *Hospital Epidemiology and Infection Control*, 3rd edition. Lippincott, Williams and Wilkins, Philadelphia, pp. 351–84.
11. Russo, P.L., Spelman, D.W., Harrington, G.A., Jenney, A.W., Gunesekere, I.C., Wright, P.J., Doutlree, J.C. and Marshall, J.A. (1997) Hospital outbreak of Norwalk-like virus. *Infection Control and Hospital Epidemiology*, 18(8), 576–9.

12. Heymann, D.L. (2004) *Control of Communicable Diseases Manual*, 18th edition. American Public Health Association, Washington, DC.

13. Pittet, D., Simon, A., Hugonnet, S., Silva, C.L.P., Sauvan, V. and Perneger, T.V. (2004) Hand hygiene among physicians: Performance, beliefs and perceptions. *Annals of Emergency Medicine*, 141(1), 1–8.

14. Roy, M.-C. (2003) Modern approaches to preventing surgical site infections, in R.P. Wenzel (ed.) *Prevention and Control of Nosocomial Infections*, 4th edition. Lippincott, Williams and Wilkins, Philadelphia, pp. 369–84.

15. Scanlon, E. (2003) Wound care, in J. Lawrence and D. May (eds) *Infection Control in the Community*. Churchill Livingstone, London, pp. 225–50.

16. Rubin, R.J., Harrington, C.A., Poon, A., Dietrich, K., Greene, J.A. and Moiduddin, A. (1999) The economic impact of *Staphylococcus aureus* infection in New York City hospitals. *Emerging Infectious Diseases*, 5(1), 9–17.

17. Fairclough, S.J. (2006) Infection control. Why tackling MRSA needs a comprehensive approach. *British Journal of Nursing*, 15(2), 72–5.

18. Centers for Disease Control and Prevention (1997) *Morbidity and Mortality Weekly Report Update: Staphylococcus aureus with Reduced Susceptibility to Vancomycin – United States*. Centers for Disease Control and Prevention, Washington, DC, p. 46.

19. Hsueh, P.-R., Teng, L.-J., Chen, C.-Y., Chen, W.H., Yu, C.J., Ho, S.W. and Luh, K.T. (2002) Pandrug-resistant *Acinetobacter baumannii* causing nosocomial infections in a university hospital, Taiwan. *Emerging Infectious Diseases*, 8(8), 827–32.

20. Whitby, M., Pessoa-Silva, C.L., McLaws, M.-L., *et al.* (2007) Behavioural considerations for hand hygiene practices: The basic building blocks. *Journal of Hospital Infection*, 65, 1–8.

21. Adrie, C., Alberti, C., Chaix-Couturier, C., Azoulay, E., deLassence, A., Cohen, Y., Meshaka, P., Cheval, C., Thuong, M. and Troche, G. (2005) Epidemiology and economic evaluation of severe sepsis in France: Age, severity, infection site, and place of acquisition (community, hospital, or intensive care unit) as determinants of workload and cost. *Journal of Critical Care*, 20(1), 46–58.

22. Sheng, W.H., Wang, J.T., Lu, D.C.T., Chie, W.C., Chen, Y.C. and Chang, S.C. (2005) Comparative impact of hospital-acquired infections on medical costs, length of hospital stay and outcome between community hospitals and medical centres. *Journal of Hospital Infection*, 59(3), 205–14.

23. Department of Parliamentary Services, Parliament of Australia (2005) *Influenza – Is Australia a Sitting Duck?* Australian Government, Canberra.

24. Office of Health Protection, Department of Health and Ageing (2006) *Australian Health Management Plan for Pandemic Influenza*. Department of Health and Ageing, Australian Government, Canberra.

25. *Public Health Act 2005* (Qld).

Chapter 7

Disaster planning and management

Paul Arbon

Introduction

This chapter introduces the principles of disaster and emergency management, provides information about current Australian arrangements for the provision of health care during disasters and discusses emerging trends in disaster health care. The disaster health care principles discussed in this chapter remain constant and are applied to the prevention, response and recovery efforts of health care in any disaster situation. More detailed information on the health aspects of disaster can be accessed through the resources listed at the end of this chapter.

The educational requirements of health professionals for disaster health care include:

- General disaster and emergency health awareness including basic knowledge of Australian and jurisdictional arrangements for disaster and emergency response
- Awareness of health care practitioner roles and lessons learnt from previous disasters and emergencies.
- Development of specific clinical skills that help practitioners to prepare for disaster, including primary and secondary assessment, triage, basic life support and minor injury or illness care.
- Knowledge of basic emergency management principles incorporating risk assessment, prevention and mitigation, the comprehensive approach and the all-hazards approach.

Many people associate the health response to disaster with emergency care, surgery and the urgent treatment of life-threatening injury. Often our experience of disaster and disaster health care is limited to the images and stories that we see in the mainstream media. Australian teams have responded to these dramatic events and the television footage is usually focused on the work of surgical teams at the site of temporary field hospitals. The surgical and emergency care response to disaster, however, has relatively limited impact on the health and recovery of affected communities. Surgical teams generally arrive too late to save life and generally cease to have much influence on survival and longer term recovery a few days or weeks after the impact of disaster. The real work in preparing for and recovering from disaster is done by community members and health practitioners who have an important role to play in developing the capacity and resilience of communities. When disaster strikes, community members and health practitioners work to re-establish health care services and provide the rehabilitation and ongoing care that is required by survivors. It is these inputs that have the greatest impact on the survival and recovery of affected populations. As a result, the role of community nurses during all phases of disaster should not be underestimated.

Defining disaster

There is no widely accepted definition of disaster. A study by Debacker *et al.* [1], for example, found over 100 definitions in general use. In the context of health care planning and response in Australia, the definition provided by Emergency Management Australia (EMA) [2], the Australian government agency responsible for coordinating the Commonwealth's response to disaster, is appropriate.

> A serious disruption to community life which threatens or causes death or injury in that community, and damage to property which is beyond the day-to-day capacity of the prescribed statutory authorities and which requires special mobilisation and organisation of resources other than those normally available to those authorities [2].

All disasters are related to specific hazards and may be categorised into:

- Natural.
- Mixed (natural + man-made).
- Man-made [3].

Natural disasters result from seismic causes and include events such as earthquake, volcanic eruption and tsunami or arise from climatic causes including high winds, high rainfall, erosion and drought.

Mixed disasters arise from a combination of human activity and environmental impacts and may include floods, landslides and fire.

Man-made disasters arise from technological causes such as the catastrophic release of harmful chemicals, transport or structural failure, explosion or from human conflict. Human conflict is a complex cause of disaster and includes war, civil conflict, terrorism and the negative impacts of sanctions and embargoes.

It is estimated that in the past 50 years more than 10 000 disasters have occurred, more than 5 billion people have been affected and more than 12 million persons have been killed, at an economic cost of more than US$4 trillion. By comparison, Australia's GDP in 2006 was only US$0.75 trillion. Disasters continue to occur and the frequency of these catastrophic occurrences is increasing [4]. In addition, the impact of disaster is becoming more severe as more people live in close proximity to possible impact zones (such as locations near the coast), in more crowded situations and with greater reliance on the community for essential services. Table 7.1 provides a snapshot of major world disasters that occurred in the month of January 2006 [5].

Background

A wide variety of current and emerging threats can be identified in the Australian context. Threats such as bush fire and flood are considered most significant in many

Table 7.1 Major world disasters that occurred in January 2006 [5, p. 5].

Jan. 2,	Sago, WV, USA: thirteen coal miners were trapped in the Sago Mine, 12 died and 1 survived.
Jan. 2,	Bad Reichenhall, Germany: a heavy snowfall caused the roof of an ice skating rink to collapse, killing 15.
Jan. 4,	Cijeruk, Indonesia: a mudslide buried 200 homes and killed at least 200 people.
Jan. 5,	Mecca, Saudi Arabia: a hotel collapsed in Mecca, killing at least 76 pilgrims on the annual hajj.
Jan. 12,	Mecca, Saudi Arabia: a stampede by pilgrims on the annual hajj killed at least 360.
Jan. 20,	Northern Hungary: a Slovak military plane, AN-24, en route to Slovakia from Kosovo, crashed soon after taking off, killing 43, most of them Slovak soldiers.
Jan. 23,	Bioce, Montenegro: a train derailed and plunged into the Moraca canyon, killing 46 and injuring 19.
Jan. 28,	Katowice, Poland: 67 people died from the collapse of the roof of the International Exhibition Hall. There had been 500 people inside at the time.

communities, although other emerging threats such as pandemic influenza and terrorist attacks are also important. Comprehensive risk assessments assist health care organisations to identify those threats that have the greatest likelihood of occurrence and the greatest risk of significant harm in their community or region. Identified threats should underpin the development of specific plans that will assist health care organisations in undertaking work to prevent or mitigate the impact, to prepare and plan for a response, and in the recovery of the community. In Australia substantial work has been undertaken at national, state, territory and local levels to prevent and respond to specific threats, notably building fires, wildfire and pandemic influenza. However, evidence shows that more generic (all-hazards) approaches should be adopted and that these provide the foundation for building the capacity and resilience of communities in responding to any threat, current or future [6].

Disasters and catastrophic emergencies will overwhelm the capacity of emergency services and acute health care agencies, at least in the short term, and it is necessary for communities to have some capability to manage through these situations until other services can recover the ability to respond. Recent workshops conducted jointly by the Attorney General's Department and St John Ambulance, Australia, to consider the 'Lessons Learned from the 2005 London Bombings' have highlighted the fact that communities will be required, regardless of whether they themselves are impacted directly, to manage: acute illness, fear and concern within their community, and other demands, such as supply, on their own for some period of time. For example, during the response to the London bombings, London Ambulance Service was unable to receive urgent (911) calls from other locations for a period of time and the community had to fend for itself [7]. Other evidence, particularly that emerging from the experience of health and aged care providers during the aftermath of Hurricane Katrina, supports the view that facilities, local communities and individuals need to be relatively self-reliant and capable, irrespective of planned support from external agencies [8]. Such a disaster overwhelms the resources of established emergency care providers.

International experience of the kind described above leads to the conclusion that even in metropolitan locations served by sophisticated health care services, communities need to be prepared, capable and resilient, and this requires training and resources that can be provided only through collaboration between emergency management and disaster health specialists and other health care providers. Additionally, it is recognised that the health care workforce is generally poorly prepared to work in disaster situations. Access to, and uptake of, basic education to increase workforce capability is poor and there is an urgent need for accessible, basic and relevant education and resources.

Training in emergency management

There are a number of difficulties associated with training in emergency management regardless of the professional discipline involved in the training. These include the problem of linking, transferring and retaining the knowledge and skills developed during training programmes with the 'real' situation that frequently occurs some significant time after training has been completed. It is also difficult to incorporate individual skills and efforts into a coordinated emergency response, and even after extensive training, practitioners may face unexpected challenges due to unforeseen situational demands [9].

For example Silverman *et al.* [10] describe the experience of a 500-bed, long-term care facility in the USA, which provided housing and nursing care units for patients (ranging from independently ambulatory to acutely ill and feeble) in preparing for, during and in the immediate aftermath of Hurricane Andrew, which struck on 24 August 1992. The problems encountered included a massive influx of evacuated elderly to the facility, facility isolation, loss of electrical power, loss of running water, special dietary needs and limited professional staffing due to personal property losses or loss of transportation. Overwhelmed county emergency medical services, limited access to hospitals and patient care, and difficulty in procuring supplies exacerbated the already complicated situation resulting from the storm. As a result of these catastrophic conditions, a number of challenges specific to the care of the elderly were identified.

Abrahams [11] considers an alert, informed and prepared community to be an integral part of any emergency management plan. Guha-Sapir [12] supports this view and regards capacity building for health responses to be best directed at the local level. Preparedness and response are dynamic processes as threats change and weaknesses are identified. Capacity is continuously built through planning, exercising, evaluating and improving [13].

Campbell [14, p. 34] cites seven main components of disaster preparedness:

1. Education and training of all health personnel (including community nurses).
2. Education and training of community members in first aid and rescue.
3. Collaboration with other key response sectors.
4. Development of plans and procedures.
5. Procurement of essential supplies and equipment.
6. Production of an inventory of resources (human and other).
7. Simulation exercises and drills.

There is no widely accepted standard or set of competencies for disaster nursing. However, the website titled 'Emergency Preparedness Competencies for Public Health Professionals' of The Centre for Health Policy at Columbia University [15] provides a starting point for discussion of the competencies that might be required by community nurses and a template to use when thinking about the roles that community nurses might play. The competencies for public health professionals are:

1. *Describe* the public heath role in emergency response in a range of emergencies that might arise.
2. *Describe* the chain of command in emergency response.
3. *Identify* and *locate* the agency emergency response plan (or the pertinent portion of the plan).
4. *Describe* his/her functional role(s) in emergency response and demonstrate his/her role(s) in regular drills.
5. *Demonstrate* correct use of all communication equipment used for emergency communication (phone, fax, radio etc.).
6. *Describe* communication role(s) in emergency response.
7. *Identify* limits to own knowledge/skill/authority and *identify* key system resources for referring matters that exceed these.
8. *Apply* creative problem-solving and flexible thinking to unusual challenges within his/her functional responsibilities and *evaluate* effectiveness of all actions taken.
9. *Recognise* deviations from the norm that might indicate an emergency and *describe* appropriate action (e.g. communicate clearly within the chain of command).
10. *Participate* in continuing education to maintain up-to-date knowledge in areas relevant to emergency response (e.g. emerging infectious diseases, hazardous materials, diagnostic tests etc.).

Community nurses need to consider the extent to which they are able to meet these requirements. Note however that these competencies focus on the response to emergency and fail to address the role of health professionals and community nurses in preparing communities and building their capacity to survive through disasters.

Principles and approaches

In Australia, four key principles or approaches underpin disaster and emergency management arrangements, which are:

1. The all-hazards approach.
2. The comprehensive approach.
3. The all-agencies (or integrated) approach.
4. The prepared community.

These approaches are utilised by organisations and governments in Australia and underpin disaster planning and response and recovery efforts.

The all-hazards approach

Even though specific countermeasures will often vary with different events or hazards, it is desirable to establish a single set of management arrangements capable of encompassing all types of hazards. In Australia, particularly in the response and recovery phases of disaster, government agencies and other organisations work within predetermined disaster management hierarchies for coordination, command and control of their operations. These are designed to be suitable in managing disaster arising from any hazard or cause. Disaster arrangements in Australia are frequently enacted and utilised in responding to smaller scale emergencies such as transport accidents or bush fire. In addition, Australian states and territories have dedicated facilities that are opened and staffed by the various agencies responding to a major emergency.

The comprehensive approach

The comprehensive approach refers to the stages of emergency/disaster management, 'PPRR', namely:

- Prevention/mitigation.
- Preparedness.
- Response.
- Recovery.

This approach advocates the development of emergency/disaster arrangements to embrace all of the stages. These stages tend to describe the sequence of events, from planning for, through to surviving through and recovering from a disaster. However some stages, notably response and recovery, actually overlap or occur in parallel with recovery activities commencing immediately after the impact of disaster.

Prevention, preparedness, response and recovery

The first stage of the comprehensive approach is to *prevent* or mitigate (reduce the severity of) any hazards.

> Effective disaster mitigation reduces or minimises the effects of disasters. In some circumstances, mitigation measures prevent disasters from occurring – hence, disaster prevention. Disaster mitigation measures act by lessening the hazard, reducing the vulnerability of a community to the hazard, or changing the environment in which hazards and communities interact. A rigorous and systematic risk management process will help communities to identify the most cost-effective combination of measures for the range of risks that they face. The plan of action for disaster mitigation will rest on priorities determined by the community and stakeholders [6].

The second stage is to ensure *preparedness* by communities and organisations through the development of disaster plans, establishment of resources and training or raising awareness. For example Australian governments have developed comprehensive plans for the risk of pandemic influenza that include training exercises to test the plans, the establishment of stockpiles of equipment and medications, and procedures for screening people who may be affected.

The third stage of the comprehensive approach is to provide an effective *response* immediately following any hazard impact. Typically, we think of the response to disaster as an activity undertaken by the traditional emergency services. However, in planning for disaster all agencies, including community health organisations, should consider how they would respond. For example, in community health we might consider how we identify and check on those who are vulnerable in our community such as the frail aged, those living with dementia or those who live alone. How will we respond to ensure that these people have access to health care, including, for example, their medications? What roles will we play during the response phase? How will we re-establish or maintain our own services?

The fourth stage is to provide for *recovery*. Recovery from disaster can be thought about as the bottom of the iceberg. The disaster that we see – the portion above water – attracts a large-scale response and is dramatic, yet relatively short lived. Recovery, on the other hand, is a long-term undertaking, which continues long after the focus of media and political interest have moved away. The recovery stage, of course, does not result in communities returning to their predisaster state but rather describes a process of rehabilitation of the community and individuals within it. This is a very complex process and our understanding of the ways that communities recover is currently quite unsophisticated. Nonetheless, community nurses will find themselves at the forefront of recovery efforts and this work will continue for a long period after the event. It is at this time that the work that community health professionals have put into building community emergency capacity and resilience prior to any catastrophic emergency will pay off.

The all-agencies (or integrated) approach

Specific arrangements for dealing with disaster vary between states and territories in Australia; however, in all cases they require an active partnership between communities, non-government organisations, statutory authorities and the state/territory and local levels of government.

Many agencies can be expected to play a role in more than one of the areas of prevention, preparedness, response and recovery, and will need to be represented in planning and management structures. As a result, committees set up throughout Australia to plan for and manage disasters inevitably comprise representatives from a wide range of organisations. This 'all-agencies' approach facilitates coordination of the plans that are developed and the responses of these many groups and also ensures that we are able to make the best use of resources and expertise that may exist within communities.

In Australia, state or territory disaster committees exist within each jurisdiction and the police assume the role of coordination or control of the various agencies during any actual event. The range of agencies likely to be involved in any aspect of disaster management is surprisingly broad, ranging across health, education, family and community services; transport, infrastructure or essential services; agriculture; emergency services; defence; media; and voluntary-aid organisations such as Australian Red Cross and St John Ambulance, Australia.

The prepared community

A prepared community is one which has developed effective emergency and disaster management arrangements at the local level, resulting in an alert, informed and active community which supports its voluntary organizations, has an active and involved local government and agreed and coordinated arrangements for PPRR [6].

Individual and community self-help often provide the most effective and decisive immediate relief. Affected communities turn first to local agencies for advice, assistance and support. Local government and organisations provide the basis for organising self-help. At the individual or family unit level, preparedness activities include developing an awareness of local hazards and plans and developing skills in areas such as first aid, which may be required in an emergency. Community health practitioners, including community nurses, have a role to play in assisting community members to access information and knowledge that will bolster their capacity to survive well through a disaster situation, should this be required. Activities might include teaching of basic first-aid skills, promoting immunisation and raising awareness about looking out for neighbours who may be more vulnerable. Frequently, however, preparation for disaster or major emergency is overtaken by the day-to-day responsibilities and work of community nurses and their organisations. Community nurses need to ask themselves, does their nursing organisation have a strategy in place to bolster the resilience of the communities in which it works? Do they spend any of their time on this task? What could they do? What should they be doing?

Key concepts

Emergency management arrangements in Australia

Australian state and territory governments have primary responsibility under the Constitution of Australia for the protection of communities and provision of emergency response and recovery services in the event of a disaster or major emergency. Links to the disaster legislation for each state and territory are listed at the conclusion of this chapter. The Australian government undertakes to support the jurisdictions by providing assistance from within its resources. This assistance is coordinated through the Australian government agency, EMA [6].

> Prime responsibility for the protection of life, property and the environment rests with the States and Territories. However, the Australian Government is committed to supporting States and Territories in developing their capacity for dealing with emergencies and disasters, and provides physical assistance to requesting States or Territories when they cannot reasonably cope during an emergency. Under the Constitution, the Australian Government is allocated responsibility for external affairs including the provision of humanitarian assistance for emergency and refugee relief overseas. The Australian Government, through EMA, supports a comprehensive approach to emergency management. EMA pursues a cooperative and collaborative relationship with Australian Government agencies such as the Department of Finance and Administration, Geoscience Australia and the Bureau of Meteorology. In doing so, EMA seeks to encourage an 'all agencies', 'all hazards' approach to the prevention or mitigation of disasters, preparedness for their impact, response to that impact and recovery from the consequences [6].

Several national plans have been developed to support disaster response. These include:

- *Commonwealth Government Disaster Response Plan* (COMDISPLAN). To coordinate the provision of Australian Government assistance in the event of a disaster in Australia or its offshore territories.

- *Commonwealth Government Overseas Disaster Assistance Plan* (AUSASSIST-PLAN). To coordinate the provision of Australian emergency assistance, using Australian Government physical and technical resources, following a disaster in another country.
- *Australian Contingency Plan for Space Re-Entry Debris* (AUSCONPLAN SPRED). To coordinate and control the activities of Commonwealth agencies in support of state/territory authorities involved in locating, recovering and removing radioactive space debris and monitoring and neutralising any radiological contamination threat arising from re-entry of radioactive space debris.
- *Commonwealth Government Reception Plan* (COMRECEPLAN). To coordinate the reception of persons evacuated into Australia following an overseas event.

In addition, there are several specialised national hazard-related plans:

- *AUSBURNPLAN* (designed to coordinate the allocation of acute burns beds in Australian hospitals for disaster victims) – Department of Health and Ageing (DoHA)
- *National Plan to Combat Pollution of the Sea by Oil* – Australian Maritime Safety Authority (AMSA).
- *National Search and Rescue* (SAR) arrangements – Australian Maritime Safety Authority (AMSA).
- *Management of Communicable Diseases in Australia* – Department of Health and Ageing (DoHA).
- *Australian Veterinary Emergency Plan (AUSVETPLAN)* – Agriculture, Fisheries and Forestry – Australia (AFFA).

The Australian Defence Force (ADF) is able to provide immediate local support in the event of a catastrophic emergency in communities where it has a facility. However, usually ADF support must be requested through state or territory government communication with EMA. Frequently, people assume that the Australian government has extensive resources, especially within the defence forces, to respond to disaster. This is however not true and it is more likely that support will be drawn from other states and territories. Defence assets in particular are often already deployed in other parts of the world or not readily available.

Coordination, command and control

Australian health organisations are not used to the paramilitary language that emergency services use every day. However, in a disaster situation these terms and the concepts that underpin them are applied to the health response and used to ensure that each agency and health care professional understands their role and where they fit within the management of the health response. This is particularly important because in these situations many health agencies will be working together, some for the first time, and good coordination of effort is important.

Command and control – Prior to any emergency, the responsibility for overall control of the situation and for the command of each organisational element involved will need to be clearly specified in either policy or in the emergency operational plan. Decisions on these issues should not be left until an emergency has occurred and are stipulated in state or territory disaster plans and in the various organisational disaster plans. Community nurses need to be asked, does your community nursing organisation have a disaster plan? Do you know where it is? Do you have a broad understanding of the command and control arrangements for staff within your agency? Who will you report to?

Coordination of support – The authority and responsibility for assembling resources to support any emergency is specified in the disaster plan. Most major issues that arise during an emergency centre on resource management issues relate more to coordinating what is available than to a lack of resources.

Coordination is the bringing together of agencies and resources to ensure an effective response. Coordination operates vertically within agencies as a function of the authority to command and horizontally across agencies as a function of the authority to control.

Command is the direction of members and resources of an agency in the performance of that agency's role and tasks. Command relates to agencies and operates vertically within an agency. Authority to command is established in legislation or by agreement within an agency. Community nurses need to be asked, who is responsible for managing the response of your organisation and who do you take direction from?

Control is the overall direction of activities in an emergency or disaster situation. Control relates to situations and operates horizontally across agencies. Authority for control is established in legislation or in the disaster or emergency plan, and carries with it the responsibility for tasking other agencies in accordance with the needs of the situation. Generally during disaster, the police have responsibility to control the activity of the various agencies that are involved.

Information management – Effective management of information is essential to successfully managing any type of disaster event. Communication networks are needed within the organisation as well as between agencies. At times, the communication methods that we employ in our daily work will break down or be overwhelmed during an emergency. Each organisation will need to establish a contingency plan in case normal communication is disrupted. For example mobile phone networks are often overloaded during disaster situations, as community members try to contact family and friends, and it may be necessary to consider other modes of communication or to adopt a plan whereby staff respond at an agreed meeting point to receive their instructions.

Disaster plan – All organisations require an effective emergency or disaster plan. This is because the nursing organisation will need to take additional steps to maintain the continuity of its normal business, and frequently the emergency will place additional demands on the organisation. This is certainly true in the health sphere and it is likely that community nurses will play a significant role in each stage of the health response to disaster, as well as be required to sustain care services for current clients of the service. A simple, properly disseminated, regularly tested and revised plan for managing during a major emergency is essential.

Risk assessment and risk treatment

At all stages, from planning through to response and recovery, management of risk is important. For this reason much of the work in preparing to confront disaster involves the principles of risk assessment and risk treatment.

There are two different approaches to dealing with risk: *the regulatory approach*, which is simply to comply with any appropriate regulations, creating them if necessary, and the *safety case approach*, which is to use the regulations to create a 'duty of care' to do all that is reasonable to secure safety [16].

The regulatory approach has the advantage of being relatively straightforward and simple in its demands – create rules and stick to them. It is clear, unequivocal and allows widespread awareness of what should or should not be done. In addition, it may be relatively cheap, although not necessarily so – measures to comply with new codes can be very expensive. On the other hand, the tendency of a regulatory approach is to manage risk, rather than to provide security against complaint. It is often minimalist and inflexible.

The 'safety case' approach involves a practical assessment of the likelihood that certain events will occur, their seriousness, possible consequences, and how resources should be deployed to respond to them. It aims to balance risks and resources and enables a management plan to be devised, which can then be reviewed by an independent party. Overall, there is a greater focus on safety through the creation of risk mitigation strategies and the promotion of collective decision making and responsibility, in preference to hierarchical declarations. A customised approach like this however might have cost implications over and above those involved in mandatory statutory code compliance. This approach also has the capacity for disputes over judgements [16] as to 'what matters' and 'what should be done about it'; disputes which the existence of rules may pre-empt. A 'safety case' approach to dealing with risk constantly challenges an organisation to act according to its analysis and to continually challenge itself to improve its practices, rather than sit comfortably behind rules.

Considering risks

There is a need to recognise that the public's perception of risk tolerance differs considerably with the circumstances. For example we are more tolerant of risk that we voluntarily accept than of risk which is imposed on us or which we passively (perhaps unknowingly) accept. Similarly, we are more tolerant of the risks of natural disaster than of human-made catastrophe, and we are more tolerant of risk that produces small occasional adverse effects than risk which has the potential to produce effects that cannot easily be accommodated, if at all [17].

A number of broad considerations have to be taken into account when assessing risk, including whether a risk can or should be 'covered'. Also, awareness needs to be developed of apparently innocuous circumstances that have the potential to become volatile and dangerous situations.

Risk is relative

The range of factors that can contribute to risk is enormous, but in assessing risk for practical purposes, what matters is the potential seriousness of the consequences of an emergency or disaster event, and the cost and feasibility of providing cover. Some events are virtually impossible to cover because the identified risk cannot be assessed at any particular location. An analysis of risk associated with disaster may be undertaken using 'frameworks'. Such frameworks consider the key features of the location and situation that might influence the outcomes. Key features to be considered fall within three areas – the biomedical, environmental and the psychosocial [18]. Biomedical factors are related to the physical and mental health profile of community members; environmental factors include weather, structures, geography, transportation and so on; psychosocial factors include community spirit, motivation and other social parameters.

A structured and logical approach to the identification and management of risks assists communities to minimise the likelihood or impact of disasters. The Australian and New Zealand standard on risk management is typically used to:

- Identify risk.
- Analyse and evaluate risk.
- Treat risk.
- Monitor risk.

This standard is available from the Australian government and provides a generic guide for the establishment and implementation of the risk management process involving the identification, analysis, evaluation, treatment and ongoing monitoring of risks.

Hazards are sources of risk. Consider the community as an element at risk and risk as the interactions between the community and its environment. What are the principal hazards, and subsequently the principal risks, to the well-being of a community? Do these risks arise from proximity to heavy industry, to transport routes through the community, to the demographic profile of the community (e.g. older communities and the risk of infectious disease) or to exposure to natural hazards such as cyclone or earthquake?

There are several options for dealing with risk. These are:

- Avoid the risk.
- Reduce the likelihood of the occurrence of the risk.
- Reduce the consequences of the risk.
- Transfer the risk.
- Accept/retain the risk [6].

Consider the nursing community environment. What hazards or risks can be identified? Which of the options listed above could be chosen in dealing with the risks from a community health perspective? Choices may depend on the potential severity of impact. A risk that is more likely to occur but has fairly limited impact on the health of the community will not be of great concern. However, a risk that is less likely to impact but has the potential to cause major disruption to health and to the community requires attention.

When preparing for disaster and in building the resilience of communities we require a commonsense approach to identifying and evaluating the hazards and risks in each community. To do this realistically, risks to the community need to be identified. For example, is the nursing community environment in an area exposed to tropical cyclones or where there is a seasonal bush fire threat? These threats should be evaluated against three criteria:

- What is the likelihood that the hazard will impact on the community?
- How severe will the impact be?
- What will the impact be like?

The third criterion is important because different hazards raise different scenarios and require different responses from health services and community nursing organisations. For example a serious transport accident may require a response from community health agencies that is limited to care for any community members who may be involved – often this will be during the rehabilitation or recovery phase of their care. On the other hand, a natural disaster such as cyclone or wildfire raises different issues as community members may need to be evacuated or rehoused for a period of time and the impact on their lives and lifestyle can be extensive and of long duration.

Practical concerns

When preparing for, and working through, an emergency or disaster situation community nurses should consider a number of practical issues. It is important to think about those who may be more vulnerable and less able to provide for their own health needs during the emergency. Frequently, as mentioned above, emergencies can have unexpected consequences, including loss of essential services such as electrical power and water, loss of transportation, limited access to medical services and hospitals, and difficulty in procuring food and supplies. Community members may experience difficulty achieving many basic requirements such as preparing food, obtaining medications, maintaining a safe environment, keeping warm and having shelter. While the so-called *federation effect* means that most relatively able-bodied community members will actively work to assist their neighbours, during these difficult times vulnerable community members will require specialist support [19]. The current clients of community nurses may well be members of vulnerable groups in the community including:

- Children.
- People with a disability.
- The elderly.
- Confused people.
- People with sensory impairment.
- People who are technology dependent – e.g. dialysis.
- People with specific health needs – e.g. diabetes.

In addition, a primary concern for health agencies and community nursing organisations during disaster is the need to sustain their services, often at a higher tempo as new clients present for care and current clients still require services. Sustainability depends on the work undertaken to prepare and plan for the impact of disaster. Key elements in preparation include:

- *Building community resilience* – All health agencies have a role to play in building the capability of individuals and the resilience of communities because this will assist in relieving the pressure on agencies themselves during the impact of disaster and result in better outcomes for those affected. Community capacity-building activities include community education, stockpiling of resources and assisting individuals to have a personal plan. For example the client who is dependent on technology should be advised about strategies and resources to maintain their care, and the elderly or infirm should have established links with neighbours or others who can check on their safety and assist them in the event of an emergency.

- *Managing recovery* – Recovery from disaster is a complex process and occurs over many years. For this reason, at least after the short period of immediate response by external agencies to the event, health services that are embedded in the community have a significant role to play in the ongoing care and development of affected communities. Recovery will include re-establishing your own organisation and resuming work and also supporting the recovery of staff and helping them to return to work. This will require great flexibility and understanding of the true impact of disaster on the community in which staff live, on their families and the day-to-day resources that support people in the workforce. Recovery from disaster will take many years. Recovery processes must involve collaboration with the community, be undertaken in consultation with local level management, consider the differing effects of the disaster on segments of the community and encourage empowerment, resourcefulness, accountability, flexibility and the integration and coordination of services [20]. Key considerations in community recovery include the physical, psychological and economic effects of disaster on the lives of community members.
- *Staffing* – Maintaining an adequate level of staffing will be a challenge for agencies impacted by disaster. In the first instance, some staff members may be directly affected by the emergency and be unable to attend for work. Those who are able to work will need additional support to ensure that their families remain safe and can be contacted while they are at work. Staff members will frequently be required to undertake duties outside of their usual scope of practice, such as unpacking supplies, creating and maintaining records or re-establishing damaged clinical areas. Often organisations working in disaster employ extended shift times (commonly 12 h) to allow for shift changeover and adequate rest between shifts. Some staff will need to be encouraged to take breaks and to finish their shift at the designated time. This is important because the work may continue for many days and staff will become fatigued and less effective. Occasionally, staff will be unable to return home and will need to be housed within the workplace.
- *Supplemental resources* – Additional staff and materials will probably be required and these may be brought in from other jurisdictions. As a result, briefing of new staff and orientation to the agency and the work become important activities. In addition, new approaches may be required and this is particularly true when outreach or community nursing services, such as district nursing, have difficulty in accessing clients in areas where roads are damaged or blocked.
- *Equipment* – There may be a need to consider triaging equipment to those clients with greatest need. A disaster is defined as a situation in which resources are overwhelmed and clients may not receive the complete care that is usually provided.
- *Vendors* – If other service providers are relied on for supplies or support, consideration needs to be given to whether they will be able to provide support during a disaster. Even those services that are included in a disaster plan, such as fire or ambulance authorities, may not be available in a disaster situation and community nurses should always consider ways in which they can become more independent.
- *Stockpiles* – Frequently, organisations operate a 'just-in-time' system for restocking of consumables. This system ensures that stock is used and the amount of out-of-date or expired stock is reduced. However, health agencies need to ensure that some stock lines are stockpiled in case of emergency. This is especially important if an identified 'risk' in your location is the likelihood that supply routes may be blocked as a result of disaster. For example wound care supplies with long expiry dates could

be stockpiled as well as medication supplies such as syringes, swabs and non-latex gloves.

- *Lifelines* – Consider lifelines that could be established to support and ensure the safety of staff and clients. Work to establish lifelines can be completed well before any disaster impact – indeed, often lifelines can be used in day-to-day work to ensure that those who may need support remain safe and in contact.
- *Essential services* – Water, fuel and electricity supply are among the essential services that need to be available for health services. Back-up storage of water and fuel and generators for electricity are important, especially for nurses working in rural and remote areas.
- *Communications* – Remember that communication networks are fragile and easily disrupted during emergencies. Often this is the result of overload of the system. In disaster it is best to have alternative forms of communication, such as radio or pager systems, and to remember that mobile telephone networks are likely to be the first to become unavailable. In disaster, the effectiveness of the service will depend on good coordination and communications.
- *Public relations* – In the aftermath of disaster, a common criticism is that members of the public feel that they have been poorly informed or treated badly. All organisations should consider strategies to keep their clients and other stakeholders informed, especially during the confusing and stressful aftermath of a disaster.

Issues in disaster health

Volunteers are the mainstay of Australian organisations that prepare for and respond to disaster [21]. The emergency services and non-government organisations, such as Australian Red Cross and St John Ambulance Australia, play an essential role. In addition, it should be remembered that community members will take positive steps to help each other ('the federation effect'). Building and sustaining volunteerism is an important issue in Australia, given our reliance on volunteers for disaster and emergency response, and we should all provide the support we can to assist such organisations with recruitment and training of volunteers.

Professionals with specialised skills and disaster experience are often deployed to disaster sites. However, health professional volunteers without disaster experience can do more harm than good. Responding with trained teams to a disaster site, and in overseas disasters hiring qualified disaster survivors, is much more cost-efficient practice and provides much-needed employment [22]. Self-responders should be discouraged and be asked to contact their own health service to offer assistance. Also, while specialised assistance is always welcome, local aid groups, police, firefighters and neighbours accomplish most relief and recovery efforts before external teams arrive.

Among the myths associated with disasters is the idea that disasters bring out the worst in human behaviour, and the affected population is too shocked and helpless to take responsibility for their own survival. Often isolated cases of looting or other criminal behaviour take centre stage in media reporting about the event. In fact, while people are shocked and wonder why they have survived and others have died, their resilience is often extraordinary and the stories of goodwill and support that arise from disasters demonstrate the best of the human spirit.

Another myth about disasters is that donations arrive quickly and that donations of food, clothing and household goods should be sent to disaster-affected communities. However, not all donations are helpful and at times large amounts of donated goods may worsen, or at least complicate, the disaster response effort. Donations of items such as blankets, shoes or clothing may complicate relief efforts because of the cost of shipping the items, the time required to sort, pack and ship them, and the enormous task of re-sorting and distribution when they arrive. Often those items donated by developed countries are in fact manufactured for export by these same affected countries. It is more efficient to purchase goods locally and donations of cash are a far better option [22]. Resources such as food, shelter and clothing can usually be purchased effectively within the affected region or country.

Dead bodies are not a major cause of disease and diseases that are not present normally in the affected area will not suddenly occur because of the presence of dead bodies. Even if the dead are carriers of disease, they are probably less risk to others dead than alive. Frequently, the risk of disease is the first myth to emerge in media reporting of disasters and unfortunately this has resulted in the rapid and unceremonious disposal of corpses, often without proper efforts to identify them or inform their loved ones. This of course adds to the suffering of survivors and uses resources that could be used to help the survivors.

In Australia, heatwaves have proved to be the most lethal natural hazard, having caused by far the greatest loss of life. They are also the most underrated of the natural disasters, as the bush fires that accompany – or follow – many heatwaves tend to get most of the attention. Unlike bush fires, there is generally no escaping a heatwave. While the 1939 'Black Friday' bush fires in Victoria killed 71 people and are written into our history, the accompanying heatwave – which triggered the blazes – claimed 438 lives and yet remains largely unacknowledged [2]. In this situation, preparation, and especially identification of those who are more vulnerable, and responding to provide support are important roles for community health practitioners.

Future trends

This chapter has presented general principles that are applied to manage the health aspects of disaster, regardless of the specific cause. There is however a tendency for the focus of disaster planning to follow trends determined by the most recent impact within the region or by priorities set within the political or scientific spheres. This effect can be seen if one considers the changing discussion about threats to health and disaster risk in recent years. A progression can be traced from a focus on natural disaster, especially bush fire and cyclone impacts, through to concern about the outbreak of SARS (severe acute respiratory syndrome), to the threat of terrorist attack or concern about the possibility of influenza pandemic, to planning for a tsunami and most recently concern about catastrophic emergencies at major public gatherings (mass gatherings) [23]. While these hazards do require some specific response strategies, the general principles presented in this chapter will underpin any disaster plan, including future plans as the interest of governments and media move on to new emerging threats. Perhaps global warming will provide the next driver for planning efforts.

Summary

This chapter has reviewed the principles of disaster management and the health aspects of disaster. These concepts provide the basis for thinking about the community nurse's role, the role of community nursing organisations and about training and planning for disasters that may impact on the community. This material is introductory and several links to useful resources are included below. Those interested in more detailed material should consult the web pages of the World Association for Disaster and Emergency Medicine (WADEM) and the WADEM Nursing Professional Section [24].

Useful resources

Australian Government, culture and recreation portal: Disasters and educational material at http://www.cultureandrecreation.gov.au/articles/naturaldisasters/

Department of Health and Ageing, Australian Government. Homepage of the health protection branch at http://www.health.gov.au/internet/wcms/publishing.nsf/Content/phd-health-emergency.htm

Emergency Management Australia, Lead agency in managing Australian response and preparation for disaster at http://www.ema.gov.au

Bureau of Meteorology: Warnings and weather-related advice on preparing for extreme weather at http://www.bom.gov.au/

Department of Health and Ageing, Australian Government. Pandemic preparedness pages at http://www.health.gov.au/internet/wcms/publishing.nsf/Content/phd-pandemic-resources.htm

International Center for Research into the Epidemiology of Disasters at http://www.cred.be/

World Association for Disaster and Emergency Medicine – a research and academic organisation at http://wadem.medicine.wisc.edu/

World Health Organization at http://www.who.int/topics/disasters/en/

Pan-American Health Organization at http://www.paho.org/

Wikipedia at http://en.wikipedia.org/wiki/List_of_wars_and_disasters_by_death_toll

Links to disaster legislation

Australian Capital Territory

Emergency Management Act 1999 at http://bar.austlii.edu.au/au/legis/act/consol_act/ema1999190/

New South Wales

State Emergency and Rescue Management Act 1989 at http://bar.austlii.edu.au/au/legis/nsw/consol_act/searma1989331/

Northern territory

Disasters Act at http://bar.austlii.edu.au/au/legis/nt/consol_act/da126/

South Australia

State Disaster Act 1980 at http://bar.austlii.edu.au/au/legis/sa/consol_act/sda1980168/

Tasmania

Emergency Services Act 1976 at http://bar.austlii.edu.au/au/legis/tas/consol_act/esa1976199/

Queensland

State Counter-Disaster Organisation Act 1975 at http://bar.austlii.edu.au/au/legis/qld/consol_act/scoa1975387/

Victoria

Emergency Management Act 1986 at http://bar.austlii.edu.au/au/legis/vic/consol_act/ema1986190/

Western Australia
Emergency Management Act 2005 at http://www.slp.wa.gov.au/statutes/swans.nsf/PDFbyName/
409754845EC8BE9C4825708B0028DE1F?openDocument

References

1. Debacker, M., Domres, B. and de Boer, J. (July–September 1999) Glossary of new concepts in disaster medicine: A supplement to Gunn's multilingual dictionary of disaster medicine. *Prehospital and Disaster Medicine*, 14(3), 146–9.
2. Emergency Management Australia (2007) *Definition of Disaster*. Available at http://www.ema.gov.au (viewed 20 February 2007).
3. The World Association for Disaster and Emergency Medicine (2002) The Nordic Society for Disaster Medicine. Conceptual framework of disasters. *Prehospital and Disaster Medicine*, 17(Suppl 3), 1–177.
4. Centre for Research on the Epidemiology of Disasters (2007) *EM-DAT: The International Disaster Database*. Available at http://www.cred.be/emdat (viewed 20 February 2007).
5. Fitzgerald, G. (April 2007) *Principles of Disaster*. Presentation to the Health Aspects of Disaster Colloquium. Flinders University, Adelaide, Australia.
6. Emergency Management Australia (2007) *Emergency Manual Series*. Available at http://www.ema.gov.au/ (viewed 20 February 2007).
7. Emergency Management Australia (2007) *Lessons from London and Considerations for Australia: London Terrorist Attacks*, 7 July 2005. Attorney General's Department, Australian Government, Canberra.
8. Downey, L., Andress, W.K. and Schultz, C.H. (2007) Benchmarking hospitals for hurricane evacuation. *Prehospital and Disaster Medicine*, 22(3), 259.
9. Arbon, P., Bobrowski, C., Zeitz, K., Hooper, W., Willliams, J. and Thitchener, J. (2006) Australian nurses volunteering for the Sumatra-Andaman earthquake and tsunami of 2004: A review of experience and analysis of data collected by the Tsunami Volunteer Hotline. *Australian Emergency Nursing Journal*, 9(4), 171–8.
10. Silverman, M.A., Weston, M., Llorente, M., Beber, C. and Tam, R. (1995) Lessons learned from hurricane Andrew: Recommendations for care of the elderly in long term care facilities. *South Medical Journal*, 88(6), 603–8.
11. Abrahams, J. (2001) Disaster management in Australia: The national emergency management system. *Emergency Medicine*, 13(2), 165–73.
12. Guha-Sapir, D. (2005) What have we learned? Capacity building for health responses in disasters. *Prehospital and Disaster Medicine*, 20(6), 480–82.
13. Gebbie, K., Valas, J., Merrill, J. and Morse, S. (2006) Role of exercises and drills in the evaluation of public health in emergency response. *Prehospital and Disaster Medicine*, 21(3), 173–82.
14. Campbell, S. (2005) Responding to international disasters. *Nursing Standard*, 19(21), 33–6.
15. The Centre for Health Policy (2007) *Emergency Preparedness Competencies for Public Health Professionals*. Columbia University School of Nursing. Available at http://www.nursing.columbia.edu/research/ResCenters/chphsr/erMain.html (viewed 12 April 2007).
16. Arnold, J.L. (2005) Risk and risk assessment in health emergency management. *Prehospital & Disaster Medicine*, 20(3), 143–54.
17. Chow, F.K.F. (2007) How risk assessment works with success. *Disaster Recovery Journal*, 20(1), 40–42.
18. Arbon, P. (2004) The development of conceptual models for mass gathering health. *Prehospital and Disaster Medicine*, 19(3), 208–12.

19. de Ville de Goyet, C. (1999) Stop propagating disaster myths. Editorial. *Prehospital and Disaster Medicine*, 14(4), 6.

20. Emergency Management Australia (2007) *Emergency Risk Management Applications Guide. Emergency Manual Series*. Available at http://www.ema.gov.au/ (viewed 20 February 2007).

21. Arbon, P. (1997) Volunteers in emergency services: The way forward. *The Australian Journal of Emergency Management*, 11(4), 11–13.

22. World Vision (2007) *Top 10 Myths of Disaster Relief*. Available at http://domino-01.worldvision.org/worldvision/comms2.nsf/stable/erdm_top_ten_myths_istore (viewed 11 April 2007).

23. Arbon, P. (2007) Mass gathering medicine: A review of the evidence and future directions for research. *Prehospital and Disaster Medicine*, 22(2), 131–5.

24. World Association for Disaster and Emergency Medicine – a research and academic organisation (2007) Available at http://wadem.medicine.wisc.edu/ (viewed 12 April 2007).

Chapter 8

Care of people with chronic conditions

Debbie Kralik

Introduction

Given that 77% of Australians have a chronic condition [1], it is not surprising that community nurses are concerned with knowing how they can meet the needs of this population group and what constitutes sensitive, effective and timely community nursing intervention. Community nurses who rely on the transference of acute care nursing knowledge and skills into the community care of people with chronic conditions will fail these clients. The skills and knowledge valued in the acute care system need to be extended and expanded to meet the needs of people living in the community with chronic conditions. Making a difference to this client group is not only about improved treatment options, but also about community nurses and other health professionals developing participatory and person-centred approaches to care so that the particular needs of individuals are central.

People often experience the impact of chronic conditions as life changing [2]. Adapting to life with a chronic condition involves a person learning to live with unwanted change. Chronic conditions bring many changes into a person's life, such as alterations in their capacity to earn an income, changes to relationships, changes to parenting and changes to life priorities. Working with people who are learning to adapt to such significant change and to live with chronic conditions is often a primary role for the community nurse. If nurses can understand the processes that help people to incorporate the consequences of chronic conditions into their lives, they will make a substantial contribution to enhancing clients' capacity to recognise their needs, make informed choices and effectively self-care.

The focus for this chapter is to explore ways that community nurses can work with people with chronic conditions to:

- Be at the centre of their health care with services designed around their unique health needs.
- Develop their capacity to participate fully in their own health care.
- Improve their quality of life (QoL).
- Promote self-care in order to prevent crisis situations.

The information in this chapter is not related to people with a specific medical diagnosis, but rather discusses the principles that can guide community nursing practice when working with people with chronic conditions. Much of the information will be relevant for community nurses working with people with chronic conditions across the lifespan and in urban, rural or remote areas because a person-centred approach is advocated. Care is centred on the needs of the individual. Strategies for working with clients to set self-care goals are discussed and a person-centred model to guide community nurses in their work with people in the community is presented.

Background

A chronic condition has been defined as:

> ... an illness that is permanent or lasts a long time. It may get slowly worse over time. It may lead to death, or it may finally go away. It may cause permanent changes to the body. It will certainly affect the person's quality of life [3].

The prevalence of chronic health conditions is increasing [1]; hence, prevention and management are at the forefront of government health agendas in Australia and in countries across the world. According to a report released by the Australian Institute of Health and Welfare [1]:

- Chronic diseases are common in Australia; in 2004–2005, 77% of Australians had at least one chronic condition. Most common were asthma (10.0%), osteoarthritis (7.9%), depression (5.3%) and diabetes (3.5%).
- Chronic conditions are an issue across the lifespan: in 2004–2005, almost 10% of children aged between 0 and 14 years had three or more long-term conditions; this figure increased to more than 80% for people aged 65 years and over.
- Many Australians have risk factors for developing chronic conditions. For example 54% of adults are either overweight or obese.
- There is an increased prevalence of chronic conditions in some population groups. For example compared with other Australians, Aboriginal and Torres Strait Islander persons have higher mortality from diabetes (14 times higher), chronic kidney disease (8 times higher) and heart disease (5 times higher).
- Factors associated with care and treatment of people with chronic conditions accounted for nearly 70% of the total health expenditure in 2000–2001.

The number of people with chronic conditions is growing at an alarming rate and impacting significantly on health systems and the way health services are delivered [1]. The reasons for this increasing prevalence are many, including new and advancing health treatments and technologies, improved longevity, sedentary lifestyles and an ageing Australian population [1]. Australians carry many risk factors for developing chronic conditions; for example:

- More than 85% of adults are not consuming enough vegetables on a daily basis.
- Fifty per cent of adults are not having adequate physical activity.
- Fifty per cent of adults are not consuming enough fruit.
- Twenty-one per cent of adults smoke tobacco.
- Regional areas of Australia experience higher prevalence of many of the risk factors for chronic disease, such as smoking (11% higher) and excess weight (7% higher)

when compared with city populations. Regional populations also have higher death rates for coronary heart disease, chronic obstructive pulmonary disease and diabetes.

- The least advantaged areas of Australia have higher levels of smoking, physical inactivity and obesity when compared with areas of high socioeconomic status. Least advantaged populations have higher prevalence of diabetes, behavioural problems, asthma, heart disease and arthritis and have higher mortality across most chronic conditions.
- Aboriginal and Torres Strait Islander persons have a higher prevalence of smoking, risky alcohol use and excess weight when compared with other Australians. These risk factors are associated with higher rates of asthma, arthritis and diabetes [1].

These risk factors mean that the prevalence of chronic conditions will continue to increase. However, chronic conditions may arise either as an accumulation of risk or from exposure to risk factors at critical periods in life [4]. There are often multicausal determinants of health and illness; yet individual risk factors like those listed above are often the focus, while the broader environmental, political and socioeconomic factors are neglected [5].

Another layer of complexity is that many Australians are living with several chronic conditions, including complex comorbid conditions where the individual has mental illness and chronic physical illness [1, 6]. Strategies to improve care for this population group are very slowly beginning to shift from traditional disease-specific, biomedical models towards coordinated and integrated health care framed by cultural and social sensitivity. The organisational structures inherent in the Australian health system, however, are often a significant obstruction to integrated care because of the emphasis on acute care and the fragmentation of health care due to medical and allied health specialisation [7, 8]. This results in many people with comorbid chronic conditions not receiving appropriate care due to a mismatch between their needs and the capacity of the health care system to be responsive to them [9, 10]. Prolonged waiting times in emergency departments or to be seen by a general practitioner are some indications of these issues.

Thus the way that health care is currently organised presents a significant challenge to people with chronic conditions [11]. People are often required to coordinate their own care, locate services and resources and repeat their health histories many times over when they communicate and interact with different services and health care providers. These can include general practitioners, specialists, hospital and community pharmacists, community health workers, mental health workers, allied health and community care services. Tests and procedures may be duplicated because of inadequate communication processes and lack of care coordination. This is a situation that can lead to adverse events, for example when the same medication is prescribed for a person by multiple doctors working in the acute and community health sectors, resulting in the individual taking multiple doses.

Wagner *et al.* [12] argue that successful chronic condition care needs to simplify the process of getting needs met rather than create more obstacles in the person's life. This view is echoed by Dwyer [13] who after examining the outcomes of reviews of the Australian health system over the last 10 years suggested that any government reform will not succeed unless it can make a difference for people living with chronic conditions. We are slowly coming to realise, as the World Health Organization has, that 'as long as the acute care model dominates health care systems, health care expenditures will continue to escalate, but improvements in populations' health status will not' [14].

The acute care orientation of health services is reflected in the current emphasis on disease diagnosis, patient-initiated consultations and curative and/or symptom-relieving treatments. A lack of coordination of services means that people who rely on multiple health services for ongoing care and their QoL must themselves coordinate their own care, organising and linking the services they require in the primary, community health and acute care settings [15]. For some people with chronic conditions this must be an overwhelming burden.

Care of people with chronic conditions has become a major focus for Australian community nurses [16]. One community nursing organisation in South Australia (Royal District Nursing Service, RDNS) reports that 73% of clients live with two or more chronic conditions, and of those, 49% are provided with community nursing services for longer than 6 months [16]. Working with people with chronic conditions is a large part of what community nurses do. People with chronic conditions are increasingly receiving care in the community, yet often will have minimal contact with health professionals, amounting to only a few hours each year [17]. Community nurses will often be the consistent contact that a person with chronic conditions has with a health professional; hence, they are well situated to work with people adapting to life with a chronic condition.

Community nurses working *with* people with chronic conditions

Community nurses are known and trusted as experts in providing holistic care to individuals, their families and significant others [16]. The community health sector relies on them. This credibility enables the community nurse to draw on a vast range of resources and services to meet clients' needs. They are navigators of a complex service environment, bringing a mix of multidisciplinary service providers into the person's life [16]. Community nurses are often prime movers in the client's life, getting things done and making things happen in a way that the client, family members and significant others cannot.

Community nurses are required to perform a multitude of tasks and roles relating to advocacy, information and education, self-management, health promotion, community liaison, clinical tasks, navigating and linking with community resources, empowering people, placing the person at the centre of care, case management and holistic assessment and monitoring. A holistic approach is profoundly important when working with people with chronic conditions. The experiences of health and illness are a part of life. For example an Australian Aboriginal perspective on holistic health is that:

> ... health is utterly dependant on the health of all things – tangible and intangible, ponderable and imponderable. All life, matter and energy is one united entity of which we are an inseparable part; and ... to treat any single part is insufficient to bring about the totality of health [18, p. 6].

Given that working with people who have a long-term condition constitutes much of the work that community nurses do, it is important to ask, what is important about community nursing for people with chronic conditions? That question was asked of adult clients and community nurses in a research project conducted during 2006 [16]. The findings from this research confirmed that community nurses play a central and valued role in the care of people with chronic conditions in the community. The research involved a comprehensive literature review, followed by in-depth interviews with 20 adult clients of RDNS in South Australia who had two or more chronic illness diagnoses and had been receiving RDNS services for longer than 6 months. Simultaneously, in-depth interviews were conducted with community nurses of diverse levels and specialties. All interviews were audio-taped and transcribed verbatim. The research team then analysed the data to determine themes and subsequent meanings. The outcomes of this research process informed the development of the community-nurse-led model for person-centred care detailed later in this chapter [16]. Aspects of the community nursing role that were valued highly by all participants were that it:

- Shifted the burden of illness from the person
- Provided social contact and helped to develop personal esteem
- Created a supportive environment

Let us now explore these aspects of community nursing care further.

Shifting the burden of illness

People living with severe chronic illness often spend much of their time in their home and live a life that requires help from others. In the home setting, community nurses often assume responsibility for much of the care required and are involved in the direct care or coordination of care activities.

The RDNS research [16] showed that the monitoring role undertaken by the community nurse in regular contact with people shifted part of the burden of living with chronic conditions from them. This reduced burden meant that the person and their family members could invest time and energy into other aspects of life.

Typically, people living with chronic conditions describe the constant monitoring of their symptoms and organising of their health care as a significant part of the burden of living with a chronic illness [19]. Necessarily, there is a strong constant focus on the illness and attending to its symptoms or consequences. This requires a high level of diligence and vigilance, which uses a considerable amount of precious energy [20]. The chronic condition is foremost and people often find that life becomes consumed with their loss and suffering. This results in illness management taking over other more enjoyable aspects of life. Life can easily slip out of balance [19]. When this happens, the chronic condition is likely to be experienced as overwhelming and burdensome.

The RDNS research [16] indicated that the care provided by community nurses eased the burden of having a chronic condition and brought a sense of security to people living with a high level of uncertainty. The person expected that the community nurse had an understanding of their symptoms and their impact and felt confident in the community nurse's knowledge, skills and expertise in attending to the business of their health effectively. People trusted that community nurses would know how to respond during periods of change or exacerbation of their chronic condition. When community nurses genuinely listened to the client, it promoted understanding and trust [21] Clients developed a sense of security that the nurse could coordinate whatever situation arose. Consequently, illness could be moved into the background of their perceptions where it was less overwhelming and intrusive to their life.

This is not to say that the person is not involved in their care. To the contrary, in the RDNS research community nurses actively sought partnership with the person in decisions relating to care [16]. The nurse's level of clinical knowledge and skill was not the focus of clients' responses to what is important about community nursing; however, clients had confidence that the nurse had a high level of clinical skill and competence. This confidence released the person from the cumbersome and tiring task of having to constantly monitor their health in order to stay well and identify when they needed to see a doctor or other health care worker. Essentially, this made a difference to the way illness was experienced on a daily basis.

Providing social contact and personal esteem

In the RDNS research, the client's relationship with the community nurse provided desired social contact and a sense of personal esteem for people who in many cases would otherwise be living an isolated existence. For some clients the community nurse was the only regular social contact they had. The most significant aspect of the community nurse's visit for some clients was the way that the nurse interacted with them. Not only did this provide regular enjoyable interpersonal contact but enabled the client to feel better about themselves [16].

The relationship the person with chronic conditions developed with the community nurse was one aspect of community nursing care that was most valued by people. This connection was built around trust and shared understandings about adapting to life with chronic conditions. The community nurse was present to the person and helped them to reinterpret meaning in their life [21]. What developed was a mutual understanding of the illness experience that was valued by the person.

Social isolation was frequently experienced by people living with a chronic illness and some people considered it a form of suffering. This finding is supported by other research [22]. Nurses and clients shared stories about their lives while clinical tasks were being attended to. The joking and pleasant 'chit-chat' between nurse and client brought a sense of normalcy to the person's life. Opportunity for social interaction has been identified as a vital component of building the capacity of a person to better cope with illness [23].

Equally important was the way in which a person's relationship with the community nurse contributed to a positive sense of self [16]. The manner in which the nurse approached the person in care was valued when it was respectful, non-judgemental, friendly, jovial, sensitive, caring and generous. The community nurse provided the opportunity for the person to experience a respectful relationship in which their needs and wishes were prioritised. This contributed to the person feeling a greater sense of self-worth.

Much has been written about the way that chronic illness changes perceptions and experiences of the self [19, 20, 22, 24–27]. When discussing the changes to self brought about by chronic illness, Charmaz [22] suggests that traditional medical approaches neglect an important source of suffering: the loss of self. People with chronic conditions are often sensitive to the way other people react to them, and they become aware that the community stigmatises and stereotypes people who are 'different' [28, 29].

Interactions with the everyday environment are pivotal because they provide feedback to the person – messages about themselves which are interpreted as reflections of their own value as human beings [24, 26]. The interaction with the community nurse affirms the person. Fundamentally, the person's sense of self is boosted and potentially alters the illness experience. For example the RDNS research showed that social contact with the community nurse distracted people from pain; they felt more positive about life and more resilient to the ups and downs that chronic conditions often bring. The approach taken by the community nurse has an impact on the way people feel about themselves and, given that feelings about the self are pivotal to the way people with chronic conditions cope with life, this is a critical aspect of care.

Nurses tend to take the interpersonal aspects of their care for granted because it is a fundamental part of what they do [16]. For clients with chronic conditions, contact with a friendly and respectful nurse can make a profound difference to daily life.

Creating a supportive environment

A significant proportion of health symptoms that people living with chronic conditions experience are medically unexplained and appear to have no pathological basis [30]. Even though there have been many profoundly significant technological advances, medical science does not have all the answers to questions about the human body [11]. People are greater than the sum of their functional or dysfunctional parts, so often symptoms of chronic conditions defy medical diagnosis. These are the symptoms that are never included in 'prevalence studies' or recognised by 'national initiatives'. The context in which people live with these undiagnosed and often unacknowledged symptoms and their consequences is important to the person's QoL [31]. Community nurses work effectively by acknowledging the biomedical model that dominates our health system, but also by embracing a holistic understanding of what health and illness mean to the individual person. For example the community nurse can be effective in their care by acknowledging the client's cultural background, past experiences or social and economic capacity.

Chronic conditions take many forms and there is no single pattern of experience even within the same diagnosis [11]. Maintaining a degree of wellness or keeping symptoms in remission is a juggling act of balancing treatment regimes and maintaining QoL [19]. As a consequence, people with chronic conditions are confronted with the need to coordinate and manage a range of disease-related, intrapersonal and environmental demands in order to maintain some level of quality in their life [32]. People can find it difficult to meet those demands, particularly when feeling unwell. When issues are not dealt with because of lack of energy, lack of support or knowledge about how to proceed, the person's well-being and QoL may be compromised. Here again, community nurses mediate the complex nexus between the person in their home and community services through their health promotion role. By providing information and linking the person with the services and resources that will promote their functional status and enhance their QoL, community nurses create an environment which is supportive of the person, maximising their health and well-being. This is a major part of what nurses do to enable people to live a better QoL. Bonomi *et al.* [33] and Leveille *et al.* [34] identify linkage to community resources as an essential component of providing quality care for people living with chronic conditions in the community.

The community nurse can gain knowledge about the community resources available through engaging in conversation with clients about what services and resources they have used and what they have found helpful. This will enable the nurse to be aware of people's different perspectives of illness and to keep in touch with what people find helpful and what they do not find helpful. Nurses can use this knowledge about useful and responsive services and resources to assist other clients. It can be an important starting point for meaningful chronic condition care. Population profiling takes a more formal approach and can be a useful activity for novice community nurses to undertake (see Box 8.1).

It is reassuring for the client to know that the nurse has access to a range of services and resources that can be coordinated to meet their changing needs. Drawing on their vast knowledge of services and resources in the community, community nurses assist

---

Box 8.1   Exercise in population profiling

In the community nursing role, be open to conversations with people who are learning to adapt to life with a chronic condition. Learn about their experience of living with a chronic condition and assess the resources/services utilised.

Tell the person that you are interested to learn about how they manage the chronic condition, how it impacts on their life, the changes they have made and the ways they have learnt to self-care. Ask about the services and resources they have utilised/not utilised and what has been useful information. As a reciprocal gesture, tell them that you will search for information about this particular condition and the services and resources available. Report back to them what you have found. Some prompt questions could be:

- Tell me about what it is like living with the chronic condition?
- When did you first become aware that something was wrong?
- What changes have you needed to make to your life because of this condition?
- What are some of the things that you do that help you to manage this condition?
- How have others been helpful/not helpful when learning about this condition?
- What services and resources have you used?
- Have you used health services? If so, have you found these to be useful/not useful?
- How have you learnt about your condition?
- What has been useful information? Can you recall where you found that information?

Think about the conversation. Identify the main points the person was making. Seek out information about resources that may be useful for this person. Think broadly because useful services and resources may not necessarily be those that are most obvious. Develop a resource portfolio for this individual. That is, collect information about this chronic condition depending on the needs identified by the client. Collate this information into a resource package. You could find out how many people live with this chronic condition in Australia. Identify resources (human, services and electronic information, e.g. websites) that you think may be useful for the client. Provide the client with the portfolio and discuss it with them, leaving open the possibility of further conversations.

people to navigate the complex service network and to find the appropriate supports. Clients value this aspect of community nursing practice [16].

The struggle involved in living with chronic conditions can be relentless. Community nursing can lessen the harshness of the experience and improve QoL. The ways in which community nursing is important for people reflect all the hallmarks of a person-centred care approach. Community nurses provide care that is different to that provided by other health professionals and services. They work effectively with people learning to live with chronic conditions by including the personal realm so as to create a partnership, which is highly valued by both parties.

Promoting chronic condition self-care

Self-care and self-management are terms that have been used interchangeably in the literature and have been consistently advocated as a way that the impact of chronic disease on the health system can be contained [35]. In this chapter, self-care refers to how the person adapts to the changes that are taking place in their life because of illness and learns ways to deal with all that living with a chronic condition entails, including symptoms, treatment, physical and social consequences, and lifestyle changes and disruption. Self-care decisions are informed by the personal and social context of people's lives. Medical or health advice may not always be prioritised. A type of wisdom evolves from the long-term experience of living day to day with a chronic condition. The person faces this alone, since health professionals and others are not there in everyday life situations. The process of searching for options, trailing actions and activities and experiencing the consequences equips the person with a depth of knowledge about how they respond in certain situations. Making a decision to self-care does not guarantee that this will always be the way the person approaches living with their condition. Self-care capacities and strategies fluctuate as life and the condition present new challenges [29, 36, 37].

Models of care which are prevalent in the acute sector where clients play passive roles do not work well for people who are learning to incorporate the symptoms of chronic conditions into their lives. Effective chronic condition self-care requires a team of active participants, with the client being the most important member of that team. Most chronic condition care is not provided by nurses, doctors or other health care professionals, but by the person who has the condition.

The community nurse may be the expert in clinical matters, but the client is the expert in his or her own life. The community nurse's role is to provide clinical expertise and to collaborate with the client to find solutions and to offer support. Through research [16], we have come to know that:

- Clients are usually hungry for clinical information. It is important for people to understand how their daily decisions may have a major impact on their health and well-being.
- Clients who are learning to live with a chronic condition need support to make significant and lifelong behavioural changes. One way this may be achieved is by working with people to set small, achievable self-care goals.
- The client's goals related to his or her condition or situation should be a focus when the client and nurse meet. The client's self-care goal should be documented in the plan of care.

- Nurses can help clients set goals by exploring issues they are dealing with and helping them to identify the real issues confronting them.
- Nurses can enable clients through conversation to do some problem solving of their own.

Some key points in working with people with chronic conditions are:

- Models of care, where nurses and doctors tell people what to do and try to motivate them to change, are not effective.
- Because clients' day-to-day decisions have a tremendous impact on their health, they must be acknowledged as active, informed participants in the health care process.
- Community nurses may help clients self-care by working with them to set self-care goals.

For example think about two clients who have type 2 diabetes. Focus on one client whose condition is well managed and another whose condition is not well managed. What would you say are the differences between those two people? Why is one more successful at controlling the symptoms than the other? Very often, the key difference may be the client's level of involvement in his or her own care.

Traditional models of care

Our health care systems are not always designed with the client in mind and often do little to assist clients with chronic conditions to self-care. Instead, our health care is based on an acute care model, where the client presents to health professionals to be told what to do. Hospital admissions are isolated and very brief events in a person's health care.

The health care professional is very much the authority trying to get the client to do what is needed; the client's job is simply to be obedient. The motivation to change one's behaviour however – even to take one's medication – is largely internal. In the community setting the client is responsible and will self-care within their capacity when they are enabled to take an active role in their own care. The failure of the traditional models of care for people with chronic conditions led the author to ask, what kind of approach can we use to work with people who have chronic conditions? In other words, how can we change chronic condition care so that self-care is promoted and people can better adapt to life with a chronic condition?

The client is the solution

The community nurse who is promoting chronic condition self-care will need to re-member two key points: firstly, self-care requires a team with the client at the centre. Secondly, self-care requires active, involved participants – especially an active, involved client. This model of care can be described by using various terms – empowerment, informed choice, client-centred – but they all have the same underlying premise: the client is at the centre and is actively involved in his or her own health care.

Why promote chronic condition self-care in community nursing?

There are two answers to this question. Firstly, most chronic illness care does not involve nurses and other health care professionals [38]. Instead, a large proportion of chronic condition care is actually self-care, given by the person who has the illness. On a day-to-day basis, the client is in charge of his or her own health, and the daily decisions they make have a huge impact on client outcomes and QoL. The person experiences QoL as subjective well-being. QoL refers to the difference between the hopes and expectations of a person and their present experience. The capacity of people to adapt enables people who experience adversity to maintain a reasonable QoL.

Secondly, a community nurse may know what is best for managing a wound, diabetes, asthma or congestive heart failure, but that does not mean they necessarily know how clients can best manage that condition in their day-to-day lives. Even in close relationships, the nurse will not always know the details of a client's life, such as what is most important to them, what their other priorities are, what motivates them and what their financial situation is. Each client is the expert in his or her own life.

The community nursing role is one of providing clinical expertise and information, collaborating with the client to solve his or her problems and supporting the client throughout the adaptation process. In other words, it's saying, 'Here's what I know about diabetes. How can I help you put this into the context of your life so that you can make decisions that will help you?' Community nurses consider themselves responsible to their clients – to connect with them, to inform them, to advise them, to warn them.

When clients are encouraged to be more involved and when nurses are less prescriptive, clients perceive they have better outcomes [16]. We also know that this approach does not take any more time, but can be more effective because the nurse is addressing the client's agenda first [16] – and the client's agenda is, after all, the reason they need a community nursing service. When a partnership develops between nurse and client, the way is paved for the client to make significant, lasting change in their lives.

Empowerment through education

Just as person-centred care can be more effective, person-centred education is also more effective [16]. Education programmes where people are lectured to do not work any better than telling people to 'lose 20 kilos' or 'stop smoking'. Instead, the client's needs should drive the education. For example education can be based entirely on questions from the client. The community nurse may have a checklist of topics to cover, but those topics can be addressed in the context of client questions rather than through an impersonal lecture. Clients are often not as interested in their disease from a clinical perspective as nurses are. They want to know about themselves. What does this mean to me? How is this different for me? How is it going to affect my life?

Clients with chronic conditions may find the following four points to be a useful foundation for self-care:

1. They need to learn to live with the consequences of having a chronic condition. The community nurse needs to reiterate that they are involved in a learning process.

2. Their condition is essentially self-managed. Every decision clients make throughout the day, from what they eat to whether they walk or ride on the bus, has an influence on their health. The community nurse needs to communicate to clients that they are the most important individuals in managing their illnesses.
3. They have options. There is rarely one perfect way to treat a condition. In the case of diabetes, for example, clients can be treated through diet and exercise, oral medication, insulin and so on. Clients need to understand the different treatment options available and should be encouraged to look at the personal costs and benefits of each. Only the client can decide if the benefits are greater than the costs.
4. They can change their behaviour but it may take time to do so. The community nurse needs to assure clients that they will have their support. Rarely do clients leave the doctor's office and immediately enact whatever change was recommended. Life is full of changes and fluctuations. What works one day may not work the next. The community nurse can talk with clients about significant behavioural changes that can be made by setting goals, taking that first step and figuring out what they may learn about themselves along the way.

Helping clients set self-care goals

The focus of each contact with a client is the client's agenda or self-care goals related to their condition. Ideally, the goal is clearly displayed in the client's care plan, and each person who handles the plan plays a part in supporting the client in that goal, asking, 'How did it go? What have you done this week? How can we help you do better?'

The process of setting self-care goals with the client essentially involves three steps: look, think and act. These steps have been informed by a participatory action approach to working with people [39] and are further illustrated in Figure 8.1.

1. Look... Find the issue. Rather than beginning the client encounter focused on test results begin by saying, 'Tell me what concerns you most. Tell me what is hardest for you. Tell me what you're most distressed about and what you'd most like to change.'
2. Think... When you begin to get a sense of the client's concerns, explore those issues together. Ask, 'Is there an underlying problem? Do you really want this problem to be solved? What's the real issue?'
3. Act... Develop a collaborative goal. Once you have worked with the client to identify the issue, your instinct may be to try to solve it, but don't. Don't try to fix it. Instead, validate the client's feelings and his or her capacity to deal with the issue and continue asking questions that will lead the client to his or her own solution. Ask, 'What do you think would work? What have you tried in the past? What would you like to try?'

It is always more meaningful when clients find their answers, the 'ah ha!' on their own, so community nurses need to give them that chance. They need to encourage clients to come up with ideas first and then they can offer suggestions or additional information that they may need. The nurse can say, 'This works for some people' or 'Have you tried this?' or 'Here's why I don't think that's a good idea.' The important thing is that the client is given the opportunity to say 'no' and to make the final decision on what goal to try.

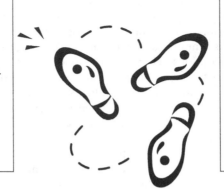

Step 1: Look

1. Talk with the client to determine the issue.
2. Ask them why they think they are experiencing the issue.
3. Find out what is important for them.
4. Identify strengths.

Step 2: Think

1. Talk with the person so as to understand the possible reasons for the issue.
2. Assist by offering informatiion or resources.
3. Work with the client to consider strategies that may address the issue.
4. Be creative and supportive so as to promote capacity.

Step 3: Act

1. Discuss the possibe strategies with the individual. Does he/she think they are helpful?
2. Find out what strategies the individual would like to try.
3. Develop a plan of action and review it on your next visit with the client. Consider documenting it.
4. Provide positive reinforcement and feedback (promoting capacity).
5. Review the action plan and modify strategies or develop new strategies as needed.

Figure 8.1 The steps in working with clients to set goals.

At the end of a goal-setting conversation, the client will be able to tell the nurse one goal he or she is going to try. It should be very specific. If the client says, 'I'm going to exercise more,' the nurse can ask what that means. Will they exercise four times a week? What activity will they be doing? How far will they walk? Help them to come up with a specific plan that they have created for themselves. It may not be the ultimate goal the nurse would have chosen for the client, but it may be one they are more likely to accomplish. At later contacts, the nurse can build on that initial self-care goal. The emphasis on self-care goals suggests that the contact with the community nurse has the client as the focus, it is the client's agenda that is being addressed and they are active participants in the outcome.

Empowering clients with information

One way to help clients focus and begin thinking about health care goals is to talk with them about their individual health measures (such as blood results, blood pressure, HbA1c) and what those numbers mean. People with chronic conditions often feel it is important for them to be informed about test results. One participant in the RDNS research [16] said, 'I find having the results and reports invaluable. I can compare my results with previous ones and know exactly whether or not I'm improving, I'm static or if my levels are dropping'. Offering explanations of what the numbers mean in the results (ideal and actual) can lead to conversations about strategies for improvement. When faced with results from tests, clients may see for themselves where they are struggling and what they can do to improve their results.

Ultimately, clients need to find their own solutions and motivation and must take responsibility for their own health. Community nurses can be an important factor in a lifelong learning process that can empower people to do just that. Community nurses can best facilitate people towards self-care by embracing new understandings of the experience of learning to live with chronic conditions. This process is enhanced when the expertise a person brings to the management of their condition is given the respect it deserves. Community nurses need to consider a practice focus that provides people with the means to grow and learn in a participative relationship.

Information needs along the chronic condition trajectory

It is important that the community nurse recognises that clients perceive their needs to be different at varying times along the trajectory of the chronic condition. It is not effective to load the client with information when first diagnosed with the condition. For example the information needs of the person when first diagnosed with a chronic, progressive condition may be different to the person's needs when nearing end of life. When the needs of the person are focused on rather than a prescriptive approach to care, the nurse is able to gauge what those shifting perspectives are. For example information needs may differ at the following phases:

1. Shortly after diagnosis the person may require 'frontline' support and information. The person may be feeling overwhelmed, confused and may want to learn as much as they can about the actual disease process.
2. In the medium term the person may get involved in reading, learning and absorbing information. Often the person begins to understand their needs and begins to build a picture of the future.
3. Finally in the longer term, the person may meet others with the same condition, may begin to locate self-help groups and may be able to negotiate resources and begin to make some longer term plans.

The community nurse needs to be flexible in order to meet the actual information needs of the person. For example there may be benefits to be gained when the community nurse links people with chronic conditions to support groups and organisations. Benefits can include meeting other affected people, expanding their horizons and appreciating the wide variety of (often positive) responses to what one might have seen initially as a death sentence.

A community-nurse-led model for person-centred care

This model was developed by merging the findings from research [16]. It draws heavily on systems theory [16] in understanding the interactions between the community nurse, the person with chronic conditions, their health network and the wider community in which the person lives. Systems theory emphasises the interconnectedness and interrelatedness of the parts of a system. Intervention in one part will have an impact on other parts. Systems theory takes a broad picture of a situation [40]. The work of the community nurse in providing care fits closely with systems thinking in that the person is seen as one part of a wider system of family, friends, the health service network and the community they live in. Nursing practice takes place in each of these parts as is deemed necessary in order to improve the person's QoL.

In the community-nurse-led model for person-centred care, the person living with chronic illness is at the centre of decision making, care and intervention. The nurse/person relationship is pivotal to the person receiving the health care and service provision that they need in order to live optimally in the community. The community nurse works in partnership with the person to determine what is important to them. The model shows interconnectedness and interrelatedness as being fundamental components of the community health system. In practice, person-centred care is demonstrated when community nurses are focused on what matters to a person. The person-centred care model is shown in Figure 8.2 and is now explained in more detail.

Structure of the person-centred care model

The person is central

The innermost circle represents the person living with chronic illness. The person is at the centre of all decision making and activity.

The community nurse circle

The community nurse occupies a unique and significant relationship with the client. This is represented by the position and strong colour of the circle. The community nurse works in partnership with the person with a chronic condition to determine what is important to them.

The circles

The circles represent the various types and qualities of care interventions that the community nurse provides to the person in a particular aspect of their life. Apart from the innermost two circles, the positioning of the circles has no significance; i.e. one circle does not indicate greater significance than another.

The three transparent supports

The three supports are a common thread running through all aspects of community nursing practice regarding the person. They are linchpins of community nursing practice and inform what happens and how it happens. They are:

- *Clinical knowledge and skills*
  Clinical knowledge and skills bring the nurse and client together. Nurses demonstrate a concern for evidence-based knowledge and skills that are being continually

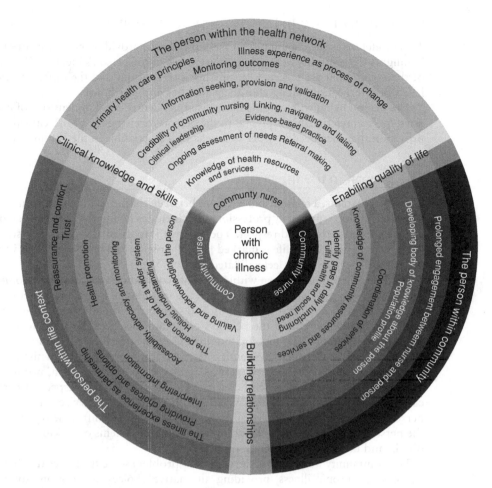

Figure 8.2 The community-nurse-led model for person-centred care.

developed. Clinical knowledge and skills provide the basis on which decisions regarding assessment and intervention rest. They also inform interactions with the client and referral to internal and external services.

- *Enabling QoL*
  This is the ultimate goal of the nurse/client partnership. It is also a key component of the nursing process. The nurse interprets and assesses a person's situation through a QoL lens and is constantly seeking to identify places where the person's QoL could be improved. All interactions are focused on enabling a better QoL.

- *Building relationships*
  Relationships are the medium through which all else happens, whether it be the relationship between the nurse and client, the nurse and family member or support person, the nurse and service provider, or the nurse and neighbour. Building relationships is considered to be pivotal to effectively working with people.

Community-nurse-led model of person-centred care

This model maps the community nursing process in providing person-centred care. It highlights the centrality of the community nurse in the person's life, the different parts of the system that are targeted for nursing interventions and the different kinds and levels of interventions along with their qualities and attributes.

The person living with chronic illness is at the centre of all dimensions of care. The nurse/person relationship is pivotal to the person receiving the health care and service provision that they need in order to live as well as possible in the community.

The person in the life context

To varying extents, a relationship develops between the nurse and the person over time. The relationship is primarily professional but includes familiarity with the person's life, the high level of trust and respect. The positive impact of this on the person's sense of self and experience of life is marked [16]. People feel acknowledged and valued for the person they are. They feel validated [16].

A holistic view of the person within their life context ensures that other components of the wider system that they are a part of are included in interventions. For example a relationship is developed with family and supportive friends to provide a basis for working together to ensure the person's needs are met. Regular visits to the person provide opportunities for ongoing monitoring of their health status and functioning. They also enable the nurse to identify when another service might assist the person to have a better QoL. The nurse acts as an advocate for the person, negotiating for the engagement of workers who can provide support with an aspect of care. They can also interpret information provided by other health care services or sought by the person in a language that is accessible and meaningful. This lifts a heavy burden from the person who may be unwell, coping with difficult systems or lacking the energy to obtain and understand information.

The community nurse assists the person to problem solve the issues that arise when living with chronic illness, providing alternative choices and options for working through them. In as much as the nurse understands chronic illness and assists the person to negotiate its consequences, there is a normalisation of the illness experience, which appears to be reassuring and comforting to the person [16]. The person trusts the community nurse and decisions are made together about how to manage their ups and downs. The illness experience is shared in partnership with the nurse.

The person within the health network

Community nursing reflects a primary health care (PHC) approach which emphasises the importance of a holistic understanding including the involvement of other services in meeting the person's needs. This approach incorporates people working together to achieve optimal outcomes for the client. Hence, emphasis is on the importance of a sound working knowledge of health resources and services.

A holistic lens enables a full assessment of the person's circumstances and identifies gaps or tensions which are obstructing an optimal QoL. There are resources available to the nurse to assist with their understanding of what is needed. Clinical leaders and specialist nurses can support the nurse to find options for the person. The person is involved in considering the options, and his or her priorities are factored into a joint decision about how to proceed. The community nurse draws on knowledge, skills and evidence-based practice in navigating the service network, making referrals and linking the person with the most appropriate service providers. The mix of service providers will change as the person's health and abilities change.

The smooth functioning of the health care network for the person is facilitated by the role that the nurse takes in liaising and communicating with the various services. The community nurse has a high level of credibility in the health care network and acts as a key reference point for the client, providing information as appropriate to services involved in their care. At all times the nurse ensures that the person has information about and understands each aspect of care.

The person within the community

The nurse is engaged with the client over a prolonged period of time. Knowledge about the person builds up to create a picture of where he or she sits in terms of the profile of the wider community. Factors such as culture, language, health status and gender make up this picture. These inform questions about how the person can be assisted to live a good QoL in their particular community. A sound knowledge of community resources and services informs the range of options that the nurse can provide to the person in ensuring that health and social needs are fulfilled.

The nurse is pivotal in identifying areas of need and coordinating access to community resources and services. There is a diversity of issues that may be dealt with in this way, ranging from, for example, organising for garbage to be collected to arranging transport to an appointment or organising a house-cleaning service from the city council. In this way the community nurse assists the person to use the resources offered by the community to enrich and improve their QoL.

Thus, the major features of the community-nurse-led model of person-centred care are:

- The person is involved in decisions about their care.
- The person is viewed as one part of a wider system.
- All parts of the system are targeted for nursing intervention.
- There is typically a close relationship between the nurse and person which is central to their working together.
- The nursing approach is humanistic and values the person.
- The nurse occupies a significant position in the person's life.
- The nurse is pivotal in connecting services with the person.
- The nurse works through relationships with the different people in the client's life.
- Evidence-based practice and sound clinical knowledge and skills inform all that the nurse does.
- Care is provided in the person's familiar environment.

Summary

Community nurses interact on a daily basis with people with chronic conditions and in so doing they facilitate a partnership that is integral to promoting the capacity of the individual to self-care. Community nurses work effectively with people with chronic conditions when they work *with* them, focusing on the needs of the person and understanding the challenges experienced by them. In summary, key principles of working with people with chronic conditions are to:

- View the person as part of a wider system.
- Engage with clients and value them as active, informed participants in the health care process.
- Develop rapport by engaging and connecting with the client and family.
- Refrain from judgement.
- Explain how the person's daily decisions may have a major impact on their health and well-being.
- Share test results and explain what they mean.
- Support people to make significant and lifelong behavioural changes utilising 'look, think, act'.
- Work with people to set small, achievable self-care goals that are meaningful to them. Always begin with what the client perceives to be important and possible.
- Enable clients through conversation to do some problem solving of their own.

Acknowledgements

I am grateful for the assistance of Kerry Telford, Natalie Howard, Lois Dennes, Anne van Loon, RDNS nurses and clients who have assisted and contributed in many ways to the development of this chapter.

Useful resources

Much of the information presented in this chapter is based on the findings of the chronic illness research programme of the Royal District Nursing Service in South Australia. Project reports and publications are available at www.rdns.net.au.

References

1. Australian Institute of Health and Welfare (2006) *Chronic Diseases and Associated Risk Factors in Australia*. Available at http://wwwaihwgovau/publications/indexcfm/title/10319 (viewed 10 December 2006).
2. Kralik, D., Brown, M. and Koch, T. (2001) Women's experiences of 'being diagnosed' with a long-term illness. *Journal of Advanced Nursing*, 33(5), 594–602.
3. Chronic Illness Alliance (2002) *Developing a Shared Definition of Chronic Illness*. Available at http://www.chronicillness.org.au/ (viewed 6 November 2006).
4. Ben-Shlomo, Y. and Kuh, D. (2002) A life course approach to chronic disease epidemiology: Conceptual models, empirical challenges and interdisciplinary perspectives. *International Journal of Epidemiology*, 31, 285–93.
5. Teschendorff, J. (2001) Does holistic medicine ignore the social causes of illness? *Diversity*, 2(4), 46–51.

6. Coleman, M.T. and Newton, K.S. (2005) Supporting self-management in patients with chronic illness. *American Family Physician*, 72, 1503–10.

7. McDonald, J. and Hare, L. (2004) *The Contribution of Primary and Community Health Services: Literature Review*. School of Public Health & Community Medicine, University of NSW, Sydney, Australia.

8. Peterson, C., Walker, C. and Southern, D. (2004) From episodic treatment to chronic disease management: Shifting the over 65 population to an alternative model of care. *General Practice Online*, 1–9.

9. Bodenheimer, T., Wagner, E.H. and Grumbach, K. (2002) Improving primary care for patients with chronic illness. *Journal of the American Medical Association*, 288(14), 1775–9.

10. Bodenheimer, T., Wagner, E.H. and Grumbach, K. (2002) Improving primary care for patients with chronic illness: The chronic care model part 2. *Journal of the American Medical Association*, 288(15), 1909–14.

11. Kralik, D., Koch, T. and Webb, C. (2001) The domination of chronic illness research by biomedical interests. *Australian Journal of Holistic Nursing*, 8(2), 4–12.

12. Wagner, E., Austin, B. and Von Korff, M. (1996) Organizing care for patients with chronic illness. *Milbank Quarterly*, 74(4), 511–44.

13. Dwyer, J.M. (2004) *Australian Health System Restructuring – What Problem is Being Solved?* BioMed Central Ltd.

14. World Health Organization (WHO) (2002) *Innovative Care for Chronic Conditions: Building Blocks for Action*. WHO Global Report. Available at http://www.who.int/mip2001/files/1986/InnovativeCareforChronicConditions.pdf (viewed August 2003).

15. Koch, T., Jenkin, P. and Kralik, D. (2004) Chronic illness self-management: Locating the 'self'. *Journal of Advanced Nursing*, 48(5), 484–92.

16. Kralik, D. and Telford, K. (2005/2006) *What Is Important About District Nursing for People Living in the Community with Chronic Illness?* Royal District Nursing Service (RDNS) Foundation of SA Inc Research Unit, Adelaide, SA.

17. Wagner, E. (2000) The role of patient care teams in chronic disease management. *BMJ*, 320, 569–72.

18. Warrawee'a, K.-D. (2000) Neetsa: An aboriginal perspective on holistic health. *Diversity*, 2(2), 2–9.

19. Kralik, D. (2002) The quest for ordinariness: Transition experienced by midlife women living with chronic illness. *Journal of Advanced Nursing*, 39(2), 146–54.

20. Corbin, J. and Strauss, A. (1987) Accompaniments of chronic illness: Change in the body, self, biography and biographical time. *Research in the Sociology of Health Care*, 6, 249–81.

21. Ohman, M., Soderberg, S. and Lundman, B. (2003) Hovering between suffering and enduring: The meaning of living with serious chronic illness. *Qualitative Health Research*, 13(4), 528–42.

22. Charmaz, K. (1983) Loss of self: A fundamental form of suffering in the chronically ill. *Sociology of Health & Illness*, 5(2), 168–95.

23. Kralik, D., van Loon, A.M. and Visentin, K. (June 2006) Resilience in the chronic illness experience. *Educational Action Research*, 14(2), 187–201. Special issue.

24. Bury, M. (1982) Chronic illness as biographical disruption. *Sociology of Health & Illness*, 4, 167–82.

25. Bury, M. (1991) The sociology of chronic illness: A review of research and prospects. *Sociology of Health & Illness*, 13, 451–68.

26. Kelly, M.P. and Field, D. (1996) Medical sociology, chronic illness and the body. *Sociology of Health & Illness*, 18(2), 241–57.

27. Kralik, D., Koch, T. and Eastwood, S. (2003) The salience of the body: Transition in sexual self-identity for women living with multiple sclerosis. *Journal of Advanced Nursing*, 42(1), 11–20.

28. Kralik, D., Koch, T. and Ashton, M. (2004) Equity and social justice issues for residents and staff of supported residential facilities. *Research, Policy and Planning*, 22(3), 15–24.
29. Telford, K., Kralik, D. and Koch, T. (2004) Acceptance and denial: Implications for people adapting to chronic illness: Literature review. *Journal of Advanced Nursing*, 55(4), 457–64.
30. Nettleton, S. (2006) 'I just want permission to be ill': Towards a sociology of medically unexplained symptoms. *Social Science and Medicine*, 62, 1167–78.
31. Taylor, B. (2005) Health, wellness, illness, healing and holism and nursing, in C. Rogers-Clark, K. Martin-McDonald and A. McCarthy (eds) *Living with Illness: Psychosocial Challenges for Nursing*. Elsevier, Australia, pp. 8–24.
32. Stuifbergen, A.K. and Rogers, S. (1997) The experience of fatigue and strategies of self-care among persons with multiple sclerosis. *Applied Nursing Research*, 10(1), 2–10.
33. Bonomi, A.E., Wagner, E.H., Glasgow, R. and Von Korff, M. (2002) Assessment of chronic illness care: A practical tool for quality improvement. *Health Services Research*, 37(3), 791–820.
34. Leveille, S., Wagner, E., Davis, C., Grothaus, L., Wallace, J., LoGerfo, M., *et al.* (1998) Preventing disability and managing chronic illness in frail older adults: A randomized trial of a community-based partnership with primary care. *Journal of the American Geriatrics Society*, 46(10), 1191–8.
35. Wilde, M. and Garvin, S. (2007) A concept analysis of self-monitoring. *Journal of Advanced Nursing*, 57(3), 339–50.
36. Kralik, D., Koch, T., Price, K. and Howard, N. (2004) Chronic illness self-management: Taking action to create order. *Journal of Clinical Nursing*, 13(2), 259–67.
37. Paterson, B.L. (2001) The shifting perspectives model of chronic illness. *Journal of Nursing Scholarship*, 33(1), 21–6.
38. Kralik, D., Telford, K., Campling, F., Crouch, P., Koch, T. and Price, K. (2005) 'Moving on': The transition to living well with chronic illness. *Australian Journal of Holistic Nursing*, 12(2), 13–22.
39. Stringer, E.T. (1999) *Action Research*, 2nd edition. Sage Publications, Thousand Oaks, CA.
40. Lilley, L.L. and Guanci, R. (November 1995) Applying systems theory. *American Journal of Nursing*, 95(11), 14–15.

Further readings

Kralik, D. and van Loon, A. (eds) (2008) *Community Nursing in Australia*. Wiley-Blackwell, Oxford.
Rogers-Clark, C., Martin-McDonald, K. and McCarthy, A. (2005) *Living with Illness: Psychosocial Challenges for Nursing*. Elsevier, Australia.

Chapter 9

Mental health

Janette Curtis, Yvonne White and Jennifer Harland

Introduction

Mental health issues affect every member of society in one way or another – from a person diagnosed with a mental illness to their relatives, friends, carers, colleagues and the health care professionals involved in their journey. This chapter provides a snapshot of current mental health statistics and focuses primarily on practical ways in which the community nurse can recognise and intervene when necessary with a person/client experiencing a mental health issue. It will be assumed throughout the chapter that the community nurse has an understanding of how to conduct a physical assessment; hence, the focus will be on conducting mental health assessments for the client. Maximising safety and reducing risk for the community nurse and the client are also covered in this chapter.

The mental health of the Australian community is highly placed on the agenda of state governments. For example, in June 2006, the Honourable Morris Iemma, premier of New South Wales (NSW), stated publicly that his government will provide more community care and early intervention so that mental health problems are identified and managed rather than escalating into acute episodes where people need hospitalisation [1]. His government has a commitment to build stronger links between private, public and the community sector, between hospitals and general practitioners (GPs), and between the state and federal governments. This means that there will be an increased role for the community nurse when interacting with and being involved in the care of people with mental illness. Box 9.1 provides a snapshot of the mental health of the NSW community.

The continuity of care between services is of major importance to people requiring treatment for mental health and mental illness. One example of collaboration between government services and the private sector is the Housing Accommodation Support Initiative (HASI) in New South Wales. This is a unique partnership between the NSW Department of Housing, The NSW Department of Health and the mental health non-government sector. Early results following 118 participants show that there has been a reduction in hospitalisation of 90%; 85% have successfully maintained their tenancy and 72% reported making new friends since joining the programme [1].

Box 9.1   A snapshot of the mental health of people in NSW [1, p. 3]

- There were approximately 1.1 million people in NSW who experienced a mental illness during 2005–2006.
- About 170 000 or 2–3% had a severe mental illness.
- Mental health units in NSW hospitals managed approximately 26 000 overnight admissions in 2004–2005.
- Community mental health services in NSW made 2.3 million clinical interventions in 2004–2005.
- The suicide rate was 8.6 per 100 000 in 2004 – the lowest in 50 years.
- In 2005–2006, the dedicated mental health recurrent budget was $854 million. Almost half the budget is dedicated to community mental health services.

Assessment and the role of the community nurse

The community nurse has an important role to play in the link between public, private and community sectors, and is often the first point of call for people who are experiencing mental health problems. The community nurse needs to be skilled in the undertaking of a comprehensive assessment of any client, including physical and mental heath assessment. One example of mental health assessment is detailed in Case Study 9.1.

Biopsychosocial model of assessment

A biopsychosocial assessment involves an assessment of all aspects of the client's problem. This includes a biological, sociological, developmental, medical, drug and alcohol, environmental, cultural and spiritual assessment.

Psychiatric assessment

The purpose of a psychiatric assessment is to develop an understanding of the person presenting for help. It involves taking a basic psychiatric history and a mental status examination (MSE). The following information is required:

- *Identifying information.* Identifying information includes name, age, sex, address, telephone number, languages spoken, marital status, children, occupation and next of kin.
- *Presenting problem.* This includes obtaining a brief description of the principal complaint and the time frame described in the client's own words. For example a brief description of the specific symptoms that are present and how long the person has been experiencing them. It is also important to ascertain any disturbances in mood, appetite or sleep as well as what current treatment the person is having. It is during this discussion where the development of a therapeutic relationship with the client can occur.

Case study 9.1

Brian is a 19-year-old university student. Following a motor bike accident, he spent 1 week in hospital for a fractured tibia and fibula. He has been referred to the local community nursing service for ongoing management. The referral letter gives details of Brian's operation and outlines the required dressing and IV antibiotic regime.

Following initial telephone contact, the community nurse allocated to Brian makes her first visit. Brian is living in a studio apartment close to the university campus. Brian's apartment is untidy and the nurse makes a joking comment that he 'will soon be out of dishes', observing the stack of dirty dishes in the sink. Brian does not laugh and looks at the nurse blankly.

Brian is not talkative. He appears distracted and the nurse asks friendly questions during the administration of the antibiotics and dressing change. Between the long silences the nurse finds out that Brian is in the first year of a law degree. Brian is from rural Australia and moved to the city to attend university.

The nurse's second visit is the day before the Easter long weekend. Brian appears more distracted, denies any pain or discomfort and is responding in monosyllables. On leaving, the nurse asks Brian what plans he has for the Easter break. Brian responds that he will be staying at home as he is the chosen one and his disciples won't be able to find him if he is not at home. The nurse is not sure how to respond and asks Brian what he means by this. Brian appears frustrated at the nurse's query but repeats in a slower, louder voice 'I am the chosen one' and closes the door behind her.

What should the nurse do?

When leaving Brian's apartment the nurse immediately rings her supervisor and reports Brian's altered behaviour. The supervisor agrees with the nurse's plan to notify the community mental health service. The community mental health team is able to assess Brian that day and he is admitted to a mental health facility. Follow-up with Brian's family establishes that he has no previous history of mental illness. The mental health team congratulates the community nurse for her action in identifying and alerting them to Brian's first episode of psychosis.

- *Mental health/medical history.* It is important to find out about any previous admissions to a mental health unit, number of previous suicide attempts or self-harm, or any history of assault. Medical history includes major medical and surgical procedures and injuries. This includes current and past medications including complementary or over-the-counter medications.
- *Alcohol and other drug history.* The nurse needs to ascertain types of drugs (prescribed and nonprescribed) used, the amount used, the frequency of use, the route of admission, how long they have been using and when they last used. For example if a person admits to drinking alcohol, ask the client what type of alcohol they drink; how many days of the week they drink; how many glasses/bottles would they have on a typical day; how old were they when they started drinking; and when was their last drink?

- *Psychosocial/relationship history*. This outlines circumstances that are significant for understanding current issues and covers aspects of the individual's life such as relationships, family background, work and school history and developmental stages.
- *Determining risk factors*. Risk factors need to be assessed. These include assessment for risk of harm to others, harm to self, suicide, vulnerability to sexual exploitation, risk to reputation and vulnerability to violence.
- *Assessment of strengths*. This looks at strengths such as support systems, education, motivation and physical health.

What to assess in a mental status examination

The MSE is a semi-structured interview used mainly as a screening tool to assess a person's current neurological and psychological status along several dimensions [2, 3]. The examination involves observation as well as an interview.

Appearance and behaviour

The aim is to observe and describe the manner and appearance of the individual at the time of the interview:

- Describe the individual's physical appearance (e.g. grooming, hygiene, clothing, nails, build, tattoos and other significant features).
- What is the individual's reaction to the present situation and the examiner (e.g. hostile, friendly, withdrawn, guarded, cooperative, uncommunicative or seductive)?
- Describe the individual's motor behaviour (e.g. psychomotor retarded, restless, repetitive behaviours, hyperactive, tremor, hand wringing or bizarre). Describe in words the actual behaviours.

Speech

The physical aspects of speech can be described in terms of rate, volume and quantity of information (e.g. slow, rapid, monotonous, loud, quiet, slurred, whispered). Some particular characteristics of speech that may be considered are:

- Mutism – the total absence of speech.
- Poverty of speech – replies to questions are brief and monosyllabic.
- Pressure of speech – speech is extremely rapid, difficult to interrupt, loud and hard to understand.

Mood and affect

Mood describes the internal feeling or emotion, which often influences behaviour and the individual's perception of the world. *Affect* refers to the external emotional response. Both aspects can provide important diagnostic information:

- Describe the individual's mood. One way is to ask the individual how they feel. They may describe themselves as sad or worried, confused or 'on top of the world'.

- Describe the individual's affect, e.g. labile (alternating between extremes), fearful, suspicious, irritable, hostile. Note whether the emotional response is appropriate, given the subject matter discussed. Some terms used are:
  - normal – expected variation in facial expression, voice, gestures or movements that are congruent with the context or content of discussion;
  - restricted – decreased intensity and range of emotional response;
  - blunted – severe decrease in intensity and range of emotional expression;
  - flat – almost complete or complete absence of emotional expression with accompanying expressionless face and monotonous voice.

Form of thought

This is assessed according to:

- Amount of thought and its rate of production (e.g. poverty of ideas, flight of ideas, slow or hesitant thinking, vagueness).
- Continuity of ideas (the logical order or flow of the ideas). Individuals may or may not be able to stick to the topic of conversation. They may digress into irrelevant conversation, completely lose their train of thought or talk 'around' the topic.
- Disturbance in language (the use of words that do not exist or conversations that do not make sense). Refer to Box 9.2.

Box 9.2   Thought disorders [2, p. 375]

Delusional thinking is a specific form of thought disorder. There are many types of thought disorder and they are usually labelled according to the pattern observed, such as thought blocking. Some types of thought disorder which may be found in people with a mental illness include:

Thought broadcasting. As the name implies, the person feels that the thoughts they have are being broadcast and therefore become available to the outside world. In thought broadcast the person can often be suspicious of all social encounters and develop the belief that people react to them in such a way as to confirm the thought broadcast. One example is a client who would interpret people smiling at him as people laughing at the thoughts being broadcast.

Thought insertion. This is where a person feels that thoughts are being inserted into the mind by someone or something else, although some clients can often be unsure who or what is inserting the thought. Thoughts inserted in this way are often at odds with the individual's related beliefs. An example is a black female client who had antiblack racist thought inserted by her neighbours.

Thought withdrawal. Thoughts being taken out of the mind wilfully by a third party. Different from thought broadcast in that a specific agent will withdraw the thought, but others will not be able to hear it.

Thought echo. Thoughts continue to sound in the mind as an echo, or repeat, either in full or part. The person feels they have no control over the process.

Made feelings. An emotion is experienced which a third party has generated.

Made actions. Can be both simple and complex actions; 'Look, see my leg twitching? It's not me doing it – it's the freak getting me to look like a fool'.

Thought content

Assess for:

- *Delusions.* False beliefs that are firmly held despite objective and contradictory evidence and despite the fact that other members of the culture do not share the same beliefs. There are numerous types of delusions, some of which tend to be associated with different disorders.
- *Suicidal thoughts.* This is addressed later in this chapter.
- *Other.* This includes obsessions, compulsions, antisocial urges, phobias, intentions, hypochondriacal symptoms and preoccupations. Refer to Box 9.3.

Box 9.3   Delusions [2, 4]

Delusions. A delusion is a false impression or belief that any person can experience from time to time. Within mental health, additional factors may distinguish it as a symptom of mental disorder. The belief is fixed and held with compelling conviction and is resistant to modification [5].

Delusional mood. The individual feels that his or her familiar environment has changed in some way, which is puzzling. The individual may not be able to describe this change clearly.

Delusions of reference. The belief that events or other people's actions or words refer specifically to the individual and have a special meaning for the individual. This does not include being overly self-conscious as in social phobia. (*Note:* Ideas of reference are false beliefs which are not held as firmly as delusions and for which the individual may see an alternative point of view.)

Delusions of control, influence or passivity. The belief that one's feelings, impulses, thoughts or actions are not one's own, but are controlled by an external force. The individual must acknowledge that they no longer have a will of their own, but are being controlled by another force (other than God or fate).

Somatic delusions. Somatic means a physical manifestation or feeling. Hence, a person can feel that they have cancer when they do not, or a part of their body has died while they continue to exist.

Grandiose delusions. Exaggerated belief of one's importance, power, knowledge or identity. The person may think they have special powers such as being able to heal the sick or change world events.

Religious delusions. The individual believes they have a special link with God/Christ. This excludes intense religious or cultural beliefs.

Nihilistic delusions The individual believes that the self or part of the self does not exist, or is dead, or that others or the world does not exist. This is often associated with depressive episodes.

Fantastic delusions. The belief that the individual has had an amazing adventure or experience. This is often associated with manic episodes.

Delusions of jealousy The belief, without good reason, that one's partner is unfaithful. This may be associated with a delusional disorder.

Sensorium and cognition

Assess for:

- *Level of consciousness*. Impairment of consciousness usually indicates organic brain disease.
- *Memory*. The three main areas are immediate, recent and remote.
- *Orientation*. Obvious disturbances in orientation usually indicate organic brain disease.
- *Concentration*. Concentration may be assessed by asking the individual to subtract serial 7s from 100.
- *Abstract thought*. Abstract thinking involves the ability to:
  - deal with abstract concepts,
  - extract common characteristics from groups or objects,
  - juggle more than one idea at a time and
  - interpret information.

Abstract thinking may be assessed by asking the individual to interpret the meaning of common proverbs, such as 'don't put all of your eggs in the one basket'. The mini MSE is the most commonly used screening tool for assessing cognitive impairment such as dementia or head injury [2].

Perception

This area assesses for hallucinations, which are false sensory perceptions in which the person sees, hears, smells, tastes or feels something that other people do not. Hallucinations are the most common form of perceptual disturbances [2]. There may be a physical cause for hallucinations, such as a head injury, brain tumour, epilepsy, drugs and/or alcohol. If the client is experiencing perceptual disturbances, it is important to check for underlying medical or physical causes. Although hallucinations are described as false, they are real to the individual experiencing them. They can affect any of the five senses [2] as referred to in Box 9.4.

Insight

Insight refers to the individual's awareness of his or her situation or illness. There are varying degrees of insight. For example someone may be aware that they have a problem, but may regard it as the fault of someone else [4].

Safety for the community nurse

During everyday nursing practice, the community nurse needs to be assessing for risk and actively reducing risk. Risk can come in many forms; it may include assessing for risk to the client, themselves and/or others.

Box 9.4	Perceptual disturbances	
Sense	**Hallucination**	**Notes**
Hearing	Auditory hallucination	Most commonly reported. Can be an individual voice, a combination of voices or simple noises
Sight	Visual hallucination	Can be definite shapes such as faces of people or lights and flashes
Smell	Olfactory hallucination	Often linked to other symptoms. Can be indicative of a physical problem such as a tumour or epilepsy
Taste	Gustatory hallucination	Often linked to other symptoms. Can be indicative of a physical problem such as a brain tumour or epilepsy
Touch	Tactile hallucination	Often linked to other symptoms. Can be indicative of a physical problem such as a brain tumour or epilepsy

Reducing risk

Suicide and self-harm

Self-harm may be distinguished from suicidal behaviour in that self-harm is often an impulsive, non-lethal attempt by a person to alleviate emotional distress, where the person deliberately inflicts injury on him or herself. A person may self-harm without having suicidal intent [6, 7]. However, research demonstrates that there is an increased risk of suicide in the year following an incident of self-harm [8]. Some people view deliberate self-harm and suicide on a continuum [9] as indicated in Table 9.1.

It can be very confronting for community nurses when they are faced with a person who deliberately self-harms. The reasons for this may be due to anxious feelings that are provoked or frustration that results in the community nurse feeling ambivalent, making it difficult to develop a therapeutic rapport and to empathise [10].

Assessment for self-harm

When assessing the person who self-harms, it is important to focus on the person's strengths as well as their needs. This approach provides a more accurate and comprehensive overview of the person rather than simply view their behaviour from a pathogenic or illness perspective [11]. The nursing skills required when caring for a person who self-harms are detailed in Box 9.5.

Assessment for suicide

If the community nurse suspects that a person may be suicidal, it is important that a suicidal assessment is conducted by talking directly with the person. If the nurse does not ask, they will not know. Discussing suicide will *not* make the person more likely to

Table 9.1 Deliberate self-harm – suicide continuum [9, p. 751].

	Any client may have suicidal thoughts, feelings or plans whether or not they actually self-harm										
	Behaviours that may be socially acceptable, but cause harm and could result in accidental or premature death						Behaviours with varying risk of completed suicide. Remember to consider the client's view of whether an act might be lethal				
Deliberate self-harm	Tattoos, body piercing, tribal cuts or scarring	Risk-taking: driving too fast, unsafe sex	Smoking or drinking to excess	Illicit drug use or excessive use of prescribed drugs	Deliberate self-harm as a coping mechanism for psychological distress	Cutting or overdosing without suicidal ideation	Binge eating or starvation	Non-lethal cutting or overdosing with the intent to kill oneself	Overdoses, hanging, cutting or immersion with suicidal intent	Attempted suicide with lethal method resulting in death	**Completed suicide**
	Boredom, thrill seeking, frustration, experimentation, socialisation, self-expression				Feeling 'out of control', angry, guilty, low self-esteem, need to punish or purge oneself			Depressed, hopeless, unable to see a future, guilty, angry, resolved to die or apathetic about living			

Box 9.5   Nursing skills with the person who is self-harming [12]

- Approach the person with an open mind and a supportive attitude.
- Be non-judgemental in your approach.
- Encourage the person to discuss their thoughts and feelings regarding their self-harm.
- Remove any potentially harmful objects such as knives, glasses, razors and/or lighters.
- Assess for risk of suicide.
- Convey a sense of calm, control and safety to the person.
- Explore alternative coping methods for expressing negative feelings.
- Refer to the community mental health team for ongoing assessment and interventions.

---

attempt suicide; rather it is more likely that the person will realise that there is another solution to their problem(s) [3].

During the assessment, the nurse needs to ask questions of the person as to whether they have ever felt like killing themselves and how strong the feeling is. The nurse will also need to ask if the person has a plan for how they would kill themselves (such as taking pills, hanging, jumping off a bridge). They will also need to find out whether the person has the means available to carry out their plans. (For example have they stockpiled their pills? Do they have a rope or other device?) The time frame of the suicide attempt also needs to be elicited. Is it something that they plan to do immediately? Is it a future plan? It is also important to find out whether the person has attempted suicide before, as research demonstrates that if a person has attempted suicide previously, they are at greater risk of attempting again and being successful [11]. The assessment of the suicidal intentions of a person is detailed in Box 9.6.

Following completion of the suicide assessment, if the community nurse is concerned for the person's safety, it is important that they stay with the person (as much as practicable) until a mental health nurse or someone such as a medical officer attends

---

Box 9.6   Assessment of suicidal ideation: direct questions [12]

Examples of questions that may be used for assessing suicidal ideation:
- Have you been feeling 'down' or depressed for a few days at a time?
- Do you ever feel that life is not worth living?
- When you feel like this, have you ever had thoughts of killing yourself?
- Have you taken steps towards doing this (e.g. buying pills)?
- Have you thought about when you might kill yourself?
- What has stopped you from doing this so far?
- What would make it easier to deal with your problems?

---

to assess the person thoroughly and who may arrange for the person to be admitted to a mental health facility. For nurses practising in remote areas, phoning a colleague, the person's GP or the community mental health nurse is imperative.

Many community nurses, like others, feel unsure of how a person with a mental illness will react. The next section deals with some practical ways to recognise and diffuse a potentially aggressive situation.

Managing aggression

De-escalation of behaviours

De-escalation refers to the processes by which a client's expressed anger or aggression are defused so that a calmer state occurs. There are several stages in the application of skills to de-escalate behaviours. These stages involve immediate risk assessment together with verbal and non-verbal communication skills [3].

The individual's specific situation must be considered. What are the underlying reasons for aggression? Has something specific happened? Is the nurse or others involved with (or perceived to be involved with) restriction or control, irritating or personally criticising the client? If we listen to what the client is saying, then incidents can often be dealt with before they escalate into something bigger. Common behaviours linked to escalating aggression are listed in Box 9.7.

Non-verbal communication

Non-verbal communication is as important as verbal communication when communicating with people. Practice strategies for monitoring safety are listed in Box 9.8. However, if the person's behaviour begins to 'escalate' (e.g. becoming agitated, argumentative, elevated, aggressive, angry), there are some helpful non-verbal communication strategies that can be used, which have been outlined by Sookoo [13, p. 736]:

Box 9.7   Behaviours linked to escalating aggression [12, p. 58–64]

- Rapid, loud or profane speech
- Sudden change in the client's level of consciousness, e.g. increased disorientation and confusion
- Clenched fists, gritted teeth, reddened face, widened eyes, flaring nostrils, rapid breathing
- Motor agitation, such as pacing and inability to remain still
- Hallucinations, which can be auditory or visual and may be benign or command oriented
- Sudden change or extremes of affect
- Sudden loss of affect in someone who was previously very agitated and threatening

---

Box 9.8   Practice points for monitoring safety [1, p. 736]

- Don't isolate yourself – check that colleagues know your whereabouts.
- Check that you are familiar with mechanisms for calling for help and that you have access to these.
- Check escape routes – avoid corners.
- If isolated when a violent incident occurs, the priority is to get away from the situation and summon help. Do not tackle a violent person alone, whatever your or the client's gender or size.
- Make a visual check of the immediate area for potential weapons (e.g. there may be chairs, glasses, cups in the dining room; if in a kitchen, there may be knives or boiling water; in the bathroom, there may be a razor or aerosols). If identified, the priority is to maintain distance and offer the option to the person to leave the area and continue the discussion elsewhere.

- Maintain an adequate distance. Closeness may be interpreted as a threat or may increase tension.
- Stand at an angle to the client to avoid appearing confrontational and to allow for defence (put weight on back foot). Do not point and do not touch the person.
- Maintain normal eye contact – staring can be perceived as threatening, while avoiding can seem dismissive.
- Be aware of your own reactions, which may be fear or anger, and try to consider the client's point of view – which may be anxious as well as angry. Do not feel that you have to win an argument or that you have to deal with the situation alone and effectively in order to 'be a good nurse'.

Verbal communication

The verbal communication we use when someone is becoming agitated is very important. Early intervention may de-escalate the situation [14]. It is important to remain calm and speak softly and slowly using clear and short sentences. However, avoid being patronising (e.g. avoid telling the client to calm down). Be courteous and use the person's name [3]. The following strategies may be useful when dealing with an aggressive or angry person:

- Use non-judgemental communication and be aware of the client's feelings. Remain in control of your own feelings.
- Attempt to uncover the source of distress and engage the client in questions that might help identify the problem area.
- Ask the person to sit down and talk with you.
- Do not try to talk when they are shouting or talking loudly, and do not argue or become defensive.
- Use reflective listening to acknowledge concerns. This is not simply stating the obvious or parroting what the client has said. Be specific; for example 'I can see you are disappointed and upset that we are unable to do your shopping for you'.

- Use open-ended questions to elicit additional information from the client, but do not attempt to interrogate.
- Attempt to help the client identify ways to deal effectively with the situation.
- Convey that you want to help the person find a solution; e.g. 'Give me 20 min to find out what has happened'.
- Most importantly, know when you need help, and when you do need it, call for it and/or leave the situation if there is no one immediately available [3, 13].

Medication

The management of mental illness involves a collaborative approach based on good case management. Major treatment strategies are based on a biological, sociological and environmental model [14]. The treatment of mental illness involves the use of many medications in either single or combined therapies.

Community nurses should be aware that it may take time for the right medication to be found, which will have the best outcome for the individual client. 'A feature of most psychiatric medications is that they may only begin to have a beneficial effect over several weeks' [15, p. 1]. Therefore patience is required whilst awaiting the effect to be optimal. A community nurse should request the following medication-related information regarding psychiatric medications:

- The name of the medication and its purpose.
- How long it will take until the effect is optimal.
- What special considerations are required (e.g. what foods, medications, activities should be avoided).
- Potential adverse reactions and side effects of the specific medications.
- What other prescription or non-prescription medications the client is taking.
- Whether the client has a history of or is currently a substance abuser.
- Whether the client is pregnant or breastfeeding.
- Whether the client is taking their medications as prescribed by the medical practitioner on a regular basis [14, p. 1].

The community nurse should be aware of the general categories of psychiatric medications. These include antipsychotic medications, mood stabilisers, antidepressants and antianxiety agents.

Antipsychotics are generally used for schizophrenia and substance-induced psychosis, and the optimal improvement in mental health may take a few months to be overt [14, p. 2]. Side effects related to these medications include 'parkinsonian' movements and tardive dyskinesia (involuntary movements). It has been reported that after approximately 5 years of treatment with antipsychotics, 3–5% of people will have tardive dyskinesia [15]. These involuntary movements include chewing movements, tongue protrusion and lip puckering [14, p. 2]. Anticholinergics are given to counteract the severe side effects of psychotropic medications [14, p. 2]. Tardive dyskinesia has been described as the 'most humiliating movement' as it is associated with the stigma of mental illness. This stigma leads to social isolation and a poorer perception of quality of life [16].

Mood stabilisers are used for acute manic and depressive states, and again may take several weeks to be optimally effective [14, p. 3]. It is important that regular serum levels of these medications are taken and the levels monitored as side effects are related to therapeutic levels. Each medication has its own specific adverse events and side effects and the community nurse should be aware of these for the individual client.

Antidepressants are used in the treatment of depressive states and yet again take several weeks to have the best effect [14, p. 4]. The selective serotonin uptake inhibitors are the most common. These medications should never be ceased suddenly, as this may lead to withdrawal effects. Monoamine oxidase inhibitors (MAOIs) which are one family of antidepressant medications may result in a hypertensive crisis if foods with tyramine are not excluded from the diet [14, p. 4].

Antianxiety medications are prescribed for people with anxiety disorders. The majority of these people have a high risk of developing dependence on these medications [14, p. 5], and clients' doses should be reduced gradually so as not to induce withdrawal symptoms. Consultation with the prescribing medical practitioner is advised.

Due to the expected therapeutic effects of psychiatric medications, it is important for the community nurse to undertake regular mental health assessments, as well as a comprehensive physical assessment. The community nurse should also collect information specific to the psychiatric medications that their individual clients are prescribed. This knowledge will enable the nurse to understand their responsibility in specific observations and monitoring and interpretation of observations and monitoring data, and to implement appropriate nursing actions to maintain the safety of the client, the nurse and others.

Legal considerations

Mental health acts

Each Australian state and territory has its own mental health act [17]. The acts vary slightly in content between states; however, they have all been designed to protect individuals with mental illness from inappropriate treatment, to direct the provision of mental health care and the facilities in which it is provided and to instruct the practice of mental health professionals in principles of treatment and care. The various mental health acts involve the care of both voluntary and involuntary clients. For further information refer to the mental health act for each state or territory.

Guardianship Act

The NSW Guardianship Act [1987] was created to protect the legal rights of people over the age of 16 years who have a disability which affects their capacity to make decisions. (Similar acts are found in all states.)

The NSW Guardianship Act [1987] provides for the appointment of a guardian to make substitute decisions on behalf of a person who meets the criteria documented above. A guardian must be aged over 18 years and can be an enduring guardian (one whom the person has appointed to make personal or lifestyle decisions for them in the event that the person is not capable of doing this themselves) or a guardian appointed by the Guardianship Tribunal or the Supreme Court. A guardian can only make decisions in areas for which they have been appointed and must make those decisions in line with the Guardianship Act. Some examples include decisions about accommodation (deciding where the person may reside), medical and dental treatment, health care and services. A guardian does not make financial decisions.

Conclusion

This chapter provides the knowledge and skills base that will assist the community nurse to meet the challenges of caring for clients who are managing their mental health. Knowledge of how to effectively work with clients with mental health issues may lead to an enhanced quality of life for the client and better health outcomes for the community. The role of the community health nurse is important in the treatment of a person who is experiencing mental illness. It is especially important to regularly assess and document the client's mental condition even when they appear to be stabilised on a treatment regime. Because the side effects of medication can be very unpleasant, clients are often reluctant to continue taking their medication. Very often the community nurse is the first person in a position to assess the client as he/she might be the only regular visitor that a client may have, especially for those clients living alone or residing in rural/remote areas of Australia. Mental health, like all areas of health, is moving increasingly towards community care. This may mean that people who were once treated in an inpatient environment are now treated in the community. It is thus important to possess assessment skills and to refer to the appropriate sources or services when a person is suspected of becoming mentally unwell.

Whilst only a very small percentage of people who are mentally ill are violent, the nurse must be prepared to deal with someone who may be agitated. Risk assessment should be undertaken during every contact with the client – a risk assessment that includes the client's safety as well as that of the nurse. Lifelong learning and developing creative nursing practice skills for use in an uncontrolled environment are the greatest challenges for the community nurse.

Useful resources

NSW Guardianship Tribunal at http://www.health.wa.gov.au/mhareview/resources/legislation/NSW_Guardianship_Act_1987.pdf

NSW: A new direction for mental health at http://www.health.nsw.gov.au/pubs/2006/pdf/mental_health.pdf

The NSW government's plan for mental health services at http://www.health.nsw.gov.au/aboutus/pdf/mental_health_services.pdf

Mental Illness Fellowship of Australia at www.mifellowshipaustralia.org.au

Mental Health Research Institute at www.mhri.edu.au

National Action Plan for Mental Health 2006–2011 at http://www.coag.gov.au/meetings/140706/docs/nap_mental_health.pdf

National Alliance of the Mentally Ill (NAMI) (USA) at www.nami.org

National Practice Standards for the Mental Health Workforce at http://www.aasw.asn.au/adobe/publications/mental/MH_endorsed_prac_standards.pdf

Australian Nurse Supply Recruitment and Retention Report 2003 at http://www.health.nsw.gov.au/amwac/pdf/menhealth_20032.pdf

National Health Workforce Action Plan at http://www.health.nsw.gov.au/amwac/pdf/NHW_action_plan.pdf

National Review of Nursing Education: Our Duty of Care Available at http://www.dest.gov.au/archive/highered/nursing/pubs/duty_of_care/duty_of_care.pdf

Australian State and Territory Mental Health Acts at http://www.austlii.edu.au

Suicide risk assessment and management protocols. Community Mental Health Service at http://www.cs.nsw.gov.au/mhealth/documents/suicide_com_mh_protocols.pdf

References

1. NSW Department of Health (2006) *NSW: A New Direction for Mental Health*. Available at http://www.health.nsw.gov.au/pubs/2006/pdf/mental_health.pdf (viewed 14 April 2007).

2. Brennan, G. (2004) The person with a perceptual disorder, in I. Norman and I. Ryrie (eds) *The Art and Science of Mental Health Nursing: A Textbook of Principles and Practice*. Open University Press, Berkshire, pp. 365–88.

3. Usher, K., Luck, L. and Foster, K. (2005) The patient as person, in R. Elder, K. Evans and D. Nizette (eds) *Psychiatric and Mental Health Nursing*. Elsevier, Marrickville, pp. 359–78.

4. Project, T.P. (2000) *Management of Mental Disorders*, 3rd edition. World Health Collaborating Centre for Mental Health and Substance Abuse, Sydney.

5. Ryrie, I. and Norman, I. (2004) The origins and expression of psychological distress, in I. Norman and I. Ryrie (eds), *The Art and Science of Mental Health Nursing: A Textbook of Principles and Practice*. Open University Press, Berkshire, pp. 3–34.

6. Gallop, R. and Tully, T. (2004) The person who self harms, in P. Barker (ed.) *Psychiatric and Mental Health Nursing: The Art of Caring*. Arnold, London.

7. Weber, M. (2002) Triggers for self-abuse: A qualitative study. *Archives of Psychiatric Nursing*, 16(3), 118–24.

8. Department of Health (2002) *National Suicide Prevention Strategy for England*. Available at http://www.dh.gov.uk/en/Publicationsandstatistics/Publications/PublicationsPolicyAndGuidance/DH_4009474 (viewed 17 November 2007).

9. Noonan, I. (2004) Therapeutic management of self harm, in I. Norman and I. Ryrie (eds) *The Art and Science of Mental Health Nursing: A Textbook of Principles and Practice*. Open University Press, Berkshire, pp. 747–69.

10. Smith, S. (2002) Perception of service provision for clients who self injure in the absence of expressed suicidal intent. *Journal of Psychiatric and Mental Health Nursing*, 9(5), 595–601.

11. McAllister, M. and Estefan, A. (2002) Principles and strategies for teaching therapeutic responses to self harm. *Journal of Psychiatric and Mental Health Nursing*, 9(5), 573–83.

12. Distasio, C. (2002) Protecting yourself from violence in the workplace. *Nursing*, 32(6), 58–63.

13. Sookoo, S. (2004) Therapeutic management of aggression and violence, in I. Norman and I. Ryrie (eds) *The Art and Science of Mental Health Nursing: A Textbook of Principles and Practice*. Open University Press, Berkshire, pp. 729–46.

14. Delaney, J., Cleary, M., Jordan, R. and Horsfall, J. (2001) An explanatory investigation into the nursing management of aggression in acute psychiatric settings. *International Journal of Mental Health Nursing*, 11(3), 77–84.

15. Mental Illness Fellowship of Australia (2005) *Mental Illness Fact Sheet Series: Understanding and Managing Mental Illness.* Psychiatric Medication. Mental Illness Fellowship, Victoria, pp. 1–6.

16. Antai-Otong, D. (2003) Adverse drug reactions associated with antipsychotics, antidepressants and mood stabilisers. *Nursing Clinics of North America*, 38, 161–76.

17. Australian State and Territory Mental Health Acts (2007) Available at http://www.austlii.edu.au (viewed 17 November 2007).

Chapter 10

Addiction and homelessness

Janette Curtis, Jennifer Harland and Yvonne White

Introduction

No one ever plans to become homeless. No school career information day has a booth displaying how to develop a drug addiction and become homeless. Unfortunately, despite paving our plans with good intentions, many Australians become homeless for a variety of reasons and many will develop addictions that often lead to homeless periods during their lives. Many of their individual stories feature common elements.

This chapter explores the impact of addiction and homelessness and highlights the challenges they present for community nurses. It offers practical solutions and presents a variety of assessment tools.

Case study 10.1 illustrates one person's life experiences which led him to a period of homelessness.

Case study 10.1

Five days after Christmas, Jerry is observed asking people for money at a seaside tourist attraction. Although his approach is polite, even friendly, the responses are consistently abrupt. Apparently, the season for giving is not a reason for giving and few passers-by are keen to hand over the requested $5 train fare to Jerry. But eventually he finds somebody willing to share and – in return – shares his story.

Jerry does not present himself as a victim. Instead he mentions the positives of the surroundings – the beach, the waves, and the fact that it has finally stopped raining. In a jigsaw of questions and answers, Jerry's story is revealed. He grew up on the south coast of New South Wales and loved surfing; he even spoke of fun times when the surf was flat, playing cards on his floating board. Following a 2-year period of alcohol abuse, he reunited with his parents in Queensland for a clean break. Jerry spoke with pride of his 6 months being sober and the joy of having his son come to live with him. Like all proud parents, he was quick to pull out a folded A4 size school photo of his 6-year-old son, speaking knowledgeably of the price of school uniforms, particularly the cost of replacing the school caps his son was always losing.

So what went wrong? How did Jerry now find himself in such a desperate situation? The details were sketchy, not only for the quiet listener but also for Jerry, who spoke of how things started going wrong after 'just a couple of beers'. He seemed bewildered that as soon as he confessed those 'couple of beers' to his father, his son was returned to his mother and he himself was heading south in search of his life.

Jerry recalled flashes of his previous 5 days. He outlined some of the events of Christmas, spending the day with his family in a local park, falling asleep, waking up to find his wallet had been stolen and how he had been trying to get home since then – although he did not specify where home was.

Jerry was street smart. He spoke of how he had been sleeping on the beach for several nights, as the local shelter for men was fully occupied. He knew the process at the men's shelter and complained about walking a long distance every day, just to be turned away. He also said that the local police had been helpful, stopping regularly as he wandered the streets to see if he was okay – but he wryly joked about the fact that the police had not been there when he was 'belted by four blokes'.

Jerry appeared homeless, wearing layers of stained clothes on a warm summer's day and with hair and skin that did not have the just-washed gleam. To a trained observer, Jerry displayed signs of a person with a history of alcohol abuse accompanied by early signs of alcohol withdrawal. Jerry's experience is in common with many homeless people in Australia.

Points to be considered:

- What are the main priorities for Jerry at this time?
- What are some of the potential problems that Jerry may face?
- What symptoms would Jerry exhibit if he was experiencing early signs of alcohol withdrawal?
- If Jerry was to present to an emergency department within the next 24 h, outline a management plan.
- What could you do for Jerry as a community health nurse?
- What services may be available to Jerry?
- Discuss some of the problems Jerry may face accessing services.

Homelessness

Australian census data in 2001 estimated that 100 000 people were homeless across Australia [1] and that many of the homeless move from one temporary form of accommodation to another. Many definitions of homelessness exist (see Box 10.1); however, there is agreement that homelessness is more than just houselessness [2]. Aspects of homelessness include isolation and marginalisation and among these are people experiencing problematic use of substances. There is also evidence that strongly indicates that there is a much higher prevalence of mental illness, including dual diagnosis (mental illness and problematic substance use), among people who are homeless [2].

Being homeless can affect young and old, women and men and even whole families. Recent research suggests that there is a new group of people experiencing homelessness who, although they have had very little income and have lived close to the poverty line, have never previously experienced homelessness. However, as they age they are more likely to be unable to adapt to changes in availability of low-cost housing and find themselves homeless for the first time [4].

A significant number of the homeless are young people (12–24 years) and are more likely to be male, although the numbers of females becoming homeless is increasing [1].

> **Box 10.1   Definitions of homelessness [3, p. 8]**
>
> *Primary homelessness.* People without conventional accommodation such as those who 'sleep out' or use derelict buildings, cars and railway stations for shelter.
> *Secondary homelessness.* People who frequently move from temporary accommodation such as emergency accommodation, refuges and temporary shelters. People may use boarding houses or family accommodation just on a temporary basis.
> *Tertiary homelessness.* People who live in rooming houses, boarding houses medium or long term, where they do not have their own bathroom and kitchen facilities and tenure is not secured by a lease.
> *Marginally housed.* People in housing situations close to the minimum standard.

In 2001, families represented 9% of the homeless (comprising 9543 parents and 13 401 children) and 60–70% of people had been homeless for 6 months or longer [1]. The population of homeless people is not evenly spread in Australia. The Northern Territory continues to have the highest rate of homelessness (288 per 10 000), largely due to Indigenous people living in improvised dwellings [1]. In New South Wales, South Sydney and Sydney have the highest concentration of homeless people. In the area covered by the South Eastern Sydney Illawarra Health Service (SESIH), 4236 people have been identified as homeless in 2001 [1].

Risk factors for homelessness

The causality between risk factors and homelessness is multifaceted. Substance dependence, social isolation and mental illness may be contributing factors or may even be the consequence of homelessness. Homelessness can occur for many reasons including childhood experiences, mental health and/or substance-use issues, unemployment, as well as any combination of these factors [5, 6].

Addiction

Addiction is a term which is widely used, but not always useful, as the word conjures up an emotional response for many people. For the purpose of this chapter, addiction will refer to addiction to certain substances (drugs and/or alcohol) and exclude other substances and activities such as gambling, tobacco, coffee and food. For a more detailed classification please refer to Box 10.2. A person with a drug addiction, or dependence, is defined as having at least three of the following signs:

- Having a tolerance for the drug (needing increased amounts to achieve the same effect).
- Having withdrawal symptoms, taking the drug in larger amounts than was intended or over a longer period of time than was intended.
- Having a persistent desire to decrease or the inability to decrease the amount of the drug consumed.

Box 10.2   DSM-IV-TR diagnostic criteria for substance dependence [7]

A maladaptive pattern of substance use, leading to clinically significant impairment or distress, as manifested by three (or more) of the following, occurring at any time in the same 12-month period.

1. Tolerance, as defined by either of the following:
   - a need for markedly increased amounts of the substance to achieve intoxication or desired effect;
   - markedly diminished effect with continued use of the same amount of the substance.
2. Withdrawal as manifested by either of the following:
   - the characteristic withdrawal syndrome for the substance;
   - the same or a closely related substance taken to relieve or avoid withdrawal symptoms.
3. The substance is often taken in larger amounts or over a longer period than was intended.
4. There is a persistent desire or unsuccessful efforts to cut down or control substance use.
5. A great deal of time is spent in activities necessary to obtain the substance (e.g. visiting multiple doctors or driving long distances), use of the substance (e.g. chain smoking) or recovering from its effects.
6. Important social, occupational or recreational activities are given up or reduced because of substance use.

- Spending a great deal of time attempting to acquire the drug.
- Continuing to use the drug even though the person knows there are reoccurring physical or psychological problems being caused by the drug [7].

Addiction to alcohol and/or drugs, however, refers to a very small percentage of people who have problems with substance use [8]. It is more advisable to classify problematic substance use in different ways. The terms used are on a continuum that extends from abstinence to hazardous use and dependence [9]. In general, the greater the frequency of use and the greater the amount of substances consumed per occasion, the more severe the consequences for the individual's health, the psychosocial consequences and the risk of dependence [10].

Risk levels of alcohol use

The Australian Alcohol Guidelines developed by the National Health and Medical Research Council outline the level of risk associated with patterns of alcohol consumption:

- *Low risk* – Up to two standard drinks per day for females and up to four standard drinks per day for males. This includes at least two alcohol-free days per week for both males and females.

- *Risky* – Three to four standard drinks per day for females and five to six standard drinks per day for males.
- *High risk* – Five or more standard drinks daily for females and seven or more drinks for males [11].

Note: The Australian Alcohol Guidelines are currently under review at the time of writing this chapter.

Hazardous use is a form of repetitive pattern of use that poses a risk of harmful physical and psychological consequences (potential problems). Some examples are at-risk behaviours such as sharing needles and using substances when operating machinery.

Harmful use is when the pattern of substance use is actually causing harm.

Substance abuse is a term often associated with the term addiction and as such is considered to be value laden and has limited use in contemporary addiction literature [5]. The focus needs to be on the social, interpersonal, legal and failure in role obligations consequences of the individual's substance use.

Dependence is the persistent use of a substance despite negative consequences. Dependence can be both physical and psychological and is discussed in the section on addiction in this chapter.

Alcohol withdrawal

People who use large amounts of alcohol on a regular basis may experience withdrawal symptoms when they stop or reduce their drinking. Alcohol withdrawal is a syndrome of central nervous system (CNS) hyperactivity characterised by symptoms that indicate the severity of the withdrawal. Withdrawal can be classified as mild, moderate or severe [12].

Mild withdrawal from alcohol

The following signs and symptoms may occur within 24 h and subside 48 h after stopping or substantially reducing alcohol intake:

- Mild sweating.
- Mild anxiety.
- Mild dehydration.
- Headaches.
- Mild hypertension.
- Insomnia.
- Tachycardia.
- Dyspepsia.
- Malaise.
- Slight tremor [12].

Moderate withdrawal from alcohol

The following signs and symptoms may occur within 24 h and subside 72 h after stopping or substantially reducing alcohol intake:

- Moderate anxiety (will respond to reassurance).
- Dehydration.
- Hyperventilation and panic attacks.
- Moderate sweating.
- Diarrhoea.
- Dyspepsia.
- Anorexia.
- Headaches.
- Mild-to-moderate hypertension (diastolic reading of 100–110 mm Hg).
- Insomnia.
- Nausea and vomiting.
- Mild tremor.
- Weakness [12].

Severe withdrawal from alcohol

The following signs and symptoms may occur within 24 h or may be delayed until 48 h after stopping or substantially reducing alcohol intake. Further delays in onset may be caused by the administration of other CNS depressants (opioid analgesia or anaesthetics). The usual course of withdrawal is 3 days, but may be up to 14 days.

- Acute anxiety (may not respond to reassurance).
- Hyperventilation and panic.
- Agitation.
- Convulsions.
- Dehydration.
- Excessive sweating.
- Diarrhoea.
- Disorientation (for time and place).
- Fever.
- Hallucinations (auditory, tactile or visual).
- Sensory hyperacuity.
- Moderate-to-severe hypertension (danger sign is diastolic pressure greater than 120 mm Hg) or hypotension.
- Tachycardia.
- Marked tremor.
- Withdrawal seizures can be lethal. They are preventable [12].

Delirium tremens

The most serious withdrawal involves the individual experiencing delirium tremens (DTs). The community nurse needs to be able to recognise symptoms and intervene or refer on appropriately, when necessary.

DT is the most severe form of alcohol withdrawal syndrome and is a medical emergency. It usually develops 2–5 days after stopping or significantly reducing alcohol consumption, but may take 7 days to appear. The usual course is 3 days, but it can take up to 14 days. Symptoms include:

- Exaggerated symptoms of simple alcohol withdrawal (in 75% of cases).
- Autonomic instability (e.g. fluctuations in blood pressure or pulse), disturbance of fluid balance and electrolytes, hyperthermia.
- Extreme agitation or restlessness – the patient may require restraining.
- Gross tremor.
- Confusion and disorientation.
- Paranoid ideation typically of delusional intensity.
- Hallucinations affecting any of the senses, but typically visual (highly coloured, animal form) [12].

People with a mental illness and problematic drug and/or alcohol use

It is becoming increasingly difficult to separate those who are homeless related to their drug and/or alcohol use and those who are homeless because of an existing mental illness and also problematic drug and/or alcohol use. We do know that people with problematic drug or alcohol use and schizophrenia are less likely to remain in stable accommodation than those without drug and alcohol problems [13]. The terms 'dual diagnosis', 'comorbidity' or 'coexisting disorder' are used interchangeably to describe someone who has a mental illness and a substance-use disorder [7]. The prevalence rates for dual diagnosis vary significantly, but it is generally agreed that approximately 50% of individuals with a severe mental illness have a dual diagnosis [14, 15]. There is national evidence to suggest that people with a serious mental illness, including those with a dual diagnosis, have poor physical health and poor levels of health treatment [16, 17], which in term means that the community nurse is more likely to be involved in their care. These findings have also been demonstrated in international studies [18, 19].

What can be done to minimise the risks associated with homelessness?

There are several strategies that have proved to be successful and some of these are presented in the following section.

Health promotion approach (early intervention)

One obvious intervention to prevent homelessness is to assist people, before they lose their accommodation, through financial counselling, emergency relief or application for public housing.

Drug and alcohol management programmes

Studies reveal that if community mental health services or primary health services are accessible, homeless people will use and benefit from such treatment and support [6, 20, 21]. Accessible treatment options for substance use are critical, but have been found to be not readily available or accessible. Treatment services need to reflect the experiences and needs of the homeless person. Underlying the success of treatment to these vulnerable groups is the need for comprehensive service provision, which includes a range of housing options with flexible support [6, 20, 21].

Community impact programmes

Supportive networks including care and community integration (look at models of intersectoral collaboration). For example community detoxification programmes involve the community drug and alcohol services as well as the hospital sector (emergency departments) and the relevant general practitioners.

Brief intervention

Intervention at an early stage of a person's alcohol or drug use aims to prevent the development of serious drug-use problems. A brief intervention is defined as 'a treatment strategy in which a short structured therapy is offered (between 5 min and 2 h), on one occasion or spread over several visits. It is aimed at helping a person to reduce or stop substance use' [12, p. 87]. There is strong evidence of the effectiveness of using brief intervention for alcohol and tobacco use, and the evidence for its effectiveness for other substances is growing [10, 22]. Although brief intervention is generally not designed to treat serious substance abuse or dependence, it can be a very valuable instrument for encouraging people into more intensive treatment [23].

During the past 20 years, there have been numerous randomised clinical trials of brief intervention in a variety of health care settings. Studies have been conducted in Australia, Bulgaria, Mexico, the United Kingdom, Norway, Sweden, the United States and many other countries. Evidence for the effectiveness of brief intervention has been well researched and widely published [22].

One of the earliest review articles published about brief intervention [24] was a meta-analysis of 32 controlled studies involving over 6000 patients. The report indicated that brief intervention was often as effective as more extensive treatments and suggested that harmful alcohol use can be effectively altered in relatively brief-contact contexts, such as in primary health care settings [24]. These initial findings have been supported by other researchers [25–27].

Types of brief interventions

One of the easiest brief interventions that can be undertaken is through the use of a self-report screening tool, such as the Alcohol-use disorders identification (AUDIT) screening instrument. It takes only a few minutes to complete and score. It has reliability across cultural groups and a range of specific populations including women, psychiatric patients, university students and the unemployed [28].

The AUDIT is a self-report measure comprising ten items, which are scored by adding each of the items. Items 1–8 are scored on a 0–4 scale and items 9 and 10 are scored 0, 2 or 4. A score of 8 or above is used to indicate the presence of alcohol problems, but it may be advisable to have a lower cut-off point of 4 for women. The AUDIT is in the public domain and is reproduced in Box 10.3. A copy of the AUDIT and guidelines are available free of charge from the World Health Organization (WHO) website http:www.who.int/publications/en/.

Box 10.3   Alcohol-use disorders identification test [28, p. 1]

AUDIT screening instrument

Please circle the answer that is correct for you.

1. How often do you have a drink containing alcohol?
   Never
   Monthly or less
   Two to four times a month
   Two to three times a week
   Four or more times a week

2. How many drinks containing alcohol do you have on a typical day when you are drinking?
   One or two
   Three or four
   Five or six
   Seven to nine
   Ten or more

3. How often do you have six or more drinks on one occasion?
   Never
   Less than monthly
   Monthly
   Weekly
   Daily or almost daily

4. How often have you found that you were not able to stop drinking once you had started?
   Never
   Less than monthly
   Monthly
   Weekly
   Daily or almost daily

5. How often during the last year have you failed to do what was normally expected of you because of drinking?
   Never
   Less than monthly
   Monthly
   Weekly
   Daily or almost daily

6. How often during the last year have you needed a first drink in the morning to get yourself going after a heavy drinking session?
   Never
   Less than monthly
   Monthly
   Weekly
   Daily or almost daily

7. How often during the last year have you had a feeling of guilt or remorse after drinking?
   Never

Less than monthly
Monthly
Weekly
Daily or almost daily

8. How often during the last year have you been unable to remember what happened the night before because you had been drinking?
Never
Less than monthly
Monthly
Weekly
Daily or almost daily

9. Have you or someone else been injured as a result of your drinking?
No
Yes, but not in the last year
Yes, during the last year

10. Has a relative or friend or a doctor or other health worker been concerned about your drinking or suggested you cut down?
No
Yes, but not in the last year
Yes, during the last year

Although cut-off points are indicative of risk, they are not based on sufficient evidence to be normative for all groups or individuals. Clinical judgement must be used to identify situations in which the AUDIT score might not represent the full level of risk [22]. However, guidelines serve a useful starting point (see Box 10.4).

How can the community nurse keep accurate records of a homeless client?

Information systems are important to community health. The Community Health Information Management Enterprise (CHIME) is an example of a clinical information

Box 10.4   AUDIT cut-off scores[a] [22, p. 2]

Risk level	Intervention	AUDIT score*
Zone I	Alcohol education	0–7
Zone II	Simple advice	8–15
Zone III	Simple advice plus brief counselling and continued monitoring	16–19
Zone IV	Referral to specialist for diagnostic evaluation and treatment	20–40

[a] The AUDIT cut-off scores may vary slightly, depending on the country's drinking patterns, the alcohol content of standard drinks and the nature of the screening programme. Consult the AUDIT manual for details. Clinical judgement should be exercised in the interpretation of screening test results to modify these guidelines, especially when AUDIT scores are in the range of 15–20.

system designed to improve service delivery, outcome measures and productivity through improved capture and management of community-based health service (CBHS) information. It is also intended to improve the mechanisms for reporting at the local area, state and national levels, thereby improving the quality of available community health information and the efficiency with which it is produced. The CHIME project was initiated in 1996 and is a joint venture between NSW Health, Queensland Health, the South Australian Department of Health and ACT Health and Community Care [29].

Benefits for service providers and community nurses

Information systems have many potential benefits. They enable community-based health care staff to accurately document the assessment of clients, develop individualised management plans based on best-practice principles, monitor outcomes of clinical care and generate reports for client and management reporting.

Through the use of an information system such as CHIME, the community nurse can:

- Assist with the development of efficient processes for recording client information across the health system. These processes help to eliminate duplicated recording of demographic data for clients.
- Track referrals, appointments and service contacts.
- Provide real-time information, by storage and retrieval of client case management information. This enables information to be transferred to other community-based health professionals who are consulting with a client and enables staff to spend more time on case management.

Information systems can also:

- Enable community-based health staff to develop 'clinical practice norms' and case management guidelines and measures to assess the effectiveness of their services.
- Enable the collection of workload indicators for community-based health staff. This provides measures to assess service efficiency and costs to assist in resource allocation and management.
- Facilitate the introduction of a 'case-mix-type' classification system and benchmarking for CBHS [30].

Benefits for health authorities

Adopting information systems with this client group brings benefits for health authorities and ultimately for the community nurse and the client. These benefits include:

- A reduction in clinician time dedicated to clerical work.
- Rapid responses to changing health care needs.
- Provision of multidisciplinary service delivery.
- Improved service planning and targeting.

- Improved understanding of the health and needs of the community.
- Minimisation of duplicated effort and functionality.
- Best-practice pathways (clinical practice guidelines).
- Improved management of information between (and within) each health authority.
- Outcome measurement [30].

What can the community nurse do to help homeless people?

Community nurses need to recognise that homeless people are 'fringe dwellers' – i.e. they are on the fringes of society – and they are a marginalised group. It is also important that nurses do not lose sight of the care aspect in nursing this group, as nursing procedures become more technologically based [31, p. 309].

The primary aim of nursing care for those who are homeless should be to support the individuals in developing self-efficacy and confidence, as this will enable them to identify their individual health needs and have the confidence to accept health care. Care needs to:

- Be person focused.
- Have the ability to integrate multiple services.
- Have fluid targets.
- Be open to individualised learning styles.
- Be aimed at the normalisation of the individual [32, pp. 212–15]. Normalisation infers the ability to function within society norms, for example the ability to maintain personal hygiene, eat regular nutritious meals, maintain accommodation in a clean manner.

This requires that community nurses be extremely flexible in their approach to, and management of, the health issues of the homeless person. Many homeless people have nocturnal habits and a high participation in risky behaviours such as prostitution, crime and substance abuse. For example it has been reported that homeless youth will sell sex to enable themselves to buy food [33]. The homeless are also 'generally isolated, poor and unwell' [33, p. 34]. The community nurse needs to be resilient to deal with the homeless person's chronicity of health and social issues. A clinician's story is detailed in Box 10.5.

The WHO has identified 'poverty as the greatest threat to health ... [and] ... the overall level of illness is much higher among the poor' [34, p. 75]. An individual's health behaviour is determined by many factors including sociological, psychological and environmental influences. It has been reported that lower socioeconomic groups have lower expectations of health and a fatalistic attitude to health and therefore take more risky health behaviours and choices [34, p. 77].

If one refers to Maslow's hierarchy of needs [35], the need for food and shelter is the base on which all else is built. If these needs are not met then an individual cannot develop, and this will have a major impact on their biopsychosocial health. Therefore the community nurse should develop an awareness of the common health problems of the homeless, the barriers to their accessing basic health care services and the development of alternative methods of health care delivery for them. The commonest health issues related to homelessness are [36]:

- Lack of access to facilities to maintain good basic hygiene.
- Feelings of despair and hopelessness.
- Poverty.
- Lack of education.
- Poor diet and nutritional intake.
- Seizure disorders.
- Diabetes.
- Upper respiratory tract infections.
- Dermatitis and skin disorders and infections.
- Disorders of the feet.
- Fungal infections.
- Sexually transmitted infections.
- Substance abuse.
- Mental health issues.
- Hepatitis.
- Inadequate shelter.
- Poor dental health.
- Trauma.
- Pregnancy.
- Physical and sexual victimisation.
- Social isolation.
- Chronic wounds, wound infection and wound infestations (e.g. maggots).
- Parasites such as lice, fleas and scabies.

The basic need for shelter and food is severely compromised within the homeless population. The lack of food security leads to an increased risk of disease and is strongly linked to poverty in Australia [37]. Many homeless people depend on charitable organisations to provide them with a daily meal, as they may have insufficient

---

Box 10.5   A clinician's story

Whilst working in a remote area of New South Wales where the majority of the population were Indigenous persons, I was the early childhood health nurse. The usual clinics ran Monday to Friday from 0900 to 1630 h. I found there was a poor attendance at the clinics and my observation was that there were many Indigenous children who had ear problems, were not adequately immunised and had issues with gastrointestinal parasitic load. I discussed these issues with the local Indigenous health worker. She pointed out that the clinic hours were mostly in the day when temperatures soared to above 40°C and therefore the Indigenous people would not come out (sounded good to me). Therefore I approached the health service manager to alter my clinic hours to run 3 days a week from 1500 to 2100 h. This was agreed to and a local general practitioner was also available during these hours if needed. This small change resulted in a marked increase in attendance at the early childhood health clinic and improvements in ear problems, immunisations and parasitic management.

funds to purchase food. This lack of food and resulting poor nutrition may have serious implications for young women who may be pregnant and their subsequent children. The homeless person may not have skills in purchasing food or the preparation of food. Therefore the community nurse may be responsible for seeking out and referring homeless individuals to support services which will develop these skills.

Homelessness is also associated with an increased risk of communicable diseases. Immunisations are now available for many communicable diseases and therefore would reduce the risk of illness in those who are homeless. However, access to immunisation programmes may be difficult for the homeless. One way to address this may be to develop outreach immunisation programmes to improve the immunisation level of homeless people, particularly for those living in remote areas of Australia. Such a programme has been found to be successful in Vancouver [38].

Barriers to health care

Barriers to health care for the homeless include financial considerations, bureaucratic processes, programmatic issues and personal behaviour and beliefs. Daiski (2007) reported that the homeless person has a very negative perspective in relation to their health [39]. The homeless have identified specific barriers to health care. These include access to and cost of transport, lack of transport, fear of having possessions stolen and inconvenient clinic hours [39]. Community nurses and health care services have to be flexible to facilitate better access to health care by the homeless or other marginalised groups.

A qualitative study involving 24 adults in a Canadian city was undertaken to investigate the homeless person's perspective on their health and health care needs [39]. Data were collected via a semi-structured interview. The reported findings included:

- Health problems, mainly chronic illnesses, were exacerbated by poverty and the homeless lifestyle.
- Having an adequate and sustainable income was a great concern.
- Lack of privacy led to low self-esteem.
- Participants feared for their safety.
- All participants reported emotional distress.
- Many participants felt socially isolated, excluded and invisible.

Recommendations from this small study were that nursing education should include care of marginalised persons and that the goal of nursing care should be the reintegration of homeless individuals into the community [39].

Homeless people have reported the need for health care professionals to treat them with respect and dignity, to maintain confidentiality, avoid the use of jargon and be non-judgemental [34, 35]. These expressed feelings from homeless people support the need for community nurses to be 'culturally' competent and for policies for the homeless to involve input from homeless individuals themselves.

With the development of technological advances to support health care such as telemedicine, there are now options available to enable services to be taken to people and ensure a high standard of care. One such option is mobile vans which take health care to the community and these have been utilised with great benefit to the homeless.

One such service in Connecticut in the United States was utilised to assess the effectiveness of human immunodeficiency virus (HIV) and sexually transmitted infection (STI) screening. A total of 712 people visited the van over a period of 8 months, with a total of 1177 occasions of service. Occasions of service included HIV-related concerns, substance-abuse concerns, STIs, respiratory problems, hypertension, TB testing and immunisations [40]. The majority of people attending the van were non-white, unemployed, poorly educated and homeless [34].

In Australia, the Greens political party has called for the development of mobile medical clinics especially in relation to rural and remote communities and low-income groups. They further suggest that these mobile medical clinics target health issues such as mental health, substance-abuse issues, dental services and Indigenous health [41].

Recommendations for research and practice

- Maximise any current positive health care behaviour in the homeless person.
- Recognise that the period in early substance-abuse recovery is an optimal time to promote healthy behaviours, such as lifestyle modification and health screening.
- Investigate the need to educate those who work with the homeless in health-promoting skills.
- Acknowledge and implement strict confidentiality in any dealings with the homeless person in relation to their health care [42].
- Focus on primary health care.
- Provide a therapeutic relationship which builds trust with the homeless.
- Provide screening and education services.
- Recognise that there is a need for both drug and alcohol and mental health first-aid education for community nurses.
- Recognise the need for good triage and assessment skills for community nurses as substance-abuse/psychiatric disorders may mask other medical conditions/events.

Conclusion

The homeless population has a multitude of health issues; they do not trust health professionals and they have nocturnal habits. All of these factors impact on the ability of health service providers to deliver basic health care to this population. However, it is possible to deliver a high standard of health care which is appropriate to the needs of the homeless as long as the nurse has flexibility in the delivery of services and has the resilience to cope with the chronicity of the health and social issues which plague the homeless person. Community nurses should recognise that assessment, interpretation of assessment findings and the implementation of sustainable and appropriate nursing care are essential elements of caring for the homeless.

From the information presented in this chapter, it is clear that even in a country such as Australia that has a universal health care system, a comprehensive social security system and is internationally known as an affluent and democratic society, a large number of the population are homeless or have insecure housing. Homeless people are amongst the most marginalised in society and most are marginalised because of their mental illness, alcohol and other drug issues or because of being an Indigenous Australian.

Homelessness affects all ages and is a difficult and complex issue. The prevention of homelessness and the provision of adequate housing and access to appropriate health care are crucial social and health policy challenges facing Australia. Federal, state and territory governments have responded to this challenge, and since May 2000 The National Homelessness Strategy has developed a framework for future policy. As a community nurse there is still much to do. It is hoped that some of the suggestions and information presented here will be helpful in going some way towards meeting the needs of this complex and vulnerable group.

Useful resources

Alcohol Audit Screening Test at http://www.therightmix.gov.au/pdfs/HealthProviderAUDIT.pdf
Guardianship Act at http://www.health.wa.gov.au/mhareview/resources/legislation/NSW_Guardianship_Act_1987.pdf
Rehabilitation and recovery services at http://www.health.nsw.gov.au/policy/cmh/publications/pdf/rehabilitation.pdf
South Eastern Sydney and Illawarra Health demographics at http://sesiweb/PPPdatainformation/demography/census/census_summary.asp

References

1. Chamberlain, C. and Mackenzie, D. (2003) *Counting the Homeless 2001*. Australian Bureau of Statistics, Canberra. Cat. no. 2050.
2. Department of Health and Ageing (2006) *Homelessness and Mental Health Linkages: Review of National and International Literature*. Commonwealth of Australia, Canberra.
3. Chamberlain, C. (1999) *Counting the Homeless: Implications for Policy Development*. Australian Bureau of Statistics, Canberra.
4. Lipmann, B., Mirabelli, F. and Rota-Bartlink, A. (2004) *Homelessness Among Older People: A Comparative Study in Three Countries of Prevention and Alleviation*. Wintringham. Available at http://www.vaada.org.au/resources/items/2007/03/140088-upload-00001.pdf (viewed 16 April 2007).
5. Hussein Rassool, G. (2002) *Dual Diagnosis, Substance Misuse and Psychiatric Disorders*. Blackwell Science, Oxford.
6. Herman, H. and Neil, C. (1996) Homelessness and mental health: Lessons from Australia, in D. Bhugra (ed.) *Homelessness and Mental Health*. Cambridge University Press, London, pp. 244–64.
7. American Psychological Association (2000). *Diagnostic and Statistical Manual of Mental Disorders*, 4th edition. American Psychological Association, Washington DC.
8. Blume, A. (ed.) (2005) *Treating Drug Problems*. John Wiley and Sons, New Jersey.
9. Saunders, J. and Young, R. (2002) Assessment and diagnosis, in G. Hulse, J. White and G. Cape (eds) *Management of Alcohol and Drug Problems*. Oxford University Press, Melbourne.
10. Curtis, J. (2005) Substance-related disorders and dual diagnosis, in R. Elder, K. Evans and D. Nizette (eds) *Psychiatric and Mental Health Nursing*. Elsevier, Marrickville, pp. 304–23.

11. National Health and Medical Research Council (1999) *A Guide to the Development, Implementation and Evaluation of Clinical Practice Guidelines*. National Health and Medical Research Council, Canberra.

12. NSW Health Department (2000) *Alcohol and Other Drugs Policy for Nursing Practice in NSW: Clinical Guidelines 2000–2003*. Better Health Centre – Publications Warehouse, Gladesville.

13. Caton, C., Shrout, P., Eagle, P., Opler, L. and Felix, A. (1994) Correlates of co-disorders in homeless and never homeless indigent schizophrenic men. *Psychological Medicine*, 24, 681–8.

14. Alverson, H., Alverson, M., Drake, R.E. (2000) Addiction services: An ethnographic study of the longitudinal course of substance abuse among people with severe mental illness. *Community Mental Health Journal*, 36(6), 557–69.

15. Brunette, M., Drake, R., Woods, M. and Hartnett, T. (2001) A comparison of long-term and short-term residential treatment programs for dual diagnosis patients. *Psychiatric Services*, 52(4), 461–4.

16. Jablensky, A., McGrath, J., Herman, H., Castle, D., Gureje, O. and Morgan, V. (1999) *National Survey of Mental Health and Wellbeing: Report 4. People Living with Psychotic Illness: An Australian Study*. Commonwealth Department of Health and Aged Care, Canberra.

17. Lawrence, D., Coghlan, R., Holman, D. and Jablensky, A. (2001) *Duty to Care: Physical Illness in People with Mental Illness*. University of Western Australia and Department of Public Health, Perth.

18. Chafetz, L., White, M., Collins-Bride, G. and Nickens, J. (2005) *The Poor General Health of the Severely Mentally Ill: Impact of Schizophrenic Diagnosis*. University of California, California.

19. Jones, D., Macias, C., Barreira, P., Fisher, W., Hargreaves, W. and Harding, C. (2004) Prevalence, severity and co-occurrence of chronic physical health problems of persons with serious mental illness. *Psychiatric Services*, 55, 1250–57.

20. Buhrich, N. and Teesson, M. (1996) Impact of a psychiatric outreach service for homeless persons with schizophrenia. *Psychiatric Services*, 47(6), 644–6.

21. Herman, H. (1999) Homelessness in mentally ill people: Understanding the risks and service needs. *The Journal of the Mental Health Foundation of Australia*, 1(1), 7–16.

22. Babor, T.F. and Higgins-Biddle, J.C. (2001) *Brief intervention for Hazardous and Harmful Drinking: A Manual for Use in Primary Care*. Department of Health and Substance Dependence, World Health Organization, Geneva.

23. Henry, S., Humeniuk, R., Ali, R., Monteiro, M. and Poznyak, V. (2003) *Brief Intervention for Substance Use: A Manual for Use in Primary Care* (Draft version 1.1 for Field Testing). World Health Organization, Geneva, Switzerland.

24. Bien, T.H., Miller,W.R. and Tonnigan, S. (1993) Brief interventions for alcohol problems: A review. *Addiction*, 88, 315–36.

25. Kahan, M., Wilson, L. and Becker, L. (1995) Effectiveness of physician-based interventions with problem drinkers: A review. *Canadian Medical Association Journal*, 152(6), 851–9.

26. Moyer, A., Finney, J., Swearingen, C. and Vergun, P. (2002) Brief interventions for alcohol problems: A meta-analytic review of controlled investigations in treatment seeking and non-treatment seeking populations. *Addiction*, 97(3), 279–92.

27. Wilk, A. and Jensen, N.T.H. (1997) Meta-analysis of randomized control trials addressing brief interventions in heavy alcohol drinkers. *Journal of General Internal Medicine*, 12, 183–274.

28. World Health Organization (1992) AUDIT: The alcohol use disorders identification test. *Guidelines for Use in Primary Health Care*. World Health Organization, Geneva.

29. The Community Health Information Management Enterprise (2007) Available at http://www.health.nsw.gov/au/asd/chime/chime/overview/index.html (viewed 17 April 2007).

30. NSW Department of Health (2006) *A New Direction for Mental Health*. Available at http://www.health.nsw.gov.au/pubs/2006/pdf/mental_health.pdf (viewed 14 April 2007).

31. Wright, C. (2005) Tomorrow's world: Our youth a global issue. *Community Practice*, 78(9), 309–11.

32. Crome, S. and Barton, S. (2003) The lighthouse foundation. *Contemporary Nurse*, 14(2), 211–16.

33. Tschirren, R., Hammett, K. and Saunders, P. (1996) *Sex for Favours: On the Job Youth Project*. Sex Industry Network, Adelaide.

34. Swinnerton, S. (2006) Living in poverty and its effects on health. *Contemporary Nurse*, 22(1), 75–80.

35. Maslow, A. (1954) *Motivation and Personality*. Harper, New York.

36. O'Sullivan, J. and Lussier-Duynstee, P. (2006) Adolescent homelessness, nursing and public health policy. *Policy Politics and Nursing Practice*, 7(1), 73–7.

37. Booth, S. and Smith, A. (2001) Food security and poverty in Australia – challenges for dieticians. *Australian Journal of Nutrition and Dietetics*, 58(3), 150–56.

38. Weatherill, S., Buxton, J. and Daly, P. (2004) Immunisations in non-traditional settings. *Canadian Journal of Public Health*, 95(2), 133–7.

39. Daisk, I. (2007) Perspectives of homeless people on their health and health needs. *Journal of Advanced Nursing*, 58(3), 273–81.

40. Leibman, J., Lamberti, M. and Altice, F. (2002) Effectiveness of a mobile van in providing screening services for STDs and HIV. *Public Health Nursing*, 19(5), 345–53.

41. Greens Party (2007) Available at http://nsw.greens.org.au/media-centre/news-releases/state-of-the-art-mobile-medical-clinics-for-rural-nsw (viewed 15 March 2007).

42. Swigart, V. and Kolb, R. (2004) Homeless persons' decisions to accept or reject public health disease-detection services. *Public Health Nursing*, 21(2), 162–70.

Chapter 11

Continence

Norah Bostock and Carolyn Roe

Introduction

Stigma and shame surround adult incontinence, so it can be devastating for a person to live with the threat of being publicly incontinent. Community nurses however can make a profound difference in the lives of people who are living with continence issues. The aim of this chapter is to identify the essential elements for continence promotion when working with people experiencing incontinence, including assessment and management of incontinence across the human lifespan, and to determine intervention points for the community nurse that will enhance a client's quality of life (QOL). This chapter concludes with discussion on future trends likely to impact on the provision of continence care for Australian populations with a specific focus on community clients.

Background

Incontinence is a common health issue that affects many Australians [1]. Prevalence data vary, but a 2006 report revealed that 24% of Australians experience urinary incontinence and 35% experience faecal incontinence [1]. Approximately 65% of these people were living in the community [2]. Continence is a major community health issue and continence promotion a common community nurse role.

More common in older people [3], urinary incontinence is a mortality factor [4] and predictor for institutionalisation [5–7]. Myths and misconceptions abound regarding incontinence [8], especially in older people. However, the impact of incontinence on health-related QOL is undeniable [5, 6, 9] and fiscal expenditure on incontinence can be evaluated in terms of economic, physical, psychosocial and relational terms [1, 9]. Incontinence occurs across the lifespan, across socioeconomic and cultural groups and in both genders [1]. There are social implications and stigma attached to incontinence [10], which can be reasons that people do not seek help [11]; hence, underreporting may be a factor in prevalence data.

Children, teenagers and young adults living with incontinence or enuresis require additional support, nurturing, understanding and encouragement to tackle multiple issues relating to identity, peer pressure and physical/psychological development, to ensure that they are well equipped to mature to their full potential and self-manage into the future.

Examining contributing factors in help-seeking behaviours allows health professionals to target interventions appropriately [12]. Some of these behaviours extend from:

- Concerns about discussing intimate issues with a general practitioner (GP) of a particular gender.
- The freedom to choose not to treat incontinence.
- Difficulties in accessing designated services in rural/remote areas where clients may consider travel to the city too expensive or time consuming.

With global refugee, immigrant and Indigenous migrations, community nurses will be sensitive to ethnic, cultural and environmental diversity [13] and how these factors impact on help-seeking behaviours. Often social norms in culturally and linguistically diverse minority groups lead to a natural reticence to discuss incontinence outside of the home especially when unusual life events occur [14], disturbing the balance of family relationships [15–17], e.g. younger-generation migrant children wishing to pursue independent lives instead of caring for parents in a traditional fashion. Traditional perceptions of the expected patterns of continence are based on generations of beliefs, fears, expectations and myths [18–22].

With the Western world experiencing an increasing trend in caring for people at home, caregiving can become extremely stressful, yet the caregiver burden specific to continence has not been quantitatively or qualitatively measured on any test or scale [9, 10]. Nursing practice models that are cognizant of all community environments are needed to ensure equity of continence care not only across the human lifespan but also across the geographical/environmental landscape [23–25].

Anatomy and physiology

Urinary system

The aims of this section are to revise normal bladder and bowel function and system dysfunction. It is vital for community nurses to understand bladder dysfunction as it may be the key to a number of underlying comorbidities, e.g. diabetes, pelvic tumours or hormonal imbalances.

The urinary system is responsible for secretion, conveyance, storage and excretion of urine [2, 5, 26, 27] (see Figure 11.1).

- The kidneys lie retroperitoneal and secrete urine via functional units called nephrons. The ureter, blood vessels, lymphatics and nerves congregate within the renal sinus.
- Ureters are thin hollow tubes 25 cm long, commencing at L2 and descending retroperitoneal. They enter obliquely into the posterior bladder wall, which prevents urinary backflow during the bladder-filling phase. Peristaltic-like contractions transport urine via the ureter to the bladder.

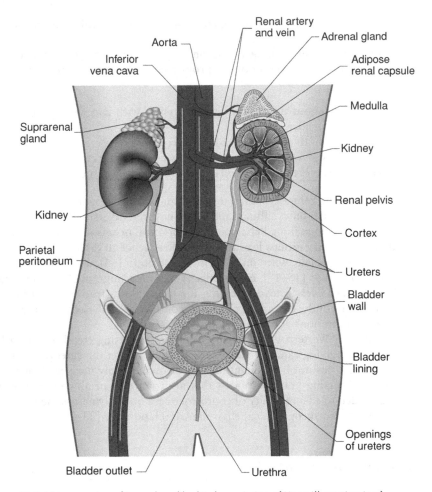

Figure 11.1 Urinary system. [Reproduced by kind permission of Kopp Illustration Inc.]

- The bladder is a smooth collapsible sac situated in the true pelvis, posterior to the pubic symphysis but in front of the other contents, acting as a urinary reservoir (approximately 500-mL capacity, which may be palpated externally when full). The bladder comprises:
  - outer serous coat (peritoneal extension),
  - detrusor muscle,
  - submucosal coat and
  - mucosal lining (transitional epithelium), which collapses when empty into folds known as rugae that disappear as the bladder fills.

Parasympathetic fibres, arising from S2 to S4, infiltrate the detrusor via the pelvic splanchnic nerves acting as a relay centre, providing information about the bladder. This is called the spinal micturition centre, which is vulnerable to dysfunction due to its low siting.

Central nervous system control of bladder function is directed from three main areas:

- Cortical – inhibits detrusor contractions.
- Pontine micturition centre – integrates detrusor contraction and urethral relaxation, potentially acting as a form of 'neural' switch between storage and voiding.
- Sacral centre – spinal reflex mechanisms are usually only found in babies or adults where a spinal cord injury above S2–S4 has occurred; failure of the detrusor – sphincter coordination is termed 'dyssynergy'.

The urethra is innervated via the somatic nerve, with the pudendal nerve conveying motor and sensory impulses to the sphincter to act during micturition. It is different for males and females:

- Female urethra is 3–4 cm long: tightly bound to the anterior vaginal wall exiting via the urethral orifice.
- Male urethra is 20–23 cm long, comprising:
  - prostatic 4–5 cm long;
  - membranous 1–2 cm long;
  - spongy/penile 15–16 cm long.

Control of micturition is usually learnt during childhood. The act of micturition (the balance maintained between urinary storage and voiding) depends on the transmission of 'bladder fullness' sensation via sensory nerves, which are sensitive to stretch. As urine accumulates, stretch sensitive sensory nerves trigger 'stretch receptors' that send signals via afferent nerves to the spinal micturition centre to:

- Increase detrusor inhibition keeping the internal sphincter temporarily closed.
- Transmit impulses to the brain creating an urge to void.
- Activate the pontine micturition centre.

Once voiding impulses are urgent and voiding is desirable, pelvic floor and urethral sphincter voluntary muscles relax followed by detrusor contraction, allowing urine to flow. Normal voiding suppression occurs via pathways from the cortical and pontine centres. After normal micturition a postvoid residual of 20–50 mL is left [5].

Gastrointestinal system (Figure 11.2)

The gastrointestinal system comprises the mouth, pharynx, oesophagus and stomach. Usually containing approximately 50 mL, the stomach can distend to accept over 4 L: potentially extending as low as the pelvis. As food enters the stomach, a response termed the gastrocolic reflex is activated, which further stimulates the peristaltic evacuation response. Gastric motility and emptying is accomplished by a unique bidirectional peristalsis [26].

The small intestine is a 2- to 4-m-long muscular tube extending from the pyloric sphincter to the ileocaecal valve. The small intestine is adapted for nutrient absorption, with microscopic anatomy comprising mucosal folds called plicae circulares, villi and microvilli designed to amplify the absorptive surface by a factor of 600 (equating to floor space in a two-storey home).

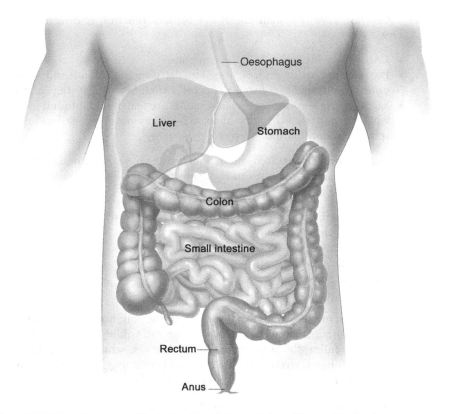

Figure 11.2 Digestive system. [Reproduced by kind permission of Terese Winslow.]

The large intestine extends 1.5 m from the ileocaecal valve to the anal sphincter. It is structurally similar to the stomach and small intestine but contains excreting or goblet cells instead of villi. The large intestine incorporates:

- Caecum.
- Appendix.
- Colon.
- Rectum, which is the lowest 13 cm containing three transverse folds (rectal valves) that prevent faeces being passed along with gas.
- Anus, which is the final 3 cm containing internal (smooth muscle) and external sphincters (skeletal muscle); both are normally closed except during defaecation.

The colon is not designed for further nutrient absorption, but to absorb sufficient fluid, form stools and propel the resultant mass towards the anal canal in preparation for defaecation (usually within 12–24 h). Food eaten today enters the stomach, stimulating colonic peristalsis, propelling yesterday's residue into the pelvic colon; this stimulates strong peristalsis and perianal sensation, intra-abdominal pressure increases, diaphragm and abdominal muscles contract, glottis closure occurs, the anal sphincter relaxes and passage of stools occurs.

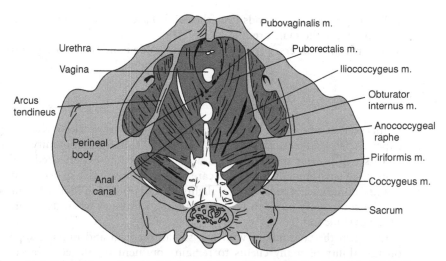

Figure 11.3 Pelvis. [Reproduced by kind permission of Professor LeRoy Heinrich, SUMMIT, Stanford.]

Pelvic floor

The pelvic floor (see Figure 11.3) is a sling-like structure comprising two paired muscles and is composed of muscles, ligaments and fascia stretching from the coccyx to the pubic bone [5, 6, 26, 27]. It plays a role in bladder/bowel control and sexual sensation. The pelvic floor supports:

- Bladder, uterus and bowel posteriorly, and urethra and vagina anteriorly in females.
- Urethra and rectum posteriorly in males.

The two paired muscles are:

- The levator ani – a broad muscle extending inferomedially around the prostate or vagina and anorectal junction. This supports the pelvic viscera during periods of supreme abdominal downward thrust, e.g. coughing, and lifts the anal canal during defaecation. It is innervated via the inferior rectal nerve (pudendal branch) via S4, comprising:
  ○ Pubococcygeus
  ○ Iliococcygeus
  ○ Ischiococcygeus
- Coccygeus is a small triangular muscle forming the posterior floor and supporting pelvic viscera; it pulls the coccyx forwards after posterior reflection incurred during childbirth and defaecation. It is innervated as above through S4 and S5.

The perineal muscles are the:

- Deep transverse perineal muscle – stretches from the ischial rami in females.
- External urethral sphincter muscle – encircles the urethra/vagina and constricts the urethra.
- Ischiocavernosus muscle – stretches from the pelvic base.

- Bulbospongiosus – extends from the penile base and deep to the labia and assists in emptying of the male urethra.
- Superficial transverse perineal – a paired muscle band lying posterior to the urethra.

Common causes of dysfunction

In this section we explore the community nurse's role in working with people who are experiencing bladder and bowel dysfunction. Within the community nurse role many factors will present themselves that are unlikely to be experienced within the more controlled environment of an aged care facility or hospital, e.g. need to mobilise without assistance, negotiating several flights of stairs or living alone. It will be necessary for the community nurse to be cognizant of such issues when determining the cause of the dysfunction.

Living in the community with few social, medical and nursing supports impacts on the ability of many clients to remain continent or indeed to access services to improve their continence status, especially clients living in rural or remote areas [5, 28, 29]. Incontinence may be acute, chronic or transient, depending on the underlying dysfunction. However, no dysfunction is exclusive of another [6] and many are not specific to age.

Factors that cause incontinence include:

Weakened pelvic floor

- Primary tissue or pudendal nerve damage associated with multiple or traumatic births affecting fascial supports and bladder/anal sphincter tone through diminished sensation and loss of movement [2, 5, 26].
- Chronic constipation and straining at stool [6].
- Hormonal imbalances (less likely to occur in women who have not had a hysterectomy), affecting urethral connective tissue volume and cell structure changes [5].
- Surgical procedures causing depletion of muscle strength [2].
- Anorectal dysfunction (anismus) contributing to constipation through pelvic floor dyssynergia (failure of pelvic floor muscles to relax during defaecation) [5].

Impaired neural pathway

Neurons are highly irritable (conductive) and when adequately stimulated will generate an impulse along the length (axon) and consequent interruption potentially causes dysfunction [26]:

- Suprapontine/cerebral lesions, e.g. dementia, cerebrovascular accident, tumours, cerebral palsy, Parkinson's, leave spinal–bulbar–spinal reflexes (S2–S4 control) intact, preserving normal micturition. However, micturition inhibitory reflexes may be lost, resulting in detrusor hyperreflexia. Despite an awareness to void, bladder contraction is unable to be inhibited, potentially resulting in urge incontinence [5]. Also, lowered rectal sensation and lack of cerebral voluntary control potentially

result in constipation and incontinence, because the person is unable to determine when it is socially acceptable to toilet and may withhold or deny the call to stool [6].
- Suprasacral lesions, e.g. multiple sclerosis, compression, injury, myelitis, spina bifida, result in detrusor-sphincter dyssynergy (simultaneous contraction of the detrusor and bladder neck causing retention).

Autonomic dysreflexia

This is a widespread reflex action following uncontrolled stimulation below T6 [5, 6]. Variable bowel effects will predominate, depending on the site of injury [2, 5, 30]:

- High cord produces reduced colonic motility causing constipation.
- Low cord produces increased motility, reduced compliance and rectal instability.
- Sacral lesions, e.g. cauda equina, sacral agenesis, diabetes, surgery, childbirth and pudendal nerve damage produce dual loss of motor supply causing detrusor and rectal areflexia (incomplete emptying), loss of urethral/anal sphincter tone and potential for organ prolapse [5, 6].

Impaired functional/mobility/environmental capacities

This may occur in people who:

- Experience impaired mobility/function/dexterity.
- Experience loss of independence within their home/local community.
- Are environmentally at risk.

These people can develop incontinence, especially if they are unable to readily access or locate toileting facilities or cognitively request directions. For example parents with a child with special needs may be hampered by a lack of facilities to clean and change a child of 6 or 7 years if the child experiences an incontinent episode when shopping. On occasion, the home environment may be a causative factor in an older person's continence issues because of poor lighting, large cluttered furniture and small furry companions underfoot. The community nurse has a role to play in determining whether or not the elderly person is able to care adequately for the animal or if the environment can be modified to include the animal and a clear path to toileting facilities.

Health conditions

Conditions that impact on normal bladder/bowel function may potentiate episodic incontinence especially if linked to any of the conditions discussed in the above section. Elevated economic constraints in the management of multiple medical conditions may lead to community clients, of any age, experiencing challenges in providing appropriate routine self-care, which may exacerbate the medical condition and incontinence.

The community nurse is ideally placed to review and assess environmental, physical and intellectual client self-management and the ability to cope with everyday needs to remain healthy and maintain an optimal QOL. Disease processes affecting organ epithelia and surrounding structures carry higher risk factors and include [2, 5, 6, 31] diabetes, colitis, neoplastic tumours, polyps, diverticular disease, enlarged prostate, urinary tract infection and cystitis or interstitial cystitis.

Endocrine disorders

Postmenopausal decline in oestrogen levels may result in atrophic vaginitis. Thinning and inflammation of the genitourinary tract [28, 32] culminates in urinary incontinence due to urethral incompetence [26].

Diminished antidiuretic hormone (vasopressin) production at night causes poor renal response to water reabsorption resulting in nocturnal enuresis and diabetes insipidus [22, 26]. Nocturnal enuresis or bed-wetting is particularly noticeable in children aged between 5 and 12 years but can persist in young adulthood. Community nurses may assist in the process of regaining continence by ensuring that when referrals are received for people in the young adult age group, they discuss the issue with the person rather than a third party, e.g. parent, carer or support worker, as individual perceptions vary and it is vital to incorporate the person's perspective. Assessments for this group are ideally conducted within the home as subtle nuances relating to family interaction may be missed if the environment is more clinical.

People with diabetes may also be at risk of incontinence because excessive blood glucose levels (BGLs) act as a bladder/bowel irritant and osmotic diuretic causing polyuria and increased colonic motility [5, 6, 26]. It is important not to discard the idea of young children, teenagers and adults being incontinent due to poorly controlled or undiagnosed diabetes. A baseline BGL will exclude this, and it is the authors' practice on home visits to complete this as part of the assessment. All community nurses should have access to, and make use of, a blood glucose monitor to exclude latent diabetes.

Pharmacology

Some classes of drugs potentially cause dysfunctions [33]; therefore, a thorough review of the medication routine of all clients is essential. Review of all medications is particularly important with older people who may purchase over-the-counter products but have little knowledge about medication interactions. For example:

- Antacids – the chalky residue may cause constipation.
- Iron decreases colonic motility.
- Anticholinergics inhibit acetylcholine action on smooth muscle, causing retention due to bladder neck constriction and constipation due to decreased colonic motility.
- Antidepressants have anticholinergic effects.
- Opioids increase colonic resting time, resulting in constipation.
- Diuretics promote fluid loss from the body and increase bladder-filling rate, potentially causing incontinence, dehydration and constipation.

- Antihypertensives promote sphincter relaxation, resulting in loss of anal/urethral sphincter resting tone.
- Sedatives cloud consciousness and mask sensation.
- Caffeine and alcohol enhance detrusor or colonic irritability and lower central inhibition, potentiating diarrhoea and urinary incontinence.
- Excessive aperients taken over extended periods of time potentially slow gut motility, interrupt peristalsis and cause constipation.

Congenital malformations

During the embryonic phase people with Hirschsprung's disease, nerve cells stop growing before maturity, causing reduced gut motility and constipation. Anal atresia is congenital absence or obstruction of the anal opening.

Assessment and continence promotion

In the 'uncontrolled' community environment where clients may make many health and lifestyle choices each day, locating the potential causes of incontinence is important because incontinence can profoundly impact on the health and well-being of the individual, creating social isolation.

Assessment involves working with a client to identify reversible factors, ascertaining presenting symptoms, noting challenging environments/behaviours and developing evidence-based management plans aimed at restoring continence [5, 34–37]. Assessment contains subjective (client perspective) thoughts and objective (assessor) observations to promote a holistic viewpoint. When management plans are developed utilising the principle of working *with* the person, the client can participate in decision making and is cognizant of their role in the plan, melding with their lifestyle and be achievable within the home environment.

A continence assessment aims to identify factors that will lead to intervention that will improve the clients' QOL, decrease the health burden and fiscal expenditure and support help-seeking behaviours [11]. Intolerance and misperceptions (or possibly embarrassment and taboos) regarding incontinence can be extended to people who have less control over bodily functions [7, 8, 14, 18]. Also a range of circumstances including childhood sexual abuse, rape, brutalisation and cognitive, dissociative, social and functional conditions may increase the risk of incontinence exponentially [21]; thus, community intolerance towards incontinence needs to be challenged [23–25]. The community nurse can play a role in this by including general assessment questions about continence issues when a client is admitted to their service. Where the nurse has access to GP rooms or community centres a display of posters or general continence information may be displayed. The community nurse must be cognizant of the movement of special needs groups into the community away from facility-based care, for example people living with mental health disorders (including dementia) and intellectual and physical disabilities [18, 19, 21]. Their approach to continence assessment must remain flexible and prepared to meet a range of social, sexual and psychological issues not traditionally met in facility-based care.

Considerations in assessment are:

Consent

A community nurse must obtain consent to enter the client's home or their presence may be construed as trespass. Clients with cognitive deficits or special needs and culturally diverse groups who may have English as a second language may require additional time and patience at the front door for explanation and interpretation as to the purpose of the nurse's visit [6, 34]. Any nurse who is declined entry into the home should not enter. Conversely, those nurses who have gained entry but are then asked to leave by the client should do so, as consent to remain has been withdrawn and the same interpretation of trespass may be implied. Consent applies to all aspects of the community nurse's visit, as this is the client's home environment. (Further information about this issue is in Chapter 3.)

As an absolute minimum informed consent consists of the following:

- Detailed explanations and clear documentation in the medical notes; otherwise abuse could be construed [34]. Clients declining or unable to sign/comprehend consent are advised that assessment cannot proceed [38].
- Prior to invasive procedures requests for verbal consent should be reiterated and if not provided or if doubt exists examinations should not proceed [5, 6].
- Linguistic variations of consent forms should be made available.
- Cultural diversity extends beyond race and may include religion, gender and generational values. It cannot be overstressed how important it is to ascertain an individual's needs in reference to their cultural background, as people born into one culture or ethnicity may choose or be relegated later in life to adopt secondary values. At the initial assessment the community nurse is unlikely to be aware of people's past history and must approach with tact and caution.
- Children of any age who decline examination or assessment must have their concerns validated and accepted even if parental consent has been given. Potential long-term psychological effects of an examination far outweigh the short-term gain made at assessment [21, 22].

Quality of life

Community clients will find ways to manage their incontinence and still retain what they believe is an excellent QOL. Therefore, what may bother the family may in fact not bother the client, especially if they live alone and the family rarely visits. It is important to discover what elements of the issue bother who and why [2, 6].

Organ dysfunction

Assessment of dysfunction must be detailed because incontinence is deemed a symptomatic illness occurring due to organ/system failure, not a result of ageing [37, 39, 40].

Drug interactions

Certain medications may cause or exacerbate incontinence [41–43]. Ascertain all medications consumed, including over-the-counter, prescribed and home-brewed [44–46].

Community nurses may consider developing alliances with local pharmacists, as home medication reviews (HMR) (a Medicare rebatable service available via selected pharmacists) will provide reassurance that medication interactions are therapeutic.

Continence data

Consideration should be given to the client's ability to maintain records. Obtaining accurate records from some clients may be challenging, as they may not lead regulated or routine lives and may combine data across time periods or days to fit in with their record-keeping abilities. Community clients may, in fact, choose to maintain records in a variety of ways and on a variety of papers so that the community nurse can be intellectually challenged during interpretation, as clarity may not necessarily be optimal.

- Duration/frequency of incontinence may be acute, chronic or transient and indicative of underlying causes [5, 28].
- Elimination patterns [47] may be ascertained objectively via bladder and bowel charts (Figures 11.4 and 11.5) in conjunction with a stool recognition chart (Figure 11.6) and will enable the community nurse to examine and interpret data in meaningful ways [5, 43, 48–50].
- Symptomology may include pain, burning, bleeding, urgency, pre/postelimination loss [23, 24], stool/urine volume, colour/consistency and detrimental triggers [2, 6, 51], indicating pathology and a need for a medical review.

Simple in-home diagnostics can enable the community nurse to establish baseline records [2, 49, 50]:

- Determine postvoid residual using either bladder ultrasound [5, 52, 53] or intermittent catheterisation [5, 28]. The use of an in-home bladder ultrasound is routine and an expectation for all clients in need. It is important to ensure that policies and procedure guiding the safe use of the ultrasound are current and the home environment is conducive to the use of the machine. The same expectation guides the following:
  - Obtain the client's BGL to exclude covert diabetes [6, 28, 52].
  - Check the client's blood pressure to exclude cardiac disease or undiagnosed/long-standing hypertension with potential renal damage [5, 52].
  - Perform a urinalysis to exclude infection, diabetes and renal insufficiency [5].

Complex diagnostics

An abdominal X-ray ordered by the client's GP may confirm impaction or pathology indicating the need for investigation, e.g. colonoscopy [6]. When the community nurse builds a relationship with the GP, it is demonstrated to clients that they have a supportive health team involved in their care and that they may place faith in the relationship, ensuring the best possible outcomes are achieved.

Cognition/language

Issues relating to language barriers and literacy are considerations for the community nurse [34, 42]. A lack of comprehension might impede a client's ability to clarify

✖RDNS
Royal District Nursing Service of SA Inc.

BLADDER CHART

Gender................. PID NUMBER
Title.................
Surname ....
First name ....
Date of Birth...........................*(Affix sticker)*

Instructions

Date: /   /

Choose a day when you plan to be at home. Commence this chart when you first get up in the morning. Complete for 24 hours including:

1. What time you pass urine and how much you pass. Record if you had the urge to pass urine (yes or no)
2. Note if your pad or pants are dry, damp, wet or soaked. Record if you changed your pad or pants
3. What time you have a drink, how much you drink and what you drink
4. In the **COMMENTS** column write down anything that affects your continence such as medications, constipation, running water or physical activity
5. When you finish a 24 hour period, rule it off and start a new day
6. If possible, complete the chart for three full days. They do not have to be consecutive days.

Time	Amount of Urine	? Urge	Damp Wet Soaked	Time	Type of Drink	Amount of Drink	Comments

BLADDER CHART

CR 10.08

NLR0057 02/06

Figure 11.4 Bladder chart. [Reproduced by kind permission of the Royal District Nursing Service – SA Inc.]

BOWEL DIARY/ FREQUENCY AND TYPE

✪RDNS
Royal District Nursing Service of SA Inc.

Gender..................   PID NUMBER

Title..................

Surname ....

First name ....

Date of Birth...........................(*Affix sticker*)

(Using Bristol Stool Scale)

DAY	Record every evacuation & DESCRIPTION (using Bristol Stool Scale 1–7)							Comments/aperients taken etc.
	Before breakfast	After breakfast	Before lunch	After lunch	Before Dinner	After Dinner	Over night	
Mon								
Tue								
Wed								
Thur								
Fri								
Sat								
Sun								
Mon								
Tue								
Wed								
Thur								
Fri								
Sat								
Sun								

Instructions:

1. Check bowel result against the Bristol Stool Scale as illustrated below and determine which number corresponds most closely to the stool result to be recorded.
2. Record this number in the appropriate column alongside the day and date the stool occurred.
3. Record any aperients taken, or relevant comments pertaining to bowel symptoms in the comments column alongside the relevant day and date.
4. If no bowel action, record this in the comment column.

BRISTOL STOOL SCALE

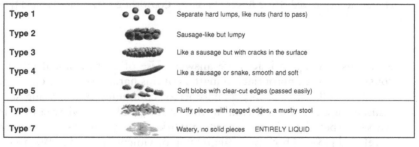

Type 1		Separate hard lumps, like nuts (hard to pass)
Type 2		Sausage-like but lumpy
Type 3		Like a sausage but with cracks in the surface
Type 4		Like a sausage or snake, smooth and soft
Type 5		Soft blobs with clear-cut edges (passed easily)
Type 6		Fluffy pieces with ragged edges, a mushy stool
Type 7		Watery, no solid pieces ENTIRELY LIQUID

NUR0057

BOWEL CHART

CR 10.08

Figure 11.5 Bowel chart. [Reproduced by kind permission of the Royal District Nursing Service – SA Inc.]

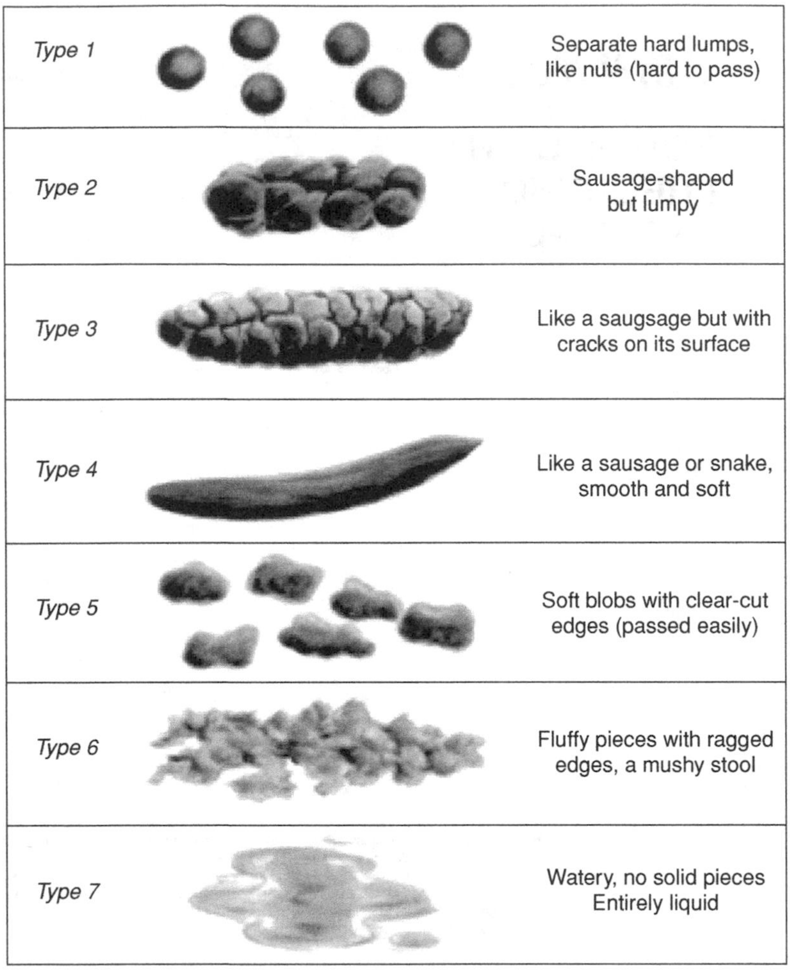

Type 1		Separate hard lumps, like nuts (hard to pass)
Type 2		Sausage-shaped but lumpy
Type 3		Like a saugsage but with cracks on its surface
Type 4		Like a sausage or snake, smooth and soft
Type 5		Soft blobs with clear-cut edges (passed easily)
Type 6		Fluffy pieces with ragged edges, a mushy stool
Type 7		Watery, no solid pieces Entirely liquid

Figure 11.6 Bristol scale stool recognition chart. [Reproduced by kind permission of Dr K.W. Heaton, reader in medicine at Bristol University. Copyright 2000 Norgine Limited.]

questions, leading to inaccurate answers. Use of a professional interpreter is often considered more appropriate in matters of this nature to ensure clear comprehension and data collection [6, 34]. A number of community interpreting services may be utilised for a small fee. Mental health issues should be reviewed by a mental health worker, especially if issues regarding worker safety have been identified at the time of referral [15–17] because of aggression or violent behaviour. Where possible advise family members to attend interviews with a client who has dementia [10, 18, 19]. The presence of a family member can provide support to the client and assist with providing a health history. Occasionally, a professional worker may attend if the client has no near family.

Containment

Through a conversational approach, the community nurse can gain an understanding of the client's perspective of being wet or dry and how they obtain their supplies of items such as pads [31, 34, 37]. The ability of clients to individually access funding schemes may be limited, so the community nurse should refer clients to appropriate schemes to supplement economic resources. The schemes/eligibility vary from state to state but options to explore include the Department of Veterans Affairs, Continence Aids Appliance Scheme, Special Equipment Programme (SA) and the ParaQuad Association.

Function/environment

Assessment of the environment can include [48, 49, 54]:

- Dexterity.
- Free access to toileting facilities.
- Limb strength.
- Walking distance to toilet.
- Transferring abilities [42, 44, 55–57].
- Disrobing abilities – clients who cannot remove underwear or access a toilet will find it difficult to remain continent.
- Ancillary aids/appliances should be assessed for usability/reliability [46]; a functioning piece of equipment potentially differentiates between regaining and modifying incontinence.
- Review, with consent, toileting facilities and house layout [46], seeking potential impediments to continence [34, 42, 58] including lack of privacy, poor toilet facilities (essential for adequate elimination) [56, 57] and access hazards, e.g. lack of grab rails, steps and poor lighting [42, 48, 57, 58].

Physical assessment

A physical assessment is always approached by the community nurse with sensitivity and caution. Use of a chaperone may be needed, especially for children and culturally diverse groups who may decline examination for a variety of reasons [5, 6]. Physical examination may become more challenging in the home due to low beds, poor lighting, lack of privacy and varying levels of hygiene. Clients may feel more empowered to decline examination in their home environment than they would in a more clinical environment.

Physical assessment may include:

- Abdominal – exclude faecal impaction, masses, tenderness [5, 34, 56, 57].
- Perineal/vulval – exclude age-related changes, scrotal and vulval abnormalities [6, 42, 59].
- Rectal – determine pelvic strength, prostate health, constipation, tenderness, masses, fissures, haemorrhoids and anal gape (low resting tone associated with passive soiling) [6, 34, 42, 48, 56, 57].

- Vaginal – establish pelvic strength and detect rectocele, prolapses, cystocoele. Exclude age-related changes, e.g. vaginitis [42, 48, 50, 59]. The symptoms of vaginal thrush and vaginitis are very similar in postmenopausal women; therefore, it is essential that clients are encouraged to attend their GP for a vaginal swab to confirm diagnosis. Older people may be reluctant to discuss these issues with others and continue to self-treat with limited success. The role of the community nurse is to encourage, nurture and support these clients to attend their GP or have a home visit in an atmosphere that engenders trust and builds therapeutic relationships.
- Neurological – ascertain loss of reflexes potentially affecting continence status especially at the lumbar-sacral juncture [48, 59].

Clients confronted with a nurse who demonstrates impatience and clock watching or who makes value-laden statements are unlikely to form therapeutic relationships with clients [5, 6, 42]. The creation of safe environments and a non-judgemental approach that shows acceptance of a client's situation is vital [43, 52].

Completed continence assessments do not guarantee continence and clients will vary in their ability to change or adapt to new ways of living [34]. Clients may view the option of doing nothing as their right. Nurses must support this view even if they have invested many hours of time and energy in education and intervention [48, 49].

Planning and management

The underlying principles of continence management may be applied in any setting. Client-centred collaborative care plans incorporating elements of the client's lifestyle and their ability to adapt should be developed in collaboration with the client [34]. Impaired health and ecosocial and psychological well-being should be considered so that clients derive the full benefit from any plan [60, 61].

Learning principles, incorporating written, visual and interpretive aids, commensurate with the client's literacy, age, gender and cognitive ability, and cultural and ethnic group should be followed [62]. For example community assistance in the management of enuresis is limited due to high demand; however, lifestyle changes can help to ameliorate the effects of this condition; for example reducing soft drink and fast food consumption may reduce bladder irritation, resolve constipation and engender calmer behavioural patterns.

The community nurse may consider the following themes when working with a client to plan ways to manage incontinence:

Fluids

A client living at home who has never been a good drinker will not necessarily change just because the community nurse has advised that it is ideal to drink more. A drinking plan may be developed that is amenable to the client and their lifestyle. Some guidelines are:

- Adults require approximately 2 L daily (unless contraindicated). Children commensurately less [2, 5, 42].

- Caffeine-based drinks such as coffee, tea, coke, Pepsi, Milo, chocolate and Ovaltine ideally no more than three cups per day and consumed before 1600 h to avoid urine concentration overnight [48, 49].
- Soft drinks and alcohol are bladder irritants; therefore, advise the client to consume them in moderate quantities and gradually decrease if taking excessive amounts.
- Decrease fluid intake approximately 1 h before bed to diminish nocturia.
- Balance fluids evenly across the day to maintain hydration, prevent constipation and rapid bladder filling, which potentially lead to episodes of urgency and incontinence.

Diet

Ideally, a well-balanced diet considers all food groups with low fat, low sugar and low salt [63]. The Heart Foundation recommends five vegetables and two fruit per day [6]. Consider soluble and insoluble fibre equally (approximately 25–35 g daily):

- Soluble fibre contains no obvious stringiness, e.g. fruits, psyllium, cereals, oats and barley.
- Insoluble fibre absorbs water and is bulkier, e.g. vegetables, nuts, bran, brown rice and fruit seeds.
- For people lacking dietary fibre, gradually increase the daily amount to within an appropriate level. Be creative and ingenious – substitution of foods may not be appreciated, affordable or meet cultural needs. Clients who are on very low incomes or who have limited intellect or cognition to make good food choices may need to be linked to an agency that can provide shopping or dietitian assistance.
- Bowel retraining makes use of the gastrocolic reflex (at its strongest postprandial) [6]. Adoption of correct toileting posture assists in evacuation, prevents straining and develops improved bowel habits [6]. In the initial stages of the programme, trial toileting after each meal but aim to have an evacuation at approximately the same time each day.

The following morning programme may be adapted according to the client's particular functional and cognitive capabilities. Carer assistance may be required for clients with special needs:

- Get up.
- After rising, consume a piece of fruit, e.g. orange or kiwi fruit.
- Have a warm drink with breakfast.
- Sit on the toilet 15–30 min later and adopt an appropriate toileting posture.
- Remain for approximately 10 min as the gastrocolic reflex diminishes with time.

Recommended toileting posture is to:

- Sit firmly on the toilet/commode seat, buttocks to the centre.
- Relax shoulders, arms and legs.
- Breathe normally.
- A small footstool may be used to bring the knees higher than the hips.
- Feet should be flat and slightly apart.

- Lean forwards as if skiing, with the elbows resting on the upper thigh. (A pillow may be used for support.)
- Brace the abdominal muscles.
- Relax the anal sphincter.

Scheduled toileting (bladder retraining)

The aim is to increase bladder capacity and deferment intervals [2, 5]. This approach is ideal for stress incontinence, urgency and postprostatectomy dribble. Community nurses can encourage clients not to go 'just in case' even when they are planning an outing, as this may contribute long term to reduced bladder capacity. Encourage clients to toilet as per the planned programme that has been developed from their bladder chart with the community nurse and locate toileting facilities when out.

Scheduled toileting will require the community nurse to review the client's bladder diary and calculate the current baseline interval without an incontinence episode:

- First week – Routinely void at the baseline interval regardless of the desire to void.
- Second week – Increase the interval by 5 min. Utilise deferment techniques to achieve this. Do not go beyond the set time as principles of bladder retraining rely on regularity.
- Once the goals of the second week are mastered sufficiently, gradually increase by 5–15 min each week to a maximum of 3–4 hourly.

Continue the plan during the waking hours and advise clients not to resist voiding urges overnight.

Deferment techniques

Learning to defer urgent voiding signals takes time and practice [5, 48]. Repeat exercises until the urge lessens and comes under client control. Deferment techniques are useful in conjunction with a scheduled toileting programme:

- Stand still and focus on another activity.
- Sit down if the urge increases and engage in another activity.
- Sit on the arm of a chair or press a rolled towel against the perineum – this supports pelvic muscles and improves urethral closure pressure.
- Concentrate on squeezing vaginal/rectal muscles tightly inwards and upwards.
- Make a phone call or write a letter.
- Count backwards in 3 s from 100.
- Squeeze the tip of the penis gently between thumb and forefinger.

Prompted toileting

Ideal for clients with intellectual, cognitive or mental health conditions [2, 5, 6, 10, 18]. Carers may find a sense of relief in a more routine programme as it provides structure and aims to prevent incontinence episodes. Observe clients for elimination cues, e.g. repeated gestures or words and incorporate them into the plan. Encourage an association with elimination by using the same facility where possible.

Double voiding

Ensurés effective bladder emptying, but requires patience. Ideal for clients who have postmicturition dribble or a sensation of incomplete emptying postvoid:

- Initially empty the bladder until the sensation to void has gone.
- Wait a few moments longer and then relax and perhaps focus on a book or magazine. This allows pelvic relaxation to occur and residual urine to flow. Continue until the bladder empties itself – never force or strain.
- Try rocking gently backwards and forwards to promote complete bladder emptying.

The success of any toileting programme is reliant on the client's understanding, capacity, perseverance and skill. Promoting any small gains made will build self-esteem and confidence in the client. Routine visits by the community nurse will provide support and encouragement, allowing the client to monitor their own progress. The value of these visits should not be underestimated from the client's perspective as potentially they mean the difference in continence status.

Clean intermittent catheterisation

The act of passing a clean catheter into the bladder (by client or carer) at regulated intervals to ensure complete emptying [64–66]. Clean intermittent catheterisation (CIC) is ideal for clients with a neurogenic bladder or urethral stricture. Within the community environment there can be challenges to maintaining healthy bladder function. For example if hygiene is not maintained, then the potential for infection is increased, particularly when the client is using public facilities. Clients performing this technique in isolation must be routinely reviewed to ensure the process remains effective. Additional telephone support may be required to those clients living in rural/remote areas, as access to specialised clinical facilities may be limited. Benefits include:

- Reduced incidence of urinary infection.
- Improved renal health.
- Fewer complications than an indwelling catheter.
- Improved sense of body image.
- Greater independence.
- Continence.

Urethral catheterisation

Considered a standardised management procedure for intractable incontinence and should be used as a last option [5]. Despite providing indispensable benefits, indwelling catheters are not entirely benign interventions [67]. Management remains primarily a nursing responsibility [5]; therefore, evidence-based principles should be applied to ensure that risks to the client are minimised. Clients with cognitive deficits are unsuitable candidates for catheterisation because there may be potential for forcible removal causing trauma [5]. Community clients will need the functional ability to:

- Open and close the valve on a leg and night bag.
- Maintain perineal hygiene.
- Change the leg bag weekly.
- Wash and connect the night bag daily.
- Troubleshoot complications.
- Recognise signs of urinary tract infection.
- Order supplies as required.

If the client is unable to perform these tasks independently then the intervention may not be appropriate. Risks associated with this intervention can include:

- Hypersensitivity to product material [68].
- Bladder spasms.
- An increase in sedimentation, potentiating stone formation [69].
- Chronic uroepithelial inflammation, leading to scarring, necrosis, stricture and cancer [69].
- Altered body image and decreased QOL.
- Increased pathogenesis [70].

Pharmacotherapy

Should not be used as a first line of defence [33]. Ease of access to aperients is recognised in community nursing and abuse of these substances noted [6]. Medication interactions are possible because aperients are not simplistic interventions, so GP liaison is critical.

Bowels

- Antidiarrhoeal – such as loperamide – slows gut transit time and increases water absorption.
- Bulking agents such as Nulax and Metamucil need to be used with caution because these products require sufficient hydration to precipitate a therapeutic response.
- Softeners such as arachis oil and Coloxylcan assist in water penetration to the stool. Oil coats the colon and lubricates the passage of stools.
- Stimulants such as senna, Coloxyl and bisacodyl precipitate stimulation of the colonic nerve endings, causing an increase in peristalsis and secretion of fluid into the colon.
- Osmotic laxatives such as lactulose and Movicol retain fluid by osmotic pressure within the stool; however, prolonged usage can lead to dehydration and electrolyte imbalance.

Bladder

- Anticholinergics such as oxybutynin, Toltolderone, propantheline and solifenacin increase detrusor stability and urethral sphincter control. Caution is advised prior to commencement – an ultrasound is performed to exclude urinary retention. For people with cognitive disorders the neural pathways are fragmented and hence messages are interrupted and disjointed, which means control of the bladder may become imperfect due to lack of recognition of bladder signals and toileting facilities [70].

- Alpha-adrenoceptor blockers such as tamsulosin and terazosin decrease smooth muscle tone by blocking alpha-adrenoceptors – indicated in cases of prostate disease and associated male urinary retention.
- Tricyclic antidepressants such as amitriptyline and imipramine may cause constipation due to decreased gut motility.
- Hormonal supplements such as desmopressin act by inhibiting the reuptake of noradrenalin, causing detrusor relaxation and outlet resistance. Useful in nocturnal enuresis, but not recommended for children aged under 6 years.
- Oestrogen supplements such as Vagifem and Ovestin administered vaginally two to three times weekly. Useful in treating postmenopausal women experiencing symptoms of stress or urge incontinence and overactive bladder syndrome, e.g. epithelial irritation, inflammation and urogenital atrophy.

Pelvic floor (Kegel) exercises

Designed to improve diminished pelvic muscle tone, bulk and strength in cases of stress incontinence or postprostatectomy dribble [2, 5]. Trained physiotherapists (who may be accessed privately or through the local hospital) or continence nurses can be useful resources to provide information and education to clients about pelvic floor exercises. It may take some weeks after the commencement of the pelvic floor exercises before experience results; however, perseverance will produce effects. The role of the community nurse is to support, nurture and monitor progress during this phase so as to promote client self-awareness and confidence.

The exercises may be performed at any time when the person is sitting, standing or lying comfortably. Without using abdominal muscles, ask the client to breathe regularly and then squeeze the anal muscle upwards and inwards (as though trying to prevent the passage of wind):

- Repeat with the front muscles (harder to accomplish and takes time and practice).
- Once mastered, try lifting and holding the anal muscles (continue to breathe) for a count of five. Repeat with the front muscles.
- Repeat a series of five exercises, three to five times per day.
- Exercise all muscles correctly. Alternate both quick 1-s flicks and then longer slow holds.
- Gradually extend the hold time of the slower exercise by 1 s per week until 10 s have been achieved.

Weighted vaginal cones are a conservative method of increasing pelvic tone and resilience [5]. The sensation of the cone potentially slipping from its location causes the pelvic muscles to contract and support it. Oxford grading 3 (see below) must be attainable prior to treatment commencing:

Oxford Grading Scale

1. Nil.
2. Flicker only with muscle stretch.
3. Weak squeeze with 2-s hold.
4. Fair squeeze with definite lift.
5. Good squeeze, good hold, a few contractions able to be repeated.
6. Strong squeeze, good lift, repeatable.

Containment products

Pads may be considered by some people to be bulky, demeaning and expensive (expenditure exceeds millions of dollars annually) [9], yet they can have a role to play [37, 48, 71, 72]. The use of pads is not considered a first option however and is discontinued as soon as practicable [37, 38]. For some people, a nurse advocating the wearing of pads implies that nothing further can be done to treat incontinence [28]. Containment products include panty liners, all in one pads, Kylies, anal plugs and urinary sheaths, which can be purchased through the local supermarket, wholesaler or chemist. Limited funding may be available to people in some states and territories to partially cover costs. The community nurse's role is to ensure that clients who meet the criteria are connected with the following schemes to reduce the economic burden:

- Continence Aids Appliance Scheme (CAAS).
- Special Equipment Programme (SEP).
- Department of Veterans' Affairs (DVA).
- Private health insurers.

The needs of people living in rural and remote areas must be carefully considered because access to wholesalers, chemists or sensible product pricing may be impossible for this group.

Aids and equipment

Maintain and supplement diminished functional capacity, e.g. urinal, commode, grab rails, toilet raise, walker and bedpan [10, 19, 31, 37, 73]. Equipment may be obtained through local domiciliary care departments, chemists, wholesalers, independent living centres and manufacturers. An occupational therapy assessment is recommended prior to obtaining most equipment to ensure it meets the client's functional and dexterity capabilities.

Queens Square Bladder Stimulator

A small hand-held device for clients with neurological dysfunction to promote complete bladder emptying or to initiate voiding [74]. The device is painless, non-invasive and is activated by pressing it against the suprapubic line.

Environmental considerations

Include assessment of toileting facilities that should be conducive to a relaxed, comfortable experience [75]. Clients who have declining cognitive abilities may become disorientated or resist using facilities that are dirty, poorly lit or inadequately maintained [10]. Similarly people with physical disabilities may experience difficulty accessing facilities that are unable to accommodate a wheelchair or provide sufficient space, privacy or ambience to disrobe and manoeuvre over a toilet [10, 18].

Management should be consultative, recognise a client's gender, culture, ethnicity, literacy level and age, and incorporate all aspects of the client's health, lifestyle and environment and yet recognise a client's desire for change [2].

Clinical interventions

The aim of this section is for the nurse to develop an understanding of the interventions which aid diagnosis and management of incontinence that may occur outside of their usual scope of practice. These clinical interventions should not be viewed in isolation, as technology continues to advance and more sophisticated procedures are developed. This section does however provide a broad overview of the current interventions.

Bladder

Urodynamics aims to study the pathophysiology of bladder and urethra dynamics, comprising [5, 76]:

- Uroflometry measures the urine-voiding rate. Peak results should be at least 15 mL/s for a 150-mL volume.
- Cystometrogram (CMG) assesses bladder pressure during filling and voiding and during a series of provocative manoeuvres, e.g. coughing, laughing and standing up, but does not view the bladder neck.
- Urethral pressure profile determines the intraurethral pressure from the bladder neck to the external urethral meatus.
- Videocystometry is carried out in an X-ray department as radio opaque dye is used as a filling medium [5, 76]. The test is similar to a CMG, but views the bladder neck and urethra during filling and voiding.
- Cystoscopy is an examination of the urethra, prostate and bladder epithelium for biopsy and diagnostic purposes using a flexible cystoscope introduced via the external urethral meatus [5].
- Injectable biomaterials involve injecting bulk-enhancing agents, e.g. collagen, Botox and polytetrafluoroethylene into the bladder neck or submucosal anal plane to improve urethral resting tone through closure of the bladder neck or to restore anal sphincter symmetry [2].

Bowel

- Anal ultrasound (endosonography) is performed via a transducer to image the final 3–4 cm of the anal canal and sphincters to diagnose clinically undetectable defects and lesions [6, 51].
- Anal manometry assesses anal canal sphincter function through measurement of resting pressure via a specialised catheter inserted into the anal canal, which is attached to computerised soft wear used for data interpretation [6].
- Rectal compliance testing allows investigators to determine intraluminal rectal pressure using a barostat, which provides indirect measurement of variable rectal tone and pressure [6].
- Perineal descent testing observed during straining can be quantitatively assessed using a periometer – an external device placed against the ischial tuberosities when the client is requested to bear down [6].
- Colonoscopy is an examination of colonic tissue for biopsy and diagnosis.

Standardised procedures

Occasionally, amelioration or restoration of continence requires surgical intervention; however, this should be explored as a last line of management, where conservative interventions are ineffective or inappropriate. These procedures have potential complications that may outweigh the long-term benefits of the procedure and leave a client unable to continue functioning independently at home, placing them at risk of institutionalisation. Potential complications are infection, voiding dysfunction, urinary retention, urogenital fistula, unresolved QOL issues, pain (groin/suprapubic), dyspareunia (painful intercourse), prolapse rectal/vaginal, rectal mucosal leakage and impotence (male/female).

Bladder

- Mitrofranoff procedure – a catheterisable stoma formed from appendiceal tissue to link the bladder and abdomen creating a urinary diversion [5].
- Transurethral resection of prostate is performed when enlargement of the gland obstructs the bladder neck outlet causing urinary retention. A portion of the gland is gradually sliced away to relieve urinary symptoms [2, 5, 77].
- Artificial urinary sphincter – an implantable device designed to control urinary incontinence that is affecting QOL [2]. The cuff is placed around the bulbar urethra; the pressure-regulating balloon and scrotal pump are inserted inguinally and filled with fluid. The device is operated by squeezing the scrotal pump which transfers fluid from the cuff to the balloon, releasing urethral tension and allowing urine to flow. A reverse process will allow the fluid to return to the cuff sealing the bladder neck.
- Anterior colporrhaphy – an anterior vaginal repair with bladder buttress designed to resolve urodynamics stress incontinence. Creation of an endopelvic fascial layer provides additional support [2, 5].
- Coloposuspension aims to elevate the bladder neck through insertion of two to four long-term absorbable sutures from the paravaginal fascia to the iliopectineal ligament [2, 5].

- Pubovaginal slings vary in material and insertion technique but aim to augment bladder/pelvic organ support and consequently outlet resistance [5].
- Tension-free vaginal tape is inserted midurethrally (to the point of maximal urethral closure pressure) and aims to compensate for pubourethral ligament inefficiency and resolve urinary stress incontinence and prolapse [2].
- Marshall–Marchetti–Krantz procedure aims to resolve urinary stress incontinence through removal of two segments of bladder neck tissue and suturing the bladder neck to the periosteum at the back of the pubic bone [5].
- Suprapubic catheter (SPC) removes all risk of urethral and prostate trauma and complications by inserting a catheter via a suprapubic cystostomy (a tunnel between the abdominal wall and bladder). Although the catheter carries a degree of risk, the procedure has become accepted practice due to a lowered risk of infection and renal damage [69]. Care of the SPC is a shared nursing and client/carer responsibility [78]. Clients and carers may be taught management principles and troubleshooting skills, with emphasis on hygiene, sexual health and health promotion to ensure self-care and improved QOL [79, 80].

Bowel

- Sphincteroplasty (anal sphincter musculature repair) is a standard surgical procedure for anal sphincter dysfunction [2].
- Artificial anal sphincter is an implantable device designed to replicate normal function with use of an occlusive inflatable cuff, pressure-regulating balloon and control pump inserted into the perineal/anal region [6].
- Sacral nerve stimulation involves implantation of a permanent electrode and neurostimulator into the sacral region to improve anal/urethral sphincter closure pressure and tone. A pulse generator is placed into the abdominal or gluteal area to moderate impulses [2, 5, 6].
- Colostomy is used only as a last line of defence for faecal incontinence to assist in the restoration of dignity and QOL [2, 6].
- Posterosagittal anorectoplasty is the commonest paediatric surgical procedure performed for congenital malformations. Creation of a stoma from the ileae segment or appendix is used to provide a conduit to wash the bowel, resolve constipation and restore continence [6].
- For anal atresia the infant should undergo evaluation for other anomalies, especially genital, urinary and spinal. Surgical reconstruction of the anus is required. If the rectum connects with other organs, repair of these organs will also be necessary. A temporary colostomy is often required.

Future trends and predictors

Healthy life years lost due to incontinence to people aged under 50 years is expected to increase by 17% between 2003 and 2031, due to population health issues such as the increasing prevalence of diabetes and obesity [9]. The ageing population will also impact, with the prevalence of incontinence estimated to increase by 110% between 2003 and 2031, with 53% of this increase occurring in the 85+ age group, 27% in the 70–84 age group and 20% in the under 70 age group [9]. Total government and consumer expenditure for incontinence is projected to increase by 201% from $1.5 billion in 2003–2004 to $4.5 billion in 2030–2031 [9]. Factors driving this increase include population growth, demographic ageing and increasing health costs.

Conclusion

This chapter has identified the role of community nurses in continence promotion by highlighting areas of impact that incontinence may have on the lives of individuals and communities; the economic, emotional and social costs; and predictions for incontinence to 2031. Community nurses can make a difference in the lives of people living in the community by working with them to promote continence. The knowledge and skills the community nurse will require have been outlined in this chapter.

References

1. Hawthorne, G. (2006) *Measuring Incontinence in Australia*. National Continence Management Strategy. An Australian Government Initiative. Monash University, Australia. Available at www.ag.gov.au/cca (viewed 16 June 2008).
2. International Continence Society (2005) *Incontinence*, Vols. 1 and 2. Health Publication Limited, France.
3. Holroyd-Leduc, J., Mehta, K. and Covinsky, K. (2004) Urinary incontinence and its association with death, nursing home admission and functional decline. *Journal of the American Geriatrics Society*, 52(5), 712–18.
4. Nakanishi, N., Tatara, K., Shinsho, F., Murakam, S., Takatiruge, T., Fukuda, H., *et al.* (1999) Mortality in relation to urinary and faecal incontinence in elderly people living at home. *Age and Ageing*, 28(3), 301–6.
5. Getliffe, K. and Dolman, M. (2003) *Promoting Continence: A Clinical and Research Resource*, 2nd edition. Balliere Tindall, UK.
6. Norton, C. and Chelvanayagam, S. (2004) *Bowel Continence Nursing*, 2nd edition. The Alden Press, UK.
7. Philippe, T., Ingrand, P., Lallone, F., Hanif-Thomas, C., Billion, R., Vieban, F., *et al.* (2004) Reasons for institutionalising dementia patients previously living at home. The Pixel Study. *International Journal of Geriatric Psychiatry*, 10, 127–35.
8. Sprecht, J. (2005) 9 myths of incontinence in older adults. *Australian Journal of Nursing*, 105(6), 58–68.
9. Australian Institute of Health and Welfare (2006) *Australian Incontinence Data Analysis and Development*. A/HW cat. No. DIS 44. Australian Institute of Health and Welfare, Canberra.
10. Bostock, N. and Kralik, D. (2005) Incontinence and dementia: Providing innovative family care. *Australian and New Zealand Continence Journal*, 12(1), 16–20.
11. Shaw, C. (2001) A review of the psychosocial predictors of help-seeking behaviour and impact on quality of life in people with urinary incontinence. *Journal of Clinical Nursing*, 10, 15–24.
12. Landi, F., Cesari, M., Russo, A., Onder, G., Lattanzio, F. and Bernabei, R. (2003) Potentially reversible risk factors and urinary incontinence in frail older people living in the community. *Age and Ageing*, 32, 194–9.

13. McMurray, A. (2003) *Community Health and Wellness: A Sociological Approach*. Mosby Publishers, Sydney.
14. Tan, L., Fleming, A. and Ledwidge, H. (2001) The care-giving burden of relatives with dementia: Experiences of Chinese-Australian families. *Geriaction*, 19(1), 10–16.
15. Zhan, L. (2004) Caring for family members with Alzheimer's disease: Perspectives from Chinese American families. *Journal of Gerontological Nursing*, 30(8), 19–29.
16. Papalia, D. and Olds, S. (1996) *Issues and Theories of Human Development: Lifespan Development*, 2nd edition. McGraw-Hill, Australia, pp. 3–41.
17. Powell, A. (2002) On issues pertinent to Alzheimer disease and cultural diversity. *Alzheimer Disease and Associated Disorders*, 16(Supp 2), S43–5.
18. Stenson, A. and Danaher, T. (2005) Continence issues for people with learning disabilities. *Learning Disability Practice*, 8(9), 10–14.
19. Koch, T., Ashton, M., Kelly, S., Kralik, D., Howard, N., Wrigley, J., *et al.* (2002) *Continence Management for People Living in the Community with Mental Illness*. A Commonwealth Government Initiative. Australia.
20. Nijman, R. (2000) Classification and treatment of functional incontinence in children. *BJU International*, 85(Supp 3), 37–42.
21. Bower, W.F., Moore, K.H., Shepard, R.B. and Adams, R.D. (1996) Normative and clinical information gained from an epidemiological study of incontinence in Australian children. *The Australian Continence Journal*, 2(4), 6–8.
22. Butler, R. and Stenburg, A. (2001) Treatment of childhood nocturnal enuresis: An examination of clinically relevant principles. *BJU International*, 88, 563–71.
23. Jones, T. and Bunner, S. (1997) Approaches to urinary incontinence in a rural population: A comparison of physician assistants, nurse practitioners and family physicians. *Journal of the American Board of Family Practice*, 11(3), 207–15.
24. Glasser, M., Holt, N., Mueller, B., Norem, J., Pickering, J., Brown, K., *et al.* (2003) Meeting the needs of rural populations through interdisciplinary partnerships. *Family and Community Health*, 26(3), 230–45.
25. Dougherty, M., Dwyer, J., Pendergast, J., Tomlinson, B., Boyington, A., Vogel, W., *et al.* (1998) Community based nursing: Continence care for older rural women. *Nursing Outlook*, 46, 233–44.
26. Marieb, E. and Hoehn, K. (2007) *Human Anatomy and Physiology*, 7th edition. Pearson Benjamin Cummings, New York.
27. Pearce, E. (1975) *Anatomy and Physiology for Nurses*, 16th edition. Faber, UK.
28. Parsons, M. and Cardozo, L. (2004) *Female Urinary Incontinence in Practice*. Latimer Trend and Company, UK.
29. Sampselle, C. and DeLancey, J. (1998) Anatomy of female incontinence. *Journal of Wound, Ostomy and Continence Nursing*, 25(2), 63–78.
30. Winge, K., Rasmussen, D. and Werdelin, L. (2003) Constipation in neurological diseases. *Journal of Neurosurgery Psychiatry*, 74, 13–19.
31. Dillion, L. and Fonda, D. (2000) Medical evaluation of causes of lower urinary tract symptoms and urinary incontinence in older people. *Topics in Geriatric Rehabilitation*, 15(4), 1–15.
32. Kaschak-Newmann, D. (2001) Urinary incontinence and overactive bladder: A focus on behavioural interventions. *Advanced Practice Nursing* [serial online]. Available at http://www.medscape.com/viewarticle/408405 (viewed 23 May 2002).
33. *MIMS Annual*, 21st edition. Tien Wah Press, Singapore, 1997.
34. Hughes, M. (1998) Continence and the community nurse. *Journal of Community Nursing*, 12(10), 30–35.
35. Courtney, M., Rickard, C., Vickerstaff, J. and Court, A. (2005) *Evidence-Based Nursing Practice*. Elsevier, pp. 3–33.

36. Austin, L., Luker, K. and Martin, R. (2005) Clinical nurse specialists and the practice of community nurses. *Issues and Innovations in Nursing Practice.* The Authors' Journal Compilation. Blackwell, UK, pp. 542–52.

37. Cheater, F. (1996) Promoting urinary incontinence. *Nursing Standard*, 10(42), 47–54.

38. Dorey, G. (2001) *Conservative Treatment of Male Urinary Incontinence and Erectile Dysfunction.* Whurr Publishers, UK.

39. Goode, P., Burgio, K., Halli, A., Jones, R., Richter, H., Redden, D., *et al.* (2005) Prevalence and correlates of faecal incontinence in community dwelling adults. *American Geriatrics Society*, 53, 629–35.

40. Bharucha, A., Locke, G., Seide, B. and Zinsmeister, A. (2004) A new questionnaire for constipation and faecal incontinence. *Alimentary Pharmacology and Therapeutics*, 20(3), 35–41.

41. McGhee, M., O'Neill, K., Major, K. and Twaddle, S. (1997) Evaluation of a nurse led continence service in south-west of Glasgow, Scotland. *Journal of Advanced Nursing*, 26, 723–8.

42. Pretty, L. and Telfer, R. (1996) *Quality Continence Management – A Resource for Carers.* Resource 4.1. Resthaven Inc, Australia.

43. Sterling-Fisher, C. and Narayan, M. (2004) OASIS M0520 Incontinence? Is leaking really leaking? *Home Healthcare Nurse*, 22(9), 612–21.

44. Culligan, P. and Heit, M. (2000) Urinary incontinence in women: Evaluation and management. *American Family Physician*, 62(11), 2433–9.

45. Betts, A. (2004) Developing a continence service the Bradford way. *Primary Health Care*, 14(4), 39–41.

46. Minkler, P. (1996) Assessment of incontinence. *Journal of Urological Nursing*, 15(3), 1380–84.

47. Wallis, M., McKenzie, S., Rayner, J., Ellern, F., Gass, E., St John, W., *et al.* (2003) *Help Patients Win the Constipation Battle.* Griffith University Research Centre for Clinical Practice Innovation, Australia.

48. Thompson, D. and Smith, D. (2001) Continence nursing: A whole person approach. *Holistic Nursing Practitioner*, 16(2), 14–31.

49. Rigby, D. and Whelan, L. (2001) Parkinson's disease and the nurse's role in continence assessment. *Nurse Times Plus*, 97(20), 64–5.

50. Beheshti, P. and Fonteyn, M. (1998) Role of the advanced practice nurse in continence care in the home. *American Association of Critical Care Nurses*, 9(3), 389–95.

51. Butcher, L. (2004) Clinical skills: Nursing considerations in patients with faecal incontinence. *British Journal of Nursing*, 23(13), 760–67.

52. Palmer, M. and Newman, D. (2006) Bladder control: Educational needs of older adults. *Journal of Gerontological Nursing*, 32(1), 28–32.

53. Mathuru, G., Assassa, R., Williams, K., Donaldson, M., Matthews, R., Tincello, L., *et al.* (2004) Continence nurse treatment of women's urinary symptoms. *British Journal of Nursing*, 13(3), 140–43.

54. de Rekeneire, N., Visser, M., Peila, R., Nevitt, M., Cauley, P., Tylavsky, F., *et al.* (2003) Is a fall just a fall: Correlates of falling in healthy older persons. The health, ageing and composition study. *Journal of the American Geriatrics Society*, 51, 841–6.

55. Bradway, C. (2003) Urinary incontinence among older women. *Journal of Gerontological Nursing*, 29(7), 13–19.

56. Wilson, L. (2005) Understanding bowel problems in older people: Part one. *Nursing Older People*, 17(8), 25–9.

57. Wilson, L. (2005) Understanding bowel problems in older adults: Part two. *Nursing Older People*. 17(9), 24–9.

58. Gray, M. (2005) Assessment and management of urinary incontinence. *Nurse Practitioner*, 30(7), 32–43.

59. Pearson, B. (1996) Urinary incontinence: Treatments, interventions and outcomes. *Clinical Nurse Specialist*, 10(4), 177–82.

60. Hagan, T. and Ashworth, P. (1996) Psychological management of incontinence. *Journal of Community Nursing*, 10(10), 26–32.

61. Gallo, M., Fallon, P. and Staskin, D. (1997) Urinary incontinence: Steps to evaluation, diagnosis and treatment. *Nurse Practitioner*, 22(2), 21–6.

62. Billings, D. and Halstead, J. (2005) *Teaching in Nursing: A Guide for Faculty*, 2nd edition. Elsevier Saunders, USA.

63. Stanton, R. (1998) *Find Out About Fibre*. Allen and Unwin, Australia.

64. Woodward, S. and Rew, M. (2003) Patients' quality of life and clean intermittent self-catheterisation. *British Journal of Nursing*, 12(18), 1066–74.

65. Bennett, E. (2002) Intermittent catheterisation and the female patient. *Nursing Standard*, 17(7), 37–42.

66. Barton, R. (2000) Intermittent self-catheterisation. *Nursing Standard*, 19(9), 47–52.

67. Achmetov, T. and Gray, M. (2005) Adverse reactions to latex in the clinical setting: A urologic perspective. *Infection Control Resource*, 2(2), 1–5.

68. Young, W. (2005) Suprapubic cystostomy vs urethral catheterisation. *CareCure Community*. Available at http://carecure.rutgers.edu (viewed 16 June 2008).

69. Traunter, B. and Darouiche, R. (2004) Catheter associated infections. *Archives of Internal Medicine*, 164, 842–50.

70. Ancelin, M., Artero, S., Portet, F., Dupay, A.M., Touchon, J. and Ritchie, K. (2005) Non-degenerative mild cognitive impairment in elderly people and use of anti-cholinergic drugs: A longitudinal study [Online]. *British Medical Journal*. Avaliable at bmj.com (viewed 16 June 2008). File No: doi 10.1136/bmj38740.439664.DE

71. Chutka, D., Fleming, K., Evans, M., Evans, J. and Andrews, K. (1996) Urinary incontinence in the elderly population. *Mayo Foundation for Medical Education and Research*, 71(1), 93–101.

72. Thomas, S. (2000) Good practice in continence services. *Nursing Standard*, 14(47), 43–5.

73. Pearson, B. (1996) Urinary incontinence: Treatments, interventions and outcomes. *Clinical Nurse Specialist*, 10(4), 177–82.

74. Murray, M. and Cockerell, R. (1995) Incontinence in the cognitively impaired – a functional evaluation. *The Australian Continence Journal*, 1(3), 16–18.

75. Oats, J. (2005). *Clinical Practice Guidelines: Urodynamic Assessment*. Royal Women's Hospital. Australia. Available at http://www.rwh.org.au (viewed 16 June 2008).

76. Commonwealth of Australia (2001) *You and Your Prostate*. Union Offset Printing, Australia. Available at http://carecure.rutgers.edu/spinewire/Reasearch/Suprapubic.htm (viewed 16 February 2003).

77. Mercer-Smith, J. (2003) Indwelling catheter management: From habit based to evidence based practice. *Ostomy/Wound Management*, 49(12), 34–45.

78. Robinson, J. (2005) Clinical skills: How to remove and change a supra pubic catheter. *British Journal of Nursing*, 14(1), 30–35.

79. Bostock, N. and Kralik, D. (2006) *Sexual Health and Living with an Indwelling Catheter: A Continuum of Life*. The Pursuit of Excellence. Australia. Issue 40. Available at www.rdns.org.au/research_unit (viewed 16 June 2008).

80. Hall, J. and Taylor, R. (2003) Health for all beyond 2000: The demise of the Alma-Ata Declaration and primary health care in developing countries. *Medical Journal of Australia*, 178(1), 17–20.

Suggested readings

Billings, D. and Halstead, J. (2005) *Teaching in Nursing: A Guide for Faculty*, 2nd edition. Elsevier Saunders, USA.

Getliffe, K. and Dolman, M. (2003) *Promoting Continence: A Clinical and Research Resource*, 2nd edition. Balliere Tindall, UK.

Hawthorne, G. (2006) *Measuring Incontinence in Australia*. National Continence Management Strategy. An Australian Government Initiative. Monash University, Australia.

International Continence Society (2005) *Incontinence*, Vols. 1 and 2. Health Publication Limited, France.

McMurray, A. (2004) *Community Health and Wellness: A Sociological Approach*, 2nd edition. Mosby Publishers, Australia; Chapter 11.

Norton, C. and Chelvanayagam, S. (2004) *Bowel Continence Nursing*, 2nd edition. The Alden Press, UK.

Chapter 12

Diabetes care

Jane Giles, Kate Visentin and Pauline Hill

Introduction

The aim of this chapter is to identify key elements of working effectively with people who have diabetes and the associated management issues for nurses working in community health care contexts. We assume that nurses working in the community have some knowledge of the pathophysiology of diabetes and an understanding of the broad principles of diabetes management. We seek to build on this knowledge and provide specific information relevant for nurses working within a community health care context.

The term *diabetes* refers to a group of conditions in which the insulin supply is inadequate, inefficient or absent and this results in too much glucose in the blood [1]. Diabetes requires daily management by the person and/or their significant other. In the longer term, diabetes can cause physical complications such as blindness, renal failure, large-vessel disease and lower-limb amputation [2].

At the end of the twentieth century, two major longitudinal research studies, the United Kingdom Prospective Diabetes Study (UKPDS, 1998) and Diabetes Control and Complications Trial (DCCT, 1993), demonstrated the significance of near-normal blood glucose control in delaying and preventing diabetes-related complications [3, 4]. It is thus important that health care providers, including community nurses, work collaboratively with clients to achieve mutually agreed blood glucose targets [5].

In Australia, there are systems in place to assist people with diabetes to work with health professionals to achieve mutually agreed blood glucose levels. For example general practitioner (GP) systems provide consumers with access to management plans and team care arrangements. GPs and allied health professionals are able to claim Medicare rebates for these services. These plans financially support education and support for the person with diabetes. Diabetes management requires an interdisciplinary-based approach with the person/client central to the team. The person's capacity for self-management should be recognised by health professionals [6]. The National Health and Medical Research Council (NHMRC, 2004) guidelines for diabetes state that all people with diabetes should have access to [2]:

- Information about their condition.
- Access to education for self-management.
- Clinical care which aims for optimal blood glucose control.
- Screening and treatment for complications.

Despite the NHMRC recommendations for access to diabetes services, a 2006 government report highlights that whilst Australia compares well to the rest of the world in many areas of diabetes care, deficiencies can be seen in:

- The detection and diagnosis of diabetes.
- The coordination between services being provided.
- The ability to provide ongoing and proactive education and support for self-management.
- The ability to provide evidence-based care.
- The ability to manage psychosocial issues [6].

We believe that these deficiencies cannot be addressed through specialist diabetes services alone. With so many people at risk of diabetes or living with diabetes, it is evident that the provision of diabetes education needs to be shared across a range of health professionals and health worker groups. It is important that community nurses have the necessary skills and knowledge to carry out assessment, advice and referral. Community nurses have a pivotal role to play in the management of diabetes, including prevention and early detection of the condition. Management strategies for diabetes are best developed in partnership with the person. We hope this chapter provides insight and direction for community nurses wishing to expand and build on existing diabetes skills and knowledge.

Background

There are two main types of diabetes: type 1 diabetes and type 2 diabetes. Type 1 diabetes affects approximately 10–15% of all people with diabetes, while type 2 diabetes accounts for the remaining 85–90% [6]. Preceding type 2 diabetes is a condition which has now been labelled as 'prediabetes'. It affects about 16.4% of Australian adults [7]. There is also a type of diabetes that occurs in pregnancy. Gestational diabetes occurs in 4.2% of all pregnancies [8] and resolves after the baby is born.

Type 1 diabetes

Type 1 diabetes is one of the most common chronic diseases of childhood, with about half of the people with type 1 diabetes developing the disease before age 18 years. Type 1 diabetes is thought to be caused by a combination of genetic and environmental factors [1]. The incidence of type 1 diabetes is increasing by 2–4% each year [9]. Although diagnosis most often occurs in childhood or adolescence, it can occur at any age.

Type 1 diabetes is an autoimmune condition where the beta cells which produce insulin are destroyed [6]. Consequently, the person does not produce any insulin and insulin therapy is required for survival. Individuals with type 1 diabetes can never stop or withhold insulin therapy. Lifestyle recommendations for a person with type 1 diabetes are the same as for the general population.

Type 2 diabetes

Type 2 diabetes usually occurs in adults, but is becoming more common in teenagers and children [6, 10, 11]. The Australian Diabetes Obesity and Lifestyle Study (Aus-Diab) found an overall prevalence in the Australian population of type 2 diabetes to be 7.4% [12].

In type 2 diabetes, there is a relative insulin deficiency as well as insulin resistance and this results in high blood glucose levels (hyperglycaemia) [7]. Initially, diet and exercise may lower blood glucose levels but as the disease progresses, oral medication and insulin are added to maintain blood glucose targets [2, 3, 13].

Type 2 diabetes is a significant risk factor for cardiovascular disease. Research has now provided strong evidence that cardiovascular risk factors such as hypertension, dyslipidaemia, lack of physical activity, poor dietary habits and smoking should be targeted in addition to blood glucose in people with type 2 diabetes [3, 14].

Prediabetes

Prediabetes is considered to be a precursor to type 2 diabetes. Blood glucose levels are elevated to above normal but have not reached the diagnostic range for diabetes. The terms 'impaired fasting glucose' and/or 'impaired glucose tolerance' are often used to describe this condition. People with prediabetes are at an increased risk of developing diabetes, as well as cardiovascular and other macrovascular complications [7]. Management of prediabetes is similar to that of diabetes and aims to prevent or delay the onset of diabetes through weight loss, increasing activity levels and healthy eating. Cardiovascular risk factors are a priority, such as blood pressure and lipid control as well as counselling for cessation of smoking [7]. Monitoring capillary blood glucose levels (through finger pricking) is not recommended until there is a diagnosis of diabetes [7]. Annual screening using a fasting venous plasma glucose is recommended [15].

Gestational diabetes

Gestational diabetes is temporary and subsides after delivery. The management of gestational diabetes is guided by the Australasian Diabetes in Pregnancy Society (ADIPS) guidelines [16]. Having gestational diabetes puts women at an increased risk of developing type 2 diabetes later in their lives [17]. It is important that gestational diabetes management is in line with ADIPS guidelines to reduce risks to both the woman and the infant. More detail about gestational diabetes is provided later in the chapter.

Risk factors and prevention

Researchers have not been able to successfully prevent type 1 diabetes. However, there is strong evidence that people can delay or prevent the development of type 2 diabetes

[6]. With the prevalence of type 2 diabetes expected to double by 2010, the primary prevention of diabetes is a national priority [6].

Community nurses are well positioned to recognise those who may be at risk of type 2 diabetes and can initiate strategies for preventing or delaying its onset. Nurses working in community settings can have a significant role in encouraging people to make healthy lifestyle choices, for example encouraging clients to set realistic and achievable goals when talking about the importance of healthy weight, being active and healthy eating. It is important to [6]:

- Consider strategies that are tailored to the individual; e.g. consider how socioeconomic or cultural factors may impact on implementing lifestyle changes.
- Target only one risk factor at a time; e.g. smoking cessation may be the initial priority.

An approach used in general practice called SNAP (smoking, nutrition, alcohol, physical activity) is designed to assist clients to set healthy lifestyle goals. Contact information about SNAP and the QUIT smoking programme can be found in the resource list at the end of this chapter.

Community nurses also have an important role in assisting with the early diagnosis of diabetes. Many people with type 2 diabetes do not have symptoms or their symptoms go unnoticed for many years (e.g. tiredness) [6]. The 2002 AusDiab study confirmed that for every known case of diabetes, there was one undiagnosed case [12]. Early diagnosis of type 2 diabetes is important because it can prevent and/or slow the progression of long-term complications [6].

Screening for diabetes using capillary testing (a blood glucose meter) is not currently recommended [18, 19]. Instead the emphasis should be to identify those at risk and refer them for venous glucose testing (ideally fasting). A screening tool can be found on the Diabetes Australia National website www.diabetesaustralia.com.au.

It is recommended that the following high-risk groups be tested for undiagnosed type 2 diabetes [6]:

- People with impaired glucose tolerance or impaired fasting glucose (prediabetes).
- Aboriginal and Torres Strait Islander people aged 35 years and over.
- People aged 35 years and over *and* whose origins are in the Pacific Islands, the Indian subcontinent or China.
- People aged 45 years and over who are obese or have hypertension.
- All people with clinical cardiovascular disease.
- Women with polycystic ovarian syndrome who are obese.
- Women with a history of gestational diabetes.
- People aged 55 years and over.
- People aged 45 years and over, with a first-degree relative with type 2 diabetes [15, 17].

Assessment

Assessment is the cornerstone of any nurse's role regardless of their work setting. The person's home is an ideal environment for observing and talking with clients about their diabetes, lifestyle and self-management practices. Nurses who see clients in their own homes can gain more insight into how the person lives than a nurse who is seeing a client in a clinic situation. Utilising a primary health care approach which emphasises social justice, equity and participation can help people to make decisions about what they can do to address their own health needs [20].

Discussion with the client could include current health care needs (e.g. diabetes, wound management, foot care and medication administration). Asking if people can demonstrate how they use their equipment or their medicines can help to ascertain the person's level of knowledge, skill and understanding in self-management of their diabetes.

Psychosocial issues

Prior to embarking on any clinical assessment, it is important to consider the psychosocial issues that may impact on the client accessing and utilising health services. It is known that the prevalence of diabetes is higher among socially disadvantaged groups [21]. Furthermore, people who live in socially disadvantaged areas are more likely to be faced with multiple barriers when trying to implement the many lifestyle changes that are required when preventing or managing type 2 diabetes. Issues such as low income, level of education, area of residence and language barriers will all impact on the way in which a person accesses services [21]. For example an individual who is unable to find work and pay the rent will be unlikely to see lifestyle changes as a priority.

Depression and anxiety have also been found to be more prevalent amongst people with diabetes and this can adversely affect quality of life [6]. When talking with clients the community nurse should assess for signs of anxiety or depression. The use of a depression-screening tool, such as the K6 Psychometric Measure, can assist in identifying those people who are at risk [22]. Referral to appropriate services is recommended.

Types of diabetes

It is important to ask a client whether they know what type of diabetes they have as this can reveal understandings about their condition and any specific issues relating to self-management. The type of diabetes and the person's individual goals will direct the care planning process and identify appropriate areas for education updates. For example care planning with a person with type 2 diabetes will identify the individual's goals and priorities, such as achieving a healthy weight through increasing activity and healthy eating. Alternatively, a person with type 1 diabetes may identify that they are unsure how to manage their insulin during sick days.

Diagnosis

Diagnosis of diabetes is made when a fasting plasma glucose level is ≥ 7.0 mmol/L on two separate occasions or the person is symptomatic with one elevated reading. An oral glucose tolerance test (OGTT) may be performed to confirm a diagnosis if the fasting blood glucose is unclear [15].

Screening for gestational diabetes is usually done at 26–28 weeks' gestation. However, if the woman has had gestational diabetes in a previous pregnancy, screening is also done at 12 weeks.

The diagnosis of any type of diabetes is a significant event in a person's life. It is important not to underestimate the physical and psychological impact the diagnosis of a lifelong condition can have on an individual and their family. This initial impact can influence the client's approach to their diabetes education and management.

Listening to the person's story of diagnosis can provide the community nurse with information about the person's psychological state, their motivations and capacity to self-manage diabetes. The community nurse is well placed to build a relationship where they can support the person to make lifestyle changes. It is also important for community nurses to work closely and communicate with specialist diabetes health professionals and the client's GP.

Signs and symptoms

Initial signs and symptoms of diabetes can differ, depending on the type of diabetes and the level of hyperglycaemia. Type 1 diabetes usually causes young people to become ill quickly and symptoms such as excessive thirst, frequent drinking, frequent urination and weight loss are common. Clients may present with diabetic ketoacidosis (DKA), which if left untreated can result in coma and death [6].

Conversely, in type 2 diabetes the onset tends to be gradual, with many people unaware that they have the condition. Symptoms such as lethargy and polyuria may be attributed to other causes. Consequently, people may actually present with a long-term complication (e.g. myocardial infarction), without even knowing they have diabetes [6]. People with type 2 diabetes are also prone to slow healing of cuts and a higher prevalence of skin/wound infections [15].

Long-term complications

Long-term complications of diabetes present as either microvascular or macrovascular complications. Macrovascular complications result from damage to major blood vessels and can result in:

- Coronary heart disease.
- Cerebrovascular disease.
- Peripheral vascular disease.

In some cases, this group of complications can already be present in people with type 2 diabetes at diagnosis.

Microvascular complications result from damage to smaller blood vessels and nerves and can result in:

- Neuropathy (damage to the nerves of the feet and lower limbs).
- Nephropathy (impaired renal function).
- Retinopathy (damage to blood vessel in the eye).

In some cases microvascular complications can be more common in those with type 1 diabetes; however, people with type 2 diabetes are also at risk [23].

Community nurses are well placed to reinforce education about the need to have a medical review to ensure that complication risk reduction strategies are in place. Reviews will also enable the early diagnosis of complications and therefore allow the best chance of establishing strategies to delay progression.

Hyperglycaemia

For people with type 1 diabetes, hyperglycaemia can be a transient state, but can also progress to DKA. To assist with early identification the person with type 1 diabetes can monitor ketones in capillary blood or urine.

Hyperglycaemia and dehydration in people with type 2 diabetes can also progress to a condition called hyperglycaemic hyperosmolar state (HHS). Both DKA and HHS are best managed in an acute care facility, with rehydration and insulin therapy a priority [23]. A person will be most at risk of hyperglycaemia during illness.

Within a community setting, nurses have a role in reinforcing the education people receive about the home management of sick days. Instructions are based on the Australian Diabetes Educators Association sick-day guidelines [24]. For example:

A client is febrile and has lost their appetite. The community nurse can make an assessment as to the person's capacity to self-manage at home. Key questions that can be asked include:

- Can the person self-monitor their blood glucose and respond to low and high blood glucose readings?
- Does the person have a friend or family member who can assist (e.g. to take them to the doctor)?
- Is the person able to maintain fluid and carbohydrate intake?
- Is the person able to continue their diabetes medications, e.g. self-administer insulin?
- If the person has type 1 diabetes, can they monitor the blood or urine ketones? Are the strips in date? Do they know what to do if a test is positive?
- Does the person know when to discontinue home management and seek medical review?

All the above questions can be used to determine if the person can self-manage at home or if a medical review should be sought.

Hypoglycaemia

Hypoglycaemia can occur in any person with diabetes who is treated with insulin or a particular group of oral medications (e.g. sulphonylurea). A response plan is most commonly developed by the person in partnership with their diabetes team and should include [23]:

- The blood glucose level at which to treat hypoglycaemia.
- Self-treatment options (e.g. glucose drink).
- Risk-reduction strategies (e.g. check blood glucose before driving).

An example of a response plan:

1. Blood glucose less than 4 mmol/L or symptomatic.
2. Have 90-mL Lucozade, wait 10 min and retest blood glucose.
3. If blood glucose still under 4 mmol/L, repeat step 2; if 4 mmol/L or above, have some slowly digested carbohydrate, e.g. slice of bread or piece of fruit.
4. Monitor blood glucose in 1 h and then 4-hourly for 24 h in case of repeat hypo.
5. If you have one severe or more than three mild hypos in 1 week, please see your medical practitioner or diabetes educator.
6. Always test before driving or walking for more than 1 h.

Mild hypoglycaemia is when a person is able to self-treat based on a blood glucose reading or recognition of symptoms. Severe hypoglycaemia is when the person requires assistance from another person. They may or may not be unconscious. If the person is unable to swallow or is unconscious they will require emergency treatment. Call an ambulance [23].

Some clients will be prescribed a glucagon injection, particularly those with type 1 diabetes and with insulin-treated type 2 diabetes. In this situation, friends or relatives can be taught to inject glucagon to reverse the symptoms. It may be appropriate for there to be a standing order for a community nurse to administer glucagon in an emergency. This should be documented in the person's care plan [23].

Nurses working in community settings can play an important role in identifying people at greatest risk, such as those [6]:

• With hypoglycaemia unawareness.
• With a history of severe hypoglycaemia.
• Who have had a rapid improvement of their blood glucose levels.
• Who are on medication, such as non-selective beta blockers.
• With autonomic neuropathy.
• Who use and abuse alcohol.

Community nurses are in a position to contribute to the education and reinforcement of safety measures, such as advising the person to always carry fast-acting carbohydrates (such as glucose tablets or jelly beans). Nurses can also contribute to:

• Community-wide awareness about the acute complications of diabetes.
• Ensuring that people with diabetes and their significant others have access to information about identification and management.
• People with diabetes having information about follow-up, support services and self-care [6].

Self-management

Self-management describes the activities carried out by the individual with diabetes to manage their condition. It can include physical activity, healthy eating, being part of the health care team, managing any psychosocial aspects and daily tasks such as blood glucose monitoring (BGM) and medication administration [6].

Working with a client to self-manage diabetes involves the community nurse working alongside the client to identify needs regarding education and information, and is based on a shared responsibility for the person's health and lifestyle choices. Self-management strategies can change as the person progresses along the illness trajectory and develops diabetes skills and knowledge which enhance their capacity to self-care. The key to success at any of these levels is in the negotiation and communication between the health care professional and the client.

There is now a strong evidence base to support the effectiveness of healthy eating and physical activity in the management of type 2 diabetes [13]. In type 1 diabetes, balancing insulin therapy, diet and exercise therapy usually requires a collaborative effort between the person, the dietitian, the diabetes educator and the medical specialist. Foot care and managing medications are also integral aspects of self-management. The community nurse is well positioned to support people to self-manage.

Diet/nutrition

A community nurse who works with the client in their own home is in a position to assess a client's food and nutritional intake. Nurses can work with clients to encourage meals that are appropriately sized to the person's age, gender and activity levels. They can also suggest a range of high-fibre carbohydrate foods (e.g. wholegrain breads and cereals, beans, lentils), vegetables and fruits, low-fat protein foods and low-fat dairy products [25]. Nutritional advice for people with diabetes can be guided by the joint statement published by the Dietitians Association Australia and the Australian Diabetes Educators Association [26].

Discussing weight issues with clients can sometimes be awkward. It is however important to raise awareness that overweight or obese individuals will find their diabetes more difficult to manage. The use of body mass index (BMI) [27] and waist circumference [28] (Table 12.1) measurement can be useful tools for determining risk and monitoring progress.

Physical activity/exercise

The amount and type of physical activity in a person's life varies significantly over time and will depend on age and changes to health and lifestyle. People with type 2 diabetes are often carrying extra weight and physical activity and therefore have substantial benefits such as [14]:

- Improved insulin sensitivity.
- Increased energy expenditure.
- Increased feeling of well-being.
- Improved blood pressure and lipid profiles.

Table 12.1 Waist circumference [28].

	Increased risk	High risk
Men	>94 cm	>102 cm
Women	>80 cm	>88 cm

A Cochrane review concluded that exercise in type 2 diabetes improves blood glucose control even when there is no weight loss [29]. If the person has not undertaken purposeful physical activity for some time, starting slowly and at low impact is recommended and then building up to a level which is suitable for the individual. It is paramount that the nurse collaboratively works with individuals to set and document specific goals for activity.

It is recommended that all adult Australians undertake moderately intense physical activity, e.g. walking, for >150 min per week [13, 15]. It is important that community nurses encourage all clients to incorporate some physical activity into their day. Each person needs to be assessed individually to ascertain safe, achievable and mutually desirable goals. For many people incorporating activity into their usual activities can be helpful, e.g. walking to the shop instead of driving or parking their car a bit further from the entrance of the building. A person who has problems mobilising could be encouraged to do leg and arm exercises whilst sitting. Exploring with the client about what exercise is possible for them is a good starting point.

Community nurses do need to be aware of the risks associated with starting an exercise programme, particularly when a person has cardiovascular risk factors. It is important to take an accurate history and advise the person to report to their doctor any exertion-induced symptoms, such as chest pain, abdominal discomfort or syncope [15]. Suitable footwear is also important for the person undertaking activities such as walking, jogging or cycling.

Education about blood glucose level management before and after exercise is vital. People on oral hypoglycaemics (e.g. sulphonylureas) or insulin must have glucose foods available when exercising as there is an increased risk of hypoglycaemia (low blood glucose level) [15].

People with type 1 diabetes will gain the same benefits from exercise as those in the general community, but care must be taken due to the risk of hypoglycaemia and hyperglycaemia [9]. Hypoglycaemia can occur during, immediately after or many hours after physical activity. Exercising with blood glucose >15 mmol/L can cause blood glucose to rise further [9]. The management of type 1 diabetes during exercise is complex and beyond the scope of this chapter. If a client is experiencing difficulties with exercise, referral to a Diabetes Education Service is recommended.

Foot care

People with diabetes are at risk of small- and large-blood-vessel disease, nerve damage and mechanical instabilities in the foot. Foot assessment is essential in the early identification of risk and to inform self-management education.

Community nurses have a role in reinforcing foot self-care strategies for people with diabetes. It is essential that a person with diabetes knows if their feet are at increased risk of injury or infection due to [23]:

- Loss of sensation (neuropathy, e.g. unaware of soft touch, tingling or burning of feet has disappeared, signs of pressure such as corns and calluses).
- Reduced blood supply to feet (peripheral vascular disease, e.g. reduced or absent foot pulses).
- Mechanical factors (e.g. abnormal shape such as hammer toes, bunions).

- Poor skin or nail condition.
- Inappropriate footwear (e.g. if shoes are too tight, there is a risk of blisters).
- Inability to self-care (e.g. cut nails safely).

All people with diabetes should check their own feet regularly. Community nurses should refer people to a podiatrist if their assessment reveals reduced sensation, reduced blood supply or mechanical deformities [30]. If the person is unsure of their own risk profile then with the client's consent, a referral to the person's medical practitioner, diabetes educator or podiatrist should be made. Some community nurses have undertaken extra training in the area of foot risk screening and are therefore adding to the pool of health professionals with this skill.

If a client with diabetes requires assistance with nail cutting, it is recommended that they have an assessment by their medical practitioner, diabetes educator or podiatrist. Nail cutting may need to be done by the client's family or a support person (including community nurses); however, the presence of vascular disease needs to be assessed, and if present, consultation with a podiatrist is recommended [31].

Oral therapy in type 2 diabetes

There is sufficient evidence to demonstrate that elevated blood glucose can cause a number of diabetes complications. In 1998 the UKPDS confirmed that hyperglycaemia in people with type 2 diabetes is progressive due to the gradual failing of the islet B cells' insulin production [13] and increasing insulin resistance [14]. By explaining to clients that many individuals with type 2 diabetes will eventually require insulin, a community nurse can assist people to understand that the commencement of insulin is not their fault [32].

Metformin and sulphonylureas are usually recommended as first-line medications for the management of type 2 diabetes unless contraindicated [13]. Results from the UKPDS support the use of metformin in all overweight people with type 2 diabetes and it is therefore recommended as the first oral medication to be initiated [13].

Sulphonylureas are used when metformin alone can no longer control blood glucose levels [13].

Metformin has been shown to significantly reduce the risk of diabetes-related morbidity and mortality in overweight people [3]. Metformin works by increasing insulin sensitivity in the liver, has positive effects on body weight and on its own will not cause hypoglycaemia [33]. Renal impairment is a contraindication for the use of metformin because it can cause a rare complication called lactic acidosis [13].

Sulphonylureas are insulin secretagogues and therefore increase insulin secretion. This in turn reduces glucose levels through the day [33]. The main side effect of these medications is hypoglycaemia and those with renal impairment are at an increased risk [13].

Acarbose is the only alpha-glycosidase inhibitor on the market in Australia. It inhibits the digestion of a form of carbohydrate (sucrose) and thus slows the rate of glucose delivery into the circulation. It needs to be taken at the time of starting the meal. Dosage needs to start low and increase gradually to avoid flatulence and abdominal discomfort. On its own, acarbose will not cause hypoglycaemia. If combined with a sulphonylurea or insulin and if hypoglycaemia occurs, it is important that glucose is used as treatment instead of sucrose [15, 33].

Thiazolidendiones are used to reduce insulin resistance in fat, muscle and, to a lesser degree, the liver. They are effective in reducing blood glucose levels throughout the day [15, 33]. Thiazolidendiones can be used with insulin or oral agents but are contraindicated in clients with heart failure or liver impairment [33].

Repaglinide is a meglitinide and is the only one available in Australia. It is a non-sulphonylurea insulin secretagogue that can be used on its own or with insulin sensitisers to control hyperglycaemia [33]. It should not be used in combination with sulphonylureas. Due to its rapid onset it should be taken immediately before each meal. Clients need to be aware that meals cannot be delayed or omitted and must contain adequate carbohydrate. Absence of carbohydrate will increase the risk of hypoglycaemia.

Many people with type 2 diabetes find themselves having to take a number of different medications. It is now understood that the more medications a person takes, the more likely there are to be errors [6, 34]. The following list of nursing interventions may assist community nurses to identify issues with medication:

1. Ask the client when and how they are taking their tablets or insulin.
2. Ask the client if they are experiencing any side effects from the medication; e.g. gastrointestinal side effects are common with metformin and acarbose.
3. Check that food intake is adequate and timely when they take their tablets or insulin.
4. Assess for risk of hypoglycaemia:
   a. Does the client have any renal impairment?
   b. Is the medication known to have hypoglycaemia as a side effect?
   c. Alcohol can increase the risk and severity of hypoglycaemia. Ask about alcohol consumption and assess risk.
   d. Does the client know how to prevent and manage hypoglycaemia?

Insulin therapy

Insulin is the only treatment for type 1 diabetes and is commonly used as the treatment in type 2 diabetes and gestational diabetes. Evidence-based guidelines recommend commencing insulin for people with type 2 diabetes when glycosylated haemoglobin (HbA1c) is greater than 7.5% [13]. HbA1c is a measure of the average blood glucose levels from the previous 4–6 weeks.

Research has highlighted that it is best to start insulin therapy in type 2 diabetes before insulin deficiency has progressed too far. It is usual for some oral agents to continue to be used in conjunction with insulin [13]. Starting insulin can cause anxiety, and support and education will be required. A diabetes education service can provide education for insulin initiation and stabilisation. A community nurse may be required to provide further support and supervision as needed. With the support of a medical practitioner and diabetes educator, a community nurse can provide education and primary care support of the person, depending on the skills and experience of the nurse. Refer to the Australian Diabetes Educators Association National Standards for the development and quality assessment of services initiating insulin therapy in the ambulatory setting [35].

As part of self-management education, people with diabetes can be taught to titrate their own insulin doses. In some circumstances the person may need assistance and a shared care arrangement between the community nurse, medical practitioner and diabetes educator can be set up.

There are a number of insulins available in Australia, which are listed below. Community nurses may learn more about the different types of insulins by obtaining a copy of the manufacturer's consumer medicine information.

Eli Lilly   www.lilly.com.au
NovoNordisk   www.novonordisk.com.au
Sanofi-aventis   www.sanofi-aventis.com.au

In type 1 diabetes, multiple daily injections of both basal insulin and meal-time (quick-acting) insulin are required and insulin is essential for survival. Some people may use an insulin pump that provides a continuous infusion of insulin. The use of various regimens and their benefits are described clearly in the NHMRC guidelines for type 1 diabetes [9].

In type 2 diabetes the evidence recommends [36, p. 39]:

- A basal insulin such as insulin detemir, insulin glargine or NPH (NPH has a higher risk of hypoglycaemia than detemir or glargine) *or*
- Twice daily premixed insulin *or*
- Multiple daily injections, e.g. meal time and basal (may be required in time)

There has been a substantial change in the types of insulins available now. Consequently, community nurses need to keep abreast of information about all medicines. This is best done by referring to information from the manufacturer in the medicine packaging, the *MIMS Handbook* and the *Australian Medicines Handbook* website, http://www.amh.net.au/.

Nurses who are visiting clients in the home are advised to check the following [9, 37]:

1. Insulin in use is stored at room temperature.
2. Insulin not in use is stored on its side in the fridge (between 4°C and 8°C).
3. If insulin is clumpy or frosting or if it shows signs of precipitation, discard as this can cause loss of potency.
4. Check manufacturer's guidelines for discard date once opened.
5. Check manufacturer's guidelines for mixing insulin. (Long-acting analogues should not be mixed with any other insulin.)
6. Check manufacturer's guidelines for storage of predrawn syringes.
7. Check client's technique when administering insulin.
   - Do they rotate within the abdomen area each time? (Abdomen is preferred site.)
   - Do they ensure complete delivery of the dose by keeping the needle embedded in the skin for 5 seconds after administration is complete (especially with insulin pens)?
8. The timing of quick-acting insulin with food is critical. Assess client to ensure that timing of insulin and food intake is appropriate.
9. When using insulin pens/device:
   - Refer to the manufacturer's instructions prior to using the insulin device.

- Manufacturers recommend that pen needles are not reused, as this practice can increase the risk of infection or the tip could break off.
- Ensure person checks for insulin flow before every injection when using these devices.
- All health care agencies should have in place specific protocols regarding the safe use of all available insulin delivery devices.

Capillary blood glucose monitoring

Blood glucose meters are available for capillary testing in the home and are available at some hospitals, community health services or pharmacies and Diabetes Australia in each state. The meters can be operated by the person, and rely on a single drop of blood from the finger. Strips for the meters are sold at a subsidised cost via the National Diabetes Services Scheme (NDSS). This scheme is operated out of Diabetes Australia offices in each of the states and territories, and in some states via selected pharmacies. A GP or credentialed diabetes educator can arrange registration for the client.

The frequency and timing of capillary BGM will vary depending on the type of diabetes and how stable the person is at the time (e.g. medication change or unwell). Frequency, timing and targets for capillary BGM should be discussed with the client's GP, diabetes educator and the client (see Table 12.2). It is also important that appropriate diabetes self-management education be provided to those wishing to/recommended to self-monitor, as this has been shown to provide the best outcomes (clinical and quality of life) for people [39].

Table 12.2 A general guide to capillary BGM in a community setting [23].

Type 1 diabetes	<ul><li>Fasting and premeals daily[a]</li><li>Any time person suspects either hypo- or hyperglycaemia</li><li>2–4 hourly if unwell</li></ul>
Gestational diabetes [38] Pregnant type 1 or type 2 [16]	<ul><li>Fasting</li><li>2-h postprandial[b]</li><li>Any time person suspects either hypo- or hyperglycaemia</li><li>2–4 hourly if unwell (if on insulin)</li></ul>
Type 2 diabetes – Insulin treated – Sulphonylurea treated – Metformin/glitazones/acarbose[c] – Lifestyle only[c]	<ul><li>Fasting</li><li>Pre-meals depending on type of insulin[a]</li><li>Fasting</li><li>Pre-meals[a]</li><li>Fasting</li><li>Pre-meals[a]</li></ul>

[a]Pre-meal test can vary during the week.
[b]Postprandial monitoring is defined as 2 h from start of meal.
[c]There is limited evidence to support clinical outcomes for capillary monitoring in this group.

Times when the community nurse would be required to perform extra capillary BGM include [36]:

- If the client is unwell (e.g. hypoglycaemia, fever, infected wound, gastrointestinal upset, not eating/drinking).
- If there are changes to treatment, such as increased hypoglycaemic medication or commencement of/changes to insulin.
- If the client has been recently discharged from hospital.
- Any time the nurse is concerned about the person or accuracy of results.

Why test?

The purpose of BGM in diabetes is to monitor and evaluate the capillary blood glucose level and the effect of diabetes management for an individual. Capillary blood glucose measurements enable the assessment and adjustment of therapy in a timely manner, such as identifying aberrations in blood glucose levels that may put the person at immediate or long-term risk [40]. BGM can be a useful tool in monitoring progress and managing fluctuations in blood glucose levels. Community nurses can be pivotal in discussions about how various lifestyle measures or medications can affect blood glucose. Encouraging clients to record their blood glucose levels as well as any comments about diet or exercise can help clients to develop better problem-solving skills.

Who should test?

There is evidence of the benefits of capillary BGM for clients with type 1 diabetes and those with gestational diabetes [4, 38]. It is recommended that BGM be available to clients when it is used to [13]:

- Provide information about hypoglycaemia.
- Assess how glucose levels are affected by medication and lifestyle.
- Monitor changes during intercurrent illness.

Targets

In partnership with the person, BGM targets are developed by the GP or diabetes specialist. It is important when setting targets to consider the person's age, living circumstances (e.g. lives alone) and their capacity to respond to hypoglycaemia (e.g. physical or mental impairment). Nurses need to know general blood glucose targets (see Table 12.3) whilst being aware that some people will require modification of targets.

Importance of quality control

Quality control refers to both the accuracy of the meter and the operator's technique.

Nurses working in the community are advised to check the following with their clients who are self–blood glucose monitoring [41]:

- Blood glucose meters and strips should be protected from extreme heat and cold.
- The strips must be in date and secure in the packaging. (Exposure to air/moisture can cause incorrect readings.)
- Calibration codes/code sticks must be consistent with each new pack of strips.

- Meters used by individual clients should be quality control checked, with control solution as outlined by the manufacturer.
- The person's finger-pricking device should have the lancet changed regularly and disposed of in a sharps container.
- All sharps should be disposed of in a sharps container (ridged-sided containers available from local councils, Diabetes Australia, some health services).
- Ensure the person's finger is clean prior to testing (handwashing).
- The person should be able to demonstrate correct technique as per operator's instructions.

Organisations should ensure that [41]:

- Meters used by the health care team are quality control checked, with control solution as outlined in their health service policy.
- Finger-pricking devices used by the community nurse must be single use and have a retractable lancet and be fully disposable.

Aims of diabetes management

The focus of care in diabetes management may differ depending on the type of diabetes (type 1, type 2 or gestational), the time since diagnosis and existing comorbidities. Clients and their health care team should design a management strategy to prevent, delay and reduce the impact of any complications. Community nurses have a key role in reinforcing management strategies that have been developed by the person in partnership with their diabetes team. Table 12.4 summarises the general targets that underpin management strategies.

Table 12.3 General targets for capillary BGM.

Type of diabetes	Fasting and premeal (mmol/L)	2-h postprandial (mmol/L)	Comment
Type 1 and type 2 diabetes [15]	4.0–6.0	4.0–7.7	Normoglycaemia
	6.1–6.9	7.8–11.0	Minimises microvascular problems
	≥ 7.0	≥ 11.1	Associated with micro- and macrovascular complications
	>8.0	>20.0	Consider more active treatment Generally prompts further and more active treatment
Gestational diabetes [38]	4.0–5.5	<7.0	At least one or two postprandial levels obtained each day
Pre-existing type 1 or type 2 diabetes in pregnancy [16]	4.0–5.5	<7.0	

Table 12.4 Aims for diabetes management (type 2 diabetes focused but can be adapted for type 1 diabetes) [15].

	Target
BGL	4–6 mmol/L (fasting)
HbA1c	≤ 7%
LDL-C	<2.5 mmol/L
Total cholesterol	<4.0 mmol/L
HDL-C	>1.0 mmol/L
Triglycerides	<1.5 mmol/L
Blood pressure	≤ 130/80mm Hg
BMI	<25 kg/m^2 where practicable
Microalbuminuria	<20 mg/L spot collection
	<20 mg/min timed overnight collection
Smoking	Review yearly
Alcohol intake	Review
Physical activity	Review yearly
Healthy eating	Review yearly
Medications	Review yearly
Self-care	Review yearly
Feet examination	Referral if problem requiring review
Eye examination	At least 2 yearly

Community groups with specific needs

Pregnant women

About 4.7% of pregnancies will be complicated by diabetes mellitus (0.5% in women with pre-existing diabetes – type 1 or type 2 – and 4.2% gestational diabetes) [8].

Women who have either pre-existing type 1 or type 2 diabetes benefit from having access to preconception counselling and are advised to try for close-to-normal blood glucose readings and HbA1c in the months prior to conception.

An education update is recommended before and during pregnancy when diabetes management is usually altered and intensified. For example women with pre-existing type 2 diabetes will usually have oral hypoglycaemic agents stopped prior to or as soon as conception is realised. Insulin therapy remains the most frequently used medication [16]. Women with type 1 diabetes will usually have a change in insulin requirements. It is therefore necessary for such women to have regular contact with their treating medical practitioner, diabetes educator and dietitian.

Because of the changing insulin needs throughout pregnancy, the ADPIS recommends regular BGM (approx four tests per day), but this will be dependent on the type of insulin therapy.

In gestational diabetes or pre-existing type 1 or type 2 diabetes, the aim of treatment is to maintain the fasting blood glucose value <5.5 mmol/L and 2-h postprandial <7.0 mmol/L [40]. If glucose targets are not being met, insulin therapy can be commenced/modified depending on the type of diabetes. Insulin therapy is safe to commence in a community setting with the support of the medical practitioner and diabetes educator. A community nurse can provide reinforcement of education and primary care support for the women. As part of self-management education most people are taught to titrate their own insulin doses. In some circumstances the person may need extra support, and a shared care arrangement between a community nurse and the diabetes team can be set up for this purpose.

After delivery, the insulin requirements will change for both women with type 1 diabetes or women with insulin-treated type 2 diabetes. Women who decide to breastfeed may have decreased insulin requirements and increased energy requirements. Continuing to see a dietitian or diabetes educator can assist in this transition.

Community nurses can remind women who have had gestational diabetes that they should continue with a healthy diet and lifestyle and also aim for a healthy weight. Women with gestational diabetes should receive counselling about the risks of developing type 2 diabetes and/or gestational diabetes in subsequent pregnancies. There is no need for ongoing self-monitoring if the mother's blood glucose level is normal after delivery. Women should know that symptoms such as polyuria, polydipsia, polyphagia, thrush and blurred vision may indicate the development of type 2 diabetes [40].

Rural and remote communities

Thirty four per cent of Australians live in either a rural or remote area [42]. It is important to acknowledge that rural and more so remote communities have less access to health care, suffer more preventable morbidity and mortality and have lower numbers and diversity in specialist health professionals per population [43]. The above factors can contribute to barriers in access to necessary services for the community.

Community nursing in a rural or remote area brings with it the challenges of distance, isolation and limited access to specialist support services. In the context of diabetes there are a number of strategies that can assist community nurses in providing evidence-based care for people with all types of diabetes. These strategies include:

- Develop networks with local/regional diabetes education health professionals and those in the cities where clients are sent or referred to. Having access to the local/regional diabetes team is essential.
- Use distance communication technologies in rural and remote areas which can facilitate communication with other members of the diabetes team and assist with access to diabetes professional development.

A significant number of rural and remote centres now have videoconferencing technology and this can be used to facilitate consultation with specialists. It can also be used as a means to link multiple sites to enable case conferencing and problem solving.

As new research emerges and information about the management of diabetes changes, it is important to have in place continuing education strategies to assist with 'keeping up to date.' In some Australian states this has been addressed by setting up either regional or statewide networks to assist with access to peer support and specialist health professionals [44]. Diabetes resource nurse positions have also been established in some areas. These positions can be located in acute or community care and have become effective providers of diabetes information in primary health settings.

Indigenous communities

'Diabetes is a significant cause of excess morbidity and mortality among Aboriginal and Torres Strait Islander people' [45]. Type 2 diabetes also occurs at a higher rate and at a younger age than for non-Indigenous people [46].

In Australia, state-funded health services provide services to the community. In some areas the Aboriginal-Community-Controlled Health Services (ACCHS) are also providing primary health care services specific to Indigenous communities. Community health nurses are employed in a range of settings, including ACCHS, and can contribute significantly to the health of these communities and to the support and education of Aboriginal health workers. The roles of Aboriginal health workers within the community health team are integral when working with Aboriginal people with diabetes. Some Aboriginal health workers are also trained as diabetes educators and assist with providing care.

Culturally and linguistically diverse community groups

It is well recognised that many culturally and linguistically diverse (CALD) community groups have a high prevalence of diabetes compared with the non-Indigenous Australia-born population. This has been attributed to a combination of genetic, biological, behavioural and environmental risk factors [47]. Ethnic background is also an important risk factor in the development of gestational diabetes [48].

For some migrants adopting a 'Westernised' lifestyle, such as increased consumption of energy-dense foods, in conjunction with a more sedentary lifestyle leads to excess weight gain and thus increases their risk for type 2 diabetes [47]. A systematic review has highlighted that communities from CALD backgrounds are also at a high risk of diabetes complications because of the many barriers they face when accessing health services. Barriers identified include [49]:

- Language.
- Literacy (in English and native language).
- Stigmatisation.
- Lack of access to culturally specific care.
- Religious beliefs and cultural practices.

Religious beliefs and cultural practices can affect the person's ability or desire to self-manage. There may be different perceptions of what actions will have a positive effect on health across various cultures. For example Muslims wishing to fast during Ramadan will require community nurses to work with them to ensure that blood glucose levels do not become too low [50, 51]. A systematic review has identified that strategies to address diabetes health care needs should [49]:

- Be culturally specific.
- Incorporate the diet, beliefs and attitudes of the cultural group.
- Foster increased understanding, interest and participation.

Culturally specific resources can help with these situations and Diabetes Australia does provide a national multilingual internet resource for consumers and health professionals [52].

Children and adolescents

Type 1 diabetes is by far the most common type of diabetes in childhood and adolescence [53], though the incidence of type 2 diabetes in this age group is increasing [10].

Children with type 1 diabetes will be treated with insulin from diagnosis. Their insulin schedules will be expected to change as they grow into adulthood. There are a range of insulins covering both basal and meal-time (bolus) insulin needs, as well as a range of insulin delivery devices such as syringes, pens and insulin pumps. It is now more common to commence children with type 1 diabetes on insulin pump therapy as a standard insulin administration strategy. Community nurses visiting schools will see a range of insulin and devices used. In children with type 2 diabetes, lifestyle education remains the foundation of management. It is essential that the education be done as a whole-of-family approach.

Any child with type 1 or type 2 diabetes will need access to a specialist diabetes team. This team (including the parents or carers) will oversee insulin dosage and timing of insulin. However, medications such as metformin and insulin are also prescribed in some cases. A community nurse may be required to provide support to a child at school if insulin injections or BGM is needed within school hours. Working closely with the parents and school staff is essential.

The management of diabetes may be more difficult during the adolescent years and it has been documented that glycaemic control deteriorates [54–56]. Puberty is associated with insulin resistance and therefore young people at this time may require more insulin than specified for body weight [53]. Important issues such as alcohol and illicit drug use, dating, sex, contraception, driving, employment, study and sport must be discussed in a non-judgemental way with the client. It is important that community nurses identify adolescents at risk and provide appropriate support and referral to specialists as required, e.g. a credentialed diabetes educator.

People with mental health/illness issues

There is a higher prevalence of diabetes amongst individuals who live with psychotic disorders and other mental illness as compared with the rest of the population [57]. A diagnosis of diabetes has also been shown to double the odds of depression [58]. Increased prevalence of diabetes in people with depression relates to the illness itself, poor dietary habits, lack of exercise and the direct or indirect effects of antipsychotic and other psychotropic medications [57, 59].

Second-generation antipsychotic (SGA) medications are widely used in conditions such as schizophrenia, bipolar disorder, dementia and psychotic depression. In many individuals these medications can be the difference between leading an engaged and fulfilling life and being severely disabled [60]. The use of SGA medications has been associated with reports of dramatic weight gain, diabetes and changes in lipid profiles [60]; hence, all people taking antipsychotic medication should be screened by their GP for diabetes risk factors [57].

Nurses caring for clients with mental illness can encourage healthy eating and activity, as these can improve metabolic parameters even when there is no weight loss

[57]. Assessing clients for signs and symptoms of diabetes as well as being aware of the possibility of DKA in clients taking SGA medication is also important [60]. Furthermore, knowledge of diabetes has been demonstrated to be lower in populations with mental illness when compared to the general population [61]. Frequent repetition of important information can be beneficial for all persons with diabetes but is deemed critical in clients with a psychotic illness.

An Australian guide about diabetes for consumers and their carers has been produced and may be useful for community nurses who are caring for clients with a psychotic condition who are at risk of diabetes or already have been diagnosed with diabetes (see 'Useful resources').

Summary

Diabetes is a condition which requires the response of a dedicated interdisciplinary team that is committed to providing person-centred care. A diagnosis of diabetes places a huge responsibility on the person to manage a multifaceted treatment programme [6]. In addition, people have to cope with the knowledge that diabetes complications are a possibility, and for many, complications are already present at diagnosis. It is not surprising that psychosocial and mental health issues may arise.

Due to the self-managing nature of diabetes there is a significant role for nurses who work in community settings. Firstly, they can identify clients who require more information or support for their diabetes and assist to link them into appropriate services. Secondly, the community nurse is in an excellent position to reinforce information around lifestyle measures, acute complications, medications and screening. All health professionals who have a point of contact with people with diabetes have a responsibility to ensure that they are linked into appropriate services. We contend that community nurses are pivotal in connecting such people with acute and community-based diabetes services.

Useful resources

Australian Diabetes Educators Association (ADEA) at http://www.adea.com.au/index.aspx
  Provides information and support for health professionals interested in diabetes care
Beyond Blue at www.beyondblue.org
  A national organisation that works to address issues associated with depression, anxiety and substance misuse in Australia
Diabetes Australia (DA) at http://www.diabetesaustralia.com.au/home/index.htm
  Provides a full range of fact sheets for the person with diabetes and their support person. There are also a number of links to resources for health professionals on the DA website
Diabetes, psychotic disorders and antipsychotic therapy at www.psychiatry.unimelb.edu.au/open/diabetes_consensus/
  Includes a consensus statement as well as a guide for consumers and carers
Dietitians Association of Australia at http://www.daa.asn.au/
  Provides up-to-date information about nutrition
Indigenous people at http://www.healthinfonet.ecu.edu.au/
  For people interested in improving the health of Indigenous Australians

National Evidence-Based Guidelines for the Management of Type 2 Diabetes Mellitus at http://www.diabetesaustralia.com.au/education_info/nebg.html
  Guidelines endorsed by the NHMRC and can be found on the DA website
National Diabetes Supply Scheme (NDSS) at http://www.diabetesaustralia.com.au/ndss/index.html
  An Australian government programme that provides blood- and urine-testing strips, syringes and needles at a subsidised cost
National Service Improvement Framework for Diabetes at www.health.gov.au/internet/wcms/publishing.nsf/Content/pq-ncds-diabetes
  Part of the National Chronic Disease Strategy and provides a national approach for improving health services and care for people with diabetes
Quality of use of medicines at www.health.gov.au/internet/wcms/publishing.nsf/Content/nmp-quality.html
  Australian Government Department of Health & Ageing, National Medicines Policy
Royal Australian College of General Practitioners' Diabetes Guidelines at http://www.racgp.org.au/guidelines/
SNAP (Smoking, Nutrition, Alcohol, Physical Activity) at www.racgp.org.au/guidelines/snap
  A population health guide to behavioural risk factors in general practice
QUIT smoking at www.quitnow.info.au

References

1. Australian Institute of Health and Welfare (2002) *Diabetes: Australian Facts* 2002. AIHW Cat. No. CVD 20 (Diabetes Series No. 3). Australian Government, Canberra.
2. Australian Centre for Diabetes Strategies, Diabetes Australia Guideline Development Consortium (2004) *National Evidence Based Guidelines for the Management of Type 2 Diabetes: Part 5 Prevention and Detection of Macrovascular Disease*. National Health and Medical Research Council, Canberra.
3. UK Prospective Diabetes Research Group (1998) UK Prospective Study 24: A 6 year, randomized, controlled trial comparing sulfonylurea, insulin and metformin therapy in patients with newly diagnosed type 2 diabetes that could not be controlled with diet therapy. *Annals of Internal Medicine*, 128(3), 165–75.
4. The Diabetes Control and Complications Trial Research Group (1993) The effect of intensive treatment of diabetes on the development and progression of long-term complications in insulin-dependent diabetes mellitus. *The New England Journal of Medicine*, 329(14), 977–86.
5. Linekin, P. (2003) Home health care and diabetes assessment, care and education. *Diabetes Spectrum*, 16(4), 217–22.
6. National Health Priority Action Council (2006) *National Service Improvement Framework for Diabetes*. Australian Government Department of Health and Ageing, Canberra.
7. Twigg, S., Kamp, M., Davis, T., Neylon, E. and Flack, J. (2007) Prediabetes: A position statement from the Australian Diabetes Society and Australian Diabetes Educators Association. *Medical Journal of Australia*, 186(7), 461–65.
8. Chan, A., Scott, J., Nguyen, A. and Sage, L. (2004) *Pregnancy Outcomes in South Australia*. Epidemiology Branch, Department of Health, Adelaide.
9. Australasian Paediatric Endocrine Group for the Department of Health and Ageing (2005) *Clinical Practice Guidelines: Type 1 Diabetes in Children and Adolescents*. Australian Government and National Health and Medical Research Council, Canberra.
10. McMahon, S., Haynes, A., Ratnam, N., Grant, M., Carne, C., Jones, T., *et al.* (2004) Increase in type 2 diabetes in children and adolescents in Western Australia. *Medical Journal of Australia*, 180(9), 459–61.

11. Diabetes Australia (2007) *What is Diabetes?*. Fact Sheet. Available at http://www. diabetesaustralia.com.au/education_info/sheets.html (viewed 21 April 2007).

12. Dunstan, D., Zimmet, P., Welborn, T., De Courten, M., Cameron, A., Sicree, R., *et al.* (2002) The rising prevalence of diabetes and impaired glucose tolerance: The Australian Diabetes, Obesity and Lifestyle Study. *Diabetes Care*, 25(5), 829–34.

13. Clinical Guidelines Task Force (2005) *Global Guidelines for Type 2 Diabetes*. International Diabetes Federation, Newcastle on Tyne, UK.

14. Campos, C. (2007) Treating the whole patient for optimal management of Type 2 diabetes: Considerations for insulin therapy. *Southern Medical Journal*, 100(8), 804–11.

15. The Royal Australian College of General Practitioners (2007/8) *Diabetes Management in General Practice*. Diabetes Australia and The Royal Australian College of General Practitioners, Sydney, NSW.

16. McElduff, A., Cheung, N.W., McIntyre, H.D., Lagstrom, J.A., Oats, J.J.N., Ross, G.P., *et al.* (2005) The Australasian Diabetes in Pregnancy Society consensus guidelines for the management of type 1 and type 2 diabetes in relation to pregnancy. *Medical Journal of Australia*, 183(7), 373–7.

17. Australian Centre for Diabetes Strategies, Diabetes Australia Guideline Development Consortium (2004) *National Evidence Based Guidelines for the Management of Type 2 Diabetes Mellitus: Part 3 Case Detection and Diagnosis of Type 2 Diabetes*. National Health and Medical Research Council, Canberra.

18. Australian Diabetes Educators Association (2005) *Use of Blood Glucose Meters: Position Paper*. Available at http://www.adea.com.au/public/content/ViewCategory.aspx?id=37 (viewed 18 November 2007).

19. Welborn, T. (1996) *Position Statement; Screening for Non-Insulin Dependent Diabetes*. Available at http://www.racp.edu.au/ads/posstate_archive.htm (viewed 18 November 2007).

20. Wass, A. (1998) *Promoting Health: The Primary Health Care Approach*, 2nd edition. Harcourt Australia, Sydney.

21. Diabetes Clearing House (2007) *Diab Info Newsletter: Diabetes and Social Inequalities*. Department of Health, Adelaide.

22. Kessler, R., Barker, P., Colpe, L., Epstein, J., Gfoerer, J., Hiripi, E., *et al.* (2003) Screening for serious mental illness in the general population. *Archives of General Psychiatry*, 60(2), 184–9.

23. Diabetes Outreach (2006) *Diabetes Manual: A Guide to Diabetes Management*, 5th edition. Diabetes Outreach, Adelaide, Australia.

24. Australian Diabetes Educators Association (2006) *Sick Day Guidelines: Guidelines for Sick Day Management for People with Diabetes*. Available at http://www.adea.com.au/public/content/ViewCategory.aspx?id=39 (viewed October 2007).

25. National Health and Medical Research Council (2003) *Dietary Guidelines for Australian Adults*. Canberra.

26. Dietitians Association Australia, Australian Diabetes Educators Association (2005) *Joint Statement on the Role of Accredited Practicing Dietitians and Diabetes Educators in the Delivery of Nutrition and Diabetes Self Management Education Services for People with Diabetes*. Dietitians Association Australia and Australian Diabetes Educators Association, Canberra.

27. National Health and Medical Research Council (1997) *Acting on Australia's Weight: A Strategic Plan for the Prevention of Overweight and Obesity*. National Health and Medical Research Council, Canberra.

28. Heart Foundation (2004) *Hypertension Management Guide for Doctors*. Available at http://www.heartfoundation.org.au/Professional_Information/Clinical_Practice/Prevention. htm (viewed 25 November 2004).

29. Thomas, D., Elliot, E. and Naughton, G. (2006) Exercise for type 2 diabetes mellitus. *The Cochrane Database of Systematic Reviews*, 3.
30. National Association of Diabetes Centres, Podiatry Council (2001) *National Foot Care Training Manual*. ACT, Braddon.
31. Australasian Podiatry Council (1997) *Australian Podiatric Guidelines for Diabetes*, 2nd edition. Australasian Podiatry Council, Victoria.
32. Eskesen, S., Kesberg, G. and Hitchcock, K. (2006) What is the role of combination therapy (insulin plus oral medication) in type 2 diabetes? *Journal of Family Physicians*, 55(11), 1001–3.
33. Phillips, P. and Braddon, J. (July 2002) Oral hypoglycaemics. *Australian Family Physician*, 31(7), 637–43.
34. Cramer, J. (2004) A systematic review of adherence for diabetes. *Diabetes Care*, 27(5), 1218–24.
35. Australian Diabetes Educators Association (2004) *National Standards for the Development and Quality Assessment of Services Initiating Insulin Therapy in the Ambulatory Setting*. Australian Diabetes Educators Association, Canberra.
36. Walker, R. (2004) Capillary blood glucose monitoring and its role in diabetes management. *British Journal of Community Nursing*, 9(10), 438–40.
37. American Diabetes Association (January 2004) Insulin administration. *Diabetes Care*, 27, S106.
38. Hoffman, L., Nolan, C., Wilson, J.D., Oats, J.J.N. and Simmons, D. (1998) Gestational diabetes mellitus – management guidelines. *The Medical Journal of Australia*, 169(2), 93–7.
39. Martin, S., Scheidener, B., Heinemann, L., Lodwig, V., Kurth, H. and Scherbaum, W. (2005) Self-monitoring of blood glucose in type 2 diabetes and long-term outcome: And epidemiology cohort study. *Diabetologia*, 49(2), 271–8.
40. Australian Diabetes Educators Association (September 2005) *Position Statement: Use of Blood Glucose Meters*. Australian Diabetes Educators Association, Canberra.
41. Australian Diabetes Educators Association (2004) *Minimum Standards for Use of Capillary Blood Glucose Sampling Devices in a Health Care Setting*. Australian Diabetes Educators Association, Canberra.
42. Australian Institute of Health and Welfare (2006) *Australia's Health*. Available at http://www.aihw.gov.au/publications/index.cfm/title/10321 (viewed 21 April 2007).
43. Muula, A. (2007) *How Do We Define 'Rurality' in the Teaching on Medical Demography?* Rural and Remote Health. Available at http://www.rrh.org.au/articles/showarticlenew.asp?ArticleID=653 (viewed 23 November 2007).
44. Giles, J. and Phillips, P. (2006) *Diabetes Outreach Report*. Diabetes Outreach, Adelaide.
45. Couzos, S. and Murray, R. (2003) *Aboriginal Primary Health Care: An Evidence Based Approach*, 2nd edition. Oxford University Press, Oxford.
46. De Courten, M., Hodge, A., Dowse, G., King, I., Vickery, J. and Zimmet, P. (1998) *Review of the Epidemiology, Aetiology, Pathogenesis and Preventability of Diabetes in Aboriginal and Torres Strait Islander Populations*. Commonwealth Department of Health and Family Services, Canberra.
47. Thow, A. and Waters, A. (2005) *Diabetes in Culturally and Linguistically Diverse Australians*. Australian Institute of Health and Welfare, Canberra.
48. Beischer, N., Oats, J., Henry, O., Sheedy, M. and Walstab, J. (1991) Incidence and severity of gestational diabetes mellitus according to country of birth in women living in Australia. *Diabetes*, 40(Suppl 2), 35–8.
49. von Hofe, B., Thomas, M. and Coligiuri, R. (2002) *A Systematic Review of Issues Impacting on Health Care for Culturally Diverse Groups Using Diabetes as a Model*. Australian Centre for Diabetes Strategies & Multicultural Health Unit, Sydney.
50. Burden, M. (2001) Culturally sensitive care: Managing diabetes during Ramadan. *British Journal of Community Nursing*, 6(11), 581–5.

51. Naeem, A. (2003) The role of culture and religion in the management of diabetes: A study of Kashmiri men in Leeds. *The Journal of the Royal Society for the Promotion of Health*, 123(2), 110–16.

52. Diabetes Australia (2002–2005) *Multilingual Internet Resource*. Available at http://www.diabetesaustralia.com.au/multilingualdiabetes/index.htm (viewed 27 March 2007).

53. Pickup, J. and Williams, G. (2004) *Handbook of Diabetes*, 3rd edition. Blackwell Publishing, UK.

54. Bryden, K.S., Peveler, R.C., Stein, A., Neil, A., Mayou, R.A. and Dunger, D.B. (September 2001) Clinical and psychological course of diabetes from adolescence to young adulthood: A longitudinal cohort study. *Diabetes Care*, 24(9), 1536–40.

55. Frank, M. (September 1992) Rights to passage: Transition from paediatric to adult diabetes care. *Beta Release*, 16(3), 85–9.

56. Silink, M., Clarke, C., Couper, J.J., Craig, M., Crock, P., Davies, R., *et al.* (2003–2004) Chapter 3: Medical management. *Australian Clinical Practice Guidelines: Type 1 Diabetes in Children and Adolescents*, pp. 41–7.

57. Lambert, T. and Chapman, L. (2004) Diabetes, psychotic disorders and antipsychotic therapy: A consensus statement. *Medical Journal of Australia*, 181(10), 544–9.

58. Anderson, R., Freedland, K., Clouse, R. and Lustman, P. (2001) The prevalence of comorbid depression in adults with depression. *Diabetes Care*, 24(6), 1069–79.

59. Sokal, J., Messias, E., Dickerson, F., Kreyenbuhl, J., Brown, C., Goldberg, R., *et al.* (2004) Comorbidity of medical illnesses among adults with serious mental illness who are receiving community psychiatric services. *The Journal of Nervous and Mental Disease*, 192(6), 421–7.

60. American Diabetes Association (2004) Consensus development conference on antipsychotic drugs and obesity and diabetes. *Diabetes Care*, 27(2), 596–602.

61. Dickerson, F., Goldberg, R., Brown, C., Kreyenbuhl, J., Wohlheiter, K., Fang, L., *et al.* (2005) Diabetes knowledge among persons with serious mental illness and Type 2 diabetes. *Psychosomatics*, 46(5), 418–24.

Chapter 13

Vascular access device management in the community

Lisa Turner

Introduction

Management of vascular access devices (VAD), commonly referred to as intravenous therapy, is an emerging nursing specialty. The development of devices designed to ensure long-term venous access for a client results in the community nurse's involvement in their management. Community nurses are involved in the care of clients with VADs who are discharged from the acute care sector and those who are managed by general practitioners (GPs). Confusion occurs regarding the management of these devices because each organisation has policies and procedures which at times contradict each other. National guidelines for the management of VADs in Australia are under development but are well established in the United States of America [1–6]. The purpose of this chapter is to identify the principles that underpin the management of VADs in the community setting. This will enable the community nurse to effectively maintain venous access and develop the ability to troubleshoot difficulties that may be encountered.

The management of VADs remains controversial because of differing organisational protocols and procedures. The evidence found in the literature explores issues surrounding almost every aspect of VAD management but also describes prescriptive, localised protocols and procedures. Clinicians need to be comfortable with all aspects of this information spectrum to effectively manage these devices. A potential complication of any device inserted into the venous system is infection, either local catheter infection or bloodstream infections [1, 7]. Regardless of the type of infection, it can lead to the need to remove the device prematurely [8, 9], thus impacting on the successful or timely completion of intravenous therapy. Exploration of the broader information and the debate concerning VAD management is important because of:

- The increasing diversity of the types of access devices.
- The evolving evidence surrounding various components of VAD management.
- The diverse settings where VADs are managed mean that rigid protocols and procedures will not remain current or relevant for long.

Community nurses need to be able to consider appropriate options for managing a VAD, in any given context, based on the current collective knowledge. It may be difficult for the individual community nurses to obtain a level of expertise with VAD management if they are infrequently required to care for clients with VADs. The importance of a dedicated VAD team for the effective management of these devices is supported by the evidence [10, 11]. The relevance of this approach to the management of VADs will be discussed further in this chapter.

What are VADs?

A VAD is a sterile, thin, flexible catheter inserted into a vein or artery to provide short- or long-term vascular access for the administration of medication, total parenteral nutrition, fluids, blood products and chemotherapeutic agents or aspiration of blood for analysis [12]. The most commonly encountered VADs in the community are:

1. Peripherally inserted venous catheters (PIVC) – often referred to as
   a. Jelcos
   b. Bungs
   c. Cannulas
2. Mid- or long lines
3. Peripherally inserted central catheters (PICC)
4. Central venous catheters (CVC) – tunnelled or non-tunnelled
5. Port-a-caths or infusaports – referred to as 'ports'

The terminology used to identify different types of catheters can be confusing because clinicians and researchers utilise components of the catheters to describe the catheter in use. The Centre for Disease Control and Prevention [1] recommends using systematic criteria for identifying VADs. The criteria and descriptions of VADs are detailed in Table 13.1.

Overview of VADs

A basic understanding of the anatomy and physiology of the vasculature is an important underpinning principle for the community nurse who is required to utilise this knowledge in the everyday management of all VADs. This knowledge also assists the nurse to educate clients about VADs. For example many clients are not aware that a PICC line is a catheter that has its tip terminating in the superior vena cava (SVC) or very close to their heart. If the nurse is not aware of the importance of this from a management perspective then the client cannot be educated appropriately about their responsibilities in caring for their PICC.

As with any medical device there are advantages and disadvantages that come with specific device properties. Catheter material is an important consideration when exploring the appropriate device to be used. An understanding of catheter properties provides additional knowledge to be drawn upon when troubleshooting catheter issues. Table 13.2 identifies commonly encountered catheters and their properties.

Table 13.1 The criteria and descriptions of VADs.

Catheter type	Entry site	Length	Comments
Peripheral venous catheter	Usually inserted in veins of forearm or hand	<7 cm, rarely associated with bloodstream infections	Phlebitis with prolonged use
Midline catheters	Inserted via the antecubital fossa into the proximal basillic or cephalic veins: does not enter central veins	>7 cm, <19 cm	Lower rates of phlebitis than short peripheral catheters
Non-tunnelled central venous catheters	Percutaneously inserted into central veins (subclavian, internal jugular or femoral)	>8 cm depending on patient size	Account for majority of CRBSI
Peripherally inserted central catheters	Inserted into basillic, cephalic or brachial vein with the tip residing in the superior vena cava	>30 cm depending on patient size	Lower rate than non-tunnelled CVC
Totally implantable	Tunnelled beneath the skin and subcutaneous port accessed with a needle: implanted in the subclavian or internal jugular vein	>8 cm depending on patient size	Lowest risk for CRBSI: improved patient self-image, no need for catheter site care, need surgery to remove

Adapted from [1, p. 3].

Table 13.2 Catheter properties.

Catheter material	Teflon	Polyurethane	Silicone	Antimicrobial coating

		Firm, not stiff, material that softens and becomes more pliable in the vein in response to core body temperature
		1. Exceptional tensile strength which allows a catheter to be constructed with a thinner wall and greater internal diameter
		2. Smaller external diameter, thus causing less trauma on insertion
		3. Increased biocompatibility and thus less adherence of fibrin to the catheter
		4. Used for short- and long-term devices
			Flexible material that causes less damage to the intima and allows the catheter to float within the vein
			1. Offers increased biocompatibility and thus less adherence of fibrin to catheter material
			2. Used for long-term access devices
				These catheters are coated with a substance that gives them an anti-infective quality.
				These catheter types can be broadly categorised into:
				1. Antimicrobials
				   a. Cephalosporins
				   b. Penicillin
				   c. Vancomycin
				   d. Rifampin
				2. Antiseptics
				   a. Chlorhexidine
				   b. Silver sulphadiazine

Advantages	Ease of insertion			
Disadvantages	Stiff material that causes damage to the vein intima (inner lining) during insertion	Catheter is either cut prior to insertion or a choice is made with regard to catheter length according to client size and vasculature, thus relies on the clinician to correctly estimate catheter length	Requires special insertion technique due to flexibility of material	Clients are at risk for allergic reactions

Adapted from [11, pp. 3–4].

Principles of VAD management

The care and maintenance of VADs becomes the role of the community nurse in partnership with the client on discharge from a hospital or other facility. Regardless of the device used to access the venous system, an understanding of the 'principles' underpinning VAD management is the foundation for best-practice-based VAD management [6, 13–15]. VAD management in the community practice context are identified below:

1. VAD identification
   a. PIVC
   b. PICC types (open or closed)
   c. Other CVADs (port-a-caths, peripheral intravenous catheters)
2. Insertion site care and maintenance
   a. Dressing technique
   b. Securement
   c. Add-on devices
   d. Flushing techniques
3. Infection control principles
4. Implications for infusion therapy
5. Removal
6. Troubleshooting

These principles are discussed further in this chapter.

Appropriate VAD selection – pre-insertion

The choice of catheter depends on the type of therapy, the length of therapy, vascular anatomy, and client comprehension and client choice of device [1].Device selection is an important consideration and should occur prior to commencement of treatment, rather than when all other alternatives have been exhausted. Although this aspect of VAD management is not usually a choice made by the community nurse, it is important that a basic understanding of appropriate device selection is gained. Criteria for VAD selection are detailed in Figure 13.1.

Appropriate device selection occurs in the acute care sector, where insertion often takes place. The community nurse however can play an important role in the identification of inappropriate device selection for intravenous therapy via utilisation of Figure 13.1. Poor device selection may result in delay in completion of therapy which may lead to compromised client outcomes.

When are VADs indicated?

VADs for intravenous therapy can be indicated for the delivery of:

- Long-term therapy – weeks, months, even years
- High concentrations of fluids and medications, including:
  - Vesicant chemotherapy
  - Parenteral nutrition solutions
  - Hyperosmolar antibiotic solutions

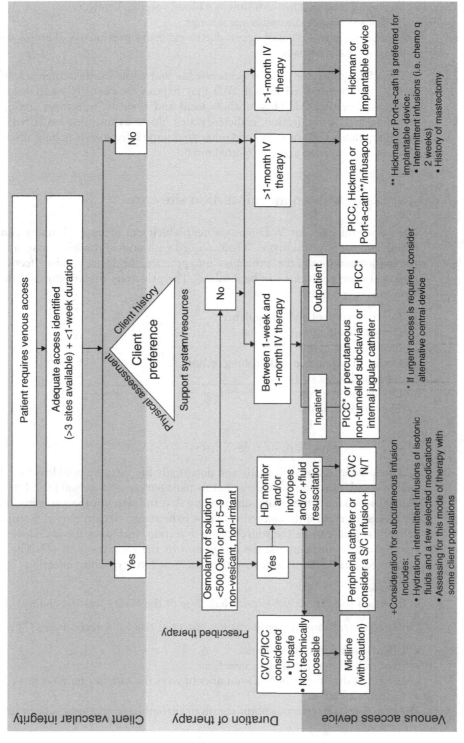

Figure 13.1 Vascular access device selection. [Used with permission from the Australian Vascular Access Advisory Group (AVAA).]

- Frequent blood product infusion and blood specimen collection.
- IV fluids in outpatient and home settings.
- Limited peripheral venous access due to extensive previous IV therapy, surgery or previous tissue damage.

The CDC guidelines [1] also acknowledge that while intravascular access is a necessity, the potential risk that a VAD may expose the client to once inserted must not be underestimated. These include local and systemic infectious complications, including local site infection, catheter-related bloodstream infection (CRBSI), septic thrombophlebitis, endocarditis and other metastatic infections (e.g. lung abscess, brain abscess, osteomyelitis and endophthalmitis).

VAD care and maintenance: insertion site care

There are principles for VAD management which can be applied in any community setting and for any VAD type. When coupled with critical thinking, assessment skills and implementation of the 'principles' into practice, the device can be effectively managed and most problems can be resolved. The principles of care can be listed under seven themes/strands:

1. Infection control and surveillance.
2. Device identification.
3. Insertion site care.
4. Device maintenance and flushing techniques.
5. Add-on devices.
6. Device securement.
7. The 'at-risk' client.

Infection control and surveillance

VAD-related infections are costly and potentially life threatening. However, there is a lack of standardisation of evidence in the management of infection [16]. Infection can be localised to the catheter site, surrounding skin and systemic (bacteraemia and sepsis) [7]. It is important for the community nurse to be aware that any part of the intravenous delivery system can be the source of the infection, including the accessories used to administer the medications, the bung/ports or the catheter itself [7]. The activities associated with VAD management that are most likely to cause infection [7] include:

- Insertion.
- Insertion site care or subsequent handling of the VAD (dressing changes, bungs).

Other considerations in identifying the potential risk for infections are [7]:

- Client's immune system status.
- Client's health at the time of insertion.
- Length of dwell time of VAD (number of days the catheter remains in situ).
- Catheter material.
- Adherence of bacteria to fibrin sheath or thrombus formation inside or around the catheter.

Many VAD-related complications can be reduced or limited by:

- Inserting the smallest gauge VAD and in centrally located VADs (CVAD), with the least number of lumens possible for the client's treatment [17].
- In the case of a CVAD, verifying the catheter tip location regularly over the treatment period.
- Regular and, more importantly, consistent maintenance of the device utilising a strict aseptic technique.

Paramount to the reduction of incidence of infection is basic handwashing: [1] VADs are no exception to this fundamental infection control practice. Skin preparation at and around the insertion site is also imperative in the management of all VADs [7, 9, 14, 18–20]. Surveillance of the incidence of CRBSIs is fundamental to effective VAD management. Without monitoring of CRBSIs and occlusion rates, it is difficult to identify poor VAD management practices. It is universally accepted that CRBSIs are reported in catheter days rather than percentages of infection rates.

Regardless of the device used the goals for care remain the same [21]:

- Prevent infection.
- Maintain a closed 'intravascular' system or limit amount of times device is accessed.
- Maintain a patent device.
- Prevent damage to the device.

Device identification – prior to undertaking care of the device

Before any VAD can be effectively managed, the community nurse is required to identify the type of device in use. This can be difficult in the community setting, as often this level of detail is not received with the information shared by the referring agency. Ideally, the following information should be sought prior to the first visit to the client:

1. Type of device
   a. PIVC
   b. Midline
   c. PICC
      i. Open ended
      ii. Close ended
   d. CVC
   e. Port-a-cath
2. Insertion history, including:
   a. Number of attempts
In the case of PICC:
   b. Length of catheter from insertion site to catheter hub
   c. Arm circumference
   d. Radiological confirmation of catheter tip location (should terminate in the SVC)
(*NB.* This also applies to CVCs)
3. Client risk factors
4. Reason for referral
   a. Care and maintenance of VAD
   b. Administration of intravenous therapy

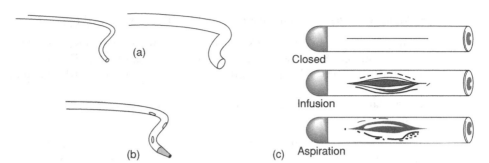

Figure 13.2 Commonly encountered catheters and their properties [29]. (a) Open-ended single and double lumen; (b) open-ended staggered exit; (c) closed-ended distally located.

Obtaining this information allows the community nurse to have a baseline to work from and directs the type of management approach required depending on the device type.

Types of devices and indications for use

- PIVC: A cannula is a flexible tube containing a needle (stylet) which may be inserted into a blood vessel [22]. Cannulae are usually placed in the peripheral veins in the lower arm but may also be placed in the veins of the foot (an area particularly used in paediatric care) [23]. However, veins of the lower extremities should not be routinely used in adults due to the risk of embolism and thrombophlebitis [3].
- Midline catheter: A midline catheter can be defined as one that is between 7.5 and 20 cm in length [3, 24–26]. It provides vascular access in a larger peripheral vein without entering the central venous circulation. It is inserted into an antecubital vein and the tip is extended into the vein of the upper arm up to 20 cm, but is not extended past the axilla [4, 25–27]. Dwell time for a midline catheter is 2–4 weeks, provided no complications occur.
- PICC: A PICC can be defined as a central venous catheter inserted via a peripheral vein, with the tip terminating in the SVC [28, p. 60]. The dwell time for these devices varies with some studies showing that safe use can be sustained for a year or longer. It is generally acceptable that these devices are chosen for therapies of weeks to months in duration. These devices can be divided into two categories: open-ended or closed-ended, according to the type of catheter tip of the VAD. Figure 13.2 shows examples of 'open-ended' and 'closed-ended' catheter tips.

Identification of the device at this level determines the flushing regimen required to maintain catheter patency. Broadly speaking, open-ended PICCs require heparin flushing or locking, whereas closed-ended PICCs require saline-only flushing.

There is limited evidence regarding the specific heparin concentrations required for flushing of the open-ended PICCs [8, 11]. The technique used for flushing should be the priority of care rather than the type of flush used (see 'Device maintenance and flushing techniques').

- Central venous catheters

    1. *Tunnelled.* A large-diameter catheter, frequently with multiple lumens, surgically tunnelled through subcutaneous tissue to an exit site on the chest or abdominal

wall; the catheter tip terminates in the SVC [30, p. 61]. The dwell time for this device can be several years, provided that no complications occur.

2. *Percutaneous non-tunnelled.* A large-diameter catheter, often with multiple lumens, inserted percutaneously through the subclavian, jugular, or femoral vein, with the catheter tip terminating in the SVC [28, p. 60]. This device is considered a temporary VAD with a dwell time of up to 30 days.

3. *Port-a-caths.* A surgically implanted reservoir, usually placed in the chest or arm, attached to a catheter that terminates in the central circulation. Medication is delivered to the reservoir via an external non-coring needle and extension tubing [28, p. 61]. This device has a dwell time of several years, provided no complications occur.

Dressing changes

Regardless of the VAD type there is evidence suggesting that dressing changes should occur at 7-day intervals for midlines, PICCs and CVCs, unless the dressing has become loosened, or exudate is seen under the transparent dressing, or it becomes soiled [1]. The properties of the transparent dressing should include a high-moisture vapour transfer rate (HMVTR) [1, 2, 6]. This ensures that any moisture present under the transparent dressing is quickly transferred away from the insertion site. The evidence supports a reduction in infection rates for all VADs utilising a transparent dressing with these properties [6, 7, 9, 18, 19, 31].

Whilst a sterile technique should be adopted for the insertion of all centrally located VADs, an aseptic technique is acceptable for peripherally inserted cannulae. Generally, any procedure which exposes (opens) the insertion site or the end of the catheter should involve an aseptic technique with sterile gloves. Any procedure which maintains a closed system requires an aseptic technique with clean gloves [12].

In the case of centrally located devices (PICCs, CVCs and newly placed port-a-caths), dressings should be changed 24 h after insertion, and if gauze is required due to localised bleeding or exudate, then the dressing should be changed every 48 h. Adherence to this regime will help to reduce the incidence of infection [1].

The procedure associated with a dressing change for PICCs and CVCs is a dexterous task and requires practice to ensure that the principles suggested above are achieved. It is through regular practice that the community nurse will develop a systematic approach to dressing changes. This is particularly important to the community nurse practising in isolation. Client education is also important prior to commencement of insertion site care. Asepsis may be compromised by an 'eager' client if the time is not taken to explain the procedure prior to commencement. It also helps the client if the community nurse explains that although each community nurse may undertake the procedure slightly differently, it is the maintenance of asepsis that underpins the principles of insertion site care.

Add-on devices: positive displacement valves, bungs and tubing

The use of a positive pressure displacement device negates the need to use heparin flushes or heparin locks [9, 13, 20, 29, 32, 33]. Historically, heparin use (to decrease thrombus formation) has been controversial with no standardisation of its use evident in the literature reviewed. There is mention of heparin-induced thrombocytopenia [13, 32, 34] and the use of add-on devices to reduce occlusion and infection rates. All add-on devices should be routinely changed every 7 days while insertion site care is undertaken [1].

Flushing techniques

Patency of the line for the duration of therapy is the focus of VAD care and maintenance. Agreement on flushing solutions is not found in the literature, but rather flushing technique [2, 6, 7, 9, 18, 20, 33–37]. Utilisation of a 'push–pause' or 'pulsatile' technique is seen by the literature as the cornerstone in ensuring continued catheter patency, thus ensuring long-term vascular access. This technique results in the creation of turbulence within the catheter walls and decreases the potential for build-up of infusate precipitates or formation of small blood clots. There is a relationship between catheter occlusion and poor flushing techniques. Maintenance of positive pressure while removing the syringe – achieved by continuing to apply pressure on the syringe plunger whilst removing the syringe from the bung – also assists in reducing reflux of blood into the catheter tip as a result of pressure changes. A useful method for maintaining a consistent approach to flushing is described below:

Open-ended catheters

A S A S H

Aspirate: Attach 10-mL syringe and aspirate until blood is returned in the syringe (discard).
Saline: Flush device with normal saline (N/S) via a 10-mL syringe utilising a 'pulsatile' technique.
Additive: Administer intravenous medication or infusion if required.
Saline: At completion of IV medication, flush device with another 10 mL of N/S utilising a 'pulsatile' technique.
Heparin: Flush or lock the device with heparin (concentration dependent on organisational protocols).

Close-ended catheters

A S A S

As for open-ended catheters without the heparin flush or lock.
   Special note. Provided a 10-mL syringe is used for all flushing, catheter damage is unlikely as the PSI (pounds per square inch) exerted via a syringe 10 mL or greater in size will not create enough pressure to cause catheter rupture.

Securement

Device securement is essential to ensuring longevity of the VAD. There is overwhelming evidence in the literature [27, 31, 35], suggesting that excellent securement results in reduction of mechanical phlebitis caused by 'pistoning'– the catheter moving in and out of the vein. There are a variety of securement options (Statlock, tapes and sutures), all of which achieve adequate patient outcomes. The Statlock and tapes should be treated as additional devices and for this reason should be changed every 7 days or more often if securement is compromised.

VAD complications

The goal of VAD management is the completion of therapy without complications. In reality, this is an idealistic goal. The community nurse has an important role in the appropriate care and maintenance of VADs to ensure that the ideal becomes the reality. Understanding the signs and symptoms of common complications assists in early intervention and successful completion of therapy. Broadly speaking, VAD complications can be described in three categories:

1. Client risk factors.
2. Device factors.
3. Infusate factors.

Prevention of CRBSI, explored earlier in the chapter, and phlebitis, thrombus formation and occlusions are the focus for the management of VAD complications.

Phlebitis

Phlebitis is inflammation of the vein which may be associated with pain, erythema, oedema or a palpable cord [4]. Prevention of this most common complication is related to sufficient vessel size to accommodate catheter size, haemodilution, non-traumatic insertion and infusing non-irritating solutions. Hand veins have a lower risk of phlebitis than veins on the wrist or upper arm [17, 23]. Phlebitis can have different causative factors usually associated with prolonged dwell time and from mechanical or chemical irritation [38]. The risk factor for phlebitis also increases with age [39].

Mechanical phlebitis is common following a traumatic insertion of a VAD and can be treated with the use of a heat pack over the insertion site. If the phlebitis is caused by chemical irritation, it is very important to have an understanding of the properties of the infusate. Is it an irritant or a vesicant? Vesicants cause tissue necrosis and cell death (commonly referred to as an extravasation injury). This is why it is important to confirm blood return prior to commencement of infusion therapy with a vesicant [11]. The infusion must be stopped immediately and the client treated according to the organisation's policy.

Occlusions

Catheter occlusions in VADs are common and 60% of occlusions are caused by thrombosis [30]. The community nurse becomes aware of occlusions when there is an inability to infuse medications or withdraw blood. Aspiration should always occur prior to utilising the VAD to ensure catheter patency [3]. If no blood is returned or resistance is met, the community nurse must take steps to assess catheter patency. This is particularly important if a vesicant intravenous medication is to be administered. Determining the most probable cause of a catheter occlusion requires first assessing whether the problem is mechanical, non-thrombotic or thrombotic. The initial check of the catheter should include the assessment for mechanical obstruction within the tubing, withdrawal occlusion, pumps problems, catheter kinks, clamps, catheter insertion site or sutures. Assessment must also include identification of the last medication infusion and the type of flush. A sluggish flow or inability to infuse fluids or withdraw blood is the first indication of an occlusion. The entire infusion plan should be assessed to determine whether drugs and fluids are being given appropriately and that the device is being maintained correctly [30].

Treatment of catheter occlusions by the community nurse is dependent on the cause. Often it requires the client to be referred back to the acute care organisation where the insertion took place. Hospital avoidance is a goal of community nurses, hence the need to prevent occlusions by utilising consistent management practices. Delay in treating the occlusion impacts directly on the likelihood of successfully restoring catheter patency.

Intraluminal blood/fibrin forms within the catheter lumen(s) resulting in catheter occlusion. Client factors (see 'Identifying the "at-risk" client') and flushing technique impact on this type of occlusion [11, p. 15].

Fibrin sheaths or tails occur when fibrin adheres to the tip of the catheter and external surface, acting as a one-way valve permitting infusion but not aspiration of blood [11, p. 15].

Identifying the 'at-risk' client

The community nurse should be knowledgeable about client and device factors that increase the risk of VAD occlusion or infection. Ongoing assessment and evaluation of all of these factors and communication with the multidisciplinary health care team are essential to improve client outcomes [6, p. 33].

Client risk factors

- Disease processes and/or medications that may alter the circulation and/or coagulation status.
- History of clots such as deep vein thrombosis (DVT) and pulmonary embolus.
- Poor history of device occlusions.
- Client compliancy to catheter care protocols.
- Alterations in intrathoracic pressure caused by persistent coughing, retching or vomiting, heavy lifting and vigorous exercising [6].

Device risk factors

- Appropriate device selection for the therapy.
- Choose valve technologies that are designed to minimise blood reflux and thrombus device occlusions [6, 8, 30].

- Monitor clients for altered tip position
- Be knowledgeable of incompatibilities between infusates to ensure correct choice of locking and flushing techniques

Infusate risk factors

Certain intravenous solutions can also increase thrombus formation and device occlusion. These include:

- Irritants whose pH lies outside the normal range (7.35–7.4).
- Vesicants with pH less than 5 and greater than 9, and/or osmolarity greater than 500 Osmol/L.
- Medications that have the potential to precipitate and cause occlusions. Flush with adequate volumes of normal saline prior to locking, administering or infusing another medication in order to clear the lumen of any residual build-up [6, p. 32].

Documentation

Clear, concise and accurate documentation supports the management of VADs. Development of organisational policies which address components of vascular access therapy to ensure positive client outcomes is paramount [6, p. 11]. The management of VADs can be accurately documented utilising the following headings:

1. Insertion procedure
   a. Type of VAD
   b. Location of insertion site
   c. Method of catheter securement
   d. Number of attempts at insertion
   e. Confirmation of catheter placement and patency (radiological confirmation if required)
2. Follow-up care
   a. Contact number and equipment for emergencies
   b. Activity restrictions if necessary
   c. Follow-up appointment
   d. Supply details (if required)
3. Care and access of VAD
   a. Record of VAD use, i.e. medication administration or maintenance only
   b. Dressing change including site assessment and patient-reported symptoms
   c. Add-on device changes
4. Use of VAD
   a. Evaluation of device functionality
   b. Any complications noted when using the device and who was contacted
   c. Strategies used to manage the complications
   d. Evaluation of effectiveness of implementation of strategies
5. Malfunction or complications of VAD
   a. Note date and time when complication was identified
   b. Describe complication

    c. Strategies used to manage and other health care professionals contacted

    d. Completion of appropriate organisational surveillance tool (e.g. client incident form)

6. Removal of VAD

    a. Indications for removal (e.g. completion of therapy, CRBSI, total catheter occlusion)

    b. Date, time and type of device removed

    c. Procedure used to remove device

    d. Confirmation that device was intact once removed

    e. Complications of removal

    f. Client reaction to removal

Consistency in recording of information in the documentation assists all community nurses involved with the care of VADs to make clinical decisions based on accurate information. Recorded information is also an important communication tool for all those involved in the care of clients with VADs in the community. Without it assumptions can be made that may result in poor management of VADs which may result in poor client outcomes.

Education

Education is the key to successful treatment completion. All nurses involved with VADs require education on the principles and practice of infusion therapy. Evidence-based education should be available on a continuing basis, included in staff orientation for new employees and made available via continuing professional development opportunities. Clients and their family/caregivers must not be forgotten in the education process. Care of VADs should be viewed as a partnership between the community nurse, members of the health care team, the client and the family/caregivers.

Client and family/caregiver education

Client and family/caregiver education should occur regularly throughout the duration of the VAD's life. Education on the care of the device, its potential complications and, more importantly, the symptoms of these complications directly impact on client outcomes [3, 6, 40]. Equally as important to client education is the assessment of the client's and/or family/caregiver's ability to assimilate this new information. Nurses work effectively with people in the process of education when they are available to them and provide support to enable the transfer of education throughout the duration of the treatment. Clarification of the transfer of education can be determined by establishing if the client/caregiver can:

- Describe the VAD and the rationale for its use.
- Verbalise the signs and symptoms of VAD-related complications.
- Demonstrate how to manage any aspect of care of the VAD that has been deemed their responsibility.
- Verbalise their understanding of what to do and whom to contact should any issues arise [40, p. 6].

The ability of the client or family/caregiver to identify complications in the early stages of VAD management assists the clinician to implement the appropriate intervention in a timely manner. This will often negate the need to delay therapy or the need to remove the device.

Community nurse education

Ideally, the community nurse should participate in annual or biannual education opportunities which will assist in the maintenance of knowledge and clinical competence in VAD technology. Community nurses require education in the following areas:

- Information about specific devices.
- Basic understanding of insertion and access procedures.
- Care and maintenance.
- Potential complications and interventions.
- Essentials of client and family/caregiver education [11, p. 80].

Nursing best-practice guidelines can be successfully implemented only where there are adequate planning, resources, organisational and administrative support as well as appropriate facilitation [11, p. 11].

Benefits of a dedicated team for the management of VADs

Clinical excellence and competence in VAD management requires that the nurse have regular exposure in the clinical setting to such devices. It is well recognised that a dedicated individual or team, tasked with the management of VADs, impacts on improved client outcomes [11, pp. 10, 11].

Primary drivers of the PICC service's continuing success include consistent applications of technique and technology, a data-driven approach to assessing the programme's progress and appropriately managing customers' expectations and needs [10, p. 1].

It is through regular exposure to the management challenges of the community client with a VAD that the community nurse develops the skills and experiences underpinning effective care and maintenance of the VAD. Hence if a dedicated individual or team is implemented as the first 'port of call', management of VADs is streamlined and efficiencies are increased. Once the care of a client with a VAD is established, the dedicated VAD team member or an individual highly skilled in the management of these devices can hand over the care to the less experienced nurse, hence building capacity amongst the community nursing team.

Research gaps and future implications

There is limited Australian research in terms of randomised controlled trials and/or cohort studies to support current practices regarding VAD care and maintenance in the community nursing context. The information available to clinicians involved in VAD management is not consolidated in one area or guideline and so it may be a challenge for community nurses to access evidence that will inform education and upskilling.

The author has identified the following research priorities.

Interventions

- Effectiveness of various flushing techniques and solutions and their impact on VAD complications in the community nursing context.
- Effectiveness of heparin versus normal saline for locking.
- The use of positive pressure displacement devices (or valved VADs) in the community nursing context.
- Effectiveness of various types of dressings and securement devices for the community nursing client.

Education

- Targeted client education and its effectiveness in reducing VAD complications.
- Effectiveness of different education models/approaches in developing critical thinking skills of the community nurse.
- Effectiveness of increasing the community nurse's knowledge of the importance of identifying 'at-risk client' types and disease processes and their impact on improved client outcomes.

Monitoring and evaluation

- Development and validation testing of audit and surveillance tools for monitoring of VAD complications in the community setting.

Community nurses should play an important role in identifying the importance of addressing the research gaps. Management of VADs in the community setting is influenced by complex client conditions, the changing home environment in which community nurses practice and the importance of fostering independent clients. This requires research that confirms or denies the well-established 'acute care' guidelines that are currently used to support practice. The assumption should not be made that these guidelines are transferable to the community nursing setting.

A word on 'critical thinking'

Critical thinking is defined as the 'intellectually disciplined process of actively and skilfully conceptualising, applying, synthesising, or evaluating information' [41, p. 162]. In nursing, critical thinking is crucial to the outcomes of clients. Critical thinking is the ability of the nurse to think reasonably, purposefully and with a specific goal in mind. Although intertwined with clinical reasoning and clinical decision making, it is contextual and changes depending on circumstances. Critical thinking skills are imperative in all aspects of nursing but especially so in VAD management. It is unusual that two clients with a VAD are ever the same. The nurse is required to utilise critical thinking skills to 'troubleshoot' problems in often differing clinical situations.

Conclusion

The management of VADs requires skilled clinicians utilising knowledge in assessment, planning, implementation and evaluation in all aspects of VAD care. It is acknowledged that this is a challenging aspect of community nursing. Client complexities contribute to these challenges. However, a collaborative best-practice-based approach to the management of VADs ultimately results in improved client outcomes – a goal of all community nurses.

References

1. CDC (2002) Guidelines for the prevention of intravascular catheter-related infections. *Morbidity and Mortality Weekly Report*. CDC.
2. Infusion Nurses' Society (INS) (2002) *Policies and Procedures for Infusion Nursing*, 2nd edition. Infusion Nurses' Society Incorporated.
3. INS (2006) *Infusion Nursing Standards of Practice*. Lippincott Williams & Wilkins, Philadelphia.
4. Royal College of Nursing (2003) *Standards for Infusion Therapy*. Royal College of Nursing, London.
5. Registered Nurses' Association of Ontario (RNAO) (ed.) (2004) *Assessment and Device Selection for Vascular Access*. Registered Nurses' Association of Ontario, Toronto, Canada.
6. RNAO (2005) *Care and Maintenance to Reduce Vascular Access Complications*. Registered Nurses' Association of Ontario, Toronto, Canada.
7. Department of Health (2001) Guidelines for preventing infections associated with the insertion and maintenance of central venous catheters. *Journal of Hospital Infection*, 47(Suppl), S47–67.
8. Gorski, L.A. and Czaplewski, L.M. (2005) Managing complications of midlines and PICCs. *Nursing*, 35(6), 68–9.
9. Fitzpatrick, L.M. (November/December 1999) Care and management issues regarding central venous access devices in the home and long-term care setting. *Journal of Intravenous Nursing*, 22(65), S5–40.
10. Burns, D. (2005) The vanderbilt picc service: Program, procedural, and patient outcomes successes. *The Journal of the Association for Vascular Access*, 10(4), 1–10.
11. Camp-Sorell, D. (2004) *Access Device Guidelines: Recommendations for Nursing Practice and Education*, 2nd edition. Oncology Nursing Society, Pittsburgh.
12. Leaver, D.D., Annette, and Boland, M. (2005) *Central Venous Catheter Manual*. The Canberra Hospital, Canberra.
13. Rummel, M.A., Donnelly, P.J. and Fortenbaugh, C.C. (2001) Clinical evaluation of a positive pressure device to prevent central venous catheter occlusion: Results of a pilot study. *Clinical Journal of Oncology Nursing*, 5(6), 261–5.
14. INS (2006) *Infusion Nursing Standards of Practice*. Infusion Nurses' Society.

15. Yamamoto, A.J., Solomon, J.A., Soulen, M.C., Tang, J., Parkinson, K., Lin, R., *et al.* (2002) Sutureless securement devices reduces complications of peripherally inserted central venous catheters. *Journal of Vascular and Interventional Radiology*, 13(1), 77–81.

16. Camp-Sorell, D. (2004) Implanted ports; skin erosion. *Clinical Journal of Oncology Nursing*, 8(3), 309–10.

17. O'Grady, N.A.M., Dellinger, E.P., Gerberding, J.L., Heard, S.O., Maki, D.G., Masur, H., *et al.* (August 2002) Guidelines for the prevention of intravascular catheter-related infections. *Centre for Disease Control and Prevention, Morbidity and Mortality Recommendations Report.*

18. Arrow International (2000) Peripherally inserted central catheters. *Continuing Education Program.* Arrow, Reading, PA.

19. Cope, D.G., Ezzone, S.A., Hagel, M.E., McCorkindale, D.J., Moran, A.B., Sanoshy, J.K., *et al.* (2004) *Access Device Guidelines: Recommendations for Nursing Practice and Education*, 2nd edition. Oncology Nursing Society, Pittsburgh.

20. Moureau, N. (2004) *Focus on Prevention of Vascular Access Device Complications* [series of titles]. Available at (viewed 2 August 2004).

21. Hospital, T.R.M. (2007) *Vascular Access Devices: Insertion and Management.* Available at http://www.mariecurie.org.uk/thestaffroom/nursingprocedures/content/mars44.htm#c044-sec2-0014 (viewed 5 November 2007).

22. Anderson, K.N.A. and Anderson, L.E. (eds) (1995) *Mosby's Pocket Dictionary of Nursing, Medicine and Professions Allied to Medicine.* Mosby, London.

23. Weinstein, S. (2001) *Principles and Practice of Intravenous Therapy*, 7th edition. Lippincott, Philadelphia.

24. Carlson, K.R. (1999) Correct utilisation and management of PICCs and midline catheters in the alternate care setting. *Journal of Intravenous Nursing*, 22(Suppl 6), S46–50.

25. Hadaway, L. (2000) *Self Study Workbook. Peripheral IV Therapy in Adults.* Hadaway Associates, GA.

26. Perucca, R. (2001) Obtaining vascular access, in J. Hankin (ed.) *Infusion Therapy in Clinical Practice.* W.B. Saunders, Philadelphia.

27. Frey, A.M. and Schears, G.J. (2006) Why are we stuck on tape and suture?: A review of catheter securement devices. *Journal of Infusion Nursing*, 29(1), 34–8.

28. Halderman, F. (2000) Selecting a vascular access device. *Nursing*, 30(11), 59–61.

29. States RNCEU (2001) *Exam & Evaluation (PICC Line Care and Maintenance).* Available at https://www.rnceus.com/secured/rnceus_exam.asp?exam_id=17 (viewed 2004).

30. Haire, W.D. and Herbst, S.F. (2000) Consensus conference on the use of alteplase (t-PA) for the management of thrombotic catheter dysfunction. *Journal of Vascular Access Devices*, 5(2), 28–35.

31. Gabriel, J. (2003) PICC dressings: Not just a decision based upon clinical performance. *Journal of Association of Vascular Access*, 8(4), 41–3.

32. Crnich, C.J. and Maki, D.G. (15 May 2002) The promise of novel technology for the prevention of intravascular device-related bloodstream infection. II. Long-term devices. *Clinical Infectious Diseases*, 34, 1362–8.

33. Lenhart, C. (2001) Preventing central venous access device occlusions with saline only flush by use of an adapter. *Journal of Vascular Access Devices*, 6(6), 34–5.

34. Rosenthal, K. (2004) Type II heparin-induced thrombocytopenia: Toward developing a strategy to determine the role of routine vascular access device heparinsation. *Journal of Association of Vascular Access*, 9, 221–5.

35. Aston, V. (2000) Community management of peripherally inserted central catheters. *British Journal of Community Nursing*, 5(7), 318, 20–25.

36. Beacock, B. (2004) A new vein for nursing. *Australian Nursing Journal*, 12(2), 27.

37. Lenhart, C. (2000) Prevention vs. treatment of VAD occlusions. *Journal of Vascular Access Devices*, 5(4), 34–5.

38. Campbell, L. (1998a) IV-related phlebitis, complications and length of hospital stay: 1. *British Journal of Nursing*, 7, 1340, 6, 8, 10–12.

39. Campbell, L. (1998b) IV-related phlebitis, complications and length of hospital stay: 2. *British Journal of Nursing*, 7, 1364, 6, 8–70, 72.

40. Cancer Nurse Society of Australia (2007) *Central Venous Access Devices: Principles for Nursing Practice and Education.* Cancer Nurse Society of Australia, pp. 4–26.

41. Zunkel, G., Cesarotti, E., Rosdahl, D. and McGrath, J. (2004) Enhancing diagnostic reasoning skills in nurse practitioner students. *Nurse Educator*, 29(4), 161–5.

Chapter 14

Child and maternal health

Gay Edgecombe, Creina Mitchell and Irene Ellis

Introduction

Maternal and child health nursing in the community is the cornerstone of primary health care for mothers, infants, young children and their families. Every state and territory within Australia has a universal maternal and child health (MCH) service. These services provide support for families and provide care for children from birth or before to 8 years. This chapter provides an overview of a selection of MCH services, programme standards and nurse competencies. Health promotion principles and examples will be integrated throughout. The chapter also provides examples of some guidelines relevant to key areas in child, family and community health nursing, namely:

- Antenatal care and support.
- Postpartum care and support.
- Breastfeeding.
- Child development assessment.
- Immunisation.
- Mental health.
- Vulnerable children and families.

Leaders in early years' research, policy development and practice refer to Bronfenbrenner's ecological model of human development as being the most useful to consider as a foundation for MCH work. This model argues that 'families belong in a complex web of relationships within the community and larger social systems' [1, p. 204].

Key definitions and concepts

Health promotion

Health promotion is 'the process of enabling people to increase control over the determinants of health and thereby improve their health. Participation is essential to sustain health promotion action' [2, pp. 1–2]. Strategies for health promotion range from those with an individual focus, for example child health surveillance and providing health information to parents, through to strategies with a population focus, for example social marketing and regulatory activities. In practice, the MCH nurse may most commonly use strategies with an individual or family focus. This approach, however, does not preclude involvement in community-level strategies (community development work) or policy-related strategies (public policy advocacy or submission writing). Breastfeeding support, immunisation advocacy and well-child checks are all examples of nurses' health promotion work with children, families and communities.

Primary health care

Primary health care has been defined as:

> ... essential health care based on practical, scientifically sound and socially acceptable methods and technology made universally available to individuals and families through their full participation and at a cost that the community and country can afford to maintain at every stage of their development in a spirit of self reliance and self-determinism [3, p. 245].

Primary health care is underpinned by a number of interconnected key principles. McMurray [4, p. 33] has broadened them to include accessibility, appropriate technology, increased emphasis on health promotion, intersectoral collaboration and public participation.

Evidenced-based practice

Evidence-based practice is based on the work of Sackett [5]. Muir Gray [6, p. 9] describes this approach to practice as clinical decision making based substantially more on research findings than in the past. McMurray further explains that evidenced-based practice integrates three elements: (1) the best available research, (2) the clinicians' knowledge and experience and (3) the individual client's values and belief systems [4, p. 356].

Family centred practice

In family centred practice, the family is central to all decision making, including choices of service. Control over the goals and content of individual support strategies always remains with each child [7].

Working with diversity

Maternal and child health nurses work with families from a broad range of cultures. It is critical for the nurse to be aware of the different values and customs of each family [4, p. 40].

Strengths-based practice

McCashen [8, p. 9] notes that the emphasis on a strengths approach to practice is founded on the following:

- All people have strengths and capacities.
- People can change.
- People change and grow through their strengths and capacities.
- People are experts in their own situation.
- The problem is the problem; the person is not the problem.
- Problems can blind people from noticing and appreciating their strengths and capacity to find their own solutions.
- People have good intentions.
- People are doing the best they can.
- The power for change is within us.

Maternal and child health: programmes, service delivery, standards and nursing competencies

Maternal and child health programmes and service delivery

Each state and territory in Australia delivers a universal MCH service to children and their families. Across Australia the names of programmes and how they are implemented vary; however, their ultimate aim is to promote the health and well-being of children and their parents (see 'Useful resources' at the end of this chapter). For example the goal of the Victorian Maternal and Child Health Programme is 'to promote a comprehensive and focused approach for the promotion, prevention, early detection and intervention of physical, emotional or social factors affecting young children and their families in contemporary communities' [9, p. 6]. There is a huge range of issues which impact on families with young children. Within most policy documents that focus on population outcomes, there is a section which addresses childhood. The issues identified may include nutrition (prevention of obesity), safety (reduction in non-intentional injury) and immunisation (reduction of vaccine-preventable disease).

It is imperative that child, family and community nurses understand how MCH services are organised and delivered in their state or territory. There is usually a key document that outlines the programme and services delivered. State or territory child and family professional nursing bodies can direct nurses to the current practice and programme guidelines. For example each year, in Victoria, a *Maternal and Child Health Program Resource Guide* is produced to assist service providers to manage, deliver and monitor the MCH service [9]. This guide outlines the MCH policy context; the vision, mission, goals and principles guiding the service; service activities; and service performance measures and targets [9].

It is also important to understand the interplay between the MCH programme and other programmes. Very often, it is the MCH programme which is responsible for implementing key public health messages from other programmes. This cross-programme interaction can be confusing for practitioners, and is another reason it is vital for them to understand their policy and service context.

MCH service standards

Most states and territories have programme standards relevant to their own MCH service which are available from the local professional child and family organisation.

The Commonwealth Department of Health and Ageing funded a project to develop national standards for maternal and infant care services [10]. The project produced a module which highlighted the core concepts that underpin service provision as well as standards that services should meet. These standards are generic and may be a useful reference for practitioners working in a small programme or service which does not have its own standards.

Maternal and child health nurse competencies

Community nurses need to adhere to the professional competencies or standards relevant where they work, for example national nursing and midwifery competencies. There may also be state or territory competencies that are relevant to MCH nursing, for example paediatric, community or MCH nursing competencies. Most competency documents highlight the requirement for community nurses to function in accordance with legislation, standards and policies pertinent to their practice. Hence, if working in Victoria, nurses must be registered appropriately with the Nurses Board of Victoria, practice within relevant federal and state legislation, adhere to the programme standards of the Victorian Maternal and Child Health Service [11] and abide by the Standards of Professional Practice for Maternal and Child Health Nurses [12] (for an example refer to Table 14.1).

MCH nursing

There are a number of principles that underpin MCH clinical practice [12], for example evidence-based practice [5, 6], primary health care [4], family centred practice [7], health promotion [4], working with diversity [4] and strengths-based practice [8]. Many of these align with the principles that underpin the MCH service delivery [13]. The following sections of this chapter provide guidelines to key areas in MCH nursing. For each topic area, community nursing practice is underpinned by the principles described above.

Antenatal care and support

The following guidelines relate to antenatal care and support service provision. They are designed to incorporate primary health care philosophies, including health promotion within a community approach to care, whilst encouraging the incorporation of client self-management techniques. The management of client care has a multidisciplinary focus and it is essential that it includes:

- Provision of information regarding the aims of antenatal care, content of visits and agreed schedule of visits through discussion with the client/carer and health care team.
- Awareness of the need for a well-developed caring attitude and support of the client to self-care, including physical safety and psychological and emotional well-being.

High-quality antenatal care of the pregnant woman contributes to the best prenatal environment for the developing fetus and, subsequently, the young child. Antenatal

Table 14.1 Standards of professional practice for maternal and child health nurses: Standard Seven [12].

Standard Seven:	The maternal and child health nurse uses health promotion and health education strategies with children, families and communities to promote optimal health
Criteria	**Interpretation**
7.1 Collaborate with the client in identification of health education and health promotion needs	7.1.1 Participate with clients in order to identify their health needs, including priorities and expected outcomes 7.1.2 Assist families to identify health education needs 7.1.3 Provide a trusting and non-judgemental environment
7.2 Undertake health promotion and health education by responding to health goals of clients	7.2.1 Inform and encourage parents to participate in health promotion and health education activities 7.2.2 Promote early intervention strategies 7.2.3 Work with clients to develop strategies to meet their identified health needs 7.2.4 Use appropriate education tools 7.2.5 Provide education which the client may use to achieve changes if required 7.2.6 Provide current education resources in appropriate language 7.2.7 Provide relevant health promotion information to parents for children 0–6 years 7.2.8 Facilitate groups as a format for health promotion activities 7.2.9 Use appropriate community resources 7.2.10 Undertake health promotion activities
7.3 Participate with multidisciplinary teams in national, state and local health promotion campaigns	7.3.1 Collaborate with other agencies on child and family health promotion campaigns 7.3.2 Work with health and municipal departments in developing programmes and services to meet the identified needs of residents 7.3.3 Contribute to the implementation of municipal and state public health program
7.4 Evaluate health education and health promotion activities	7.4.1 Use appropriate tools to evaluate program 7.4.2 Refine health education program using evaluation outcomes 7.4.3 Consult the community in evaluation program

care is provided by both midwives and doctors through a variety of models, for example shared care between general practitioner and hospital, midwife-led care through community health care centre or hospital clinic or care by a private obstetrician. In Australia, approximately 67% of women access a public hospital for maternity care [14]. Traditionally, this care has consisted of 14 visits by the well-pregnant woman to the health care professional throughout the pregnancy. In 2001, The Three Centres Consensus Guidelines on Antenatal Care Project [15] determined a reduced number of content-specific visits to reflect best practice in contemporary antenatal care. This consortium stated that the number of visits a low-risk woman needed could safely be reduced to between seven and ten [15, p. 5].

Regardless of the model of care employed, the aims of antenatal care remain consistent. During the first trimester, the objectives are to:

- Compile a comprehensive history and date the pregnancy.
- Assess maternal and fetal well-being, with particular reference to fetal abnormalities.
- Instigate health promotion strategies where indicated such as the 'QUIT' programme for cigarette smoking.

During the second and third trimesters, the focus shifts and the primary objectives become to:

- Monitor fetal growth and well-being.
- Monitor maternal well-being and detect complications such as pregnancy-induced hypertension.
- Prepare the woman for admission, labour and birth, and going home.

First or booking visit (before 12-week gestation)

Assessment and screening tests

- Identify the first day of last menstrual period (LMP) and determine nature of the woman's normal cycle.
- Using Naegele's rule or a pregnancy calculator (280-day rule) determine the expected due date (EDD).
- If the first day of LMP is not known, or if clinical features are inconsistent with the date given, consider referral for ultrasound dating.
- Measure and record maternal blood pressure to establish baseline. This is repeated at each visit.
- Abdominal palpation or symphyseal-fundal (S-F) height measurement as an indicator of fetal growth.
- Offer auscultation of the fetal heart at each visit from the time the midwife or doctor can detect a heart beat.
- Conduct blood tests including group and rhesus factor, rhesus antibodies, full blood count, syphilis, hepatitis B (HBV), hepatitis C (HCV), human immunodeficiency virus (HIV), rubella antibodies and haemoglobinopathies.
- Other screens may include a midstream specimen of urine for asymptomatic bacteriuria or a blood test, nuchal translucency scan, chorionic villus sampling (CVS) or amniocentesis for neural tube defects and Downs syndrome.

Health promotion

- Continue folate supplementation (0.5 mg/day) [16]. It is unlikely that women will take a folate supplement preconception unless specific information is given by the health care professional regarding the reduced risk of neural tube defects such as spina bifida [17].
- Diet and exercise.

- Smoking – QUIT intervention and referral. In 2004, 16.7% of mothers reported cigarette smoking during their pregnancy [18].
- Safety – consider 'Safety Plan' if family violence is disclosed. Consider ways to avoid infections such as listeriosis and toxoplasmosis.

Subsequent visit

Assessment and screening tests

- Blood pressure.
- S-F height measurement.
- Auscultation, fetal movements.
- Blood tests: Depending on results of previous tests, the following may be required:
  - For rhesus-negative woman, antibody screening is repeated at regular intervals throughout the pregnancy.
  - Haemoglobin (Hb) or ferritin levels screening is also repeated regularly, with the aim of maintaining the woman's Hb at or above 100 g/dL at term.
- Ultrasound scan, if routine, may be offered for 16- to 20-week gestation for fetal anomalies.

Health promotion

- The recommended dietary intake (RDI) of iron during pregnancy is 27 mg/day [19]. Discuss both dietary intake and oral supplementation.
- Promote breastfeeding through provision of written information and available resources.

Further visits

- Group B haemolytic streptococcus is screened for at 35–37 weeks and women positive for this are treated with intravenous antibiotics throughout labour. While group B haemolytic streptococcus is a normal vaginal commensal and vaginal carriage has been found in 15–20% of women [20], early infection of the neonate can develop quickly and be life threatening.
- Routine monitoring for the onset of gestational diabetes is still controversial, although there is an increasing incidence in Australia. For example 6% of all pregnant women in Victoria have diabetes, and 80% of these are gestational [21]. Screening with the use of either an oral glucose tolerance test (OGTT) or an oral glucose challenge test (OGCT) is performed between 24- and 28-week gestation.

Health promotion strategies

- Pregnancy-induced hypertension and preterm labour and birth remain concerns. The incidence of prematurity has not reduced (8.2%), but technological advances in neonatal intensive care have enabled the 'saving' of increasingly immature infants [18]. Pre-eclampsia (pregnancy-induced hypertension and proteinuria) accounted for 13% of maternal deaths in 1994–1996 [22].

- The occurrence of placenta praevia has increased during the last decade and this can be partly attributed to the increase of birth by caesarean section, now 29.4% [18]. Discuss the perceived advantages and disadvantages of caesarean birth with the woman.
- Preparation for admission, birth plans, change of life with a new baby.
- Discuss postnatal sleeping arrangements with reference to sudden infant death syndrome (SIDS).
- Discuss community-based support networks – suggest woman source local agencies and support groups.
- Determine available support and resources for early postnatal days.
- Discuss postnatal care plan with reference to the administration of vitamin K and hepatitis B immunoglobin, and the newborn screening test (NST).
- Emphasise the importance of skin-to-skin contact of mother and child and the timing of the first breastfeed.

This section has presented an overview only of the prenatal care of a woman. Such care must be holistic in nature and flexible to meet the needs of the individual woman and her family in all community settings. For the midwife or MCH community nurse providing antenatal care, the Australian College of Midwives has developed guidelines for consultation and referral if the woman's health or pregnancy varies from the normal [23].

Postpartum care and support

The postnatal period or puerperium is a time not only for physical recovery from pregnancy, labour and birth, but also for the emotional transition to parenting. The puerperium has been defined as 'the period from completion of the third stage of labour to the return to the normal nonpregnant physiological state, 6 weeks later' [24, p. 519]. However, for some women the physical discomforts following childbirth persist for a significantly longer period of time [25]. Also, the transition to parenting and adaptation to motherhood is unique for each mother and her family. This transition can be influenced by many factors such as a long labour, difficult birth or unexpected outcome [26].

The immediate postnatal period

In Australia, less than 1% of women give birth at home, and 4 days was the median length of hospital stay following all births in 2004 [18]. Now in 2007, following a vaginal birth in a public hospital, a mother can expect to stay 'two sleeps' before discharge and between 3 and 4 days following a caesarean birth. This does not leave much time for the midwife to achieve the traditionally accepted aims of postnatal care, which include:

- Facilitating the mother's physical recovery following pregnancy, labour and birth.
- Guiding and supporting the mother in the feeding of her infant.
- Guiding the family in the transition to parenthood.
- Educating and supporting the mother in the care of her infant.

Major concerns during the postnatal period

- Difficulties with breastfeeding (addressed later in this chapter).
- Postnatal depression (covered in detail later in the chapter).
- Urinary incontinence has been reported to affect one in every three women who has given birth [27]. Guidelines for postnatal care outline how to assess urinary problems and provide details of pelvic floor exercises [28].

Specific conditions requiring consultation and/or transfer of care during the postnatal period are listed in the National Midwifery Guidelines for Consultation and Referral [23]. During the early days following birth, the emphasis is on the woman's physical recovery so that she can feel cared for herself while learning to breastfeed and care for her infant. The midwife's role will include the following:

Physical assessment of mother
- Vital signs such as blood pressure if course of pregnancy indicates, temperature and pulse rate if infection is suspected.
- Breast and nipples.
- Uterus and lochia.
- Perineum.
- Maternal well-being.

Physical assessment of infant
- Vital signs such as temperature, heart and respiratory rate.
- Skin: colour, jaundice and bruising.
- Elimination.
- Cord condition.
- Reflexes and Ortolani's test for developmental dysplasia of the hips (DDH).
- Weight, length and head circumference.

Ongoing care of the infant
- Newborn screening test for inborn metabolic and endocrine disorders.
- Hepatitis B immunisation.

Measures to reduce any maternal physical discomfort and promote rest
- Therapeutic environment.
- Pain management.

Facilitation of mother–infant interaction
- Providing time and privacy.
- Positive feedback for infant care activities.

Health promotion strategies

Provision of information for self-care regarding:

- Uterine involution.
- Blood loss or lochial discharge.
- Breasts and nipples.

- Bladder and bowels.
- Perineum.

Provision of information for when to seek help and how to obtain appropriate help regarding:

- Mastitis.
- Any abnormal bleeding or excessive bleeding.
- Signs of infection, e.g. offensive vaginal discharge.

Identification of community support agencies and resources
- Domiciliary service from hospital of birth.
- Family and friends.
- MCH service.

Prevention of sudden infant death
- Review SIDS and kids recommendations and provide written information

Continuity of care from maternity to maternal, child and family health services will ensure that the maternal, child and family health nurse is aware of any complication or concern regarding the new mother, her infant and family [29]. Domiciliary care provided by either the hospital of birth or the Royal District Nursing Services (RDNS) will transfer postnatal care to the specific state maternal and infant health service.

The MCH nurse, or child and family health nurse, will continue health promotion as part of her core activities; for example the Victorian service focuses on:

- Breastfeeding.
- Immunisation.
- SIDS.
- Communication, language and play.
- Injury prevention.
- Car restraints.
- Postnatal depression.
- Food in the first year of life.
- Sunsmart.
- Tooth tips.

Breastfeeding

Breastfeeding is a term that can be used to describe many different practices and patterns of infant feeding. Ever breastfed, fully breastfed, exclusively breastfed and predominantly breastfed are defined categories of breastfeeding [30].

Benefits of breastfeeding

Breastfeeding is an important public health measure which offers benefits to the infant and mother [31]. Breastfeeding should be promoted as the primary method of infant feeding and the risks of not breastfeeding should be highlighted. Exclusive breastfeeding is recommended for the first 6 months of life and breastfeeding is recommended to continue until 12 months of age [32].

Breastfeeding initiation

Breastfeeding initiation usually occurs in a hospital setting. The Baby-Friendly Hospital Initiative [33] recommends that maternity hospitals:

- Have a written policy regarding breastfeeding that is routinely communicated to all health care staff.
- Train all health care staff in the skills necessary to implement this policy.
- Inform all pregnant women about the benefits and management of breastfeeding.
- Help mothers initiate breastfeeding within 30 min after birth.
- Show mothers how to breastfeed and maintain lactation even if they should be separated from their infants.
- Give newborn infants no food or drink other than breast milk, unless medically indicated.
- Practise rooming-in to allow mothers and infants to remain together 24 h a day.
- Encourage breastfeeding on demand.
- Give no artificial teats or pacifiers to breastfeeding infants.
- Foster the establishment of breastfeeding support groups and refer mothers to them on discharge from the hospital or clinic.

Breastfeeding mothers need support to establish breastfeeding and this should occur in hospital and in the community.

Breastfeeding guidelines

The National Health and Medical Research Council (NHMRC) updated the 'Infant Feeding Guidelines for Health Workers' in 2003. These guidelines, included within the 'Dietary Guidelines for Children and Adolescents' provide information to help promote, support and encourage breastfeeding [32]. Nurses in hospitals and the community require up-to-date knowledge of ways to promote and support breastfeeding, as lack of knowledge can result in inconsistent or inaccurate advice, leading to negative support [34]. These guidelines provide information on breastfeeding, including common problems and their management, as well as guidelines on expressing and storing breast milk.

Clinical features

The Royal Women's Hospital (RWH) guidelines for breastfeeding outline how to assess a breastfeed (feel, look and listen) and provide indications of good and faulty attachment [35].

Successful breastfeeding is identifiable from the infant's condition:

- Baby is feeding frequently on demand.
- Baby is alert, active and happy.
- Baby has six to eight wet nappies in 24 h.
- Baby is gaining weight.

Principles to support breastfeeding women

The role of the community nurse is to ensure support for the breastfeeding woman. In clinical practice this may be achieved by offering advice on breastfeeding issues. If the issues are significant, referral to a community breastfeeding support organisation or secondary service may be warranted. The following principles provide a framework for clinical practice:

- Ensure correct attachment to the breast (prevent problems).
- Provide prompt attention to problems and manage them correctly.
- Provide accurate, up-to-date information to mothers.
- Refer mothers to community breastfeeding support organisations for support.
- Refer to secondary services if necessary, e.g. breastfeeding clinic or a community lactation consultant.

Drug therapy

Drugs can be prescribed to improve milk supply, for example galactogogues (e.g. metoclopramide). Appropriate antibiotics can be prescribed to treat infective mastitis (e.g. flucloxacillin). Drugs required to treat other conditions will need to be prescribed with caution. Prescribers should consult specialist drug information and/or services if unsure of appropriate drug therapy in lactating women [32, 36].

Breastfeeding maintenance

Child, family and community nurses should combine breastfeeding information with guidance and support. If necessary, home visits may be performed to assess and solve breastfeeding concerns. These strategies can extend breastfeeding duration [37].

Child health surveillance (growth and development)

Child health surveillance

Child, family and community nurses implement most primary care growth and development assessments in Australia. It is the community nurse's role to ensure that accurate and valid growth measurements and developmental assessments are performed and documented, which are in line with the programme standards of the service (for example in Victoria this would be the *Maternal and Child Health Program Resource Guide*, Department of Human Services [9]). The physical and developmental assessment of children may also be referred to as 'well-child checks' and contributes to child health surveillance in Australia [38].

Growth rates

Variations in growth are normal and shifts in growth across growth percentiles are common [39]. In general, most children's growth approaches the mean. Thus large babies tend to shift downward on the growth chart, whereas small babies tend to shift upward on the growth chart [40]. One of the key issues when monitoring growth is the ability to distinguish between normal and worrisome growth. Worrisome growth, either poor growth or excessive growth, may be an indication of undernutrition (failure to thrive) or overnutrition (obesity).

Growth monitoring: clinical practice guidelines

It is normal practice to undertake three anthropometric measures: weight, length (or height) and head circumference. In practice, it is weight that is usually a reference for growth concerns [40]. Once the anthropometric measurements are undertaken, they are usually recorded and charted on a growth chart [41]. Good measurement practice includes the following:

- Take a bare weight rather than a weight with the child dressed.
- For children <2 years, take height (length) measurements in supine position with feet flat against a foot board.
- Undertake serial measurements, rather than a single measurement.
- Take and record measurements accurately.
- Use appropriate growth charts and chart accurately.
- Adhere to any service guidelines or standards that apply to clinical practice [32, 40, 42].

The frequency of serial measurements may depend on the structure of the well-child visit schedule. For example in Victoria there are 10 key child health visits funded by the state government [9]. These visits are at 2 weeks, 4 weeks, 8 weeks, 4 months, 6–8 months, 12 months, 18–21 months, 2 years, 3.5 years and 4–5 years. In clinical practice, measurements may be recorded on the child's parent-held record, MCH clinic record card and/or in a computer program.

According to Winch, growth is the 'single most important indication of overall health and wellbeing' [42, p. 169] and it is widely recognised as an important indicator of chronic, not acute, conditions, and it is for this reason that growth is monitored. Growth continues to be monitored to detect worrisome growth issues, and to date no evidence suggests that recording growth measurements does harm [43].

Developmental milestones

Developmental milestones for children are usually reported across four domains, for example:

- Posture and large movements (gross motor).
- Vision and fine movements.
- Hearing and speech.
- Social behaviour and play.

Normal development has a sequence and it is widely recognised that although the sequence will be followed, there will be variation in achievement of developmental milestones [44]. One of the key issues when monitoring development is the ability to distinguish between normal and worrisome development. Worrisome development may be an indication of underlying pathology. Typically, advanced development is not seen as an issue, so it is developmental delay that is of concern. Developmental delay is associated with a number of syndromes, as well as the more general conditions of autism and attention-deficit/hyperactivity disorder (ADHD).

Monitoring health and development

Development is monitored in a number of ways: by history taking, physical examination [45] and observation of development. In order to assess development, community nurses need to understand the expected precursors of a skill, as well as what is expected at each age and stage.

Usually observations and questions will be directed by the use of formal screening tools or programme requirements and nurses need to be familiar with the developmental charts used for developmental assessment in their state or territory. There are now moves for greater parent involvement in monitoring of development [46]. Research by Glascoe [47] supports the validity and implementation of short questionnaires, such as the Parents' Evaluations of Development Status (PEDS), and this tool has been validated for use in Australia [48].

Monitoring development: clinical practice guidelines

As in growth monitoring, it is important to undertake serial assessments of development, which Oberklaid and Efron [49] refer to as ongoing developmental surveillance, rather than a single assessment. Development is monitored not so much for prevention but for early identification of problems. Although it may be possible to prevent some problems, many will not be preventable and will require treatment or intervention to ensure optimum child outcomes.

It may be possible to prevent delay in some gross motor areas. For example it is now widely recognised that plagiocephaly has been associated with campaigns for back sleeping [50]. There are also reports of delayed neck muscle tone and head lifting when children are not placed prone whilst awake and the literature now advocates 'tummy time' for children [51].

Referral for further evaluation/treatment

If a growth or development problem is suspected, it may be necessary to refer the family to another service for further evaluation of the child. If the problem is confirmed, an intervention plan can be developed, possibly with interdisciplinary input.

Future trends

There is a move away from child health surveillance towards child health promotion [52]. In the past, growth and development checks by child, family and community nurses were the cornerstone of child health surveillance. The health promotion approach emphasises a more holistic strategy, including family and other early years workers in the early identification of problems and early intervention to enable optimal child health outcomes. Challenges include increased participation of parents at all well-child checks, more flexible service times for working parents and greater engagement with diverse families and hard-to-reach groups, such as Indigenous remote communities.

Immunisation

Vaccinations protect the population against vaccine-preventable infectious diseases. Immunisation is a successful, effective public health initiative, and child, family and community nurses play an important public health advocacy role by promoting immunisation. They may also contribute to the health protection of the population by providing vaccinations.

Immunisation statistics

To reduce the incidence of vaccine-preventable disease in Australia, high levels of immunisation coverage are required. The national target by the year 2000 was to achieve over 90% coverage of children at 2 years of age for all diseases specified in the NHMRC Standard Childhood Vaccination Schedule [53]. According to the Australian Childhood Immunisation Register (ACIR) data, 91.3% of Australian children 12–15 months of age were fully immunised as on 31 December 2007 [54].

Immunisation policy and services

It is important for child, family and community nurses to understand the policy context of immunisation and the framework of service provision, as both these factors shape the provision of immunisation services in Australia and ultimately impact on parents. In Australia, immunisation is not compulsory. Australia has both national- and state-level policies to promote immunisation and the implementation of policy has been guided by immunisation strategies and plans [55]. Service delivery varies across the nation, utilising both public and private providers, and there are now financial incentives for both parents and providers to encourage immunisation uptake. Since 1986 Australia has had a national childhood surveillance system, the ACIR, which monitors the uptake of childhood immunisation across the nation.

Vaccine-preventable diseases

Many diseases are considered vaccine preventable. For example:

- Chickenpox.
- Diphtheria.
- Haemophilus influenzae type B.

- Hepatitis B.
- Influenza.
- Measles.
- Meningococcal disease.
- Mumps.
- Pertussis (whooping cough).
- Pneumococcal disease.
- Poliomyelitis (polio).
- Rubella.
- Streptococcal disease.
- Tetanus [56].

Immunisations schedule

The vaccines that are provided free in Australia under the National Immunisation Programme are listed in the routine schedule of vaccines [57]. The childhood vaccination schedule (current at publication) is listed in Table 14.2.

Immunisation guidelines

Child, family and community nurses play an important public health advocacy role by promoting immunisation. It is vital for nurses to remain up to date about available vaccinations and to provide appropriate advice to parents about the benefits and risks of immunisation and where to seek additional support or advice. *The Australian Immunisation Handbook* is designed for health professionals who are responsible for advising on or providing immunisations [58]. It contains details of the childhood vaccination schedule, as well as recommendations for schedule variations. It discusses commonly encountered issues, such as what to do if infants are premature; vaccine doses have been interrupted; doses have been missed; or additional vaccinations are required [58].

Child, family and community nurses can advise parents what vaccinations are required and monitor a child's immunisation status to ensure the child is up to date according to the immunisation schedule. Community nurses should be able to provide answers, source information or refer parents, in response to the following queries:

- Why immunise?
- Is immunisation safe?
- My child has a cold, should I go ahead with immunisation?
- My religious beliefs prevent me having pork; can my child complete the standard schedule?
- Where can you obtain information about homeopathic immunisation?
- What do I need to know if I choose not to immunise my child?
- What do I need to do to claim parental benefits for my immunised child?

The publication *Understanding Childhood Immunisation* is a most helpful guide to respond to such questions [59]. Community nurses also need to be able to respond to

Table 14.2 National immunisation schedule for children <6 years [58].

Birth	Hepatitis B (hepB) a
2 months	Hepatitis B (hepB) b Diphtheria, tetanus and acellular pertussis (DTPa) *Haemophilus influenzae type b* (*Hib*) c, d Inactivated poliomyelitis (IPV) Pneumococcal conjugate (7vPCV)
4 months	Hepatitis B (hepB) b Diphtheria, tetanus and acellular pertussis (DTPa) *Haemophilus influenzae type b* (*Hib*) c, d Inactivated poliomyelitis (IPV) Pneumococcal conjugate (7vPCV)
6 months	Hepatitis B (hepB) b Diphtheria, tetanus and acellular pertussis (DTPa) *Haemophilus influenzae type b* (*Hib*) c Inactivated poliomyelitis (IPV) Pneumococcal conjugate (7vPCV) e
12 months	Hepatitis B (hepB) b *Haemophilus influenzae type b* (*Hib*) d Measles, mumps and rubella (MMR) Meningococcal C (MenCCV)
12–24 months	Hepatitis A (Aboriginal and Torres Strait Islander children in high-risk areas) f
18 months	Varicella (VZV)
18–24 months	Pneumococcal polysaccharide (23vPPV) (Aboriginal and Torres Strait Islander children in high-risk areas) g Hepatitis A (Aboriginal and Torres Strait Islander children in high-risk areas)
4 years	Diphtheria, tetanus and acellular pertussis (DTPa) Measles, mumps and rubella (MMR) Inactivated poliomyelitis (IPV)

myths and sensational news items that may appear on television current affairs shows or in magazines, and refer to the Commonwealth Department of Health and Ageing publication that is designed to guide providers on how to respond to arguments against immunisation [60].

If parents choose to immunise their child, they will need to understand the benefits and risks associated with immunisation [59]. Although nurses may discuss these issues, it is up to the immunisation provider to ensure that parents understand them before the parents consent to their child being immunised. Community nurses contribute to population monitoring of immunisations by reporting adverse events possibly related to immunisations.

Parents need to understand that immunisation is not compulsory; however, if they choose not to immunise their child or conscientiously object, they will need to complete paperwork to this effect [61]. Currently, there are many entitlements and regulations that affect parents. For example parents are entitled to payment if their child has been immunised. To obtain this payment, 'conscientious objectors' must provide documentation that they have received appropriate counselling from a registered immunisation provider.

Nurse immunisers

Child, family and community nurses may also become immunisation service providers. Most states and territories have programmes which community nurses may undertake to become accredited as an immunisation provider. Accredited community nurse immunisers may provide opportunistic immunisation when a child presents or they may work in an immunisation clinic setting to provide a service to children who are due or overdue for vaccinations.

Education of vaccine providers is considered an essential component of an effective immunisation programme. The creation of the 'National Guidelines for Immunisation Education for Registered Nurses and Midwives' is an example of a key document that guides training organisations and educators on the core components necessary to ensure nurse vaccinators are trained as safe and effective immunisation providers [62].

Role of the nurse

Child, family and community nurses are respected professionals and parents look to them as a primary source of knowledge. Nurses play an essential role in the provision of immunisation services by providing evidence-based advice and by providing vaccinations.

Mental health

The following guidelines relate to mental health and support service provision and are designed to incorporate primary health care philosophies, including health promotion within a community approach to care, whilst encouraging the incorporation of client self-management techniques. The management of client care has a multidisciplinary focus and it is essential that it includes:

- Knowledge of the key, locally accessible, mental health services.
- Awareness of the need for active listening.
- Awareness that some individuals choose to self-disclose for the first time about a suspected mental health condition when they become parents.

Mental health conditions of new mothers

The most common mental health conditions of new mothers include postnatal depression, conditions already diagnosed and being treated such as depression, and disclosure of suspected mental health conditions that have not yet been diagnosed.

Postnatal depression

MCH community nurses in all states and territories have received continuing education on postnatal depression for decades. They will now receive more information through the 2007 National Plan to tackle pre- and postnatal depression [63].

Postnatal depression (PND) is the name given to the mood disorder that occurs in women, '10–15% of new mothers', following childbirth [64, p. 371]. It can develop at any time in the first year after childbirth and can develop suddenly or gradually. It may persist for months [65].

'The symptoms of postnatal depression may include some or all of the following:

- Feeling sad, irritable or unhappy most of the time.
- Loss of interest in work, hobbies or things that used to be enjoyed.
- Chronic exhaustion or hyperactivity.
- Difficulty concentrating, remembering or making decisions.
- Feeling unable to cope with daily tasks.
- Anxiety/panic attacks.
- Negative, recurring or morbid thoughts.
- Thoughts of self-harm or suicide.
- Loss of confidence and self-esteem.
- Feelings of guilt or inadequacy.
- Fear of being alone or of social contact' [65].

The Edinburgh Postnatal Depression Scale (EPDS) has been developed by Cox *et al.* [66] as a guide to identifying whether a woman has postnatal depression. The higher the score, the more likely an individual may be distressed or depressed. For a diagnosis to be made, the MCH nurse must refer the woman to her general practitioner with a referral letter containing the score, and date and time the EPDS was administered.

Other mental health conditions

It is important to ensure that any new mothers with a diagnosed mental health condition are receiving specialist support, treatment and ongoing care. When there is concern about a mother's mental health it is important to arrange a referral to their doctor or to the local Primary Mental Health & Early Intervention (PMHEI) team, who are available to provide secondary consultations to primary health care providers with the mother's permission. This support may be via internet, mail or telephone for a new mother living in rural or remote areas.

Mental health conditions of infants and young children

Hall and Elliman [67, pp. 268–74] list a number of conditions in children which they call minor psychological conditions. The characteristics of these conditions are:

- They are a source of considerable misery.
- They are relatively persistent.
- They tend to present with varying combinations of difficult behaviour (e.g. angry outbursts, feeding disorders, fads or habits).

- They may present as single problems, e.g. enuresis and separation anxiety.
- Psychological problems and physical health problems may occur together and the distinction between them may be unclear and confusing to parents and practitioners.

Hall and Elliman [67] recommend that child development programmes should be available for children wherever they live. Child, family and community nurses in Australia play a major role in this work and are a major referral source to early childhood specialist services.

Acute mental health emergency

As child, family and community nurses often work alone in isolated clinics, local halls and in the family home, they need to be aware of how to manage a mental health emergency. Each state and territory has specialist mental health teams, such as Crisis Assessment and Treatment Teams (CATT) that provide 24-h urgent community-based assessment and short-term treatment interventions. States and territories also have regionally based 24-h mental health phone triage services that are able to provide phone consultation, treatment recommendations and appropriate specialist referrals as required for both service providers and consumers.

Mental health promotion

Key points for the community nurse to consider in mental health promotion are:

- Increase awareness of common mental health conditions in the antenatal and post-natal period.
- Timely referrals.
- Group support.
- Social support.
- Meet regularly with local mental health teams to be aware of what is available locally for mental health promotion.

Vulnerable children and families

Within Australia, vulnerable families fall into a number of groups and can be characterised as unsupported teenage parents, Indigenous families, single-parent families, families living in poverty, refugee families, families suffering from drug and alcohol abuse and families where one or more parents have an intellectual disability [9]. It is important to note, however, that any family with young children may become vulnerable at any time, requiring supportive home visits and a range of specialist children's services.

The following guidelines relate to children and families at risk and are designed to incorporate primary health care philosophies, including health promotion within a community approach to care, whilst supporting families with ongoing outreach services. The management of client care has a multidisciplinary focus and it is essential that it includes:

- Provision of information through first-time parent groups.
- Provision of additional support via home visits, e.g. South Australian Child and Youth Health Services.
- Access to a range of health and community welfare services that are well integrated.

Indicators of potentially vulnerable children

The report of the Australian Health Ministers' Conference and Community and Disability Services Ministers' Conference [68, pp. 9–15] lists the following indicators as potential causes of poor developmental outcomes for young children:

- Poor emotional attachment between mother and child.
- Prenatal stress, prematurity and low birth weight.
- Growth and failure to thrive.
- Child characteristics, e.g. irregular sleep and eating patterns.
- Caregiver characteristics, e.g. age, knowledge and mental state.
- Carer depression and mental illness.
- Carer substance or alcohol abuse.
- Frequent changes to parental/primary carers.
- Carer isolation.
- Family disharmony, conflict and violence.
- Lack of stimuli.
- Low socioeconomic status/poverty.
- Harsh parenting /abuse or neglect.

MCH services in each state and territory have a range of services available for families who may have a number of these indicators. However, this is not as simple as it seems. Some services are more integrated than others. Many agencies work like isolated silos and a number of agencies have a small capacity with long waiting lists. McCain *et al.* [69, p. 113] describe early childhood programmes in Canada as 'disorganised and scattered across communities'. Examples of such disconnected programmes are health, social services, public health, early intervention, family support, education and local government. The situation is similar in Australia. It is important that nurses understand the available referral networks or vulnerable families may not get the services they need. UNICEF's 2007 report card [70, p. 2] provides a useful summary of what countries are doing for child well-being. The six categories examined are material well-being, health and safety, education, peer and family relationships, behaviours and risks, and young people's own subjective sense of well-being.

Domestic violence/family violence/intimate partner violence

Each state and territory has specialist services for prevention and management of domestic violence. Braaf and Sneddon [71, pp. 12–13] provide an overview of domestic violence and family violence in Australia, with a useful guide for the screening for family violence including:

- Whether a past or current partner is making the client feel unsafe.
- Whether a past or current partner has threatened or harmed the client, their children or their pets.
- Whether a past or current partner has hit, slapped or hurt the client in other ways.
- Whether the client has been forced to have sexual activities against their will by a past or current partner.
- Whether the client feels safe to go home.
- Whether the client would like any assistance in regard to these issues.

Health promotion

Intervening as early as possible is critical for health promotion in the area of family violence. Key strategies include:

- Provide additional family support, e.g. family health workers, home-visiting services.
- Encourage use of quality child care for children (provide 'time out' for parents).
- Make contact with other early childhood services, including kindergartens and/or schools.
- Link parents with agencies that provide groups and/or social support, e.g. parent programmes, mothers' groups.
- Make timely referrals to other services, e.g. relationship counselling, domestic violence services, drug support agencies.

Child-abuse prevention and reporting

A child in need of protection has been described as:

> A child who has suffered, or who is likely to suffer, significant harm from sexual abuse, physical injury, emotional or psychological harm, neglect or abandonment, and where the parents have not protected or are unlikely to protect them. This may be the result of one abusive or neglectful incident, or cumulative result of many instances, or a general pattern of behaviour or circumstances [72, p. 4].

Each state and territory has legislation and services in place to prevent, identify early and report suspected child abuse. In some states and territories it is mandatory to report suspected child abuse. For example Victoria, South Australia and the ACT have mandatory reporting. (See Australian Institute of Family Studies' website http://www.aifs.gov.au/nch/pubs/sheets/rs3/rs3.html for an overview of mandatory reporting by state and territory.)

The related legislation in Victoria is the *Children, Youth and Families Act 2005* [72]. This legislation is new and a range of changes specified in the new act are currently being implemented. For example new reporting and referral arrangements are being implemented during 2007. Referrals by professionals working with families through pregnancy until the child is 17 years may be made direct to child protection or child-first teams. For a referral to be made to a child-first team, the following circumstances may exist:

- Significant parenting problems.
- Family conflict such as family breakdown.
- Families under pressure due to, for example, substance abuse and mental illness.
- Young, isolated and or/unsupported families.
- Significant social or economic disadvantage [72, p. 18].

A report to a child protection team should be made in any of the following circumstances:

- Physical abuse.
- Sexual abuse.
- Emotional abuse.
- Persistent neglect.
- A child's action or behaviour placing them at risk of significant harm.
- Where a child appears to be abandoned [72, p. 18].

Child, family and community health nurses need to examine the legislation in their state and territory and be familiar with processes for reporting suspected child abuse. State and territories have guidelines to assist with this role. For example the Department of Human Services in Victoria [73] has developed the Victorian Risk Framework (see Appendix 14.1) to provide a standardised model for the assessment of significant harm to children.

Attending a children's court for a child protection case

If a community nurse is requested to attend a children's court for a child protection case, they need to be well briefed by child, family and community nurses and management who are well informed about the court processes. Preparation for court includes the recording of contemporaneous clinical notes. These notes must be accurate, succinct and non-judgemental as they may be subpoenaed by a court. McAllister *et al.* [74, pp. 105–6] point out that practitioners must have the skills to write reports, records and referrals that avoid ethical and legal pitfalls.

Future trends

Child, family and community health nurses must work towards the provision of a seamless service to families following the birth of a new baby. Many new parents are older than in the past and do not live within close reach of family members who can provide them with support. As family demography and characteristics change across communities, MCH nurses will need to re-examine their programmes to ensure they are meeting the needs of all parents.

It is likely that universal MCH services will continue to provide programmes for families with new babies, infants and young children. In order to maximise the support for parents, MCH services will need to improve their links with short- and long-term day care and kindergartens to ensure that all parents are being given the same messages and information about the early years of child development. Other future trends are likely to be:

- Additional services will be provided for vulnerable families. Child, family and community nurses will receive enhanced continuing education from employment bodies to support their work with vulnerable families. Telephone counselling services will expand to support parents, particularly after business hours and at weekends.
- Gender inclusiveness will remain an issue for all early intervention programmes. Child, family and community nurses must remain focused on the need to include fathers and other family members and caregivers in their parenting programmes. Programmes will need to have flexible hours for fathers to attend on a regular basis.
- Domiciliary midwives must ensure that they are well integrated with child, family and community nurses. Formal protocols similar to those available in Victoria need to be considered by all domiciliary midwifery and MCH services in Australia.
- Clinical supervision will become essential as a strategy to support MCH nurses and to ensure that their practice competencies are appropriate for working with vulnerable families.

Summary

This chapter has provided guidelines for community nursing practice in child and maternal health and located some of the key services and programmes for the maternal/child/family client group. As conditions which are not managed well in infancy and childhood may become serious and/or chronic problems in adulthood, the work of child, family and community nurses remains an essential universal direct access public health service worldwide.

Useful resources

National website with links to state/territory health departments at http://www.health.gov.au/internet/wcms/publishing.nsf/Content/phd-child-health-index
Antenatal websites at: http://www.rwh.org.au/rwhcpg/maternity.cfm?doc_id=3704
    http://www.health.nsw.gov.au/health_pr/mph/pdf/models_maternity.pdf
    http://www.npsu.unsw.edu.au/ps18high.htm
    http://www.health.vic.gov.au/maternity/resrch/consum06.htm
    http://www.gestation.net/main.htm
    http://www.betterhealth.vic.gov.au/

Other websites
Immunisation
ACIR statistics at http://www.hic.gov.au/providers/health_statistics/statistical_reporting/acir.htm
Immunise Australia Programme at http://www.immunise.health.gov.au/

Breastfeeding at http://www.health.gov.au/internet/wcms/publishing.nsf/Content/health-pubhlth-strateg-brfeed-links.htm

ABA breastfeeding information at http://www.breastfeeding.asn.au/bfinfo/index.html

National breastfeeding strategy at http://www.health.gov.au/internet/wcms/publishing.nsf/Content/health-pubhlth-strateg-brfeed-strategy.htm#accreditation

Royal Women's Hospital guidelines, including breastfeeding at http://www.rwh.org.au/rwhcpg/maternity.cfm?doc_id=1812

World Health Organization (WHO) at http://www.who.int/nutrition/publications/infantfeeding/en/index.html

Depression at www.beyondblue.org.au

Health promotion at http://www.who.int/hpr/health.promotion.shtml
http://whqlibdoc.who.int/euro/-1993/ICP_HSR_602__m01.pdf

Child protection at http://www.aifs.gov.au/nch/sheets/rs3.html
http://www.betterhealth.vic.gov.au/bhcv2/bhcarticles.nsf/pages/Child_abuse_reporting_procedures?OpenDocument=

Domestic violence at http://www.aph.gov.au/library/intguide/SP/Dom_violence.htm
http://www.austdvclearinghouse.unsw.edu.au/
http://www.austdvclearinghouse.unsw.edu.au/PDF%20files/Issuespaper_12.pdf

References

1. Scott D. (1992) The ecology of the family and family functions, in A. Clements (ed.) *Infant and Family Health in Australia*, 2nd edition. Churchill Livingstone, Melbourne, pp. 203–17.
2. World Health Organization (WHO) (1998) *Health Promotion Glossary*. World Health Organization, Geneva.
3. Talbot, L. and Verrinder, G. (2005) *Promoting Health: The Primary Health Care Approach*, 3rd edition. Elsevier Churchill Livingstone, Sydney.
4. McMurray, A. (2007) *Community Health and Wellness*, 3rd edition. Mosby Elsevier, Sydney.
5. Sackett, D.L., Straus, S., Richardson, W.S., Rosenberg, W. and Hayes, R.B. (2000) *Evidence-Based Medicine. How to Practice and Teach*, 2nd edition. Churchill Livingstone, London.
6. Muir Gray, J.A. (2001) *Evidence-Based Healthcare*, 2nd edition. Churchill Livingstone, Sydney.
7. Health and Community Services, Specialist Children's Service and The Australian Early Intervention Association [Victorian Chapter] Inc (1994) *Family Centred Practice*. Specialist Children's Services Unit, Health and Community Services, Melbourne.
8. McCashen, W. (2005) *The Strengths Approach*. Innovative Resources, Bendigo.
9. Department of Human Services (DHS) (2006) *Maternal and Child Health Program Resource Guide*. Department of Human Services, Melbourne.
10. Quality Improvement Council Limited (1999) *Australian Health and Community Services Standards. Maternal and Infant Care Services Module*. La Trobe University, Bundoora.
11. Edgecombe, G.A., Mackey, R., Hindell, A., Stanesby, F. and Rinaldi, M. (1995) *Maternal and Child Health Service Program Standards*. Health and Community Services, Melbourne.
12. Maternal and Child Health Nurses Special Interest Group, Australian Nursing Federation (Vic Branch) (1999) *Standards of Professional Practice for Maternal and Child Health Nurses*. Maternal and Child Health Nurses Special Interest Group, Melbourne.

13. DHS (2004) *Future Directions for the Victorian Maternal and Child Health Service*. Family and Community Support Branch, Department of Human Services, Melbourne.

14. Pairman, S., Pincombe, J., Thorogood, C. and Tracy, S. (2006) *Midwifery. Preparation for practice*. Elsevier, Sydney.

15. Southern Health and Women's & Children's Health (2001) *Three Centres Consensus Guidelines on Antenatal Care Project, Mercy Hospital for Women*. Available at http://www.health.vic.gov.au/maternitycare/anteguide.pdf (viewed 10 April 2007).

16. National Health and Medical Research Council (NHMRC) (1993) *Revised Statement on the Relationship Between Dietary Folic Acid and Neural Tube Defects Such as Spina Bifida*. National Health and Medical Research Council, Canberra.

17. Watson, L., Brown, S. and Davey, M. (2006) Use of periconceptual folic acid supplements in Victoria and New South Wales, Australia. *Australian and New Zealand Journal of Public Health*, 30(1), 42–9.

18. Laws, P.J., Grayson, N. and Sullivan, E.A. (2006) *Australia's Mothers and Babies 2004*. Perinatal statistics series no. 18. Australian Institute of Health and Welfare (AIHW) Cat. No. PER 34. AIHW National Perinatal Statistics Unit, Sydney.

19. National Health and Medical Research Council (NHMRC) (2005) Nutrient reference values for Australia and New Zealand. Australian Government Department of Health and Ageing and National Health and Medical Research Council, Canberra. Available at http://www.nhmrc.gov.au/publications/synopses/_files/n35.pdf (viewed 10 June 2008).

20. Connellan, M. and Wallace, E. (2000) Prevention of perinatal group B streptococcal disease: A screening practice in public hospitals in Victoria. *Medical Journal of Australia*, 172(7), 317–20.

21. AIHW (2007) *The National System for Monitoring Diabetes in Australia*. Available at http://www.aihw.gov.au/publications/cvd/nsmda/nsmda-c01.pdf (viewed 10 April 2007).

22. Walters, W., Ford, J. and King, J. (2002) Maternal deaths in Australia. *Medical Journal of Australia*, 176(9), 413–14.

23. Australian College of Midwives (2004) *National Midwifery Guidelines for Consultation and Referral*. National College of Midwives Inc, Canberra.

24. Beischer, N. and Mackay, E. (1986) *Obstetrics and the Newborn. An Illustrated Textbook*, 2nd edition. W.B. Saunders Company, Sydney.

25. Brown, S. and Lumley, J. (2000) Physical health problems after childbirth and maternal depression at six to seven months postpartum. *BJOG: An International Journal of Obstetrics and Gynaecology*, 107(10), 1194–201.

26. Nelson, A. (2003) Transition to motherhood. *Journal of Obstetric, Gynecologic, and Neonatal Nursing*, 32(4), 465–77.

27. Continence Foundation of Australia (2007) *Frequently Asked Questions*. Available at http://www.contfound.org.au/ (viewed 10 April 2007).

28. Bick, D., MacArthur, C., Knowles, H. and Winter, H. (2002) *Postnatal Care Evidence and Guidelines for Management*. Churchill Livingstone, Edinburgh.

29. DHS (2004) *Continuity of Care: A Communication Protocol for Victorian Maternity Services and the Maternal and Child Health Service*. Community Care Division, Department of Human Services, Melbourne. Available at http://www.office-for-children.vic.gov.au/maternal-child-helath/care

30. Webb, K., Marks, G.C., Lund-Adams, M., Rutishauser, I.H.E. and Abraham, B. (2001) *Towards a National System for Monitoring Breastfeeding in Australia: Recommendations for Population Indicators, Definitions, and Next Steps*. Commonwealth Department of Health and Aged Care, Canberra.

31. Akre, J. (1989) *Infant Feeding: The Physiological Basis. Bull World Health Organ*, Vol. 67(Suppl). World Health Organization, Geneva.

32. NHMRC (2003) *Dietary Guidelines for Children and Adolescents in Australia Incorporating the Infant Feeding Guidelines for Health Workers.* Commonwealth of Australia, Canberra.
33. WHO (1998) *Evidence for the Ten Steps to Successful Breastfeeding.* World Health Organization, Geneva.
34. Dennis, C.L. (2002) Breastfeeding initiation and duration: A 1990–2000 literature review. *Journal of Obstetric, Gynecologic, and Neonatal Nursing,* 31(1), 12–32.
35. Royal Women's Hospital (2006) *Guidelines for Breastfeeding.* Available at http://www.thewomens.org.au/BreastfeedingBestPracticeGuidelines
36. WHO (2002) *Breastfeeding and Maternal Medication.* World Health Organization, Geneva.
37. De Oliveira, M.I., Camacho, L.A. and Tedstone, A.E. (2001) Extending breastfeeding duration through primary care: A systematic review of prenatal and postnatal interventions. *Journal of Human Lactation,* 17(4), 326–43.
38. Centre for Community Child Health (2002) *Child Health Surveillance: A Critical Review of the Evidence.* National Health and Medical Research Council, Melbourne.
39. Hockenberry, M.J., Wilson, D., Winkelstein, M.L. and Kline, N.E. (2003) *Wong's Nursing Care of Infants and Children,* 7th edition. Mosby, St Louis.
40. Freeman, J.V., Cole, T.J., Wales, J. and Cooke, J. (2006) Monitoring infant weight gain: Advice for practitioners. *Community Practice,* 79(5), 149–51.
41. De Onis, M., Wijnhoven, T.M. and Onyango, A.W. (2004) Worldwide practices in child growth monitoring. *Journal of Pediatrics,* 144(4), 461–5.
42. Winch, A.E. (2001) Obtaining accurate growth measurements in children. *Journal of Specialists in Pediatric Nursing,* 7(4), 166–9.
43. Garner, P., Panpanich, R. and Logan, S. (2000) Is routine growth monitoring effective? A systematic review of trials. *Archives of Disease in Childhood,* 82(3), 197–201.
44. Sheridan, M. (1997) *From Birth to Five Years: Children's Developmental Progress.* ACER Press, Melbourne.
45. Engel, J. (2006) *Pediatric Assessment,* 5th edition. Mosby/Elsevier, St Louis.
46. Williams, J. and Holmes, C.A. (2004) Improving the early detection of children with subtle developmental problems. *Journal of Child Health Care,* 8(1), 34–46.
47. Glascoe, F.P. (1999) Using parents' concerns to detect and address developmental and behavioural problems. *Journal of the Society of Pediatric Nurses,* 4(1), 24–35.
48. Coghlan, D., King, J.S. and Wake, M. (2003) Parents' evaluation of developmental status in the Australian day care setting: Developmental concerns of parents and carers. *Journal of Paediatrics and Child Health,* 39(1), 49–54.
49. Oberklaid, F. and Efron, D. (2005) Developmental delay – identification and management. *Australian Family Physician,* 34(9), 739–42.
50. Najarian, S.P. (1999) Infant cranial molding deformation and sleep position: Implications for primary care. *Journal of Pediatric Health Care,* 13(4), 173–7.
51. Chizawsky, L.L. and Scott-Findlay, S. (2005) Tummy time! Preventing unwanted effects of the 'Back to Sleep' campaign. *AWHONN Lifelines,* 9(5), 382–7.
52. Blair, M. and Hall, D. (2006) From health surveillance to health promotion: The changing focus in preventive children's services. *Archives of Disease in Childhood,* 91(9), 730–35.
53. NHMRC (1994) *Standards for Childhood Immunisation.* Australian Government Publishing Service, Canberra.
54. Australian Childhood Immunisation Register (31 December 2006) *Coverage Report Percentage of Children Vaccinated with Highest Level Appropriate for Age Group: State Summary by Age Group* (age calculated at 30 September 2006). Available at http://www.hic.gov.au/providers/health_statistics/statistical_reporting/acir.htm#coverage (viewed 6 April 2007).

55. Australian Government Department of Health and Aging (2006) *About us – Immunise Australia Program*. Available at http://www.immunise.health.gov.au/internet/immunise/publishing.nsf/Content/about-iap (viewed 6 April 2007).

56. DHS (2007) *Vaccine Preventable Diseases*. Available at http://www.health.vic.gov.au/ideas/diseases/gr_vacc.htm (viewed 6 April 2007).

57. Australian Government Department of Health and Aging (2005) *National Immunisation Program*. Available at http://www.immunise.health.gov.au/internet/immunise/publishing.nsf/Content/nips (viewed 6 April 2007).

58. NHMRC (2008) *Australian Immunisation Handbook*, 9th edition. Australian Government Publishing Service, Canberra. Available at http://www.immunise.health.gove.au/internet/immunise/publishing.nsf/Content/5335A7AB925D3E39CA25742100194409/$File/handbook-9.pdf (viewed 10 June 2008).

59. The Commonwealth Department of Health and Aged Care (2005) *Understanding Childhood Immunisation*. Available at http://immunise.health.gov.au/internet/immunise/publishing.nsf/Content/ucibooklet (viewed 6 April 2007).

60. Commonwealth Department of Health and Aged Care (2001a) (2001) *Immunisation: Myths and Realities: Responding to Arguments Against Immunisation*, 3rd edition. Available at http://immunise.health.gov.au/internet/immunise/publishing.nsf/Content/uci-myths-guideprov (viewed 6 April 2007).

61. Medicare Australia (2007) *Immunisation Exemption: Conscientious Objection Form*. Available at http://www.medicare.gov.au/resources/acir/ma_conscientious_objection_form.pdf (viewed 6 April 2007).

62. Commonwealth Department of Health and Aged Care (2001) *National Guidelines for Immunisation Education for Registered Nurses and Midwives*. Available at http://www.health.gov.au/internet/immunise/publishing.nsf/content/5AA253E0F64E4ADECA25719D0018341A/$File/training-guide-nurses.pdf (viewed 6 April 2007).

63. Mason, B. (29 March 2007) *National Plan to Tackle Pre and Postnatal Depression* [Media release]. Parliamentary Secretary to the Minister for Health and Aging.

64. Keltner, N.L., Schwecke, L.H. and Bostrom, C.E. (2007) *Psychiatric Nursing*. Mosby Elsevier, St Louis.

65. The National Postnatal Depression Program (2007) *Post Natal Depression* [Brochure]. Beyondblue.

66. Cox, J.L., Holden, J.M. and Sagovsky, R. (1987) Detection of postnatal depression. Development of the 10-item Edinburgh Depression Scale. *British Journal of Psychiatry*, 150(6), 782–6.

67. Hall, M.B. and Elliman, D. (2003) *Health for All Children*, 4th edition. Oxford University Press, Melbourne.

68. Australian Health Ministers Conference and Community and Disability Services Ministers Conference (2006) *The Child Health and Wellbeing Reform Initiative: Supporting Vulnerable Families in the Antenatal Period and the Early Years*. Department of Health and Human Services, Tasmania.

69. McCain, M.N., Mustard, J.F. and Shanker, S. (2007) *Early Years Study 2: Putting Science into Action*. Council for Early Childhood Development, West Toronto, Ontario.

70. UNICEF (2007) *Child Poverty in Perspective: An Overview of Child Well-Being in Rich Countries*. Innocenti Report Card 7. UNICEF Innocenti Research Centre, Florence.

71. Braaf, R. and Sneddon, C. (2006) *Family Law Act Reform: The Potential Screening and Risk Assessment for Family Violence*. Issues paper 12. Australia Domestic & Family Violence Clearinghouse, Sydney.

72. DHS (2007) *Providing Support to Vulnerable Children and Families*. Every Child Everychance. Department of Human Services, Melbourne.

73. DHS (2001) *Safe from Harm: The Role of Professionals in Protecting Children and Young People*. Child Protection and Care, Department of Human Services, Melbourne.

74. McAllister, L., Hay, I. and Street, A. (2005) Writing records, reports, and referrals in professional practice, in J. Higgs, A. Sefton, A. Street, L. McAllister and I. Hay (eds) *Communicating in the Health and Social Sciences*. Oxford University Press, Melbourne, pp. 105–19.

Appendix 14.1

The Victorian Risk Framework

The Victorian Risk Framework (VRF) provides a consistent and standardised model for the assessment of significant harm to children and guides child protection workers in the key activities of information gathering, analysis and judgement. The following risk factors warning list demonstrates the complexity and thoroughness that is applied to making decisions about the safety and well-being of children.

Risk factors warning list

Research and experience has found that combinations of the following factors are commonly associated with heightened risk to children or young people. Any one factor, however, is meaningful for a particular family only when its occurrence can be demonstrated as affecting the safety of the child or young person. The purpose of the risk factors warning list within the VRF is to signal a warning to the worker, and any identified risk factor must be explained within the worker's subsequent risk analysis.

Category	Description of possible risk factors
Prior child protection history	Prior substantiated abuse reports
	Escalating concern or pattern of contact with Child Protection Service
The child	If the child:
	• Is under 2 years
	• Shows evidence of physical abuse/shaking
	• Is premature, disabled and chronically ill
	• Has difficulty feeding, sleeping, cries a lot
	• Was born underweight or drug dependent
Another child or young person in the home	If any child or young person in the home has:
	• A developmental/other disability
	• A history of self-harm/suicide (talk or attempt)
	• A history of offending
	• Violent behaviour
	• A mental health problem
	• Substance-abuse problems
	• Recent significant behaviour change
	• A history of multiple separations or no stable placement, for example no stable day programme (education/employment/other)

(continued)

(*continued*)

Category	Description of possible risk factors
Carer(s)	If a carer: • Was under 20 at birth of first child • Was abused as a child • Is not the biological parent • Has an intellectual disability • Is socially isolated or the family is severely fragmented
Parenting skills of carer(s)	If there is: • Use of excessive punishment or inappropriate discipline • A domineering parenting style (high-criticism/low-warmth family type) • A lack of motivation or realism regarding improvement of parenting skills
Response to investigation or incident by carer(s)	If a carer: • Viewed the situation less seriously than did the child protection worker • Failed to cooperate satisfactorily
Carer(s)' history of violent relationships	If a carer has: • Physically abused a child (past or present) • Been a perpetrator of domestic violence • Been a victim of domestic violence • A history of other violence
Carer(s)' current problems	If a carer has problems concerning: • Alcohol abuse • Abuse of other drugs (with or without alcohol) • Psychiatric illness • Self-esteem • Apathy or depression
Carer(s)' beliefs about the child	If a carer: • Describes (or acts towards) the child in a predominately negative manner • Has unrealistic expectations
Carer(s)' history of perpetrating sexual assault	If a carer has a history of perpetrating sexual assault: • Of children • Of adults Carers can include any parent, carer or adult in the household

Source: Department of Human Services (DHS) (2001). *Safe from Harm: The Role of Professionals in Protecting Children and Young People*. Child Protection and Care, Department of Human Services, Melbourne, pp. 59–61.

Chapter 15

Medication support

Katherine Trowbridge

Introduction

The role of the community nurse encompasses clinical knowledge, expert communication skills and the ability to practise within a variety of metropolitan, rural or remote settings [1]. Medication support by community nurses across diverse settings, including urban, rural and remote, will be the focus of this chapter. Rural community nursing practice has been defined as 'the practice of a registered nurse where no medical practitioners or allied health professionals are available full time' [1, p. 6]. Remote area nursing practice has been defined as 'not having a medical practitioner able to physically respond due to geographical remoteness' [1, p. 6].

The practice of medication support for clients in the community can be a challenging role for the community nurse because often the environment or setting in which care is provided may lack the essentials of light, running water or a clean surface on which to prepare for a procedure. There is a wide array of nursing knowledge required to meet the needs of different age and cultural client groups, for example weight dose requirements for antibiotic therapy or how to respond when a client who has dementia refuses to take their prescribed medications in the presence of the community nurse. In the face of these challenges, however, medication support has the potential to make a difference to people by facilitating a level of independence and control [2].

Medication support by the community nurse has many facets such as knowledge of relevant legislation and safety practices; collaboration with and role definitions for general practitioners (GPs), pharmacists and clients; and a team approach to care delivery. These will be discussed in this chapter. National medication support strategies and supporting guiding principles for the community nurse will be a key component of this chapter as will consideration of national nursing guidelines, codes of conduct and standards relating to medication administration and documentation. A focus on the practical approaches to care delivery in the community setting, with examples provided through case studies, will offer the reader the opportunity to process the information and relate the guidelines to their own individual clinical setting.

Definitions of some key terms include:

- A community clinical setting could include remote stations, homeless clinics, parklands, correctional facilities, schools, work sites, community centres and clients' homes [3].
- For the purpose of this chapter, all people receiving community nursing care delivery and support will be known as a 'client'. This includes infants, children, adolescents, midlife adults, older people, people from culturally and linguistically diverse (CALD) [4] communities, special needs groups (people living with a disability) and Aboriginal and Torres Strait Islanders.
- A 'community nurse' is inclusive of enrolled nurses (ENs), registered nurses (RNs), registered midwives (RMs) and nurse practitioners (NPs) working within a community setting.
- Medication is 'a substance taken to prevent and/or treat illness and/or maintain or promote health' [5, p. 1] and is inclusive of all substances administered for a therapeutic purpose as part of prescribed care. It includes all synthetic chemicals, herbal extracts, vitamins, minerals, oxygen and blood/blood products. These can be prescribed medications or those purchased 'over the counter' (OTC), such as analgesia and vitamin supplements.

Background

Medicines come in many forms and may be ingested, inhaled, injected, inserted or applied [3, 5]. Therefore, routes of administration can be described as oral, transdermal, guttae, otic, subcutaneous, intramuscular, intrathecal, epidural, intravenous, buccal, vaginal, rectal, stomal, nasogastric and inhalant [3].

The management of medications or 'medication support' is a complex process [1, 6, 7] involving a team of health workers [8], including the community nurse [9] as a coordinator of the receipt, storage, supply, administration and monitoring of medications [1]. The National Pharmaceutical Association in the United Kingdom (UK) defines medication support as 'a process that covers the process and support systems which are available to help people who administer their medication in the community to gain the optimum health benefit from their prescription' [7, p. 20]. Medication support can be described in terms of the four main relevant issues affecting the health of the community:

- *Rational prescribing and support* involves prescribing the correct medication for the client's pathological condition and assessing the efficacy and symptoms of the treatment, undertaken by a medical officer/GP or NP.
- *Client-centred medication review* is an Australian government initiative and involves the assessment of adverse events and compliance/adherence, in the form of a home medication review (HMR) [7].
- *Client information and access to medicines* involves the information (via leaflet inside the medication pack or information sheet provided by the pharmacist) provided to the client and the ability to have the medications available (delivered if the client has poor mobility or transport difficulties) and to be offered affordable alternatives to brand name products.

- *Improvements at the community care interface* involves the development of effective communication between the community nurse, GP and pharmacist, particularly when the client has had a recent acute hospital admission and the medication regime has changed [7, 10].

The above four issues and the management tactics relating to medication support can be related to the Australian environment. The community nurse and community nursing organisation can incorporate these issues into organisational policy which is inclusive of government and legal requirements in the following ways:

- Monitoring whether prescribed medications are effective for the reasons that they were prescribed (e.g. antibiotics for the resolution of an infection).
- Communication with the GP to highlight a need for an HMR, when the client's condition, home environment (safe storage of medications) or number of prescribed medications meet criteria to initiate a review of medications.
- Monitoring whether the client has received information (in a printed form appropriate for their cognitive ability and language) enclosed with prescribed medication packaging.
- Developing, documenting and making available a variety of tested effective communication processes between the community nurse, pharmacist and GP. The communication processes need to be relevant to the diverse practice settings of a community nurse (such as two-way radio communication between a community nurse and GP in a remote area).

The community nursing role in medication support

Effective medication support can be both rewarding and challenging for the nurse and the client because it is based on a person-centred approach to care. Medication support incorporates the clinical processes of assessment and documentation, which reflect an understanding of the client's goals, beliefs, wishes and concerns. A plan of care for medication support is then developed, which takes into consideration the needs, wishes and capacity of the client; the environment and social situation of the client; the care required; and the capacity and limits of the services available. This can challenge the community nurse to 'think outside the square' and develop in collaboration with the client and/or carer a plan of care that is person centred while conforming to the requirements of legislation and national standards. For example the nurse being sensitive to the particular needs and capacity of the client when making decisions about which choice of dose administration aid (DAA) to offer the client, such as a Webster's blister pack system or labelled 'yellow-top' containers. The nurse will make recommendations based on the client's lifestyle and budget, level of understanding, social support, physical abilities and the capacity of the community health services to support the client. (Refer to 'Medication safety' section of this chapter.)

Building a trusting relationship with the client, their family, parents (particularly important for child/infant clients) and carers is a basis for effective communication and the development of effective home medication planning – a plan of care to manage medications that is person centred and reflective of the client's goals [3]. The Nurses Board of South Australia describes the nurse's role in medication support as 'requiring consideration of individual, organisational, social, cultural, religious and professional factors and the exercise of professional clinical judgement' [5, p. 1]. Incorporating this role into a medication standard, the nurses boards in all states and territories collaborated to develop three national standards that represent the minimum requirements for nursing management that produce safe and therapeutic care for the client [5]. It is expected that nursing organisations adapt and integrate these standards into individual organisational policies and procedures for the nursing management of medications [5]. The following is an analysis of the three nursing standards, including evidence requirements and community nursing examples.

Standard 1 – 'The safety and well being of the client is ensured through medication support practices that reflect current knowledge, applicable law, standards and codes of nursing practice, and organisational policies and procedures' [5, p. 2].

Regardless of the setting, nurses are legally bound to provide the most reasonable or appropriate care possible for their clients [1]. To this end, a list of required evidence of nursing practices to manage medications includes [5]:

- Current knowledge of therapeutic substances and associated technology, and safe use in cotemporary health care practice.
- Nurses are authorised to administer medicines according to relevant state or territory legislation, acts and policies [3]:
  Relevant state and federal legislation, beneficence – to do good always [11]; non-maleficence – to do no harm [11]; distributive justice – the right to receive care [11]; Controlled Substances Act, Palliative Care Act and Consent to Treatment Act [2]
  Professional standards, such as National Competence Standards for Nurses – core competence standards which provide a framework for assessing competence [12]
  Codes, such as the Code of Ethics for Nurses in Australia 2005 [13] – presents ethics and ideals of the nursing profession and describes accountability, 'being answerable for one's decisions and actions' [13, p. 2] and responsibility, 'an individual assumes when undertaking to carry out planned or delegated functions' [13, p. 2]; and Code of Professional Conduct 2003 [14] – presents the minimum requirements for practice in the nursing profession in Australia
- Appropriate action in response to questionable medication orders, such as illegible prescriber handwriting [15], and decisions or behaviours of other members of the health care team, such as the dismissal of clients' concerns relating to pain management options by the palliative care specialist.
- Knowledge of and compliance with relevant organisational policies, procedures and guidelines, such as the reporting of medication errors [16, 17]; documentation requirements of medication administration [18]; or the requirement of a rural or remote community nurse to understand the need to administer and supply medications only where current protocols are in place, for example standing orders for paracetamol [1].
- Ensurance of the client's rights to comprehensive medication information and consent.
- Documenting (this will be discussed at length later in this chapter), transporting and storing medications appropriately. For example the community nurse can plan with the client a regime for the transporting of medications from the pharmacy to the point of administration and for their storage – such as a pharmacy service delivering all medications to a locked box in the client's home.

Standard 2 – 'Nursing practice promotes the quality use of medicines (QUM) and ensures a safe and therapeutic environment' [5, p. 2].

The QUM means that 'all medicines should be used judiciously, appropriately, safely and efficaciously' [19, p. 18]. The National Strategy for the Quality Use of Medicines was initiated by the World Health Organization during the late 1990s and was formally developed in 1999 [19]. Most relevant to the community nurse is the central objective to ensure timely access to appropriate quality medicines. This means that the community nurse is a key partner in implementing initiatives to achieve QUM [20], and the client should expect prescribed medicines to be affordable and available to them while being of an acceptable Australian standard [19]. Australia's National Strategy the Quality Use of Medicines is to make the best possible use of medicines to improve the health outcomes for all Australians [19]. A community nursing example is the situation of a client who has been prescribed antibiotics for an infected leg ulcer that is not responding to treatment. The community nurse could initiate a wound swab and coordinate with the GP to ascertain if the antibiotic prescribed is the most appropriate for the wound infection present in the ulcer.

Standard 2 requires the community nurse to undertake a comprehensive nursing assessment relevant to the medication therapy that may be inclusive of:

- Baseline and ongoing assessment of the client's medical history and physical, cognitive, cultural, psychological and safety needs [5, 21, 22].
- Determining the existence of known allergies. (This can be assessed by asking the client and the carers, investigating previous admission notes from your organisation (if available), and communication with the client's GP.)
- Assessing the optimum mode of administration, therapeutic goals, effects and/or side effects and interactions [5]. This includes the need to develop a complete list of client-prescribed and OTC medications in order to inform the client of potential effects and side effects to medication [23–25] and interactions with other medications. The community nurse can discuss with the client alternative routes of administration if swallowing difficulties are experienced. It may be appropriate to crush a medication or have it in a soluble form. (Discuss with a pharmacist when altering medication forms, such as crushing medications [26].)
- Client involvement in the process of care and education regarding their medication therapy. The community nurse can, through discussion with the client, ascertain their preferred level of participation and therefore tailor a care plan to suit their preferences. This may in turn enable the client to have as much control over their own medication support as physically and cognitively possible [27, 28]. Assessment of the client's ability to open a bottle of tablets, push out medications from a blister pack or pick up medicines from a saucer or egg cup will determine the type of DAA most appropriate for the client [29, 30]. Assessment should also include the client's ability to see the medication (white tablets if placed on a light-coloured saucer) and level of dexterity to manipulate medication packaging. (Clients with a physical disability or presence of plaster cast or arthritis may have impaired manual dexterity [30].) Education/information magazines called 'Medicines Talk' are available for clients with information including 'who to ask about side effects and how to manage them' through the Australian National Prescribing Service (NPS) [31, 32].

Consent – There is a legal and moral obligation to gain consent to conduct any nursing procedure, including the administration of medication, from the client. Ideally, this should be in the written form but may also be a verbal agreement from the client [33].

- Informed consent by the client or authorisation by a carer or next of kin. Within health care this refers to a person's autonomous authorisation of a specific medical intervention or participation in research [33] (also see Chapter 3 of this book).
- Recognition of a client's right to refuse a medication and the appropriate action to take when a client refuses a medication. Community nurses can encounter refusal of nursing care by clients, and many find such situations challenging and perhaps distressing. (Refer to the Chapter 3 of this book for examination of the issues relating to consent, competence and children and consent.) A discussion with the client to ascertain why they are unwilling to take their medication may prove to enlighten the nurse to specific concerns or fears that the client may have. One example is that a client may fear urinary frequency and urgency when in a public place if prescribed oral diuretic medication in the morning. The client may refuse to take that medication on the morning of when he/she goes shopping.

Administration of medicines – The community nurse needs to have an understanding of the following aspects of medication administration in order to provide safe and effective care to the client [34]:

- The safe administration of medications, including the decision to withhold medications (see 'Medication safety' section in this chapter).
- Documentation of all relevant aspects of medication therapy (see 'Documentation' section in this chapter).
- Codes that depict reasons for the community nurse not administering should be documented on the administration chart and a note describing the rationale documented in the client's medication administration forms, notes/care plan/progress notes [34]. Codes are:
  Absent   A
  Fasting   F
  Refused (by client)   R
  Vomiting   V
  On leave   L
  Medication not available   N
  Withheld   W
  Self-administering   S
- Drug schedules – The *Standard for the Uniform Scheduling of Drugs and Poisons* (SUSDP) is a document used in the regulation of drugs and poisons in Australia [35]. It is produced by the National Drugs and Poisons Scheduling Committee (NDPSC), a committee of the Therapeutic Goods Administration (TGA). The SUSDP is only a recommendation to the states however, and differences still exist in the regulation of drugs and poisons across Australian states [35]. The community nurse needs to be aware of the regulations related to the supply, storage, disposal and administration requirements for all schedules of medication prescribed for their client. The

regulations may be different in each state or territory. Some examples of schedules from the SUSDP are:

- Schedule 2 (S2) – pharmacy medicine (substantially safe, for minor ailments);
- Schedule 3 (S3) – pharmacy medicine (require pharmacist advice, e.g. salbutamol);
- Schedule 4 (S4) – prescription-only medicines (require professional diagnosis, e.g. adrenaline);
- Schedule 5 (S5) – caution poisons (low toxicity, require caution in handling, storage or use, for domestic use);
- Schedule 6 (S6) – caution poisons (high toxicity, may cause death if ingested);
- Schedule 7 (S7) – dangerous poison (extremely high toxicity, can cause death in low exposure, too hazardous for domestic use);
- Schedule 8 (S8) – controlled drugs (possession of this drug must be by without legal authority, such as via a prescribed script) dependence producing, e.g. morphine);
- Schedule 9 (S9) – prohibited substance (by law, may only be used for research purposes, e.g. heroin) [35].

Evaluation of nursing interventions

Evaluation of nursing interventions in relation to client outcomes is an important factor in medication support for community-dwelling clients. Through care planning and documentation of client goals and outcomes, the nurse can evaluate whether goals have been achieved at points along the client's journey of care. Generally, evaluation occurs at intervention points such as at 3 months or 6 months after commencing a service. Other intervention points can be after admission to an acute facility with new client goals established on return to the community service or when the client's health status has changed and previously documented goals need to be reviewed and replanned.

Example of a change or replanning in medication support: A child has accepted long-term insulin therapy support from the diabetes educator for type 1 diabetes and now has received an insulin pump and requires insulin at different intervals via the pump mechanism. The child's plan of care and support will now need to be renegotiated with the child and their family to reflect support required for management of the insulin pump. Education and support for the client and the parents/guardian may be intensive for a period of time until all parties feel comfortable with self-maintenance and monitoring of the pump and insulin delivery regime.

Standard 3 – 'Medication support requires consultation and collaboration with the client and family and other health professionals to ensure therapeutic outcomes' [5, p. 3].

Preparation and education to manage medications – It includes medication support education for community nurses to reinforce legal requirements, documentation education that includes an emphasis on the need to document all verbal communication [36], safety, practical approaches to care delivery and expected standards and procedures. Also, the use of different media to assist the nurse to learn about innovations in medication support strategies may include use of a CD-ROM program incorporating interactive learning case studies [37]. Such education assists to prepare the nurse for

---

Case study 15.1

An elderly client has been referred by the GP for non-compliance of use with a DAA. (Example is a Webster's pack.) The nurse conducts an assessment, including a safety assessment that includes the potential for the client or others to tamper with medication from easily accessible medication packaging – such as tablets in foil wrap. The assessment includes discussing goals with the client. It may become clear that the client has rheumatoid arthritis, which can inhibit manual dexterity, therefore reducing the ability to manually push tablets out of the Webster's 'blister pack'. Once a different DAA is set up – such as using labelled 'yellow-top pots'– the client may independently self-administer all medications. It is clear here that the client may not have been 'non-compliant', but simply unable to verbalise reasons why he or she was not administering their medication.

---

the complexities of medication support that can make a profound difference to the client in the variety of community settings.

Case study 15.1 illustrates the importance of assessment, documentation and care planning in a community setting.

Intentional non-compliance can also be a common referral rationale. 'Usually the result of a client's beliefs, opinions and values, as opposed to physical, mental or financial reasons, a client might believe that suffering is a part of life because this is a part of their cultural background' [28, p. 2]. Other reasons for an assessment by the health professional of presumed client non-compliance or adherence to medication regimes could be related to poor understanding of the need to complete a course of medications, such as antibiotic or antiviral therapy [38–40], cognitive impairment and forgetting to take the medication, simply being unable to see the medication – especially in the elderly population [41–44], and issues of depression and low motivation for those clients who live with a mental health condition, such as bipolar disorder or schizophrenia, and may need more support from their professional community (GP, specialist or community nurse) when mentally unwell [45, 46].

Review and management of medication incidents – including a system for the reporting of medication errors (See the section on 'Medication safety' in this chapter) and associated collaboration with other 'like organisations and nursing roles' to look for trends in errors and incidents.

Consultation – with the client, prescribing medical officer (usually the GP) and pharmacist in all aspects of the medication support process. The community nurse can communicate all concerns about prescribing (e.g. perhaps a dose of medication is causing the client unintended side effects) with the GP and supply with the pharmacist (e.g. DAA may no longer be appropriate for the client due to the client's increased vision loss associated with a chronic condition). Storage of the medication in the client's home may be of concern to the community nurse as it may continually be moved around the house making it hard for the community nurse to find. An home medicines review (HMR) [47] which aims to promote safe and effective medication use in the community [48] can be conducted and the review will cover issues such as

> **Case study 15.2**
>
> A 69-year-old woman was referred for an HMR. Her local GP listed 14 medications with symptoms 'suggestive of an adverse drug event' – nausea, vertigo, fatigue and anxiety. The client was found to be actually taking 39 medicines, of which 18 were OTC and complementary medicines. Numerous interactions and duplication of therapy were uncovered. She was seeing two GPs, a naturopath and getting her supplies from four pharmacies plus a mail order company. The woman was suffering chronic pain from polymyalgia rheumatica, asthma, stress and depression, and took everything that everyone suggested [50, p. 4].

drug interactions [42] and polypharmacy, taking more than 12 doses of medication in a day (which may increase confusion between products) [49] (see Case study 15.2).

In Case study 15.2, the role of the community nurse [51–53] is to discuss with the client the importance of:

- Choosing a single pharmacy for supply of all medication.
- Maintaining a complete list of all medications (including OTC and complementary).
- Make available the client's medication list for all prescribers for the client.
- Understanding the benefits and risks associated with the use of a DAA – for example ensuring that it is packed and fully labelled (whenever possible) by a registered pharmacist and used for solid medications only and those that are not cytotoxic in nature. Some medications can be affected during the DAA heat-sealing process (e.g. gel caps), while others may be affected by exposure to heat, light, air, moisture (effervescent, dispersible, buccal, sublingual and hygroscopic medications) or sometimes medications are prescribed on an 'as required' basis [3].

Delegation and supervision – aspects of medication support to others, for example an RN delegating aspects of medication support such as the administration of oral medications to an EN or family member, commensurate with their abilities and scope of practice. (Refer to the state and territory nurses boards to clarify delegation of medication administration roles, standards and restrictions.)

Collaboration – with clients to facilitate appropriate self-medication, for example the community midwife assessing the abilities of a woman in labour to request dosages of pain relief based on her own individual pain threshold.

The GP's role in medication support

The GP remains the central coordinator of care delivery for the client in the community. GPs can utilise the Australian Government Medicare items called enhanced primary care (EPC) services [54]. EPC services aim to improve the health and quality of life of older Australians, adult Aboriginal and Torres Strait Islander people and people of any age with a chronic or terminal condition. EPC services include:

- Health assessments for Aboriginal and Torres Strait Islander people aged 55 years and over and other people aged 75 years and over.
- Care planning for people with chronic health conditions who may also have complex care needs.
- Case conferencing for people with chronic conditions and complex care needs [54].

The GP may seek the involvement of the community nurse in all aspects of the above EPC services. The community nurse may be involved in the planning stages by way of input of clinical knowledge or in the evaluation and review stages by way of sharing assessment and planning/conferencing outcomes. The community nurse may need to negotiate with the GP and the practice nurse about how and when communication about the client will occur. This will enable the notification of planned or conducted assessments for the client and promote a 'team approach' to care. Sharing expectations of the professional relationship with other health professionals (e.g. GP, pharmacist, specialist) will encourage communication processes that are in the best interests of the client and minimise risk of errors in the prescribing, supply and administration of medications by all involved in care for the client in the community [2].

The pharmacist's role in medication support

The community or local pharmacist has a big role to play in support for the client in relation to their medications and support for the community nurse. The client receives information and advice from their pharmacist and pharmacy regarding medication effects, side effects and interactions with other medications, and may receive a home delivery or DAA service (such as weekly filling of a Webster's pack or dosette box). The client may also seek adult human interaction and conversation (for those who live alone or young single parents at home with children) and the pharmacy may be the point of community information sharing, such as through a community notice board or flyers notifying of a community event or health check service, such as blood pressure or blood glucose testing. The community pharmacist also provides information to the community nurse such as overdose signs and symptoms, brand name clarification and notification of client health concerns (such as whether the client has presented recently, showing signs of a change in affect, behaviour or grooming).

The Australian government's role in medication support

The Australian government plays a role in the provision of health care to all Australians and is a governing body in the development and monitoring of funding, guidelines and service provision by community health organisations. The list of government programmes given below provides the community nurse with a snapshot of and insight into referral information, documents for further reading and guidelines to assist with medication support in the community (see 'Useful resources' section for contact details):

- Department of Health and Ageing – National Strategy for the Quality Use of Medicines [55].

- Department of Health and Ageing – Quality Use of Medicines Evaluation Programme (2002) [55].
- Home and Community Care (HACC) programme – Jointly funded by the Australian government and state and territory governments. Services include meal on wheels, community nursing and support for people with disabilities and their carers [56].
- Home medication review (HMR) [55].
- Australian Pharmaceutical Advisory Council – Guiding principles for medication support in the community [3].
- Australian Government Department of Health [32] – Teaching packages, comprising 72-h lessons in a number of languages, provide general information about the principles of using medicines safely and wisely, taking into account the communities' cultural beliefs and practices. The activities are designed to raise family members' awareness and knowledge of QUM issues [32]. Local government health authorities can confirm the availability of these teaching packages (possibly via online tutorials or web cam) for clients or their carers.
- Therapeutic Goods Administration [55] – Assesses and monitors activities of government and non-government organisations in the development and availability of new medicines and ensures that the medicines are of an acceptable Australian standard. TGA offers advice on poisons regulations.

Medication safety

The community nurse has a major role to play in the safe administration of medications. Medications need to be prescribed, supplied, administered, stored and disposed of safely [3], and the process documented along with client risk factors, possible side effects and dose ranges [3, 57]. It is important (wherever possible and especially important with children) to document the client's weight and height as it may be required to determine doses of certain medications [34]. There is potential for medication errors when 86% of people aged 65 years and over are prescribed medications [58]. In addition, up to 400 000 adverse drug events are managed in the community by community nurses and GPs each year [59].

For optimal medication safety:

- The community nurse needs to have an understanding of organisational policy and procedure related to the supply, administration, storage and disposal of medication relevant to the particular setting. For example remote community nurses may be able to transport medications from the pharmacist to a client's remote property when the client is unable to travel long distances. During travel, the nurse will need to ensure that the medications are stored correctly in the vehicle and are signed by the client on receipt.
- The community nurse needs to have an understanding of pharmaceutical knowledge of prescribed medication dose ranges for all clients including children, especially young infants, who are at particular risk for medication misadventure because of their size, unique physiology and immature ability to metabolise medicines [60]. Older people may also be at risk due to decreased renal function, estimated to be 1% each year after 40 years of age [32]. Liver function also reduces with age [57].

- DAAs should be clearly labelled with details of the client, name, strength, form of medications, date of filling, date and day of the week the medicine is to be administered. The DAA should be packed by a pharmacist, and if medications are reviewed and changed by the GP, the DAA must be returned to the pharmacy for repacking [3].
- Telephone prescription for medication may occur on occasion. A client may need a medication administered; however, there may not be a written order available in the client's notes. An example may be simple analgesia, such as paracetamol, required for an injury sustained in a remote area when a medical officer is not physically available. In this case, a prescription can be authorised over the phone from a medical officer to two community nurses. A remote area community nursing organisation should have a telephone order protocol as to who the second witness to the phone order can be (e.g. they may be a family member of the client). Documentation for telephone orders includes the name of the medication prescribed; route of administration; dose, date and time the medicine is to be administered; name of the medical officer making the verbal order; name of both community nurses or nurse and 'other' hearing the order; and time of medication administration. A telephone order should be signed within 24 h of the verbal order (wherever practicable) [34].
- Variable-dose medications can occur when a changeable dose is prescribed, for example when medication is adjusted based on laboratory test results; as a reducing protocol which may be commonplace in the community setting; or as a client may choose to remain at home while having variable-dose treatments (e.g. variable warfarin doses to manage international normalised ratio (INR) levels) [34]. There must be clear protocols for the community nurse to follow with dose limitations, and in the case of variable doses based on laboratory results, the results of tests must be documented at each medication administration to ensure evidence of protocol compliance [34].
- Withholding medications can be appropriate if there is a known adverse drug reaction, which is 'an undesirable response associated with use of a drug that either compromises therapeutic efficacy, enhances toxicity or both' [34, p. 16]. Withholding a medication must be documented and a 'W' written on the client medication chart [34].
- The Australian 'Advanced Incident Monitoring System' (AIMS) is a computer software program which allows for incidents to be recorded electronically and data to be available centrally for analysis. This aims to promote future medication safety within Australia [59]. The function of this software is to assist staff to (1) provide easy and accessible incident reporting to all health system employees, (2) store information relating to voluntarily reported adverse incidents and near misses for management action, analysis and risk reduction activity, (3) provide a management framework for follow-up of incidents by appropriate personnel and (4) enable management of risks associated with clinical care. The community nurse needs to phone the AIMS call centre to report the incident; this should take only 4–5 min. A report is then generated and will appear on the relevant community nurse manager's incident list in their database. When you report an incident, it generates an email to the manager of the relevant area. The manager is responsible for managing and investigating the incident. Serious incidents may require mandatory reporting to the State Department of Health.

Issues associated with medication errors (such as administering medication via the wrong route or omitting to tell the client to have the medication 'with food' and gastric burning results) should have a focus on making safer systems rather than blaming individual health care providers [30]. Individual organisational incident monitoring systems (such as incident reporting forms) should be available to the community nurse for the reporting of incidents also [30].

- Medication Advisory Committees [61] or Medication Safety Committees [62] can be established in community nursing organisations to monitor the incidence of medication errors and to offer constructive suggestions to alter and improve medication administration processes, such as how nurses select a DAA for each client situation [62]. An example of a medication error could be the dose of an antiembolic medication being 'drawn up' incorrectly due to packaging confusion and consequential non-therapeutic doses of medication being given. A Medication Advisory/Safety Committee may suggest education for all nurses preparing and administering the medication to highlight any difficulties and develop a system for all nurses to follow in the future to reduce the risk of the error occurring again.

Documentation

Nursing documentation provides the evidence of clinical care provision, client progress and professional conversations. The purpose of documentation is to give an overview of the client's conditions and treatments, create continuity of care, ensure patient-safety documentation, create a basis for evaluating quality of care, support teaching and research in nursing, and to be a tool for communication between health service providers [63]. In 2004, the State Coroner of Victoria stated, 'Good documentation about medication support is an important way of delivering high quality care and maintaining patient safety: fragmented records inevitably lead to fragmented patient care' [36, p. 10].

The Nurses Board of South Australia defines nursing documentation as 'professional documentation' [18] and states that forms of documentation by a nurse recorded in a professional capacity include [18]:

- Written and electronic health records.
- Audio and video tapes.
- Emails.
- Facsimiles.
- Images (photographs and diagrams).
- Communication books.
- Any other documentation pertaining to care.

A community nursing example may be a communication book left in a client's home, used by a number of community nursing and carer agencies and the pharmacy. The information may pertain to requesting more medications to be delivered from the pharmacy or a nursing note to inform the carer that the medication regime has changed for the client.

Documentation is a tool to enhance practice. It must be clear, complete, accurate, objective, timely, legible, permanent, and be representative of professional observations and assessment and factual information. The nurse must not use white-out, must sign their name, state their designation and write their surname legibly in brackets at the end of the entry [18]. Documentation is also important because:

- It demonstrates accountability and records professional practice.
- Legislation requires specific information be recorded and maintained.
- It is a valuable source of data for health researchers.
- It provides the evidence and rationale for funding and resource management. For example the community nurse may be able to provide documented evidence that a more expensive wound management product would assist a wound to heal at a faster rate and could be left on for longer periods, therefore reducing the number of visits required to the client and the organisation's costs.

Common abbreviations

Only commonly used and understood abbreviations should be documented on medication administration forms and medication authorities/prescriptions to indicate the route of administration, frequency and time of administration and dose of medications [34]. These are listed in Table 15.1. Case study 15.3 is reflective of the importance of documenting all incidents as soon as possible following an event and shows that the inclusion of all related information is important to 'build a picture' for other health professionals who may access the notes.

Case study 15.3

Mr B had presented to the homeless nursing clinic sporadically for vitamin B injections and for continence education when his episodes of urinary incontinence became bothersome to him. Mr B also has a history of alcohol (ETOH)-induced aggression and short-term memory loss, diagnosed by a relief locum GP at an outer suburb's 24-h medical centre. On this occasion, Mr B presented to the homeless clinic, showing signs of slurred speech, unsteady gait, aggressive dialogue and smelling of alcohol. He became further agitated when the community nurse asked him to refrain from swearing at other clients who were waiting to be seen. Mr B lunged at the nurse with a clenched fist and used abusive language. The community nurse managed the situation and the man was escorted from the clinic. The outcome for Mr B's presenting need that day (administration of a vitamin injection) was that the medication was 'withheld' as the client had become aggressive. However, the community nurse was shaken by the event and was not thinking clearly, and forgot to document the incident in the client notes. The next day the nurse documented the incident, citing objective observations at the time Mr B presented, noted a plan for the administration of his medication (after a discussion with the homeless clinic medical officer) and completed the entry with a statement of why the entry had not been made at the time of the incident.

Table 15.1 Medication administration abbreviations [34, p. 1].

PO	Per oral/ by mouth
NG	Nasogastric
SUBLINGUAL	Sublingual
IV	Intravenous
IM	Intramuscular
SUBCUT	Subcutaneous
IT	Intrathecal
PR	Per rectum
PV	Per vagina
Gutt	Eye drop
Occ	Eye ointment
Top	Topical
MA	Metered aerosol
Neb	Nebulised/nebuliser
mL	Millilitre
L	Litre
g	Gram
mg	Milligram
mcg	Microgram
Unit	International unit
mane	Morning
nocte	Night
bid	Twice daily
tds	Three times daily
qid	Four times daily

Guiding principles to promote the QUM

The Australian Pharmaceutical Advisory Council (APAC) has developed a set of 12 guiding principles for medication support in the community, which aim to promote the QUM and assist community service providers (including community nurses) to develop organisational best-practice policies and practical procedures to assist older people in the community [3]. These guidelines are broad and could also guide the care provision of those clients who are not older (such as the young and the disabled and those from CALD backgrounds) and those clients living in rural and remote areas of the community [3]. The following APAC guidelines reflect the nursing role in medication support:

1. *Information resources* – Nurses should have access to current and accurate information about medicines, in a timely manner.
2. *Self-administration* – Clients should be encouraged to maintain their independence to manage their own medications in a safe and effective way.
3. *DAA* – It should only be used to help overcome specific issues for the client (such as dexterity problems with opening multiple packaging); otherwise original packaging should remain.
4. *Administration* – Clients require assistance and information to take medicines correctly. Nurses are authorised to administer medicines according to relevant state or territory legislation, acts and policies [3].

5. *Medication lists* – Clients should be encouraged to have a maintained list of medications, including any allergies and previous adverse drug reactions, previous vaccinations, name and contact details of the GP or specialist (may be specialist only in the case of an infant), pharmacy and contact details of the client [3].

6. *Medication review* – Clients are encouraged to have their medications reviewed regularly (e.g. an HMR).

7. *Alterations of oral formulations* – Clients may require assistance to guarantee that any alterations in oral formulations are managed safely and effectively.

8. *Storage of medicines* – Medication should be stored to maintain medicine quality and safeguard visitors to the home, e.g. not easily accessible by being locked away or 'out of sight', especially of young children and may include use of a locked box.

9. *Disposal of medicines* – Clients should be encouraged to return unwanted, ceased or expired medications to a local pharmacy for disposal.

10. *Nurse-initiated non-prescription medicine* – Policies and procedures need to be developed to safely manage nurse-initiated non-prescription medication.

11. *Standing orders* – Where standing orders are required in specific circumstances (such as remote areas of Australia), policies and procedures should be developed.

12. *Risk management in administration and use of medicines in the community* – Health professionals (nurses, GPs and pharmacists), clients and carers should work together to manage risks, incidents and develop care plans specific to the community and associated with medicines [3].

Summary

This chapter has examined the topic of medication support in nursing contexts with a focus on community nursing. Non-negotiable factors such as legal and nurses board standards have been examined, together with national health care guidelines related to documentation and safety challenges. The intention has been to enhance nurses' understanding of the legal and nursing frameworks that guide practice in relation to medication with people in the community health care system, including children, older people and those living with disabilities.

This chapter has demonstrated that the community nurse has an important role to play in supporting clients to safely manage their medications. Whether that is through support for use with a DAA or transfusion of intravenous blood products, the principles of safe drug administration, documentation and evaluation of treatment effectiveness have been discussed and transferred to the community setting with practical 'real-life' examples.

The community nurse in collaboration with the client, carer and other health professionals can tailor a plan of care for medication support that is client centred and relevant to the client's situation and capacity.

Useful resources

Adverse Medicines Events Line
Allows consumers and practitioners to report or receive advice on adverse medicine events. Telephone 1300 134 237

Medicines Line
Gives consumers and practitioners access to independent and up-to-date specific information about medicines, provided by experienced clinical pharmacists.
Telephone 1300 888 763

Medimate
A brochure produced by the NPS to help consumers and practitioners find, understand and use information about medicines. Medimate is available in Chinese, Greek, Italian, Vietnamese and English translations.
Telephone (02) 8217 8700
Website www.nps.org.au

Veterans Mates
A Department of Veterans' Affairs programme designed to address medicines usage by veterans and war widows and provides educational materials to veterans and their carers to assist in improving medication support at home.
Telephone (08) 8276 9666
Website www.rgh.sa.gov.au

Adverse Drug Reactions Advisory Committee (ADRAC)
Encourages the reporting of all suspected adverse reactions to medicines, including suspected reactions to new medicines. The ADRAC produces the *Australian Adverse Drug Reactions Bulletin* six times a year. The bulletin lists current drugs of interest to ADRAC.
Telephone 1800 044 114
Website www.tga.gov.au/adr/index.htm

Central Australian Rural Practitioners Association (CARPA) Standard Treatment Manual
A manual developed by CARPA as a guide to standard treatment for those working in remote and rural communities in Central and Northern Australia.
Telephone (08) 8950 4800
Website www.carpa.org.au

Australian Medicines Handbook (AMH)
Provides a source of concise, up-to-date independent drug information to facilitate effective, rational, safe and economical prescribing.
Telephone (08) 8303 6977
Website www.amh.net.au

Translating and Interpreting Services (TIS)
A 24 h a day, 7 days a week service provided by the Australian Government Department of Immigration and Multicultural and Indigenous Australia for people who do not speak English and for English-speaking practitioners needing to communicate with them.
Telephone 131 450 – local call cost

Therapeutic Goods Administration (TGA)
A unit of the Australian Government Department of Health and Ageing. TGA assesses and monitors activities of government and non-government organisations in the development and availability of new medicines and ensures the medicines are of an acceptable Australian standard. TGA offers advice on poisons regulations.
Website www.tga.gov.au

Australian Nurses Boards
Develop, monitor and update standards for medication support, professional standards and boundaries, standards for delegation to an EN or unlicensed health care worker and the professional code of ethics and code of conduct.
ACT   www.actnmb.act.gov.au
NSW   www.nmb.nsw.gov.au
NT   www.nt.gov.au/health/registrationboard
QLD   www.qnc.qld.gov.au
SA   www.nursesboard.sa.gov.au

TAS   www.nursingboardtas.org.au
VIC   www.nbv.org.au
WA   www.nbwa.org.au

Australian Nursing and Midwifery Council (ANMC)
Develops and monitors national competency standards for RNs, ENs and midwives, the code of professional conduct and the code of ethics in consultation with each state or territory nurses board.
Website www.anmc.org.au

Australian and New Zealand College of Mental Health Nurses Inc (ANZCMHN)
Develops and monitors Standards of Practice for Mental Health Nurses in Australia.
Website www.anzcmhn.org

Australian College of Midwives Inc (ACMI)
Sets competency standards, the code of ethics and guidelines for midwifery practice.
Website www.acmi.org.au

Australian Government Department of Health and Ageing (DoHA)
Provides contact information on the National Strategy for Quality Use of Medicines.
Telephone (02) 6289 8023
Website www.nmp.health.gov.au

References

1. Joanna Briggs Institute (2000) The administration and supply of medications by registered nurses in rural and remote areas. *Evidence-Based Practice Information Sheets for Health Professionals*, Vol. 4(5). Joanna Briggs Institute, Adelaide, Australia, pp. 1–5.
2. Royal District Nursing Service (2003) Executive summary, in T.K. Visentin (ed.) *What Is Current Medication Management in District Nursing Practice?* Royal District Nursing Service, SA, Adelaide, Australia, pp. 1–24.
3. Australian Pharmaceutical Advisory Council (2006) *Guiding Principles for Medication Management in the Community*. Australian Pharmaceutical Advisory Council, Canberra, ACT, pp. 1–56.
4. Disability Services Division, Department of Human Services (2004) *Cultural and Linguistic Diversity Strategy*. Department of Human Services, Melbourne, Victoria.
5. Nurses Board of South Australia (2003) *Standards for Medication Management*. Nurses Board of South Australia, Adelaide, South Australia.
6. Ashby, D. (2006) Four medication management standards to change July 1. *American Journal of Health-System Pharmacy*, 63(1), 1210–12.
7. Banning, M. (2005) Medication management: Older people and nursing. *Nursing Older People*, 17(7), 20–23.
8. Shane, R. (2006) Part 2: Evaluating the risk points in your medication management system. *Joint Commission Perspectives on Patient Safety*, 6(2), 1–2.
9. Griffiths, R., Johnson, M. and Piper, M. (2004) A nursing intervention for the quality use of medicines by elderly community clients. *International Journal of Nursing Practice*, 10(4), 166–76.
10. Banning, M. (2006) Medication review: The role of nurse prescribers and community matrons. *Nurse Prescribing*, 4(5), 198–204.
11. Harris, G. (2005) Ethical issues in community care. *Journal of Community Nursing*, 19(11), 12–16.
12. Australian Nursing and Midwifery Council (2006) *National Competency Standards for the RN, EN, RM and NP*, 4th edition. Australian Nursing and Midwifery Council, Canberra, ACT.

13. ANMC (2005) *Code of Ethics for Nurses in Australia.* Australian Nursing and Midwifery Council, Canberra, ACT.

14. ANMC (2005) *Code of Professional Conduct for Nurses in Australia.* Australian Nursing and Midwifery Council, Canberra, ACT.

15. Robbins, J. (2005) Computer-based medication management on a roll. *Australian Nursing Journal,* 13(1), 9.

16. Jarman, H. (2002) Medication study supports registered nurses' competence for single checking. *International Journal of Nursing Practice,* 8, 330–35.

17. Anselmi, M.P., Benedita, M. and dos Santos, C. (2007) Errors in the administration of intravenous medication in Brazilian hospitals. *Issues in Clinical Nursing,* 1(1), 1839–46.

18. Nurses Board of South Australia (2006) *Guiding Principles for Documentation. Standards.* Nurses Board Publishing Department.

19. Department of Communications (2002) *The National Strategy for Quality Use of Medicines – Plain English Edition.* Commonwealth Government, Canberra, ACT.

20. Gilmore, V. (2004) A nursing voice on medication management. *Australian Nursing Journal,* 12(2), 12.

21. Latter, S.Y., Rycroft, P., Malone, J. and Shaw, D. (2001) Nurses' educational preparation for a medication education role: Findings from a national survey. *Nurse Education Today,* 21(2), 143–54.

22. Orwig, D. and Gruber-Baldini, A. (2006) Medication management assessment for older adults in the community. *Gerontologist,* 46(5), 661–8.

23. Manias, E. (2005) Graduate nurse's communication with health professionals when managing patients' medications. *Journal of Clinical Nursing,* 14(3), 354–62.

24. Bolton, P. and Tasker, J. (2004) Medication review by GPs reduces polypharmacy in the elderly: A quality use of medicines program. *Australian Journal of Primary Health,* 10(1), 78–82.

25. Hamme, M. (2006) Medication management education tools for improving target outcomes: Any emergent care. *The Journal for the Home Care and Hospice Professional,* 24(2), 80–86.

26. Barnes, L., Nation, R., Gilbert, A., Paradiso, L. and Ballantyne, A. (2006) Making sure the residents get their tablets: Medication administration in care homes for older people. *Nursing and Healthcare Management Policy,* 56, 190–99.

27. Florin, J. (2006) Patient participation in clinical decision making in nursing: Study of nurses' and patients' perceptions. *Journal of Clinical Nursing,* 15(12), 1498–508.

28. Thomson, G. (2006) Solve oral medication management problems. *Case Management Advisor,* 1(1), 1–3.

29. Latter, S., Yerrell, P., Rycroft-Malone, J. and Shaw, D. (2000) Nursing, medication education and the new policy agenda: The evidence base. *International Journal of Nursing Studies,* 37(6), 469–79.

30. Metlay, J.C., Cohen, A., Polsky, D., Kimmel, S., Koppel, R. and Hennessey, S. (2005) Medication safety in older adults: Home-based practice patterns. *Journal of the American Geriatrics Society,* 53(6), 976–82.

31. Wood, R. (2007) Information for consumers and consumer groups – about using medicines wisely, in *Medicines Talk.* National Prescribing Service (NPS) Limited, Australia. pp. 1–8.

32. Wood, R. (2006) Information for consumers and consumer groups – about using medicines wisely, in *Medicines Talk.* National Prescribing Service (NPS) Limited, Australia, pp. 1–8.

33. Beauchamp, T. (ed.) (2001) *Principles of Biomedical Ethics,* Vol. 5, 5th edition. Oxford University Press, Oxford.

34. Australian Commission for Safety and Quality in Health Care (2005) *National Client Medication Chart.* Australian Commission for Safety and Quality in Health Care, Federal Department of Health Publishing.

35. Therapeutic Goods Administration (1996) *Standard for the Uniform Scheduling of Drugs and Poisons*. National Drugs and Poisons Scheduling Committee (NDPSC), Department of Health and Ageing, Canberra, Australia.

36. Aitken, M. (2006) Documentation of medication management by graduate nurses in patient progress notes: A way forward for patient safety. *Collegian*, 13(4), 5–11.

37. Schneider, P., Montanya, K., Curran, C., Harpe, S., Bohenek, W. and Perratto, B. (1 January 2006) Improving the safety of medication administration using an interactive CD-Rom program. *American Journal of Health-System Pharmacy*, 63, 59–64.

38. Aronson, B. (2005) Medication management behaviours of adherent short-term antibiotic users. *Clinical Excellence for Nurse Practitioners*, 9(1), 23–6.

39. Rueda, S. (2006) Patient support and education for promoting adherence to highly active individuals. *Cochrane Library*, 4(1), 7–8.

40. Corless, N., Davis, S., Dolan, S. and McGibbon, C. (2005) Symptom status, medication adherence, and quality of life in HIV disease. *Journal of Hospice and Palliative Nursing*, 7(3), 129–38.

41. Tangalos, E. (2006) Medication management in the elderly. *Annals of Long Term Care*, 14(8), 27–31.

42. Simonson, W. (2005) Medication-related problems in the elderly. *Drugs and Ageing*, 22(7), 559–69.

43. Van Eijken, M. Wensing, M. de Smet, P. and Grol, R. (2003) Interventions to improve medication compliance in older patients living in the community: A systematic review of the literature. *Drugs and Ageing*, 20(3), 229–40.

44. Bergman-Evans, B. (2006) Evidence-based guideline: Improving medication management for older adult clients. *Journal of Gerontology Nursing*, 1(1), 6–14.

45. Sajatovic, M. (2004) Enhancement of treatment adherence among patients with bipolar disorder. *Psychiatric Services*, 55(3), 264–9.

46. Gray, W. and Gournay, K. (2003) The effect of medication management training on community mental health nurses' clinical skills. *International Journal of Nursing Studies*, 40(2), 163–9.

47. Boothman-Burrell, L. (2004) A tough but worthy journey: Delivering HMRs in the Pilbara. *Australian Journal of Pharmacy*, 85(1), 404–5.

48. Goldney, R. (2005) Use of prescribed medications in a South Australian community sample. *Medical Journal of Australia*, 183(5), 251–3.

49. Sorensen, L., Purdie, D., Woodward, M. and Roberts, M. (2006) Medication management at home: Medication risk factor prevalence and inter-relationships. *Journal of Clinical Pharmacy and Therapeutics*, 31, 485–91.

50. Gowan, J. (March/April 2006) Home medicine reviews and the aged. *Complementary Medicine*, 1, 20–24.

51. Zhan, C.S., Bierman, A., Miller, M., Friedman, B., Wickizer, S. and Meyer, G. (2001) Potentially inappropriate medication use in the community-dwelling elderly. *Journal of the American Medical Association*, 286(22), 2823–9.

52. Johnson, R., Piper, M., Langdon, R. and Stephens, M. (2002) *Older People and the Quality Use of Medicines: Exploring the Role of Primary Health Nurses in Domiciliary Medication Review and Management*. Commonwealth Department of Health and Aged Care, Quality Use of Medicines Evaluation Programme (QUMEP), Canberra, Australia.

53. Johnson, R., Piper, M. and Langdon, R. (2005) Risk factors for an untoward medication event among elders in community-based nursing caseloads in Australia. *Public Health Nursing*, 22(1), 36–44.

54. Medicare Australia (2006) Medicare benefits schedule. Enhanced primary care (EPC) services, in *Overview of Enhanced Primary Care Services Reference Guide*. Australian Government Department of Health and Ageing, Canberra, Australia.

55. Department of Health and Ageing (2005) Executive summary, in *The National Strategy for Quality Use of Medicines*. Australian Government, Canberra, Australia, pp. 1–4.

56. Department of Health and Ageing (2004) *The Way Forward – A New Strategy for Community Care*. Australian Government, Canberra, Australia.

57. Meadows, M. (2006) Medication use and older adults. *FDA Consumer*, 40(4), 22–6.

58. Hodgkinson, B. (2006) Strategies to reduce medication errors with reference to older adults. *International Journal of Evidence-Based Healthcare*, 4(1), 2–41.

59. Joanna Briggs Institute (2005) Strategies to reduce medication errors with reference to older adults, in S. Koch (ed.) *Evidence Based Practice Information Sheets for Health Professionals*. Joanna Briggs Institute, Adelaide, Australia, pp. 1–6.

60. Leonard, M. (2006) Risk reduction for adverse drug events through sequential implementation of patient safety initiatives in a children's hospital. *Paediatrics*, 118(4), 1124–9.

61. Cheek, J., Gilbert, A., Ballantyne, A. and Penhall, R. (2004) Factors influencing the implementation of quality use of medicines in residential aged care. *Drugs and Ageing*, 21(12), 813–24.

62. Hagland, M. (September 2006) Right patient, right dose. *Healthcare Informatics*, 23(9), 52–6.

63. Throddsen, A. (2007) Putting policy into practice: Pre- and post-tests of implementing standardised languages for nursing documentation. *Issues in Clinical Nursing*, 1(1), 1826–36.

Chapter 16

Nutritional support

Elaine Tooke and Scott King

Introduction

Optimal nutrition is important to all of us because it is a basic and fundamental need for survival. The very functions of life are dependent on nutrients that are taken into our bodies and used to promote normal growth, maintenance and repair. What we ingest is converted and used by the body for growth and energy. Nutrition however goes beyond the amount and type of food we intake; it encompasses the psychological, social and emotional rituals associated with eating and preparing food. In fact a recent study found that people living with chronic disease associate the ingestion of food as only one aspect of nutrition; the person's unique historical and socio-cultural meaning given to food and eating is more important to them and is often overlooked [1].

Optimal nutrition is the mix and balance of nutrients that provide the body with the energy that it needs to function effectively. It includes a blend of grains and cereals, fruits, vegetables, legumes, nuts, dairy and meat foods, which need to be eaten each day [2]. In circumstances of altered health such as chronic conditions or disability, whether through trauma and acute injury, or disease progression and even age-related changes, nutritional requirements and abilities can change. As such clients will need to be assessed to receive additional support and supplements to meet these requirements and to maintain health.

Anatomy and physiology of the gastrointestinal tract

To understand how the human body utilises nutrients it is important to have a baseline understanding of the digestive process. The digestive system includes all the organs and glands involved in the process of eating and digesting. The gastrointestinal (GI) tract is a hollow muscular tube that extends from the mouth to the anus. Its principal function is to provide the body with fluid, nutrients and electrolytes through the:

- Ingestion of food and fluids.
- Secretion of electrolytes, hormones and enzymes used to break down large particles of food into substances that are usable by the body cells.
- Peristaltic movement of food materials through the digestive tract.
- Absorption of the end products of digestion into the bloodstream.
- Elimination of undigested material from the digestive tract by defaecation [3–5].

The digestive system is the source of intake of food for the body. It breaks down the food we consume by chemical and mechanical digestion, defined below, and supplies the cells in our bodies with energy [3–5].

Mechanical digestion consists of various movements which aid digestion, such as chewing, swallowing and movement of food particles – peristalsis.

Chemical digestion consists of the body using digestive secretions such as enzymes and bile to break down food particles into chemical compounds which are small and simple enough to be absorbed into the bloodstream and used by body cells [3–5].

The GI tract consists of the mouth, the pharynx, the oesophagus, the stomach and the small and large intestines. It is lined with a mucous membrane which aids in the protection of the lining and allows for absorption of the end products of digestion.

The mouth

The mouth is formed by the cheeks, the hard palate (front of the roof of the mouth), the soft palate (the back portion of the roof of the mouth), the tongue and the teeth. The mouth receives food and begins the digestive process by chewing and preparing food for swallowing (mastication) [6]. The functions of chewing are:

- To break food products into smaller portions
- To break down any covering around the food and allow digestive enzymes to have access to the food particles
- To prevent trauma to the mucous lining of the oesophagus by making the food smoother [3–5, 7]

Saliva

Saliva is secreted into the mouth by the numerous salivary glands, such as buccal glands (cheek), parotid glands (side of face in front of the external ear), submandibular or submaxillary glands (lower jaw) and sublingual glands (under the tongue). These glands are stimulated by the smell and ingestion of food. Approximately 1000–1500 mL of saliva is secreted in 1 day to:

- Begin the breakdown of food.
- Lubricate and soften food mass and dissolve the most soluble components of food.
- Begin the breakdown of large food particles such as starch.
- Help to facilitate chewing and swallowing.
- Assist the body to keep the teeth and mouth clean and reduce bacterial growth and debris [3–5].

The pharynx and oesophagus

The oesophagus is a hollow muscular tube which connects the pharynx (the muscular tube which extends from the back of the nasal cavity to the oesophagus) [3] with the stomach and serves as a passage for food from the mouth to the stomach. Food is pushed through the pharynx as a bolus and is then swallowed. The larynx pulls upward and covers the airway and stretches the oesophagus open and the food is therefore prevented from entering the airway. Breathing is inhibited for a short period as the respiratory passage is closed and allows swallowing to occur.

The oesophagus receives the bolus, transports the bolus through the oesophagus and propels the bolus into the stomach. The bolus of food is moved along the oesophagus (25 cm) by a process called peristalsis. Peristalsis is a wave of muscle contractions that pushes the bolus of food ahead of it. Sphincters guard the oesophagus at either end to keep the bolus of food moving in one direction [8].

The stomach

The stomach is a 'J'-shaped organ. The functions of the stomach include storage, mixing and changing the bolus of food into chime [6]. The stomach secretes gastric juice. Its major secretions are hydrochloric acid, pepsin and mucous. The secretions are regulated by nervous and hormonal mechanisms and are released when the stomach becomes distended with food. The stomach is a very acidic environment and has pH levels of 3.5–1.5. The stomach empties slowly via the pyloric sphincter, allowing the duodenum to receive and act on the contents.

Food contents usually remain in the stomach from 1 to 4 h depending on what substance was ingested. This can be much longer for certain foods. For example carbohydrates move through the stomach quicker than proteins and proteins move quicker than fats.

Abnormalities of the stomach can include ulceration (peptic ulcers), delayed emptying, vomiting and malabsorption. Some people may be taking medication to assist in the motility and emptying of the stomach contents due to a history of delayed emptying. If so, it is important to ensure that they are not being deprived of necessary nutrients if the contents are not in the stomach long enough to be absorbed. If the person is losing weight despite regular feeds, it should be reported to their health care practitioner. If the person is vomiting on a regular basis, this also needs to be investigated and treated [3–6, 8].

The small intestine

The small intestine is divided into the *duodenum*, the *jejunum* and the *ileum* [3–5].

The contents of the stomach enter the duodenum. The duodenal glands secrete certain enzymes which neutralise the bolus of chyme and therefore help to protect the duodenal lining by making the environment more alkaline in nature. The chyme is moved along through to the jejunum and then the ileum by peristalsis and propulsive activity.

The small intestine completes the digestion of food and absorbs the products of digestion along with water and electrolytes. The small intestine has an increased surface area due to villi which line the intestine wall. Absorption of up to 8 L of fluid daily occurs in the small intestine.

It is very important to balance the absorption of water with a good intake of water. This will in turn assist to prevent problems such as dehydration and constipation; 1.5–2.0 L of water is the recommended daily amount for all people except those who have a specified restricted intake as ordered by their medical practitioner.

The large intestine

The large intestine is divided into the *caecum, colon* and *rectum* [3–5]. The appendix, the anal canal and anus are also part of the large intestine. The colon is divided into the ascending colon, transverse colon, the descending colon and the sigmoid colon. The major functions of the large intestine are to absorb the remaining water, urea and electrolytes from the chyme, secrete mucous and store faeces until defaecation occurs.

The rectum is a temporary storage area for waste and the anal canal is used for the expulsion of waste. This can be either voluntary or involuntary. The longer the length of time that faeces is left in the rectum, the greater the amount of water which is reabsorbed from them.

The accessory organs

The liver, biliary tract and pancreas are known as accessory organs and are located in the upper abdominal cavity. They aid in digestion and use of nutrients by the body and also detoxify and store many substances in the body.

The liver

The liver is the largest organ in the body and has many functions including:

- The storage of glucose in the form of glycogen, and the conversion of glycogen to glucose when blood glucose levels fall.
- The formation of blood plasma proteins.
- The synthesis of urea, which is released into the blood and transported to the kidneys for elimination.
- The modification of fats so that they can be used more efficiently by cells.
- The manufacture of bile.
- The destruction of old red blood cells.
- The detoxification of harmful substances such as alcohol and certain drugs.
- The storage of some vitamins and iron [3–5].

Gall bladder and bile ducts

The bile ducts and gall bladder function as a collecting and storage site for bile. Bile is a substance used by the body to aid in the breakdown of fats so that they are able to pass through the intestinal wall [3–5].

The pancreas

The pancreas produces insulin and enzymes that aid digestion and excrete them into the duodenum of the small intestine. The enzymes neutralise the chyme which is quite acidic when it enters into the duodenum from the stomach. In doing so, these enzymes help to protect the lining of the duodenum [3–5].

Malnutrition

Malnutrition refers to any deviation from the normal adequate nutritional requirements for good health [6]. It can refer to both under- and overnutrition, although most studies refer to malnutrition as when a person has a body mass index (BMI) of under 20 kg/m^2 [6]. Overnutrition (obesity) is where the BMI is greater than 30 kg/m^2. Both these conditions occur more frequently with people with a developmental disability than in the general population [9].

Undernourishment can occur as a result of inadequate intake as well as disorders of digestion or absorption of protein and calories and social factors. It affects every organ of the body and predisposes the person to disease, delays recovery from illness, wounds take longer to heal, thus affecting body function, well-being and clinical outcome [9, 10].

Research shows that a large percentage of people who are living with chronic conditions, who are older and/or have a disability, have nutritional problems and are at risk of being malnourished [1, 9, 11]. Indigenous people have been found to be at greater risk of nutrition-based diseases due to the limited availability and the expense of nutritious foods in remote areas [12]. Added to this, detection and management of nutritional problems across health sectors, including in the community, is often poor and this can have an adverse effect on client outcomes [11]. Absence of good nutrition can be a predisposing factor for disease and illness – the effects of poor nutrition are felt within society, with the prevalence of diet-related diseases and an increased cost burden on the health system [10, 13].

Malnutrition is often unrecognised and undertreated and is typically present in 10–40% of clients admitted to hospital [14]. The onset of malnutrition can be insidious and often long term in nature. Remedies such as offering more food are often not effective and family members or other support persons sometimes feel that nothing can be done. When accompanied with chronic illness and late detection, the long-term effects of malnutrition may be difficult to recover from if at all [15]. However, with early recognition, assessment and cooperation from the client, the effects of malnutrition may be abated.

Nutritional requirements may be greater when health is compromised and yet adequate nutrition can become even less likely [1]. People with dysphagia (difficulty swallowing] [16] and those with physical limitations are more likely to be underweight and people with a developmental disability are also at risk of specific vitamin and mineral deficiencies [9]. In fact, a missed meal should be considered as important for such people as a missed medication [1].

Meeting nutritional requirements for people living in the community can be challenging. There are a multitude of issues that can inhibit good nutrition. Potential barriers to nutrition are listed in Table 16.1 and may be used as prompts to instigate further investigations or more in-depth nursing assessments.

Table 16.1 Barriers to nutrition [4–8, 10, 11].

Physical	• Poor dexterity • Poor mobility • Access to shops or transport
Cognitive changes and understanding	• Confusion • Depression • Understanding of good nutrition • Acknowledgement of the risks of malnutrition for the body
Disease process	• Arthritis • Diabetes • Emphysema • Cancer • Gastro-oesophageal reflux disease (GORD), which is common in people with scoliosis, cerebral palsy, Down's syndrome and those on anticonvulsant medications and benzodiazepines [1]
Medical factors	• Medications that may affect taste, appetite or absorption • Polypharmacy • Fatigue • Ill-fitting dentures, loss of teeth or sore mouth • Diminished sensations of taste and smell
Social factors	• Isolation, living alone • Poverty • Limited transport • Bereavement • Times meals are presented or delivered • Time allowed for eating • Use of plastic cutlery • Inappropriate texture of food • Food too hot or cold • Inability or not wanting to cook • Lifestyle (convenience foods are often cheaper and can be higher in saturated fat, salt and sugar) • Access to fresh foods in isolated areas • Availability and coping ability of carer • Economic and financial restrictions
Ageing process	Conditions that may affect the ability to digest and utilise nutrients: • Decreased salivation • Dysphagia • Delayed oesophageal and gastric emptying • Reduced gastrointestinal mobility

A challenge for community nurses is to be more aware of their role in screening, detection, assessment and health promotion in the area of nutrition. It is often assumed that people in the community have access to good nutritious fresh food, that they can get help to cook and prepare meals if they are unable to and that help is available for people who live in the community and need assistance with eating. This may not be the case for many people outside of city areas. It is important for community nurses to be aware of the community resources in the local area that provide nutrition support.

Just as important is the community nurse's development of a network of health professionals to expand the greater team in assessing specific needs of clients. This may include the engagement of and referral to speech pathologists to undertake thorough assessments to assess swallowing safety and to generate meal-time management plans that can be utilised by the client, their family and any care workers involved. Community nurses continue to play a pivotal role in the referral, selection and application of nutritional therapies [10].

Nutritional screening and assessment

It is important at this point to understand the difference between nutritional screening and nutritional assessment. Screening is often the first step in identifying clients who may be experiencing nutrition-related problems. It is the process of identifying individuals at risk and is the trigger for a more comprehensive nutritional assessment [17, 18]. For example:

> Ethel is a 76-year-old woman living alone after recently being widowed following the death of her husband of 55 years who died from complications of type 2 diabetes. Ethel has a past history of rheumatoid arthritis, type 2 diabetes and presents with a venous leg ulcer that was sustained from a knock on her leg 12 weeks ago.

A nutritional screen would identify the following risk factors for Ethel: social isolation, mobility and dexterity issues, diabetes, and a potential increase in nutritional requirements to heal her venous leg ulcer. This screening would then trigger a more formalised nutritional assessment by the nurse using an established assessment tool.

Suggested data that can be collected as part of the nutritional assessment include anthropometric measures, such as:

- Height.
- Weight.
- Ideal body weight.
- Usual body weight.
- Recent weight history including losses and gains.
- Triceps skinfolds.
- Midarm circumference (MAC).
- Midarm muscle circumference (MAMC) [17, 18].

Biochemical data can also be collected, such as:

- Serum albumin.
- Serum transferrin.
- Complete blood picture (including zinc, vitamin A and vitamin C, which are important for wound healing) [17, 18].

Clinical observations of malnutrition can be made, such as:

- Dark skin around eyes and cheeks.
- Cracked lips with lesions.
- Smooth tongue that may be swollen and atrophied.
- Dry mucosa.

- Bleeding gums that are spongy and swollen.
- Enlargement of glands.
- Dry, flaky skin.
- Brittle and ridged nails.
- Dull, brittle hair.
- Poor posture.
- Hypertension and tachycardia [17, 18].

Data collection including a food diary, food habits and choices, influences that may be cultural, spiritual or psychological, and eating behaviours, beliefs and patterns are also critical. This data can be collected from the client, family and friends [6]. Some other general questions that might be asked and discussed as part of the assessment are:

- What does food and eating mean to you?
- With whom do you usually eat your meals? What type of food do you eat? Describe what you will eat on a typical day. When do you eat?
- What do you drink during the day?
- What do you define as food? What do you believe makes up a healthy diet? Are you able to obtain the foods necessary for a healthy diet? If not, how do you think this can be remedied?
- Who shops for food? What kind of stores do you shop at? Who prepares the meals?
- How are foods prepared for you at your home (length of time cooked, type of cooking oils and seasonings used)?
- Have you chosen a particular nutritional practice such as vegetarianism or an alcohol-free diet?
- Do religious beliefs and practices influence your diet? Do you abstain from certain foods at regular intervals or at specific times determined by religious dates?
- Do you fast? What does fasting mean to you? (Define what you do and do not eat.) How long do you fast? How often?
- What exercise do you do daily?
- How do you rest and relax?
- What medications are you on? Do any of these affect how you feel about food? Do they alter feelings of hunger, taste and smell [19]?

Documentation of the nutritional assessment and conversational outcomes should always be included in the client's notes. Documentation of this information can be fundamental to effective, multidisciplinary community care.

People with high health care needs should ideally be weighed on a regular basis, such as monthly, to ensure that their correct weight is being maintained. It can be difficult to recognise slow, insidious weight loss or weight gain over time, particularly when different health care staff are providing care and so regular recording of weight taken on reliable scales provides an accurate baseline measure. The person's overall health status needs to be continually assessed, and any concerns or issues identified should be discussed with their health care practitioner with the client's consent.

It is widely thought that nurses need to view nutritional care in the same way as other health care and treatment [13]. Nutrition appears to be an undervalued aspect of client care, with the barriers for nurses being lengthy assessment tools, no extra time for assessments, scales and other equipment not being readily available, assessment tools that may not be readily available or user friendly and general time constraints [13].

However, established nutritional risk screening and assessment tools can be used and are readily available and accessible for community nurses. Clients who require additional support may benefit from referral to a dietitian or other nutritional specialist for an in-depth assessment and support [20]. Consent for referral can be obtained during discussions with the client. Nutritional screening is provided to clients by some companies that manufacture dietary formulas and supplements and is available through the local dietitian or hospital.

Thickening agents and oral nutritional supplements

To assist the person to safely intake food and fluid orally, the texture of food and drinks may need to be modified. This will assist them to swallow safely and should be under the direction of a speech pathologist or dietitian. Some general principles for preparing texture-modified foods include:

- Make sure that the food looks as appetising as possible.
- Puree meat and vegetables separately so that they look appetising.
- Use deep-coloured vegetables – broccoli and sweet potato.
- Serve foods at the correct temperature as this maximises taste.
- Ensure a variety of foods from all food groups.
- Cut food into small mouthfuls.
- Change the size of the mouthful (reducing it or increasing it according to the person's needs) if necessary.
- Encourage intake of fluids (thickened or thin as recommended by the speech pathologist) [21].

Thickening agents

For people with dysphagia (difficulty with swallowing), thickening agents can be added to drinks to aid in swallowing, subject to speech pathologist review. There are two main thickening agents used, starch and gum. Both can be added to hot and cold drinks, although there is some slight alteration to taste. Some of the newer thickening agents can be added to carbonated drinks including beer and champagne. Thickened fluids are designed to slow down the swallowing process, utilising existing muscle tone and involvement, aiding in a safer swallow. Differing amounts of thickener provide a different description for the consistency. For example Resource® describes thickened fluids as milk, nectar, honey and pudding consistency. This can be more useful practically than thin, slightly thickened or fully thickened fluids.

Texture-modified foods

Using flour, cornstarch or commercially prepared thickeners can alter the texture of foods. Pureed foods can also be placed into appropriately shaped food moulds to give the illusion that the food is whole and not vitamised. This adds to the aesthetics of the meal.

Oral nutritional supplements may be useful to add energy, protein, vitamins and minerals to the diet in smaller volumes than can be managed with food [22]. It is important to note that additional supplements will have benefit only if there is a deficiency of a particular element. For example zinc, vitamin A and vitamin C are essential for wound healing; however, current research suggests that these vitamins will aid wound healing only if the person is deficient in the first place [23]. Part of a clinical assessment may include a baseline blood profile to determine deficiencies. Calorie-boosting drinks aid healing, as the body may need a substantial increase of up to 300% in calories to aid in wound closure on top of regular caloric requirements [23].

Weight-gain powders and drinks

The most common and convenient type of supplements are weight-gain powders and drinks, which have a base of milk proteins, egg protein or soy protein [22]. They are available at supermarkets and pharmacies and whilst they are quite expensive, are an effective way of adding protein and calories to the daily diet. They can also be described as nourishing drinks. These can be as simple as milkshakes made up with skim milk, skim milk powder and flavouring. More commercially prepared nourishing drinks include preparations such as Sustagen hospital formula® and Sustagen Gold®.

Complete nutritional supplements

Complete nutritional supplements provide total nutrition and may have extra fibre or protein. These are available through the dietetics department at hospitals and chemists, for example Ensure®, Ensure plus®, Isocal® and Fortisip®. It is, however, important to remember that supplements are not meal replacements. A nutritious, well-balanced diet is still required with supplementation to boost any deficits in the client's diet.

Special nutritional supplements; modular supplements

These supplements can be added to food or drinks and usually contain only one nutrient. Carbohydrate-only supplements are made from sugars but do not taste very sweet. They are an easy way of getting more calories without really changing what you eat. Examples are Polycose®, Polyjoule®, Energy plus® and Polycal®. Protein-only supplements are used in the same way, for example Promod® and Protifar®.

Many commercial products are available to provide nutritional support. In addition to thickening agents, prethickened beverages, prepackaged puree moulds, oral liquid supplements and modular components can be added to enhance the client's caloric and protein intake. When oral intake is inadequate, enteral nutrition or parenteral nutrition may be indicated [24].

One of the most difficult challenges for community nurses is access to these supplements and aids. The client will be required to purchase the supplements and unless they are on the Pharmaceutical Benefit Scheme (PBS) list, it can become quite expensive. The PBS is a benefit provided by the Australian government to subsidise pharmaceutical costs [25]. With even the best intentions, including a thorough and comprehensive assessment and plan, the outcome is still very much reliant on the capacity of the client.

Devices – functionality and management

Equipment aids

The use of aids to assist people with self-care or to assist people at meal times is important to maintain independence and safety. Equipment such as built-up handles for forks and spoons is useful for people feeding themselves who have a poor grip. Devices such as slings and arm and finger cuffs can be useful to promote self-feeding; spoons, scoop bowls, plate guards and non-slip mats can aid in enhancing the person's oral intake. An occupational therapist, physiotherapist, independent living centre or local pharmacy can help in this area [21].

Enteral devices

At times it may be necessary for a device for the administration of nutrition to be inserted either temporarily or permanently. Enteral tubes are inserted into the stomach or the small intestine to supply liquid nutrients (water and formula) and medication directly into the body, bypassing the mouth, nasopharynx and oesophagus.

The tube may provide total nutrition for people on nil by mouth or nil orally, or supplemental nutrition for people who need to maintain or increase their weight. A risk assessment is essential prior to tube placement and ongoing assessment should continue for the duration of the placement [26]. The presence of acute illness at the time of tube placement and the presence and ability of the carer(s) to manage it may have a significant effect on client outcome [26].

There are many indications for artificial methods of nutritional support, including GI disorders, degenerative changes in anatomical structures, chronic illness states or postoperative healing.

Types of enteral tubes

There are three main types of enteral tubes: nasoenteric, gastrostomy and jejunostomy.

Nasoenteric (nasogastric, nasoduodenal and nasojejunal)

A short-term way of administering fluids, medications or nutritional support is via a nasogastric (NG) tube. A tube is passed through the nose and into the stomach. These tubes are relatively easy to insert but are often poorly tolerated by the person; they can be difficult to maintain and have significant associated risk of aspiration due to dislodgment and migration [24, 27].

Occasionally nasoduodenal tubes may be used due to problems with gastric reflux or delayed gastric emptying. Insertion of these tubes is more difficult and would only be performed by a medical practitioner in a hospital setting, and due to their fine bore, these tubes are easily blocked and difficult to keep in position [24].

There is a small risk that NG tubes can be misplaced into the lungs during insertion or move out of the stomach at a later stage (possibly after a severe coughing or vomiting episode). The most accurate method of determining their position is via X-ray, but this is not always possible for clients in the community. It is therefore recommended that a pH indicator strip/paper be used to check the position of NG feeding tubes [26, 27].

Other methods such as auscultation of air insufflated through the feeding tube (whoosh test), monitoring bubbling at the end of the tube when the end is put in water and observing the appearance of the aspirate are not recognised as safe procedures [26].

The NG tube may not be useful for all clients, as it can be readily pulled out by the young, elderly or confused. Consequently, such frequent tube extubations can interrupt treatments and prevent nutritional goals being met. There may also be possible pain and damage to the nasal mucosa. In people with disordered swallowing, the situation can be worsened by the presence of a nasoenteral tube [28].

Gastrostomy tube

A gastrostomy is an artificial tract between the stomach and the abdominal surface. Percutaneous endoscopic gastrostomy (PEG) placement is a safe procedure and an effective enteral nutrition method when oral feeding is not possible and where there is a functionally intact GI tract. It has been established as a low-risk procedure and is the access route of choice for long-term enteral nutrition [28]. A study in 2001 showed that in stable long-term elderly clients for whom enteral feeding is indicated, clients with a gastrostomy do better than those with NG tube placement; they show longer survival, fewer aspirations and better tolerance of the tube [29, 30].

There are three types of gastrostomy tubes:

- A PEG inserted endoscopically.
- A radiological inserted gastrostomy.
- A low-profile gastrostomy.

Gastrostomy tubes are secured against the stomach wall by either a retainer device or a balloon inflated with water and against the abdomen by an external stabiliser. Balloon checks are critical to ensure balloon patency and to minimise dislodgement. These checks should be performed every 7–10 days as water can evaporate from the balloon [31, 32]. The external stabiliser of the PEG tube is initially sutured to the abdomen after placement, but once the sutures are removed, the external stabiliser can be moved as the person gains weight. The external stabiliser should be positioned approximately 2–3 mm from the skin surface to minimise the risk of developing tissue necrosis and ulceration [33, 34]. Gastrostomies are contraindicated in clients with ascites and sepsis or those having undergone extensive gastric surgery, acutely ill clients,

clients with a short life expectancy and clients with severe coughing [30]. It has been reported that clients hospitalised with acute illness and those with a malignancy and low BMI are more at risk of PEG complications [26].

A low-profile gastrostomy is introduced through an established gastrostomy tract. Extension sets are required to administer the feed and are supplied when inserted. This type of tube is more expensive than a PEG tube and is indicated for young or ambulatory people [35]. It is unobtrusive and can be hidden under clothes and there is no long tube that could get caught. All low-profile tubes have an antireflux valve. Some are situated on the top of the tube, whilst others are situated at the base. The inner securing device also differs between tubes – some have a bumper and others have an inflatable balloon. The size of the low-profile tube is not adjustable; therefore, the tube will need to be replaced if the person gains weight, to prevent the external stabiliser pressing on to the stomach, potentially causing a pressure ulcer.

Jejunostomy

A jejunostomy is used when clients are at risk of aspirating, vomiting or have pancreatitis and when food delivered into the stomach causes the problems of gastro-oesophageal reflux, distention and bloating. The tube either is placed in the jejunum (first part of the small intestine) using radiologic techniques, by which it is placed through an existing PEG, or may be placed after major abdominal surgery. They pose little risk of aspiration and have the advantage of using the GI tract for absorption even if digestion is impaired [6]. The jejunostomy has a small internal bumper and is secured externally to the abdomen. The length of the tube and the security of the external fixation should be checked daily.

Positioning for nutrition via enteral tube

Prior to administering nutrition, it is important to ensure that the tube is positioned correctly by recording the measurement of the skin disc against the calibrations on the tube [36]. It is advisable that the person is sitting up, reclining at a 30° angle or propped up with two to three pillows for all formula or fluid administration [26]. People who are self-administering can stand [36]. Babies should be fed in baby seats offering firm supports in preference to bouncy chairs which can induce vomiting [26]. Never administer nutrition when the person is lying down, as there is a greater risk of aspiration (vomiting and breathing fluid into the lungs) [37]. Keep the person in a sitting position and keep their movements to a minimum for at least 30 min after administering nutrition to help prevent vomiting or aspiration.

Oral hygiene

Good oral hygiene is important to prevent tooth decay and gum disease and the development of respiratory infections. Both problems will cause unnecessary pain and discomfort for the person, may affect their ability to manage food and drink orally and can impact their social image by producing bad breath and unsightly teeth. People who are not having anything by mouth will have decreased saliva production and exchange, which may cause excessive dryness. Oral hygiene also stimulates the gums, which is important for people on soft/vitamised diets or who are on nil orally. Oral hygiene and mouth care forms an essential component to the assessment process [9, 38].

Specific medication administration and feeding guidelines

Medications can be administered via all of these tubes; however, the tube should be flushed before and after each feed/medication administration. Medications should be in liquid form and be given separately from the feed with flushing of the tube before and after [36]. Adequate flushing is required to ensure that the full dose of the drug is administered (for adults, generally 30 mL of water before and after). Each drug should be given separately, not mixed and the tube flushed with 15 mL of water between each drug [36]. Crushed tablets can block the tube, particularly if it is a fine-bore NG tube. It is important to review medications with a medical officer and/or pharmacist to seek advice that the medications can be crushed (i.e. enteric coated medications should not be crushed) and advice on what medications are the best choices for the individual client.

Stoma care

The skin surrounding the stoma should be cleaned at least daily using a face washer; during bathing is an ideal time and the tube should also be rotated 360 degree's to avoid skin adhesion. A circular motion should be used, starting close to the enteral tube and working out. This technique is used to reduce the risk of infection. After cleaning the area, it should be allowed to air dry.

The stoma site needs to be observed for signs of redness, swelling, leakage or pain. The person's medical or health care practitioner should be notified if any of the above occurs. A protective barrier cream can be applied to the skin surrounding the stoma and this should be determined by the health care practitioner and written into the care plan. Dressings under or around the tube and external stabiliser should be avoided, as this can contribute to erosion or ulceration to the abdominal skin [39].

At times the skin around the stoma can begin to overgrow and possibly migrate up the enteral tube. This is known as overgranulation of the tissue. Overgranulation of the tissue can be treated by cauterisation or surgical removal.

Complications of enteral feeding

Minor complications are common in enteral feeding and, if not resolved, can have a significant impact on well-being and quality of life [26]. Replacement tubes are required when the tube deteriorates or if there is permanent blockage or damage.

Blocked tube

Common causes of a blocked tube are:

- Milk formula left in tube to curdle.
- Medication not crushed adequately or in unsuitable form.
- The tube may be too narrow for the medication or formula.

- Tube not flushed properly after last feed.
- Pump feed given at too slow a rate.
- A problem with the type of feed and any additives reacting together.
- Kinked tube.
- Gastric reflux.

To minimise the risk of the tube blocking, try to obtain medications in liquid form or crush them finely and flush with water before and after all feeds and medications. The amount of water flushed is determined by the dietitian and will vary according to health status and age. If the tube does become blocked, it is important to use a syringe no smaller than 50 mL to unblock, as this may cause the tube to burst. Aspiration may help initially to shift the blockage. Flush the water gently into the tube and try to unblock it with lukewarm water. Do not use pineapple juice, Coca Cola or other sugary, fizzy drinks [31, 40].

Dislodged enteral tube

Seek medical advice for reinsertion of the tube. After a while the balloon can perish, causing it to deflate. Some clients accidentally pull out the gastrostomy tube.

Stomach upset

This may be evidenced by nausea, vomiting, belching, bloating, heartburn or pain.
It may be caused by:

- Infection – gastroenteritis.
- Gastric dumping syndrome (happens when the lower end of the small intestine, the jejunum, fills too quickly with undigested food from the stomach).
- Ulceration.
- Reflux.
- Intolerance to feed.
- Being too full.
- Emotional problems – stress.

What to do:

- Ensure good handwashing techniques.
- Stop feed until all symptoms subside.
- Administer feeds slowly – small, frequent feeds.
- Ensure person is in an upright or semiupright position.
- Avoid strenuous exercise or excessive movement immediately after feed.
- Do not attempt to administer a feed if a person is complaining of being nauseated or vomiting.
- Do not store feed in direct sunlight, store in fridge.
- Never add newly opened feed to old.
- Do not hang feeding formula on equipment for too long.
- Ensure the feeding equipment is cleaned adequately.
- Seek advice from medical or health care practitioner [41, 42].

Diarrhoea

This is evidenced by frequent loose and watery bowel actions and may be caused by:

- Infection – gastroenteritis.
- Overhydration.
- Stress or emotion.
- Inappropriate formula and some medications which may react together.
- Curdled formula.
- Medication, e.g. antibiotics.
- Poor absorption.
- Too much formula being administered.

What to do:

- Slow down the feeding rate.
- Keep all equipment clean; equipment for small children and babies should be soaked in antibacterial solution.
- Always wash hands prior to the feed.
- Ensure formula is always stored in the fridge once the container is opened. (Must be given at room temperature.)
- Discard formula after 48 h in fridge.
- Unresolved diarrhoea may require assessment from medical or health care practitioner as this may indicate malabsorption, infection or faecal impaction [41, 42].

Aspiration

This is the inhalation of food or fluid into the lungs, causing coughing, choking and respiratory distress. It can lead to cyanosis (blueness), fever and tachycardia (racing pulse). Pulmonary aspiration (known as silent aspiration) can occur with no obvious coughing or vomiting and pneumonia can develop insidiously. Even though a person is receiving nutrition via tube feeds, this does not exclude them from the risk of aspiration of tube formula and saliva. People who are most susceptible may have:

- NG tube in situ.
- Increased saliva production.
- Severe disability.
- Delayed stomach emptying.
- Hiatus hernia.
- Spinal deformity.
- Epilepsy.
- Impaired cough reflex.
- Gastro-oesophageal reflux.
- Swallowing disorder.
- Poor oral hygiene.
- Poor positioning.

What to do:

- Correct positioning – ensure the person is sitting up at 30–40° during the feed and for at least 30 min after.

- Administer feed slowly.
- Stop feeds if coughing or choking until symptoms subside.
- Seek advice from medical or health care practitioner [41, 42].

Constipation

This is evidenced by the difficult or infrequent passing of small, hard stools [6] and may be caused by:

- Inadequate fibre in diet.
- Inadequate fluids.
- Lack of exercise.
- Overuse of laxatives.
- Reduced muscle tone in the bowel.
- Some medications.
- Local lesions.
- Environment – lack of privacy.
- Medications.

   What to do:

- Increase fluids. (Give extra fluid at feed times or throughout the day.)
- Increase physical activity.
- Seek advice from dietitian, reincreasing fibre in formula.
- Administer aperients as required.
- Seek advice from medical or health care practitioner [41, 42].

Air in the stomach and abdominal cramping

Abdominal discomfort and bloating may be caused by excessive air/gas in the stomach. Venting or decompression is the process of releasing the air or gas. There are tubes which connect to the enteral tube designed for the release of gas. Administering feeds too quickly and feeds that are cold and receiving large volumes intermittently can contribute to cramping [41].

Education and ongoing support for clients and their carers

The insertion of an enteral tube can have a huge impact on the person and the carer, presenting many challenges in adapting to the presence of the tube to maintain a 'normal' existence [43]. There can be a period of adjustment to having a tube in place due to the social implications of tube feeding as well as the changes in self and body image. Food does not only provide nutrition; the eating and enjoyment of food can be a social, cultural and sensory experience [43]. Many of society's activities revolve around eating and drinking and there can be a period of adjustment to having a tube in place and learning how to manage it. The impact on the person's self-esteem and body image may need to be acknowledged. It is important that both clients and their carers receive appropriate written and verbal training and feel comfortable with the technique and equipment. It is very different administering a feed in a hospital where there is always someone nearby, to giving a feed in the isolation of a client's home. Ongoing

24-h support needs to be provided, even if it is over the phone. The introduction of oral foods may be important for the psychological and emotional well-being of the person [26]. Where this is safe, even a limited intake can be beneficial and promote enjoyment for the person.

Dietetics and formulas for enteral nutrition

Enteral nutrition

Some people may still eat orally and have 'top-ups' of fluid or formula through the enteral feeding tube. For others, however, the enteral tube feeds will provide the route for their total nutritional intake as determined by the person's doctor or dietitian.

Enteral tube nutrition methods of delivery

The following are methods of delivery for enteral tube nutrition:

- Bolus using a large syringe (without plunger) or a container or bottle connected to a feeding line. Fluid flows through the feeding line into the enteral tube by gravity. Generally, a 4- to 6-h volume is given four to six times per day (each feed up to 1 h long). This method is good for self-administration and for disorientated clients who require observation throughout the feed. It may cause nausea, bloating, diarrhoea, stomach distention, cramps, vomiting and the increased risk of aspiration [6]. Bolus delivery into the jejunum should be avoided.
- Intermittent – equal portions four to six times per day. Resembles a more normal pattern of intake and allows the person more freedom of movement between feeds. Tolerance is optimised by infusing the formula by slow-gravity drip or by pump over a 30- to 60-min period [6].
- Continuous over a 16- to 24-h period to maximise tolerance of nutrient absorption. This method is recommended for nutrition into the jejunum and for the critically ill. It is usually delivered by pump which reduces the incidence of diarrhoea and the line should be flushed every 6 h to clear the tubing and hydrate the client.

Formula

A dietitian can determine the type of formula to be given and the regimen for feeding and meals based on the client's weight, height, age, history of weight loss, medical conditions, activity level and present nutritional status. Formulas are available in powder form (which is mixed with liquid] and ready to use (available in cans or prefilled ready to hang containers] [36].

The goals are to:

- Find a balance so that the client does not feel bloated but is still getting maximum nutrient absorption.
- Have a complete and balanced diet.

Types of formulas

Many different types of milk mixtures are available depending on the person's dietary need. For example there are mixtures with enhanced calories, added protein, added fibre, lactose and lactose free, and formulas suitable for people with diabetes.

Components in feeds

Proteins

Protein sources vary but are considered to be the most critical component of enteral formulas. Some of these diets are similar to pureed diets, some are milk-based formulas and some are lactose-free diets. The choice of the formula will depend on the underlying health status of the client and their ability to absorb the product [3, 6, 37].

Carbohydrates

The carbohydrates that are present in the enteral formula are easily digested except for some clients who have difficulty absorbing lactose. Clients must also have a normal functioning small intestine, which is able to absorb the carbohydrate. Metabolism of carbohydrates is dependent on adequate supplies of insulin, glycagon, epinephrine, vitamin B, magnesium, chromium, zinc and pyridoxine. Non-utilisation of the carbohydrates, by an inability to either absorb or metabolise them, causes watery-diet diarrhoea, abdominal cramps, flatulence, fullness and nausea [3, 6, 37].

Fats

Fat provides concentrated calories, essential fatty acids, flavour enhancement, and serves as a carrier for fat-soluble vitamins [3, 6, 37].

Osmolality

Osmolality or ionic concentration is considered to be the most important part of formula.

Formulas with chemically simple predigested proteins have a higher osmolality. Clients receiving hypertonic formulas must be observed for delayed gastric emptying, severe diarrhoea, electrolyte depletion and severe dehydration. These problems may be further complicated by the client's clinical condition (for example by infections, drains or tracheostomy) [6, 37].

Caloric density

Enteral products' labels contain information on calorie density (the number of calories per unit volume). Calorie density has implications in terms of client management. Formulas of high caloric density provide a large number of calories in a relatively small volume; however, such formulas tend to be hypertonic, which can cause diarrhoea. Those with low caloric density, on the other hand, may cause problems for clients that must have a fluid restriction. In general, as calorie density increases, gastric motility and gastric emptying decrease [3, 6, 37].

Parenteral nutrition

Parenteral nutrition delivers nutrients directly into the bloodstream bypassing the GI tract. Nutrients can be delivered intravenously, via peripheral parenteral nutrition (PPN) and total parenteral nutrition (TPN). These routes are indicated for clients who are unable to consume enough nutrients orally or enterally, whether by altered GI function or other physical or psychological constraints. Nutrition is usually 3 L over 24 h, with fluids consisting of various strengths of sterile water, carbohydrates, proteins, fats, dextrose, amino acids, lipid emulsions, electrolytes, multivitamins and trace elements. PPN can be delivered via a peripheral vein, although great caution and care is required to ensure that the fluid is isotonic in nature to avoid extravasation and infiltration into skin cells. TPN fluids or medications can also be administered via central venous catheters (CVCs) and peripherally inserted central catheters (PICCs). It is more probable that PICCs are used in the community due to decreased risk of infection and ease of management in comparison to CVCs [6].

Nutrition through life

Nutrition and, more importantly, good nutrition is important through all the life cycle. The Department of Health and Ageing has published a number of dietary guidelines as follows:

- Dietary Guidelines for Australians [44].
- Dietary Guidelines for Older Australians [45].
- Dietary Guidelines for Children and Adolescents [46].

These provide fundamental nutrition benchmarks when examining the different needs of people as they progress through the lifespan.

Babies, children and adolescents need to receive adequate food to provide essential daily nutritional needs as they grow and develop. Breastfeeding is encouraged and is enjoying current media attention with popular slogans such as 'Each Month is a Bonus'. Children and adolescents still require a balance of all the food groups, but require greater caloric intake as their physical activity increases. The guidelines [46] also suggest that children under the age of 2 years should not be given reduced fat dairy products due to their greater demand for energy, whereas these should be encouraged for older children. Weight loss in children is not normal and should be investigated. Regular monitoring of a child's growth (height, weight and head circumference) will help to determine whether a child's food intake is meeting his or her energy needs. Young children need intake for bone, muscle, cellular development, brain development and energy. What we lay down when we are young provides a good foundation for when we get older (e.g. calcium intake prevents osteoporosis in later life). As people age they generally require less caloric intake because they become less active [46].

Adults should aim for a well-balanced diet to meet their demands for activity and daily life. Diets should be low in saturated fat, with a moderate amount of sugar or sugar-containing foods and limited alcohol. Breastfeeding mothers require a diet higher in caloric intake to balance their energy expenditure. Nutrition Australia provides a weight-for-height ratio chart that is useful in assessing the weight status of adults aged 18–64 years. People need to be able to stand upright without shoes for accurate health assessment. Another method of determining a healthy weight is by using the BMI. BMI gives a rapid interpretation of chronic protein-energy status based on an individual's height and weight [47]. A 'normal' BMI is 20–25, overweight 26–30 and morbidly obese greater than 40 [6]. A controversial discussion point in relation to BMI is that it does not take into account differences in body build and other physical limitations where height is unable to be accurately attained such as the elderly with profound kyphosis and people with multiple and severe disabilities [44].

Lifestyle factors and illness may affect a person's nutritional intake. Characteristics of disability can affect our metabolism and absorption of minerals and vitamins [1]. Older people or those with a disability can continue to access a balance of all the food groups, but may also require some supplementation. A diet low in fat and salt, high in calcium, with limited alcohol, is suggested. Frequent meals should be taken, which can include several small meals a day instead of three main meals. Activity is very important in this age group and the recommendation is still 30 min of light exercise a day, such as light walking if tolerated [45].

Community nurses working with people from diverse cultural backgrounds may need to be sensitive to ethnic groups' food traditions. Support may need to be provided to families to assist them in the modification of food and drink that may need to be thickened or pureed. Many aspects of traditional diets are beneficial; however, the Westernisation of these diets may be disadvantageous [48]. Older generations of immigrants may wish to maintain traditional eating patterns; however, diets among younger generations often change to include more sugar and fat [48].

Nutritional support of obese people

Obesity is a serious health problem and its prevalence is increasing. Community nurses can be pivotal to supporting people who are aiming to reduce weight. Obesity occurs when energy intake remains higher than energy expenditure for an extended period of time with a BMI greater than 30 [6, 48]. Environmental changes have occurred in recent years, leading to many Australians having a more sedentary lifestyle. Chronic conditions and disability may also impact on an individual's capacity to exercise, leading to obesity. Predisposition to obesity has been associated with intake of high-fat foods [48]. While dietary strategies form an important part of the treatment of obesity, they are often used in conjunction with other interventions such as behavioural therapy or surgery. Fundamental to the development of a therapeutic relationship with an obese client is a non-judgemental approach. Referral to a dietitian for advice is recommended.

Research has revealed that 89% of community nurses recognise the need for more effective primary care services to treat obesity and see obesity advice and support as part of their role [49]. However, one in five community nurses admitted that they felt awkward or embarrassed about talking to patients about obesity and only one-fifth felt they were effective when it came to helping patients to lose weight [49]. Clearly, this is a practice development area for community nurses so that a deeper understanding of weight control and problem solving among community nurses can be attained [48].

Communication and community acknowledgement

How does one find out about good nutrition? One only has to turn on the TV or open a newspaper to be aware of concerns regarding obesity, diabetes and inactivity. Obesity and associated complications are on the increase. A lot of media attention has been focused recently on getting active, including campaign slogans such as, 'Be Active'. Primary health care is a primary role of community nurses who are in a prime position to help influence clients to maintain a good health weight and to encourage regular exercise to maintain health.

Monitoring clients at risk for the presence of inadequate nutrition demands the attention and input of an alert multidisciplinary team. Knowledgeable and attentive nurses can contribute greatly to this team effort. A nutritional assessment conducted by an expert to get a more detailed overview of the person's nutritional status may be warranted. It is recommended that a nutritional assessment tool be used routinely and be repeated at intervals for clients admitted to hospital, care homes, those over 75 years of age and those in vulnerable groups and of clinical concern (frail, elderly, poor, socially isolated, with severe disease and with disabilities) [14].

As cost constraints play a major role in health care today, emphasis is placed on the ability of health care workers in all care settings to recognise and avert potential costly nutrition-related problems [10]. Nutritional screening and assessment are important in identifying potential problems and managing them as they arise instead of being complacent and having to work harder later in managing complications.

As valued members of the health team, the nurse's role is to:

- Participate in nutritional screening as a preventative approach.
- Refer to specialist.
- Link the client to community groups for further information.
- Manage plans and strategies.

In order to raise awareness, peak bodies with a vested interest in nutrition in Australia, such as Nutrition Australia, post on their website important information regarding conferences, education and training seminars, public health awareness activities as well as links for downloading the dietary guidelines previously mentioned.

Conclusion

Good nutrition is one of the most basic fundamental rights of human beings. Community nurses work with people who are at risk of or are actually malnourished or undernourished. The community nurse is in a position to initially identify clients at risk of malnutrition and initiate screening, assessment and education, to positively influence outcomes for clients in their care. Identification can be as simple as watching a client struggle with a cup, have difficulty holding a spoon or noticing an empty refrigerator. Issues regarding nutrition are individualised and complex. Nutrition is multilayered; it is more than just eating to get nutrients. Listening, observing and interacting with clients will give community clinicians the knowledge they need to support clients to promote and maintain health, recover quickly and lead long and independent lives.

References

1. Telford, K., Kralik, D. and Isam, C. (2006) Constrictions of nutrition for community dwelling people with chronic disease. *Contemporary Nurse*, 23, 202–15.
2. Shepherd, S. (2006) Good food for good health: Getting the balance right. *Geriaction*, 24(3), 13–14.
3. Marieb, E. (2003) *Essentials of Human Anatomy and Physiology*. Pearson Education Inc, San Francisco, California.
4. Marieb, E. (1992) *Human Anatomy and Physiology*, 2nd edition. Benjamin Cummings Publishing Company, California.
5. Porth, C. (1994) *Pathophysiology: Concepts of Altered Health States*. JP Lippincott Co, Philadelphia.
6. Dudek, S. (1993) *Nutrition Handbook*, 2nd edition. JP Lippincott Co, Philadelphia.
7. Richardson, M. (2006) Gastrointestinal tract part 2: The mouth and oesophagus. *Nursing Times*, 102(7), 26–7.
8. Richardson, M. (2006) Gastrointestinal tract part 3: The stomach. *Nursing Times*, 102(8), 24–5.
9. Therapeutic Guidelines Ltd (2005) *Management Guidelines Developmental Disability*, Version 2. Therapeutic Guidelines Limited, Victoria.
10. Wilson, J.M. (1996) Nutritional assessment and its application. *Journal of Intravenous Nursing*, 19(6), 307–14.
11. Torjesen, I. (2007) Malnutrition in older people. *Nursing Times*, 103, 25–6.
12. Department of Health, Western Australia (2001) *A Comparative Overview of Aboriginal Health in Western Australia*. Epidemiology Occasional Paper No 15. Department of Health, Western Australia, Perth.
13. Lecko, C. (2006) Opinion page. *Nursing Times*, 102(39), 12.
14. Elia, M. (2003) *The 'MUST' Report – Nutritional Screening of Adults: A Multi Disciplinary Responsibility – Executive Summary*. British Association for Parenteral and Enteral Nutrition, Redditch, United Kingdom.
15. Thomas, A.J. (25 February–3 March 1998) Nutrition in practice. *Nursing Times Supplement* 1, 94(8), 1–6.
16. Panaccio, J. and Carroll, L. (2004) Indications for tube feeding, in C. Barrett (ed.) *Gastrostomy Care; a Guide to Practice*. Ausmed Publications, Melbourne, pp. 1–19.
17. Barrocas, A., Belcher, D., Champagne, C. and Jastram, C. (1995) Nutrition assessment practical approaches. *Clinics in Geriatric Medicine*, 11, 675–713.
18. Edington, J. (1999) Problems of nutritional assessment in the community. *Proceeding of Nutrition Society*, 58(1), 47–51.
19. Hunt, R. and Zurek, E. (2005) *Introduction to Community Based Nursing*. Lippincott-Raven, Philadelphia.
20. Johnstone, C. (2006) Nurses role in nutritional assessment and screening. *Nursing Times*, 102(40), 28–9.
21. Cook, I., Kaatzke-McDonald, M., James, S., Simpson, S. and Risher, M. (2006) *Living with Dysphagia*. Dysphagia Working Party, Sydney.
22. South Eastern Sydney Area Health Service (2007) *Nutritional Supplements*. Available at http://www.sesiahs.health.nsw.gov.au/albionstcentre/nutrition/supplements.asp (viewed 27 August 2007).

23. Caffin, N. (2004) *Position Statement. Regulation of Food-Type Dietary Supplements.* Department of Health and Ageing, Nutrition Australia. Available at http://www. nutritionaustralia.org/News_in_Nutrition/Postition_Papers/policy_options_dietary_supplements.asp (viewed 6 December 2007).

24. Nursing and Midwifery Practice Development Unit (2003) *Nasogastric and Gastrostomy Tube Feeding for Children being Cared for in the Community.* NHS Quality Improvement Scotland, Edinburgh, Scotland.

25. Department of Health and Ageing (2007) *About the PBS.* Available at http://www.health.gov.au/internet/main/publishing.nsf/Contnet/health-pbs-general-aboutus.htm-copy2 (viewed 6 December 2007).

26. Nicholson, F., Korman, M.G. and Richardson, M.A. (2000) Percutaneous endoscopic gastrostomy: A review of indications, complications and outcome. *Journal of Gastroenterology and Hepatology*, 15(1), 21–5.

27. Camilleri, S. and Barrett, C. (2004) Nasogastric tubes, in C. Barrett (ed.) *Gastrostomy Care; a Guide to Practice.* Ausmed Publications, Melbourne, pp. 231–50.

28. Keymling, M. (1994) Technical aspects of enteral nutrition. *Gut*, 35(Suppl 1), S77–80.

29. Dwolatzky, T., Berezovski, S., Friedmann, R., Paz, J., Clarfield, A.M., Stressman, J., *et al.* (2001) A prospective comparison of the use of nasogastric and percutaneous endoscopic gastrostomy tubes for long-term enteral feeding in older people. *Clinical Nutrition*, 20(6), 535–40.

30. Schurink, C.A., Toynman, H., Scholten, P., Arjaans, W., Klinkenberg-Knol, E.C., Meuwissen, S.G.M., *et al.* (2001) Percutaneous endoscopic gastrostomy: Complications and suggestions to avoid them. *European Journal of Gastroenterology and Hepatology*, 13(7), 819–23.

31. Clinical Resource Efficiency Resource Team (2004) *Guidelines for the Management of Enteral Tube Feeding in Adults.* Clinical Resource Efficiency Resource Team.

32. The Joanna Briggs Institute (3 May 2005) Percutaneous gastrostomy tube with internal balloon, in *Aged Care Manual.* The Joanna Briggs Institute.

33. Best, C. (2004) The correct positioning and role of an external fixation device on a PEG. *Nursing Times*, 100(19), 50–51.

34. Pearce, C.B. and Duncan, H.D. (2002) Enteral feeding; nasogastric, nasojejunal, percutaneous endoscopic gastrostomy, or jejunostomy; its indications and limitations. *Post Graduate Medical Journal*, 78(918), 198–204.

35. Loan, T., Magnuson, B. and Williams, S. (August 1998) Debunking six myths about enteral feeding. *Nursing*, 98, 43–8.

36. Le Sidaner, A. (2004) *Percutaneous Endoscopic Gastrostomy*, pp. 1–11. Available at http://www.acta-endoscopica.com/a320502e.html (viewed 12 February 2004).

37. Bailey, J. (2004) Nutritional assessment and tube feeding, in C. Barrett (ed.) *Gastrostomy Care; a Guide to Practice.* Ausmed Publications, Melbourne, pp. 61–95.

38. Rogers, R. and Ryan, J. (2004) Mouth care, in C. Barrett (ed.) *Gastrostomy Care; a Guide to Practice.* Ausmed Publications, Melbourne, pp. 159–75.

39. O'Brien, B., Davis, S. and Erwin-Toth, P. (1999) G-Tube site care; a practical guide. *Registered Nurse*, 62(2), 52–6.

40. Edgar, C. (2004) Care of the gastrostomy tube, in C. Barrett (ed.) *Gastrostomy Care; a Guide to Practice.* Ausmed Publications, Melbourne, pp. 145–57.

41. Bowie, A. (2004) Troubleshooting, in C. Barrett (ed.) *Gastrostomy Care; a Guide to Practice.* Ausmed Publications, Melbourne, pp. 177–92.

42. Gebert, S. and Milner, S. (March 2005) *Tube Feeding; a Guide for Direct Support Workers.* Disability Services Division, Victorian Government of Human Services, Melbourne.

43. Hetzel, C. (2004) Living with a gastrostomy tube, in C. Barrett (ed.) *Gastrostomy Care; a Guide to Practice.* Ausmed Publications, Melbourne, pp. 97–132.

44. Department of Health and Ageing (2003) *Dietary Guidelines for Australians*. National Health and Medical Research Council, Canberra.

45. Department of Health and Ageing (2003) *Dietary Guidelines for Older Australians*. National Health and Medical Research Council, Canberra.

46. Department of Health and Ageing (2003) *Dietary Guidelines for Children*. National Health and Medical Research Council, Canberra.

47. Todorovic, V., Russell, C., Stratton, R., Ward, J. and Elia, M. (eds) (2003) *The MUST Explanatory Booklet; a Guide to the Universal Screening Tool (MUST) for Adults*. British Association for Parenteral and Enteral Nutrition, Redditch, United Kingdom.

48. Buttriss, J., Wynne, A. and Stanner, S. (2001) *Nutrition: A Handbook for Community Nurses*. Whurr Publishers, Philadelphia.

49. Brown, I., Stride, C., Psarou, A., Brewins, L. and Thompson, J. (2007) Management of obesity in primary care: Nurses' practices, beliefs and attitudes. *Journal of Advanced Nursing*, 59(4), 329–41.

Chapter 17

Caring for older people

Megan O'Donnell, Rhonda Nay and Margaret Winbolt

Introduction

The aim of this chapter is to recommend in detail how evidence-based practice can be implemented by community nurses working with older people. Links to further evidence-based guidelines and assessment tools will be provided where possible.

Of utmost importance to the care of older people is the need to assess and support their goals, their self-esteem, their need to feel worthwhile and their need to enjoy perceived control of their lives and decisions. It is not the role of health professionals to foster dependency, impose their values or assume that they know 'what is best' out of some misplaced 'duty of care'. Older people have the same rights as other people to take risks and live according to their priorities and values. Health workers' views of what constitutes cleanliness and safety, along with the tendency of families to make choices that reduce their concern, should not determine care decisions.

Age does bring with it certain changes and a reduced capacity to accommodate accumulated insults – be they physical or psychosocial. Normal age-related changes impact on how people express symptoms of illness and respond to treatments. It is essential that nurses working in the community understand these changes and how to conduct age-appropriate assessments and interventions. Nevertheless, it is also important to recognise that age brings with it accumulated experience, opportunities for further growth and continuing personhood [1]. This chapter will describe our underpinning philosophical approach, provide some relevant definitions and outline how nurses can effectively respond in common situations they will encounter.

Principles of care of the older person

The principles of primary health care [2] and those of person-centred care [3] are entirely complementary and underpin the discussion here. Both approaches to care encourage individual/community participation; both recognise the consumer/client as central to, and the driver of, care decisions; and both prescribe a role for health professionals as information sources, educators, supporters and, ultimately, providers of services to active consumers with citizens' rights. This is a fundamental change from the traditional relationships in health care. There is never an excuse for marginalising the older person who is at the centre of care.

Defining older people

In Australia, average life expectancy has leapt by nearly 30 years in the past century [4, 5] and is now the world's second highest [6]. Older people have traditionally been considered as those over 65 years of age; however, as people continue to work longer and remain healthier, this cut-off point is increasingly being shifted to 70 years or even 75 years of age. However, in Indigenous communities, these gains in life expectancy have not been replicated and old age is generally considered to commence at 55 years [7, 8].

People from culturally and linguistically diverse (CALD) backgrounds constitute a third of the ageing population in Australia, making 'older people' a diverse group with a wide range of ages, experiences, backgrounds and expectations [9, 10].

Physiological and psychosocial changes in ageing

Ageing itself is not a pathological process, and many older people in the community enjoy good health and independence until their death [11]. Ageing does however create an ever-increasing amount of wear and tear to the body and makes older people more susceptible to disease, resulting in a higher level of chronic disease. In Western societies, many common disorders are principally the result of lifestyle factors and, consequently, it is not ageing which 'creates' the disease; it is merely the time in life when the results and impact of lifestyle are most obvious [12]. Some conditions such as dementia occur most frequently in older age; however, it is vital to consider these conditions as an abnormal part of ageing, requiring assessment and intervention, and not as a frequent or natural process of maturation [13]. Some normal changes do occur in the body with ageing. Table 17.1 provides an overview of some general changes that are likely to impact on 'everyday' care provided by community nurses.

Gaining entry and establishing a relationship

When working in the community, the nurse's 'clinic' is the client's home, whether that home be a residential dwelling, local park, remote station or detention facility. Therefore it is of the utmost importance for the nurse to remember he/she is a guest in that environment. Gaining entry to the home can be a challenge with some clients. For example older people who are unwell may find visitors exhausting, so it may be best to spread out visits from various services, friends and relatives.

If a client will not let the community nurse in the door, it is important to find the root of their distrust or, failing that, try to find a family member, neighbour or other service provider who may be able to assist with gaining entry. Community nurses accessing people's residences should always wear photo identification

Table 17.1 Age-related changes [13].

Domain	Associated issues	Assessment	Possible interventions	Resources
Bowel	Slowing of colonic peristalsis and loss of smooth muscle tone may affect the bowel. Perception of anorectal distension reduced. These changes may increase the risk of faecal incontinence, constipation and confusion	Undertake a comprehensive bowel assessment. Review medications, diet and exercise habits to identify any causes of diarrhoea or constipation	Educate the client as appropriate. This may include exercise programmes or diet and fluid regimes to relieve constipation. Follow published recommendations where bowel medications are necessary	Registered Nurses Association of Ontario. *Nursing Best Practice Guideline – Prevention of Constipation in the Older Adult Population.* Available at http://www.mao.org/bestpractices/PDF/BPG_Prevent_Constipation_rev05.pdf
Buccal cavity	Some evidence suggests that taste buds are lost or their sense reduced in older people, although this is largely undetermined; however, normal age-related changes to the oral mucosa and tongue can alter enjoyment of food and result in reduced nutritional intake. Tooth loss occurs – usually due to periodontal disease. Poor dental care and no access to fluoridated water as children are linked with widespread dental problems. Infrequent dental fittings and loss of bone from gums exacerbate problems of denture fit, often resulting in ulceration and pain. In addition to pain and infection, these problems can result in weight loss and malnutrition	Assess the condition of existing teeth and gums or discuss the fit and comfort of dentures. Consider dental problems as a possible cause of weight loss. Assess swallowing ability. Dry mucosa or disease can cause swallowing difficulties. Recent research highlights a connection between dental problems and heart disease	Refer to dental services. Waiting lists are often long, so discuss with client and their general practitioner (GP) strategies to manage ulceration, dryness, dentition-related weight loss or other conditions in the interim. Educate client in the preparation of nutritious soft foods. There are various saliva substitutes, which can reduce dryness; however, they are not inexpensive and frequent sips of water and/or saline mouthwashes may be as useful. Monitor weight and body mass index (BMI)	Joanna Briggs Institute. *Maintaining Oral Hydration in Older People.* Available at http://www.joannabriggs.edu.au/pdf/BPISHyd.pdf American Academy of Peridontology. Available at http://www.perio.org/resources-products/posppr3-1.html Bouillanne, O., Morineau, G., Dupont, C., Coulombel, I., Vincent, J.-P., Nicolis, I., et al. (2005) Geriatric nutritional risk index: A new index for evaluating at-risk elderly medical patients. *American Journal of Clinical Nutrition* 82(4), 777–83. Available at http://www.ajcn.org/cgi/content/full/82/4/777

(continued)

Table 17.1 (*continued*)

Domain	Associated issues	Assessment	Possible interventions	Resources
Cardiovascular	Changes in ageing include: • Slight thickening of left ventricular wall • Arterial walls stiffen and aorta becomes dilated and elongated • Systolic blood pressure increases • Venous elasticity declines, veins become more tortuous and valves less competent • Red blood cell producing tissue in bone marrow declines • Reduced absorption of iron These changes can result in increased risk of stroke, deep vein thrombosis and pulmonary embolism. Anaemia is common in old age but is always accompanied by a causal pathology. Older people may also be less tolerant of large amounts of IV fluids	Monitor blood pressure regularly. Monitor cognition/skin colour/signs of hypoxia. Take seriously complaints of pain; older people may not experience typical MI pain; changes in cognition or vague pain may be the only signs	Refer to GP/specialist for regular check-up. Review medications (prescribed and over-the-counter) for use by dates, potential adverse effects/interactions. Educate clients and where possible develop plan for regular exercise and relaxation that suits client's lifestyle. For example some older people are happy to walk with animals or children, but they would not be involved in group exercise. If obese, initiate a plan for healthy eating	Ebersole, P., Hess, P., Touhy, T., Jett, K. (2005) *Gerontological Nursing & Healthy Aging*. Elsevier & Mosby, St Louis, USA. The Heart Foundation Guidelines for Health Professionals available at http://www.heartfoundation.com.au/index.cfm?page=45
Cognition	Normal age-related changes to cognition include: • Generalised decline in speed of processing • Slower and more cue-dependent memory performance • Learning capacity is not impaired • Decrease in learning speed and recall • No interference with daily activities, social or occupational functioning • No alteration to insight • Normal language and planning skills	Differentiate depression/delirium/dementia Assess cognitive status Recommended tools for screening (not diagnosis) include: • The Mini Mental State Examination (MMSE) for cognition assessment • The Confusion Assessment Method (CAM) for delirium. Assess for possible reversible causes; for example infection, depression, dehydration, poor nutrition and drug interactions can all produce symptoms that mimic dementia	Dependent on diagnosis. Interventions for delirium should consist of treatment of the underlying cause (often infection). Interventions for depression may include counselling, increased or more meaningful social interaction, alleviation of stressors and pharmacological intervention. It may be possible to increase interaction through the internet, where family is not located nearby. Referral to GP and/or specialist for treatment. Interventions for dementia may include environmental modification to stimulate way finding and memory, monitoring and balancing levels of stimulation. GP or specialist may recommend pharmacological intervention. Education of and support for the family is vital	Centre for Applied Gerontology (2004) *A Guide for Assessing Older People in Hospitals*. Australian Health Ministers Advisory Council, Victoria, Australia.

(continued)

				GeroNurseOnline. *Nutrition in the Elderly*. Available at http://www.geronurseonline.org/index.cfm?section_id=48&geriatric_topic_id=27&sub_section_id=208&tab=2#item_4
	Intellectual performance is maintained at the same level well into the 80s	Observe hydration and weight status. Calculate and record BMI.	Educate client regarding good diet and nutritional balance	
	Normal age-related changes to cognition do not impact on social or occupational abilities	Assess normal eating patterns and diet. Assess underlying reason for malnutrition – may be due to disease or often it is simply too much trouble to cook for one.	Encourage clients to consume frequent small meals, if they prefer, to achieve appropriate food and fluid intake.	
	Cognitive disorders (such as dementia and delirium) and depression may be observed in the older adult	Assess ability to shop for and to prepare food as functional decline may limit this. Expiry date of food is often forgotten and may require checking. Assess any changes in bowel habits or any nausea or vomiting	Suggest delivered or pre-prepared frozen meals; explore potential for social eating; for example the local RSL club may provide transport, inexpensive meals and activities	
	Impaired cognition may impact on the individual's personal safety and ability to live independently in community			
	It is of primary importance to follow accurate assessment protocols to differentiate between depression, delirium and dementia, and between these changes and other changes, as they may manifest atypically and be misdiagnosed			
	It is vital not to assume that simply because someone is old; they must have dementia			
Gastric tract	Ageing changes in the gastric tract include: • Decreased gastric secretion • Reduced absorption of vitamin B$_{12}$, calcium and iron • Change in composition of bacterial flora • Modest slowing of gastric emptying • Diminished capacity of gastric mucosa to resist damage (less mucus secretion) • Wall of large intestine becomes weaker due to gradual atrophy of tissue layers			

341

Table 17.1 (*continued*)

Domain	Associated issues	Assessment	Possible interventions	Resources
	• Gastro-oesophageal reflux more common in elderly • Prolonged gastric distension, increased feeling of fullness after meal • Less motility of intestine – decreased hunger contractions These changes can result in reduced food intake, malnutrition, dehydration, increased risk of aspiration, increased risk of peptic ulcers, development of outpockets in the large intestine, electrolyte imbalance and increased risk of constipation or incontinence			
Hearing	A high percentage of older people have some level of hearing deficit. For many it might be a mild impairment which interferes little with their functioning. In one-third of cases, hearing loss in older people is caused by a build-up of cerum, and is thus reversible. Presbycusis is also seen more commonly in old age. In the 70s, degeneration of the inner ear structures and a decrease in the number of nerve fibres occurs, affecting hearing. Loss of hearing can lead to loss of ability to communicate well, social isolation, misdiagnosis of dementia and increased risk of injury	Check ears for wax build up (using otoscope) every 6–8 weeks. Assess hearing aids if owned – they are often not worn because of discomfort, whistling or dead batteries Some older people may not realise they can acquire hearing aids free. People may be reluctant to wear hearing aids because they find magnified background noises distressing; this is especially a risk for people with severely impaired cognition	Remove or make referrals for removal of cerum. Make referrals to auditory services for hearing assessment and fitting of aids. Attend to any problems with current aids. Increase the volume settings on telephone and investigate handsets and doorbells with light alerts. Speak clearly, rather than loudly, and reduce background noise	The Cochrane Library. *Systematic Review of the Effectiveness of Ear Drops for Ear Wax Removal*. Available at http://www.mrw.interscience. wiley.com/cochrane/clsysrev/ articles/CD004326/frame.html

System	Age-related change	Assessment	Action	Reference
Liver	Via the ageing process, hepatic regeneration is delayed but not actually impaired. Volume and weight decreases and hepatic blood flow decreases, along with bile acid synthesis. This can result in elevated serum drug levels toxicity, decreased ability to metabolise certain drugs, elevation of serum cholesterol and increase prevalence of gallstones	Observe hydration (via skin turgor, oral mucosa and cognitive status) and fluid intake and output	Be aware of changes to drug metabolisation when conducting chart reviews	Ebersole, P., Hess, P., Touhy, T. and Jett, K. (2005) Gerontological Nursing & Healthy Aging. Elsevier & Mosby, St Louis, USA.
Memory	Normal ageing results in the memory becoming slower and more cue dependent. Memory loss as such is pathological. When short-term memory loss is severe, it can begin to impede on the person's ability to live independently	Memory loss is often misdiagnosed, when poor hearing, vision, confusion or other conditions exist. A number of cognitive assessment tools are available, including the MMSE. Short-term memory loss may be apparent from conversation; however, always assess to allow measurement of changes	Seek an underlying cause; review medications; test for infection; consider hearing and vision. Memory cues and use of ritual can assist greatly. Investigate the use of smart technology such as those with an automatic cut-off if left unattended. Advise use of lists, notes and diaries. Instigate habits and routines. Review medication regime and consider use of aids or services to support administration. Refer to GP or specialist for investigation	Alzheimer's Australia has numerous fact sheets and links regarding memory loss and dementia. Available at http://www.alzheimers.org.au/content.cfm?categoryid=2
Nails and hair	Many changes to hair and nails in old age are clearly observable, e.g. greying of hair due to loss of melanocytes; excessive facial hair and thinning of scalp hair in postmenopausal women; increases in coarse hair in ears, nose and eyebrows in men; decreased growth rates in hair and nails; and nails which become dry and brittle, flattened or concave with longitudinal ridges	General health assessment seeking underlying health-related causes. Assess whether these changes are causing concern (e.g. impact on social confidence and self-esteem) or other problems (such as toenails which are too hard to cut and cause pain or deformity – this is a particular cause for concern in diabetics)	Refer to GP if underlying cause suspected. Refer to podiatry services if required. Remember body image is closely linked to self-esteem	Davis, S., Nay, R., Koch, S. and Andrews, G. (In press) Practical Application of Guidelines for a Dementia Friendly Physical and Social Environment. Department of Human Services, Victoria, Australia: Body Image [serial online]. Available at http://www.elsevier.com/wps/find/journaldescription.cws.home/672932/description#description Roberts, D.T., Taylor, W.D. and Boyle, J. (2003) Guidelines for treatment of onychomycosis. British Journal of Dermatology, 148(3), 402–10.
Pancreas	The ageing process can result in reduced secretion of insulin from the pancreas, resulting in a heightened risk of type 2 diabetes mellitus	Investigate symptoms of diabetes and measure blood glucose levels (or refer to appropriate pathology service). Assess for associated pathology such as poor circulation and slow-healing wounds	Refer to GP for further assessment and treatment. Educate client in diet-based management of diabetes and preventative diets. Implement appropriate strategies for associated issues	NHMRC. Guidelines for the Management of Type II Diabetes Mellitus. Available at http://www.nhmrc.gov.au/publications/synopses/di7todi13syn.htm

(continued)

Table 17.1 (*continued*)

Domain	Associated issues	Assessment	Possible interventions	Resources
Respiratory	Changes associated with ageing include: • Reduction in amount of lung elastic tissue • Increased chest wall stiffness • Respiratory muscles weaken, diaphragm weakens • Shortening of thorax (compression of vertebral discs) • Decreased neural output to respiratory muscles • Reduction in overall alveolar surface for gas exchange • Ventilatory response to hypoxia reduced by 50% • Rate of mucociliary transport declines • Loss of effective cough reflex • Antibody response reduced These changes can result in reduced ability to clear respiratory passages, increased risk of infection and increased risk of hypoxia	Assess the client's medical history including previous disease and present symptoms Inspect skin colour, turgor, moisture, chest shape, chest expansion, capillary refill (depress nails) and presence of sputum Auscultation of breath sounds Palpate for tenderness	Encourage exercise participation. Educate clients to monitor their own respiration and take breaks if necessary during physical activity	Australian Government Health *InSite*. *Tips and Guides for Exercise for Older People*. Available at http://www.healthinsite.gov.au/topics/Exercise_for_Older_People
Sexuality and sexual expression	While old age heralds the cessation of reproductive ability and gradual slowing of libido, older people (like younger people) have a continuing need for sexual relationships and sexual expression. Social attitudes can often form barriers to acceptance of elderly as sexual beings. These societal taboos place older people at greater risk of denied sexual expression, ridicule and loneliness	Discuss sexual expression with clients once a relationship is established; be aware of the clients' reactions. They may be relieved that someone is willing to discuss sexual expression with them	Review medications to identify any that may cause issues such as impotence or vaginal dryness Discuss normal changes in ageing, changes brought about by pathology and alternate means of intimacy and expression	Practice development (2007) *International Journal of Older People Nursing*, 2(1), 62–80. Available at http://www.blackwell-synergy.com/toc/opn/2/1 Help the Aged (UK). Fact sheets. Available at http://www.helptheaged.org.uk/en-gb/AdviceSupport/HealthAdvice/HealthyAgeing/SexLaterLife/

Skeleton and bone density	Adults experience a gradual loss of bone density from the age of 30 years onwards. In women, this loss accelerates during menopause. This leads to an increased risk of osteoporosis. Older adults may have either type 1 of osteoporosis, which occurs between 50 and 70 years of age and occurs six times more in women than men; or type 2 osteoporosis, which occurs in over 70 years and occurs in twice as many women as men	Assess risk factors such as obesity, lack of exercise and poor diet	Educate clients in the benefits of diets high in calcium. Educate clients in safe, weight-bearing exercise. Refer for bone density screening	The Jean Hailes Foundation for Women's Health. *Bone Health for Life.* Available at http://www.bonehealthforlife.org.au/
Skin integrity	Skin is the body's largest organ and undergoes a large number of changes in old age, including: • Structural dryness • Roughness • Wrinkling • Laxity • Functional changes: declines in cell replacement, wound healing, immunologic response and thermoregulation • Loss of dermal thickness and a flattening of the dermal-epidermal layer – due to loss in collagen, elastin and water • Epidermal cell replacement takes longer (on average an additional 10 days compared to a younger person) • Cutaneous blood flow is reduced by about 60% • Elastin and collagen fibres become coarse and rigid (creating jowls or a double chin) • Changes in distribution of fatty tissue – decreased on face and hands and increased on thighs and abdomen (eyelids can look swollen or sunken) • Reduction in nerve endings. Reduced sensation of light touch and vibration	Observe skin condition (colour, texture and integrity). Pinch test to assess hydration and elasticity. Monitor, assess and measure wounds and ulcers	Educate client in good skin hygiene and cleansing practices. Soap is not recommended and water should be used sparingly (except for drinking). Discuss wound management with clients, including financial aspects (for example the cost of dressings). Discuss wound prevention strategies such as reducing friction from clothing, avoiding materials that do not breathe, avoiding pressure areas and good nutrition and hydration. Advise client to cover skin if outside, for example working in garden, where sunburn or trauma are likely. It is better to maintain skin integrity than try to heal old skin	Hogkinson, B. and Nay, R. (2005) Effectiveness of topical skin care provided in aged care facilities. *International Journal of Evidence-Based Healthcare*, 3(4), 65–101. Available at http://www.blackwell-synergy.com/doi/abs/10.1111/j.1479-6988.2005.00022.x?journalCode=jbr Australian Wound Management Association Inc. *Clinical Practice Guidelines for the Prediction and Prevention of Pressure Ulcers and Standards for Wound Management.* Available at http://www.awma.com.au/publications/publications.php

(continued)

Table 17.1 (*continued*)

Domain	Associated issues	Assessment	Possible interventions	Resources
	• Less sweat glands and reduced activity • Pigmentation changes (less melanocytes per unit area) • Decrease in vitamin D production These changes create a raft of effects. The most common include easy damage of skin (for example bruising or tearing), slow wound healing and itchy dry skin. The reduced production of vitamin D requires increased sun exposure; however, this should be done with caution as skin is also more susceptible to sunburn and the individual more susceptible to heat stroke			
Sleep patterns	Sleep requirements and quality change in old age. While most older people require less sleep (usually about 6 h), they may find it harder to achieve and maintain nocturnal sleep due to lower auditory thresholds and pain Less time is spent in deep (delta or stage 4) sleep and therefore sleep can be less rejuvenating and often leaves the person feeling that they have not slept at all Many older people use naps to make up for lost nocturnal sleep, or may find themselves dozing off. While this can work well for some, others may find that it interferes with their social activities, decreases nocturnal sleep further, or is just plain annoying Lack of sleep is detrimental and difficult at any age. In all age groups, sleep deprivation is associated with higher mortality, higher risk of injury, difficulty conducting ADLs and IADLs, increased confusion and lower coping threshold	Ask client about their sleep while observing their behaviour and presentation. Use sleep diaries to help assess reasons for lost sleep. Assess history and current use of medications that impact sleep. Assess pre-bedtime habits/use of 'aids' such as alcohol, milk and other drinks. Assess risk of/presence of sleep apnoea. Assess the environment, e.g. light and noise.	Encourage clients to establish and maintain bedtime rituals to cue the brain and prepare for sleep. Refer to appropriate service (e.g. sleep clinic) if client feels problems warrant this, e.g. sleep apnoea. Note that many medications taken by older people for sleep in fact reduce REM sleep and increase confusion – be sure this is assessed Advise against stimulating activity, high-caffeine drinks and alcohol prior to bedtime	Koch, S., Haesler, E., Tiziani, A. and Wilson, J. (2006) Effectiveness of sleep management strategies for residents of aged care facilities: Findings of a systematic review. *Journal of Clinical Nursing*, 15(10), 1267–75. Available at http://www.blackwell-synergy.com/doi/abs/10.1111/j.1365-2702.2006.01385.x

Temperature regulation	In older people homeostasis is less well maintained. This has the effect of making older people more susceptible to hyperthermia (including heat stroke) and hypothermia. This is also due to reduced efficacy of sweating (contributing to hyperthermia) and reduced vascular constriction, diminished perception of cold and lower body mass (contributing to hypothermia). Temperature regulation is vital for most body functions, and may cause or exacerbate confusion	Observe skin, i.e. colour, warmth and moistness Assess body temperature Assess cognition; has there been any recent change? Assess whether dressed appropriately Assess the environment to establish whether the home provides adequate heating and cooling	Explore winter heating rebates and other programmes to ensure that the client is receiving all the help they are entitled to Educate the client regarding sensible heat strategies such as staying well hydrated, staying out of direct sun and running errands or working outdoors in the cooler parts of the day Investigate with the client whether they use any heaters or fans/air conditioners that are in situ. Some older people are reluctant to use appliances due to concerns about the cost	SunSmart Factsheet. Available at http://www.sunsmart.com.au/downloads/resources/info_sheets/being_sunsmart_aust.pdf Help the Aged (UK). *Tips for Staying Warm*. Available at http://www.helptheaged.org.uk/en-gb/AdviceSupport/HealthAdvice/HealthyAgeing/StayWarmInWinter/as_staywarm_tips.htm; and *Tips for Staying Cool*. Available at http://www.helptheaged.org.uk/en-gb/AdviceSupport/HealthAdvice/HealthyAgeing/StayCoolInSummer/
Urinary tract	Impact of ageing on the urinary system include: • Decreased bladder capacity • Weakened bladder muscles • Enlargement of prostate gland • Increased alkalinity of vaginal canal • Weaker sphincters • Reduced glomerular filtration rate • Decreased urinary concentration • Thirst sensation is impaired Effects of these changes can include increased susceptibility to fluid imbalance and electrolyte or acid/base changes; higher risks of dehydration and potassium depletion; increased incidence of urinary incontinence	Assess for presence and frequency of episodes of incontinence. Assess possible causes of incontinence. Conduct bowel assessment. Assess fluid intakes and/or urinary output (fluid balance chart). Check serum potassium levels. Check blood glucose levels if other symptoms of diabetes are present. Assess for symptoms of urinary tract infection – remembering that older people often do not exhibit classic symptoms	Refer to GP or specialist continence clinic. Educate client in incontinence management; remember to discuss issues such as affording incontinence products and managing incontinence in public situations. Encourage clients to monitor their fluid intake and try to drink 2 L of fluid daily (may not be feasible in frail older person). Educate client in prevention and management strategies such as pelvic floor exercises and urge avoidance	Thomas, S., Nay, R., Moore, K., Fonda, D. and Hawthorn, G. (2006) *Continence Outcomes Measurement Suite*. Commonwealth of Australia, Victoria, Australia. Available at http://www.health.gov.au/internet/wcms/publishing.nsf/Content/ageing-continence-outcome.htm Brown, S. and Nay, R. (2007) UTI: Under treated and investigated: An examination of the nursing management of urinary tract infections in nursing home residents experiencing impaired cognition. *International Journal of Older People Nursing*, 2(1), 20–24. Available at http://www.blackwell-synergy.com/doi/abs/10.1111/j.1748-3743.2007.00049.x

(continued)

Table 17.1 (*Continued*)

Domain	Associated issues	Assessment	Possible interventions	Resources
Vision	There are normal age-related changes to vision, and conditions such as presbyopia, cataracts, dry eyes, diabetic retinopathy and macular degeneration are seen more commonly in old age. Many older people will have lifelong vision deficits that continue to require attention in older age. Good vision is needed to understand the world around us, and in older people confusion resulting from poor vision can be misinterpreted and misdiagnosed. For older people who wish to remain driving, regular vision checks are important for their and others' safety. Changes to an older person's glasses' prescription, particularly dramatic ones, can increase the likelihood of them falling as they adjust to the new glasses. This is exacerbated if they wear multifocal lenses	Preliminary vision assessment. Ask if glasses are worn and enquire when glasses were last prescribed and if they are still effective. Ask are the glasses comfortable and close to hand? Is cost preventing a new prescription? Vision may be impaired because client cannot clean glasses. New glasses may lead to increased falls	Refer for vision assessment. Educate client in the availability of low-vision aids, such as large print telephones and books or talking books. Are there environmental changes that may improve light and reduce glare? Refer to GP for assessment of structural changes such as macular degeneration or cataracts. Advise the older person of the difficulties and dangers of changing prescriptions radically and using multifocal lenses	Vision Australia Factsheets. Available at http://www.visionaustralia.org.au/info.aspx?page=795

348

(if possible), which confirms their position and employer. Media reports, police warnings and personal experience can increase the fear older people have of strangers entering their homes. Ultimately, older people have the right to deny people entrance to their homes.

It is important to form a relationship of trust and cooperation with an older person, and it is useful to have this relationship in place prior to giving professional advice.

Developing a trusting relationship within the community care setting requires the nurse to have a willingness to listen, to empathise (rather than sympathise) with the client, and to respect their wisdom, experience and ability to make decisions regarding their own life [14]. Nurses can display this by listening attentively and recording their opinions in the case notes; accepting hospitality; talking to, rather than at or about, the person; and asking for their opinions and feedback explicitly. Remember that the client–community nurse relationship should be one of communication and trust, but not dependency or reliance.

Developing a good social and medical history of the older person is a useful way of both getting to know one another and providing background to the nursing assessment. It is important to try to discover who the person is, not merely what diseases they have. Some questions to ask in order to gather this type of information may include:

- What do they enjoy?
- What do they find frustrating?
- What are their goals?
- What do they value?
- What makes them worry?
- What support do they have?
- What support could they have if needed, but would prefer not to?

In a situation where there is a carer or a group of carers, the nurse will need to find out information about them as well. Families and carers can be a great help to the community nurse; however, in some situations they can also obstruct information gathering and the development of an optimal relationship with the client. The nurse needs to bear in mind that even if a person has cognitive impairment, a community nurse's *primary* client is the older person, not the family members or carers. It may be necessary to speak to the older person alone, but this should be approached delicately as it may raise feelings of rejection or exclusion in the carer. It is important to always seek permission from the client to discuss aspects of care with family, unless the client is unable to consent.

Assessment

A key factor in assessing the health of older people is to differentiate between the changes that occur in the body as people age from changes that are caused by disease [15]. Community nurses need to take a strengths-based approach when undertaking an assessment [16] and aim to discover what the person can do, rather than what they cannot. If they are unable to complete a task alone, seek ways to incorporate what they can do into the assistance programme. Key things to remember when conducting an assessment in the community include:

Use the right tool

In the community it is useful to use tools that are designed with the community or home environment in mind; assessment tools designed primarily for an institutional environment can be inappropriate and create false readings in the community. Always use a tool that has been validated in older populations [15].

Take time

When undertaking an assessment, remember that this can be a stressful and anxious time for clients. Many older people are fearful of being placed into residential care and/or value stoicism and can be defensive about their health and abilities. This anxiety can also create an impression of less functioning than the person can manage when not under pressure. Allow the older person to take as much time as needed and to do things just as they normally would. If a client can perform a daily task, it does not matter if it takes them ten times longer than what is considered 'normal' [15].

Familiar task – familiar environment

Always assess people in their home environment, using the appliances and devices they are accustomed to. By performing an assessment that is a good replica of normal life, the nurse will gain the most accurate reading of the person's ability [15].

Optimise assessment

Limit over-assessment and duplication of assessment. This can be achieved by sharing assessment promptly and, with the client's consent, health information with other health professionals involved in the client's care. When conducting a large number of assessments, remember that they can be physically and mentally tiring for the client, so try to spread them over a few days if possible. Determine what really needs to be assessed; for example if the client receives meals on wheels routinely, is it necessary to assess their ability to cook safely? Through the assessment process, a good overview of the person's health and functioning should be achieved [15].

Refer to defined standards

When assessing older people, nurses should refer to the standards of health and safety outlined by the tool and/or guidelines being used, or by the employing organisation, rather than those of personal preference and taste. The role of the community nurse is not to impose all older people with common living standards, but rather to assess their safety and assist them in achieving their goals. Cultural and cohort factors should also be considered; for example, some older people grew up during war-time restrictions and the Great Depression and were not raised to expect daily showers the way later generations are. They may not wish to have daily showers and, with delicate older skin, a reduction in the associated friction and drying may actually be beneficial.

Determine goals

The culmination of assessment should be a combination of the person's own goals for their life and recommended health goals. Remember that lifestyle goals, such as regaining social activity, are often far more important to the older person than health goals. It should be possible to combine the goals of the nurse with the goals of the older person. However, if it is not possible, the older person's views should always take precedence. They have the right to make poor decisions about their health, just as other community members do [17].

Document

Documentation is vitally important and this remains true in the community setting, and arguably more so, as in the community setting there are generally no objective witnesses to the nurse's practice. Documentation provides a record of nursing actions, and in this regard, it is a useful protection for the nurse against litigation. However, this does not mean that it should be adopted only as a protectionist behaviour for the community nurse – documentation is first and foremost to guide communication and evaluate interventions for the older person [18].

Common issues in community aged care

Cognitive impairment, confusion and dementia

Older people may display confused behaviour for a wide number of reasons; therefore, it is vital to not assume dementia in the first instance, but rather to arrive at a suspected dementia diagnosis once all other possible causes have been excluded. Causes of confused behaviour to consider include:

- Dehydration.
- Vitamin B_{12} deficiency.
- Infection, commonly urinary tract infections.
- Drug interactions.
- Depression.
- Hearing and/or vision loss.
- Short-term memory deficits.
- Hypoxia.
- Delirium.
- Sleep deprivation.
- Other psychological disorders [17].
- Pain.
- Any acute medical condition [16].

It is important to exclude these causes (by assessment and appropriate referral and treatment) and never 'assume' dementia. Dementia-screening tools can be used to determine if referrals to community nursing organisations and other health services are appropriate. If a client is suspected or diagnosed with a dementia or other organic brain disorder, determining their level of competency becomes important. In many disorders, particularly in the early stages, people may have a very high level of function and competence. This high level of function is best maintained by remaining as close to their normal lifestyle as possible. The effects of dementia cannot be reversed; however, new medications can slow their progression and lifestyles which enhance cognition can improve day-to-day function. Lifestyles which support the individual's ability to perform activities themselves, and which provide high-quality stimulation balanced with quiet recovery periods, and which support memory by providing familiar environments and visual and other cues, all assist and support cognitive function. There is much that can be done to support people with dementia and their carers and more information is contained in the 'Further reading' section of this chapter [19].

Depression and loneliness in older people

Particularly in older people, depression, isolation, anxiety and medical comorbidities intertwine to create a situation which does not enhance health or happiness [20].

Depression can be a chronic condition requiring long-term intervention or can be the end result of many things, including:

- Early life trauma
- War-time experiences
- Incapacity
- Fear of falling
- Loneliness
- Chronic pain
- Grief and loss
- Social isolation
- Incontinence (restricting social interaction)
- Financial stress
- Loss of mobility
- Anxiety
- Fear of death
- Lack of sunlight
- Polypharmacy

For people aged over 85 years, depression and loneliness are strong predictors of mortality [20]. Social isolation is, in older populations, a better predictor for heart disease than bloodstream cholesterol or smoking habits [21]. However, depression in late life is not inevitable and, like all depressive illness, should be treated. It is important not to consider antidepressant medication as the only form of treatment of depression. Depression is a diagnosable illness, but is sometimes difficult to differentiate from sadness, a normal reaction to life events such as the loss of a life partner, constant loneliness, pain or the individual's grief for their own loss of independence and health [22]. Depression requires diagnosis by a doctor, psychologist or psychiatrist according to the standards outlined in the Diagnostic and Statistical Manual of Mood Disorders IV – TR [23]. However, depression-screening tools may be used to indicate the presence of depression.

Depression-screening tools that are validated for use in older populations include:

- The Geriatric Depression Scale (available in a short 15-item version, GDS-15, and a longer 30-item version, GDS-30).
- The Cornell Scale for Depression in Dementia (validated for use in cognitively impaired populations).

Actions which may be useful in the alleviation of depression include:

- Referral to appropriate medical or psychological services.
- Referral to appropriate counselling services.
- Assess and manage factors which may be contributing to social isolation such as poor mobility, poor continence management, lack of appropriate, affordable transport and poverty.
- Encourage the person to become involved in local groups, including CALD and interest specific groups.
- Referral for medication review.
- Referral and assessment for respite services.
- Assessment and management of pain.

It is also useful to remember that often when a client is anxious or depressed, informal carers and family members are likely to also be suffering from some level of stress, anxiety or depression. Their interaction and involvement in the above strategies can be beneficial to everyone involved.

Pain

Pain is underreported by older people and undertreated, and often serious conditions can be overlooked. Chronic pain diminishes quality of life and contributes to depression and decreased cognitive ability. Management of pain can be impaired by drug interactions excluding many forms of analgesia. Other interventions such as stretching, elevation, rest, distraction, heat or ice packs and pain-relieving creams may be useful either alone or in conjunction with pharmaceutical analgesia [24]. The client will often have their own methods of managing their pain, and can often provide good insights into what exacerbates or relieves their pain. Some older people may choose to live with a level of pain, choosing to intervene only when the pain exacerbates.

Assessment of pain in older people can be difficult. In the first instance always ask the person if they have pain. Even in people with dementia self-report has been shown to be valid, but not reliable. Visual scales and models of the body can be useful for assessing magnitude and location of pain. Proxy scales may be used to determine pain if attempts at self-report have failed [24]. It is important to discuss how the client has previously managed pain, as they may have found effective strategies.

Interventions for chronic pain may include:

- Referral to their GP for treatment or management of the cause of pain.
- Determining whether the individual is adhering to their analgesic medicines, and if not, what their reasons are. Does the medication cause unpleasant side effects? Are they concerned that it may be addictive?
- Discussion and suggesting what other methods of pain relief they use, and what might be effective.

Home environment

Assessment of the home environment is ideally conducted by an occupational therapist who can then suggest modifications, aids and improvements. However, the community nurse is generally the most frequent visitor to the house and should identify situations where further intervention is needed or may be useful.

Environmental dangers can include:

- Poorly fixed hand rails, or decorative rails and towel rails being used as grab rails.
- Showers or baths which are difficult to access or exit.
- Poorly maintained floor surfaces or loose, light rugs.
- Stairs and steps, particularly those that are steep or without rails.
- Electrical and gas appliances that are in poor repair or are too low for the person to use easily.
- Loose cords or cables crossing walkways.
- Doorways which are too narrow for the person to be able to use aids effectively or at all.
- Signs of poor hygiene which are likely to cause a health hazard, such as rotting food.
- Signs of major infestation by rodents or insects.
- Potential fire hazards.
- Footwear that increases the risk of falling.

It is important to use tact when discussing environmental modifications with older people, as some may find the cost or disruption of modification distressing. Be aware of potential funding sources for home modifications in the local area. Community nurses can work with older people to alert them to safety issues in their homes and resources in their local area.

Mobility

Arthritic changes, muscle loss and deconditioning, impaired balance, fear of falling, pain, osteoporosis and poor eyesight are some of the factors that impact on an older person's mobility. The impact of reduced mobility can be not only physically dramatic, but also psychologically and socially. Mobility may reduce social interaction, increasing depression and isolation, and feelings of entrapment (a prisoner in the home) and uselessness. Necessary assessments include:

- General assessment seeking a reversible cause.
- Mobility assessment.
- Assessment of environmental risks.
- Assessment of the condition of the client's feet – some older people have great pain and difficulty walking, simply because of ill-kept toenails or ill-fitting shoes.

With client consent, referral for podiatry assessment, mobility aids or education in the use of pre-existing aids may be useful. The client also needs to be educated regarding safe walking behaviours and potential hazards in the home and in public.

Falls

Changes or damage to the inner ear, reduced mobility, joint stiffness, pain and slowed reflexes may all contribute to falls in older people. The home environment can also add to the risk of falls. More importantly, there is an increased risk of serious and long-term injury resulting due to the impact of coexisting conditions such as osteoporosis [25]. Fear of falling can be a major contributor to anxiety and social isolation in older people.

In order to reduce the risk of falling, risk factors such as cognition, vision, hearing, mobility and balance, environment and medications need to be identified [3]. The community nurse needs to assess and refer for appropriate gait aids/training and ensure that the client is using and understands the correct use of pre-existing aids. Many medications can increase a person's risk of falling; therefore, a medication review should form part of any falls management plan.

Deconditioning

Weight loss, muscle loss and muscle atrophy can occur in old age as a result of the client's social situation, other physical pathologies or depression. Loss of weight and muscle tone can create or exacerbate mobility problems and a host of other conditions. Assessment and monitoring of deconditioning is vital as it can be insidious; therefore, measure body mass index and chart weight frequently if deconditioning is suspected. Assessment that identifies changes to normal activity or exercise patterns and ability to maintain self-care habits can be helpful in identifying the risks of deconditioning.

Exercise programmes, which may include seated exercise, stretching and weight-bearing exercise, can be useful in maintaining tone. Additionally, environmental alterations may increase the capacity of the older person to move about more independently.

Abuse

In the community setting, unlike the residential care setting, abuse is less frequently perpetrated by service, nursing or medical staff and is more commonly committed by family and friends [26]. Although stories exist of older people being attacked or abused by strangers, this is uncommon. In addition to being a heartbreaking situation, the implication of family members, friends or neighbours in abusive situations generates increased complexity. Forms of abuse in the community may be divided into abuse which is reactionary, which comes about when the carer is not coping, or exploitative, more deliberate abuse which exploits the trust and vulnerability of an older person.

Reactionary abuse may include:

- Inappropriate use of chemical and/or physical restraint.
- Overmedication (both accidental and intentional).
- Failure to provide adequate food, drink, hygiene etc.
- Rough handling.
- Ignorance, which inadvertently leads to neglect.

Exploitative abuse may include:

- Theft and appropriation of money, property and valuables (including collecting pensions against the person's wishes).
- Sexual abuse [27].
- Confinement or imprisonment.

There is a fine line between poor care and abuse. Especially in the community setting poor care may be delivered because the carer is undereducated, exhausted, or unaware of, or unwilling to accept available support.

Older people, particularly those in ill health or with a high level of incapacity, are considered easy prey. Factors which can contribute to this include:

- Perceptions that older people will not be believed ('Don't mind her! She is always losing money and saying someone stole it!').
- Loneliness making people more vulnerable to 'overtrusting' new acquaintances.
- Steady income streams (via the pension or superannuation), sometimes combined with high-value properties (due to considerable appreciation during their lifetime) or considerable accumulated wealth.
- Physical weakness and diminished capacity to flee or fight back.
- Emotional abuse ('I wouldn't do this if you weren't such a burden'.).
- Reliance on the abuser for care.

If abuse is occurring due to lack of education or as a consequence of carer exhaustion, referral for respite services should be considered and education of the carer in appropriate care strategies. It is important to ensure that the return home from respite is supported by the introduction of care services and carer support programmes [28].

The suspicion of malicious abuse is one of the hardest situations for a community nurse. If the nurse is certain that abuse is occurring, which is supported by documented or physical evidence, it may be appropriate to involve the police and the public advocate. The employer of the nurse will be likely to have policies regarding reporting and actions. If suspicions are less supported, the nurse must look for signs of abuse or neglect, including bruising and abrasion (notably those that may result from restraint use), weight loss unexplained by other conditions, poverty unexplained by circumstances, substandard housing provisions or family members who significantly resent the involvement of the nurse [29–32]. It is important to be mindful that all of these situations could occur with reasonable explanations and none 'prove' abuse.

Discussing the situation with the client is the most important way of gauging the situation. This may be difficult or impossible if the older person has a significant cognitive impairment, is unwilling to 'dob in' the abuser, is fearful of retribution or if family members and carers are always present.

Abuse can be complex and, in some circumstances, may have occurred for decades. The nurse's ability to assist in breaking the cycle hinges on motivating the person being abused to work with them. Older people, like their younger adult counterparts, have a right to refuse help – reporting abuse is not mandatory and indeed not advocated by most experts, without consent. If the person has a cognitive impairment, it may be necessary to intervene with the help of the public advocate [33].

Families

The community nurse and the client's family can offer each other additional information, practical assistance, help in educating the client and support. However, conflicts may occur within the relationship. The 'burden of care' has received extensive attention in research, and many organisations have been established to provide support to carers. Carer burden assessment tools exist, which allow greater understanding of the individual carer's experience [34]. The community nurse is in an excellent position to anticipate and prevent carer burden. Intervention may simply include listening and acknowledging that it is normal at times to experience guilt, anger and resentment, especially as caring can lead to social isolation, illness and even abuse. Some families report that the hardest thing for them is having the older person admitted to a nursing home [35]. Again, community nurses can assist with information, resources and coordination.

When working with families, remember to:

- Seek consent from the client to involve family members.
- Understand what the family wishes to do and how the community nurse can support them and/or fill the gaps where they are unable or unwilling to provide care.
- Explain medical or nursing terminology.
- Listen to family members, weigh their opinions and remain cognizant that they have known the client a lot longer and more intimately than the nurse has.
- Understand that all family members will have other pressures in their lives, other demands on their time and may feel guilt or resentment surrounding their interactions with the client.
- Discuss disputes, rather than letting them fester.
- Encourage discussion of end-of-life wishes, so all are clear on what the older person wants. If available, the nurse may be able to introduce advance care planning resources and documents to the older person and family.

Future trends

For community nurses, the changing age distribution of the population is likely to lead to an increase in the number of people who wish to receive services in their homes and who may demand a higher level of service and flexibility [36, 37]. The increasingly multicultural nature of this group will also require changes from the meals offered by council services to the way personal care is provided.

Interdisciplinary care and the use of information technology (IT) will be central to meeting care demands. Community nurses will need to develop ways of translating evidence into interdisciplinary care practices; to be far more effective and innovative in the ways IT is used to communicate, assess, diagnose and treat; and at the same time not lose the centrality of the person in this approach [18].

Older people who are able to live in the community undoubtedly account for fewer funding dollars than those living in residential care facilities [38]. Therefore, as more people reach old age and fewer people remain in the tax-paying workforce, community care is of ever-increasing importance in the provision of sustainable health care.

Summary

We have highlighted some common issues faced by older people living in the community that will be encountered by community nurses. Finally, the following key points are important to consider and implement in practice when working with older people:

- Gain consent from an older person to arrange referral, plan intervention or share information.
- Remember you are a guest in your clients' homes, as well as a professional.
- Support and assist clients to achieve *their* goals.
- Older people have the right to make their own decisions about their care – whether they are wise in your estimation or not.
- Aim for functionality and safety in the home, rather than expect every home to meet your standards.
- Work with the interdisciplinary team to ensure appropriate rather than duplicated assessment and that assessment tools are valid and reliable for older people.
- Do not assume you are observing dementia – always seek a cause for unusual behaviour.
- Remember older people present with different symptoms, underreport pain and are often overmedicated and underassessed.

Useful resources

Beyond Blue: The National Depression Initiative.

Fact Sheet 17: Depression in older people. Available at http://www.beyondblue. org.au/index. aspx?link_id=7.246&tmp=FileDownload&fid=335

Alzheimer's Australia. Depression and dementia fact sheet. Available at http://www.alzheimers. org.au/upload/HS5.3.pdf

Alzheimer's Australia. Mind Your Mind – A user's guide to Risk Reduction. Available at http://www. alzheimers. org.au/upload/MYM_book_lowres.pdf

Alzheimer's Australia website. Available at www.alzheimers.org.au

Haesler, E., Bauer, M. and Nay, R. (2006) Factors associated with constructive staff-family relationships in the care of older adults in the institutional setting. *International Journal of Evidence-Based Healthcare*, 4(4), 288–336. http://www.blackwell-synergy.com/doi/abs/10.1111/j.1479-6988.2006.00053.x

National Center on Elder Abuse (2007). *Clearinghouse on Abuse and Neglect of the Elderly (CANE)*. Available at http://www.cane.udel.edu/cane/.

Daly, J.M. (2004) *Elder Abuse Prevention*. Research Dissemination Core, University of Iowa Gerontological Nursing Interventions Research Center, Iowa City, IA.

The National Ageing Research Institute: An Australian guideline for the reduction of falls. Available at http://www.nari.unimelb.edu.au/vic_falls/vic_falls_prevent.htm

Department of Health and Ageing (2006). *A Community for All Ages: Building the Future*. Australian Government, Australia. Available at http://www.health.gov.au/ internet/wcms/publishing.nsf/Content/communityforallages-1-lp

Australian Pain Society. *Position Paper on the Management of Chronic Pain*. Available at http://www.apsoc.org.au/owner/files/dpnftp.pdf

Organisations providing information and support for carers vary from region to region. Information about organisations in individual areas is readily accessible on the internet.

References

1. Powell, J. and Wahidin, A. (eds) (2006) *Foucault and Aging*. Nova Science Publishers, Inc, New York, USA.

2. McMurray, A. (2007) *Community Health and Wellness – A Socio-Ecological Approach*. Mosby/Elsevier, Sydney, Australia.

3. National Ageing Research Institute (2006) *What Is Person-Centred Care? A Literature Review*. Department of Human Services, Victoria, Australia.

4. Australian Institute of Health and Welfare (2006) *Life Expectancy*. Available at http://www.aihw.gov.au/mortality/data/life_expectancy.cfm (viewed 19 July 2006).

5. Australian Bureau of Statistics (2004) *Year Book Australia*. Available at http://www.abs.gov.au/ausstats/abs@.nsf/0/b066d450abaaa4c7ca256dea000539dc (viewed 12 July 2006).

6. Australian Government Department of Health and Ageing (2006) The report on the findings and recommendations of the national speakers' series. *A Community for All Ages – Building the Future*. Commonwealth of Australia, Canberra, Australia.

7. Australian Indigenous HealthInfoNet (November 2005) *Summary of Australian Indigenous Health*. Available at http://www.healthinfonet.ecu.edu.au/html/html_keyfacts/keyfacts_plain_lang_summary.htm (viewed 19 July 2006).

8. Australian Institute of Health and Welfare (2002) *Older Australia at a Glance*, 3rd edition. AIHW Cat. No. 25. Australian Institute of Health and Welfare and Department of Health and Ageing, Canberra, Australia.

9. Department of Human Services (2003) *Improving Care for Older People*. Victorian Government Department of Human Services, Victoria, Australia.

10. Ward, B.M., Anderson, K.S. and Sheldon, M.S. (2005) Patterns of home and community care service delivery to culturally and linguistically diverse residents of rural Victoria. *Australian Journal of Rural Health*, 13(6), 348–52.

11. Australian Government Department of Health and Ageing (2006) *Australian Health and Ageing System: The Concise Factbook*. Commonwealth of Australia, Canberra, Australia.

12. Prime Ministers Science Engineering and Innovation Council (2003) *Promoting Healthy Ageing in Australia*. Commonwealth of Australia, Canberra, Australia.

13. Ebersole, P. and Hess, P. (1998) *Towards Healthy Ageing: Human Needs and Nursing Response*, 5th edition. Mosby, USA.

14. National Health and Medical Research Council (2006) *Tests and Treatments: Principles for Better Communication Between Health Care Consumers and Health Care Professionals*. Council on Ageing, Canberra, Australia.

15. Koch, S. and Garratt, S. (2001) *Assessing Older People*. McLennan & Petty, Sydney, Australia.

16. Ronch, J. and Goldfield, J. (eds) (2003) *Mental Wellness in Aging: Strength Based Approaches*. Health Professions Press, Baltimore, USA.

17. Garratt, S. (2004) Mental health issues, in R. Nay and S. Garratt (eds) *Nursing Older People: Issues and Innovation*. Elsevier, NSW, Australia, pp. 181–90.

18. Koch, B. (30 November 2007) Evaluation of a web enabled care planning and documentation system within aged care settings. *Electronic Journal of Health Informatics*, 2(1), 4.

19. Davis, S., Byers, S., Dorevitch, M., Andrews, G., Nay, R. and Koch, S. (In press) *Creating Dementia Friendly Social and Physical Environments*. Department of Human Services, Victoria, Australia.

20. Beyond Blue (2007) *Fact Sheet 17: Depression in Older People*. Available at http://www.beyondblue.org.au/index.aspx?link_id=7.246&tmp=FileDownload&fid=335 (viewed 24 April 2007).

21. Stek, M., Vinkers, D., Gussekloo, J., Beekman, A., van der Mast, R. and Westendorp, R. (2005) Is depression in old age only fatal when people feel lonely? *American Journal of Psychiatry*, 162(1), 178–80.

22. Centre for the Advancement of Health (2007) *Social Isolation Leaves Elderly at Risk for Heart Failure*. Available at www.hbns.org/news/lonely12-10-02.cfm (viewed 9 March 2007).

23. Beyond Blue (2007) *What Is Dementia?* Available at http://www.beyondblue.org.au/index. aspx?link_id=1.3 (viewed 24 April 2007).

24. Nay, R., Wilson, J., O'Donnell, M., McAuliffe, L. and Pitcher, A. (update) *Assessment of Pain in Older Adults with Dementia in Acute, Subacute and Residential Care*. Royal College of Nursing Australia, Australia.

25. Hill, K., Smith, R., LoGiudice, D. and Winbolt, M. (2003) Falls prevention, in R. Hudson (ed.) *Dementia Nursing: A Guide to Practice*. Ausmed, Melbourne, Australia, pp. 142–61.

26. Australian Pensioners and Superannuants League Qld Inc (2007) *Abuse of Older People*. Available at http://www.apsl.com.au/abuse.html (viewed 24 April 2007).

27. Crisp, J. and Taylor, C. (2005) *Potter and Perry's Fundamentals of Nursing*, 2nd edition. Elsevier, Sydney, Australia.

28. National Centre on Elder Abuse (2007) *Clearinghouse on Abuse and Neglect of the Elderly (CANE) Selected Annotated Bibliography*. Available at http://www.elderabusecenter.org/ default.cfm?p=cane_ea_assessment.cfm (viewed 24 April 2007).

29. American Psychological Association. *Elder Abuse and Neglect: In Search of Solutions*. Available at http://www.apa.org/pi/aging/eldabuse.html (viewed 29 November 2007).

30. Elder Abuse Prevention Unit (2007) Available at http://www.eapu.com.au/ (viewed 29 November 2007).

31. Currle, S. (2001) Assessment of elder abuse, in S. Koch and S. Garratt (eds) *Assessing Older People*. McLennan & Petty, Sydney, Australia.

32. National Guideline Clearinghouse (2007) *Elder Abuse Prevention*. Available at http://www. guideline.gov/summary/summary.aspx?ss=15&doc_id=6829&nbr=4196 (viewed 24 April 2007).

33. Office of the Public Advocate Victoria (2007). Available at http://www.publicadvocate. vic.gov.au (viewed 29 November 2007).

34. Nolan, M., Grant, G. and Keady, J. (1998) *Assessing the Needs of Family Carers*. Pavillion Publishing, East Sussex, UK.

35. Nay, R. (1995) Nursing home residents' perceptions of relocation. *Journal of Clinical Nursing*, 4(5), 319–25.

36. Victorian Community Care Coalition (2006) *Moving to Centre Stage: Community Care for the Aged Over the Next 10 Years*. NOUS Group.

37. Bartlett, D.F. (1999) The new health care consumer. *Journal of Health Care Finance*, 25(3), 44–51.

38. Cameron, I.D. (2003) Aged care issues and services in Australia. *Annals of the Academy of Medicine, Singapore*, 32(6), 723–7.

39. American Psychological Association (2000) *Diagnostic and Statistical Manual of Mood Disorders IV-TR*. American Psychological Association, USA.

Further readings

Legislation which is specifically relevant to community care:

The Aged Care Act (1997) and the Aged Care Principles which can be accessed from the Department of Health and Ageing. Available at www.health.gov.au/internet/wcms/publishing. nsf/Content

Legislation related to the changed funding of aged care after the introduction of the GST, A New Tax System (ANTS) (Goods and Services Tax) Act 1999, determinations by the minister for aged care under ANTS. Available at www.health.gov.au/internet/wcms/ publishing.nsf/Content

The nurses acts vary from state to state in Australia. Available at the Nurses Registration Board in each state.

Other recommended reading:

Kitwood, T. (1997) *Dementia Reconsidered.* Open University Press, UK.

Davis, S., Nay, R., Koch, S., Andrews, G. and Byers, S. (In press) *Creating Dementia Friendly Social and Physical Environments.* Department of Human Services, Victoria, Australia.

Nay, R. and Garratt, S. (2004) *Nursing Older People: Issues and Innovations.* Elsevier, NSW, Australia.

Ebersole, P., Hess, P., Touhy, T. and Jett, K. (2005) *Gerontological Nursing and Healthy Aging.* Elsevier & Mosby, St Louis, USA.

Nolan, M., Grant, G. and Keady, J. (1998) *Assessing the Needs of Family Carers.* Pavillion Publishing, East Sussex.

Chapter 18

Palliative care

Cathy Bennett and Dianne Roughton

Introduction

Facilitating the choice to receive care at home and being able to die at home for people with life-limiting illness involves rewards and challenges for the community nurse. Quality home-based palliative care relies on competent and skilled community nurses to meet the needs and goals of clients and their carers/families.

The focus of this chapter is to examine the issue of palliative care within community nursing contexts. Assessment, symptom management, associated complications and support for the emotional, physical, psychological and spiritual needs of the client and family will be examined. The aim of this chapter is to enhance nurses' understanding of the practicalities of nursing a person who is dying in their own home, which requires complex and considerate health care support in the community setting.

What is palliative care?

'Palliative care is the active total care of clients whose disease is not responsive to curative treatment. The goal of palliative care is achievement of the best quality of life for clients and their families' [1, p. 3]. The principal intent of palliative care is to ameliorate symptoms and maximise the quality of the person's remaining life [1]. Palliative care relates to the care of people who have a progressive, life-threatening illness, and who are confronting death in the foreseeable future or those who have a life-limiting illness [2].

Palliative care:

- Affirms life and regards dying as a normal process.
- Supports a client-centred role in decision making.
- Suggests and assists relief from distressing symptoms.
- Integrates the psychological, emotional, spiritual and social aspects of care for the client, the family and carers.
- Aims to encourage a 'death-with-dignity' approach to care.

- Recognises the need for support of the family and carers after the client's death.
- Respects the client's wishes, preferences and convictions, as a fundamental principle of autonomy.
- Aims to achieve effective symptom management according to the client's requests [3–10].

Client care has a multidisciplinary focus in palliative care and includes:

- Relief of pain and other symptoms wherever possible through discussion with the client/carer and health care team.
- Discussion of and planning for the psychological, spiritual, emotional, cognitive and social impacts of the client's illness, with the client and family/carers [11].
- Awareness that care of the carers continues after the client's death; bereavement is a part of the process [12].

Community palliative nursing operates as part of the multidisciplinary team supporting a dying person; however, the nurse is the team member who may see most of the client and family at home. This close contact gives the nurse a unique opportunity to get to know the client and the family, and is often a position of trust.

Sound communication skills together with thorough and regular symptom assessment are the cornerstone of skills required to assist the client to manage the frequently changing symptoms associated with a life-limiting illness, such as pain/discomfort, distress or fatigue [13]. Communication skills can be learnt and developed. Reflecting on experiences assists the nurse to prepare for future situations and to strengthen their confidence in managing difficult situations [14].

Social and emotional support is an important facet of the community palliative nursing experience. The need for empathy, compassion, trust building, respect and good listening skills is essential to supporting a person and family through their journey.

Holistic care of a client who has a life-limiting illness in the community should have a multidisciplinary approach. Referrals to health professionals or groups should be included in this approach and may include:

- General practitioner (GP).
- Palliative care team (medical consultant and/or pain specialist).
- Palliative care team (nursing consultant).
- Equipment service providers (for home-safety assessment and/or equipment).
- Palliative care support group (positive effects on quality of life through social support and contact) [15].
- Pastoral care worker (or chaplain).
- Social worker.
- Physiotherapist or occupational therapist.
- Stoma therapist.
- Wound care specialist.
- Volunteer.
- Complementary care therapist.

Assessment

Before commencing any formal assessments, a detailed explanation of care that is available should be given to the client in 'easy-to-understand' language. A focus should be on gaining an informed consent from the client or carer [16]. However, the assessment relies on far more than clinical information. The nurse must assess the client as a whole, taking a holistic approach to health care delivery. Fundamental issues may be:

- How ill is the client?
- Where is the client (both physically and emotionally) on their journey?
- What are the client's expectations regarding nursing care and support?
- What is the client's preferred care setting?
- Can adequate resources be provided to support the client's expectations?
- What are the client's priorities, including intervening treatments and spiritual issues?
- How does the client communicate with carers and what is the nature of the relationship?

The assessment focus may change from curative to palliative care, from the stable to the terminal phase, until 'end of life' occurs [17]. Information is gathered from a combination of active listening, noting odours, observation, skilled interviewing and an understanding of the underlying disease processes [16].

Assessment will also seek to obtain:

- Client age, sex, address, phone number, home location/map reference and other contact phone numbers (such as a neighbour when appropriate).
- Complete illness history to assist the community nurse to develop an understanding of the client's disease process and to contribute to initial care planning, in conjunction with the client, family or carers.
- Essential information about underlying pathology and disease progress, such as hospital discharge letters; reports or communication (which may include verbal information from the client or family) which may detail the person's primary diagnosis; and investigations and/or treatments which may indicate the severity and prognosis. It is important here to gain an understanding of the client and carer's knowledge of prognosis and diagnosis.
- History of other illnesses. Client medication often gives a representation of other illnesses and conditions that the client is being treated for. Be aware that particular symptoms may be attributable to another illness, and the client may have underlying conditions that may complicate the management of the presenting disease.
- Family history of other illnesses. A family history of illnesses and past deaths can enhance the community nurse's knowledge of other significant losses and alert the nurse to other family members who may be at risk of contracting the disease.

Genograms and ecomaps

Genograms and ecomaps [17] are visual documents that 'map' both family structures and support systems that create the client's environment. The mapping allows for identification of significant 'others' within this framework and assists with care planning.

Genograms also identify prior bereavements within families, which can indicate the potential risk of complicated bereavement in caregivers. A genogram looks very much like a family tree, with all terminal illness diagnoses attached to individual family members names. It is then easy to see patterns of illness at a glance.

Physical assessment

Regular and ongoing assessment of the palliative client has a focus on:

Symptoms

- Pain (including type, severity and location).
- Non-pain symptoms (such as dyspnoea, cough or haemoptysis, nausea/vomiting, fatigue, anorexia, oral or genital thrush and continence) [18].

After the initial assessment, a plan to prioritise symptom management must be developed in consultation with the client and/or carer.

General appearance

- Skin colour, integrity, oedema, redness, bruising, jaundice, tumour/swelling, fungal irritation or pruritus.
- Facial expression.
- Body language and positioning.

Psychological state

- Insomnia, anxiety, fear, depression and confusion.

Functional assessment

A component of community palliative care is the need to assess the client's functional abilities. By examining the capacity of the client to perform activities of daily living in their home environment [19, p. 143] (such as walking, weight bearing, transfers, showering and dressing), a plan of care incorporating appropriate supportive care and safety factors can be developed in consultation with the client and family. Assessment tools may be useful.

Questions to consider are as follows

- Is a referral for equipment required to facilitate showering, transfers or pressure area care?
- Is the equipment easily accessible?
- Does the client have pain when moving?

As the client's physical status deteriorates, so does functional capacity, thus requiring ongoing assessment and documentation. Changes can be sudden and unpredictable.

The need for equipment to facilitate mobility of the client, transferring and the maintenance of comfort, as well as the safety of the client, carer and visiting nurses requires assessment and documentation at each visit and when a change has occurred.

Physical environment

Another component of community palliative care is the need to assess the client's physical environment, including:

- Bed safety – height, cot sides, accessibility for nurse/carer to move/slide client, comfort and brakes.
- Floor space – room to transfer client from bed to chair (lifter possibility).
- Chair – height, mechanism to assist client to stand and comfort.
- Bathroom – shower accessibility, light, ventilation, privacy and warmth.
- Animals – restrained or locked away (a safety risk assessment needed).
- Oxygen therapy – tubing lengthy and free from kinks, no open flame near cylinder.

Ongoing assessment

Functional ability, physical environment and symptom management is assessed and documented at every visit. The nurse must consider:

- The use of a symptom assessment tool that can be utilised at each visit for thorough assessment of symptoms.
- The implementation of a terminal-phase pathway when the health status of the client deteriorates and death is impending.
- Assessment at each visit of the carer's ability to continue caring for the client at home, and the need for increased home support and/or respite, especially if the client lives in a remote area with limited face-to-face support.
- Plans of care which are continuously updated and reviewed, in consultation with the client, as management strategies are evaluated.
- Notification of changes to the multidisciplinary team (generally the GP and/or palliative medical and nursing specialist), and referrals for increased services made, as appropriate.
- The frequency of visits, guided by the physical and emotional status of the client.

Medications

In order to manage new or uncontrolled symptoms, documentation and assessment of the client's response to medications should occur at every visit. Through discussion with the client or carer, a need to change either medications or doses of medications may be concluded, which must also be discussed with the GP or palliative care specialist.

Equally important is the supply and availability of the client's medications, in order that they can be given either by nurses or by carers. Some medications are not readily available and pharmacists may need advanced warning to supply them. It is important that the nurse plans several days ahead to ensure that the supply is ongoing, particularly for client's in rural or remote areas who may not have a regularly available pharmacy service.

Planning

The following planning is necessary in community palliative care:

- Provide the client and carer with a plan of when to expect visits, and the name of the community nurse who will attend the next visit (if known).
- Provide written information in the client's spoken language at home.
- Seek consent from the client to inform their GP of the community nurse's involvement with the client and the plan of care.
- Encourage the client and carer to contact the community nursing service if they have questions related to palliative care provision.

Symptom management

Oncology in palliative care

Radiotherapy

More than 50% of radiotherapy has palliative intent to control local symptoms, such as pain, haemorrhage and obstruction [20]. Palliative radiotherapy is generally a local treatment and effects are limited to the site to which it is delivered. Certain tissues and organs are particularly sensitive to radiation and care is taken to protect these organs from the energy beam. A client's decision to utilise radiotherapy may depend on several factors, such as:

- Understanding/cognition of the process and potential side effects.
- Body image sensitivity.
- Self-management of transient symptoms (such as nausea/vomiting or incontinence).
- Previous experience of the treatment.
- Cultural or spiritual constraints or beliefs.
- Transport availability.

Radiotherapy can be effective and appropriate for the following symptoms:

- Bone pain.
- Pathological fracture.
- Spinal cord compression (SCC).
- Local haemorrhage, including haemoptysis, haematuria, vaginal or uterine bleeding and skin tumours.
- Pain due to tissue infiltration, such as hepatomegaly, splenomegaly, chest wall invasion, sacral tumours and nerve damage.

- Bronchial obstruction.
- Dysphagia from carcinoma of oesophagus or pressure from lymph nodes.
- Central nervous system (CNS) symptoms due to cerebral metastases.
- Advanced fungating skin lesions [21].

Community nurses can monitor potential side effects to radiotherapy such as fatigue and skin irritation.

Chemotherapy

Chemotherapy, the treatment of disease by chemicals [19], is a systemic treatment which affects the entire body. Chemotherapy impacts on dividing cells, such as cancer cells, normal epithelial and bone marrow cells. The use of chemotherapy in the palliative setting is restricted by its limited effect on solid tumours and the intolerance of normal tissues to the drug's toxicity. The community nurse may be involved in the management of potential post-chemotherapy reactions such as nausea, vomiting and diarrhoea management.

Surgery

Surgery can present useful control or relief of symptoms and may improve the client's quality of life; however, palliative surgery has no expectation of cure. Examples include:

- Local surgery to control symptoms due to obstruction, such as dysphagia or bowel obstruction. This may include stenting, stoma formation or insertion of a percutaneous endoscopic gastrostomy (PEG).
- Surgery to relieve compression such as spinal cord or debulking of cerebral metastasis.
- Stabilisation of pathological fractures around a bone metastasis, particularly when a long bone is involved.
- Control of bleeding such as cauterisation or cryotherapy to a bronchial carcinoma, or embolisation of blood vessels supplying a fungating breast tumour.

Neurological symptoms

People may experience neurological symptoms due to primary or metastatic disease, treatments for that disease, medication adverse effects or concurrent illnesses. In many cases these symptoms may not be easily controlled. Clients with malignant disease are at risk of tumour invasion of structures in the head or spinal cord, by direct spread or via metastasis. Signs and symptoms of cerebral tumours may vary according to the site of the tumour, and can include:

- Headache.
- Visual disturbance.
- Altered consciousness or cognitive changes.

Table 18.1 Summary of symptom management for cerebral tumours [22].

Symptom	General management	Drug therapy
↑cerebral oedema	Support and assess client	High-dose IV steroids[a]
Gross tissue growth	Surgical excision	Nil
Cerebral inflammation	Radiotherapy	Adrenal steroids
↓physical coordination and mobility	Equipment referral/support	Nil
Convulsion/seizure	Assess Dr ABC	Anticonvulsant, antianxiety or sedative medication[b]
↓physical coordination and mobility	Equipment referral/support	Nil

[a] Strong adrenal steroid medication, such as dexamethasone assists, to reduce cerebral oedema and is a common drug used in palliative care. High doses are used initially; therefore, clients on dexamethasone therapy must be monitored for undesirable side effects of excessive and/or long-term use.

[b] If seizures are recurrent, the family or carer can be taught to administer rectal benzodiazepine medication to the client in their home. Regular blood-level monitoring of ongoing dosages should occur.

- Marked personality changes, including loss of inhibitions and emotional lability.
- Motor dysfunction (such as speech and hand–eye coordination).
- Nausea and vomiting.
- Convulsions.

Personality changes can be distressing to carers and family. The nursing care and support required is often physically heavy, as client mobility and physical coordination deteriorate. Table 18.1 summarises drug and non-drug management for symptoms of cerebral tumours [22]. These include:

- Cushingoid facies (moon-faced appearance).
- Proximal myopathy (weakness of large muscles).
- Gastrointestinal (GI) bleeding.
- Opportunistic infections (particularly candidiasis).
- Weight gain/increased appetite.
- Steroid-induced diabetes.
- Psychosis/hyperactivity.
- Insomnia.
- Night sweats.

Dexamethasone withdrawal must be gradual, as a recurrence of symptoms such as corticosteroid withdrawal syndrome (desquamation, anorexia and weight loss), acute cardiovascular collapse or a decrease in adrenal response to stress may occur. Thus the client must be prescribed a reducing dose, decreased by 50% every 5–7 days [22].

Convulsions/seizures

Seizures may be caused by pre-existing epilepsy, or:

- Brain metastases or a primary brain tumour.
- Haemorrhage.
- Medication effects, e.g. neurotoxic metabolites of pethidine, alcohol or benzodi-azepine withdrawal.
- Metabolic disturbance.
- Infection, e.g. meningitis.

Pruritus

Pruritus is a generalised persistent itch, sometimes associated with malignancy (such as leukaemia or lymphoma), commonly associated with biliary obstruction or uraemia, and may also be due to:

- Skin diseases.
- Iron-deficiency anaemia.
- Opioids following spinal use.
- Hyperthyroidism.
- Psychogenic pruritus.

Itching may present as scratch marks, with no sign of a rash. Treatable causes such as scabies and allergies should be excluded before attributing the cause to generalised diseases. Management includes:

- Discuss with the client and carer alternative options to best manage the condition.
- Avoid irritating sources, e.g. overheating and rough clothing.
- Avoid self-trauma; e.g. have cotton gloves, short nails, occlusive paste bandages on limbs to limit scratching.
- Surface cooling, e.g. local emollients [22].
- Use aqueous creams for washing instead of soap.
- Offer diversional therapy, such as music or a change in the environment.

There are no specific drugs to treat itching, but the following specific measures may help with causes:

- Change opioid where an association with morphine is suspected.
- Topical corticosteroids and/or antihistamines can be offered to treat skin conditions.
- Antidepressants may be helpful in non-cholestatic pruritus [22].

Pressure areas

Pressure ulcers are caused by localised tissue death from vascular and lymphatic impairment due to compression, tension or shear forces over a critical time period. Clients receiving palliative care are severely ill and particularly vulnerable to the development of pressure ulcers. Factors which predispose palliative care clients to the development of pressure ulcers include:

- Increasing age.
- Incontinence.
- Lean-body constitution.
- Pain-predisposing reduced mobility.
- Paralysis or weakness, secondary to brain metastases, SCC, neurological injury or cerebrovascular accident.
- Ascites or oedema.
- Reduced tissue perfusion, secondary to poor nutrition, dehydration, anaemia, radiation fibrosis and low albumin levels.
- Loss of weight – bony prominences.
- Drugs, e.g. steroids causing increased skin fragility.
- Decreased spontaneous movement caused by sedation effects of medication [23, 24].

Prevention strategies

- Keep skin clean and as free as possible from contamination with urine and faeces. Urinary catheterise where necessary to reduce skin contamination.
- Minimise friction and shearing forces by use of a slippery sheet when sliding client. Covering the wound with film dressing will protect skin; however, it may not be appropriate for exuding wounds.
- Pressure relief over all bony prominences, e.g. large-cell ripple mattress or pressure-relieving mattress, sheepskins and 2- to 3-hourly pressure area care.
- Client/family education regarding the need for regular pressure area care.
- Maintenance of adequate nutrition and hydration where possible.

Lymphoedema

While oedema may have a variety of causes, it is appropriate to consider the management of all types of oedema collectively, as it is rare for oedema to exist without some degree of lymphatic involvement. Common causes of oedema are:

- Changes to cell permeability due to chemotherapy agents.
- Obstruction and/or dilatation of major veins by tumour; e.g. inferior vena cava presents by massive bilateral and genital oedema; portal vein or superior vena cava (SVC) presents by bilateral limb swelling.
- Poor lymphatic drainage, due to tumour obstruction, surgery to lymph nodes, radiotherapy (long-term effects) and lymphangitis (inflammation of lymphatic channels).
- Cardiac or renal failure causes pitting oedema.
- Drugs, e.g. steroids, non-steroidal anti-inflammatory drugs (NSAIDs) and calcium-channel blockers.
- Venous hypertension presents as varicosities or venous ulceration.
- Metabolic changes; e.g. hypoproteinaemia (low albumin) presents as massive bilateral and genital oedema.

Management of oedema

- Elevation of the limb and the use of diuretics may be effective with some types of oedema (e.g. cardiac origin) and with early lymphoedema, but it is unlikely to help hypoproteinaemia or advanced lymphoedema. Oedema in the lower limbs may predispose a client to falls and reduced mobility.
- Passive limb movements and mobilisation (with support and observation of a carer to reduce risk of falls).
- Treat the identifiable cause, e.g. cardiac failure and steroids for tumour reduction. Radiotherapy may be considered if oedema is due to tumour obstruction.
- Support, e.g. compression stockings, compression bandaging or custom compression garments. (Check arterial sufficiency prior to initiating this.)
- Gentle lymphatic massage by a trained therapist or carer. Clearing lymph channels proximally first and then gradually working distally along the limb. (Creams, oils or powders should not be used with lymphatic massage.)
- Severe oedema is a poor prognostic sign, and may indicate lymphatic failure or thromboembolus. Truncal lymphoedema is distressing and debilitating, and compression bandaging of limbs may be inappropriate due to further exacerbation of swelling.

Respiratory symptoms

Respiratory difficulties in palliative care clients are common and can be due to multiple causes. Symptoms may be chronic or acute and frequently initiate fear, panic and anxiety in the client. Symptoms are also often a source of distress to carers/family and community nurses as they can be difficult to influence.

Dyspnoea

Dyspnoea occurs in 70% of clients in the terminal phase of life at some time during the last weeks of life, and may be defined as a subjective sensation of being unable to breathe and therefore can only be determined by the person experiencing it [13, 26]. Table 18.2 shows the causes of dyspnoea [26]. If breathlessness appears, reassessment of the client is paramount.

Identifying the cause of the dyspnoea is imperative to managing the symptoms and supporting the client. Breathlessness may not necessarily be related to a malignancy. Regardless of the medical management instigated, nursing can play a vital role in assisting the client in the management of dyspnoea in the following ways:

- *Environment:* Nursing interventions aimed at reassurance, comfort (sitting the client in the high fowlers position) [19], and improving airflow in the room may assist the client greatly.
- *Reassurance:* The client is supported in a calm and reassuring manner.
- *Anxiety:* Anxiety which often leads to panic attacks is a common component of dyspnoea. While reassurance and explanation may help to alleviate some anxiety, medication for anxiety may be required, and is usually of benefit.

Table 18.2 The main causes of dyspnoea [26].

Reduction in functional lung tissue	Impaired lung expansion	Airway obstruction	Cardiovascular	Anxiety
Lobectomy	↑diaphragm ascites	Tumour fistula	CCF LVF SVC	Fear of
Pleural effusion	Enlarged liver phrenic	Oedema	Obstruction	choking
Lymphangitis	Lesion-uncontrolled pain	infection	Haemorrhage	Past
Chemotherapy		Aspiration	Pericardial	experience
Radiotherapy		Consolidation	Effusion	Emotional
Infection		Collapse	anaemia	issues
Pulmonary			Uraemia	Depression
embolis				Fear of
				suffocation

- *Complimentary Therapies:* Relaxation, massage, visualisation and/or meditation may help to influence exacerbation of dyspnoea related to anxiety.
- *Family Support:* Nurses play an important role in reassuring and offering support for carers who often feel helpless caring for their loved one who may be fighting for breath.
- *Anaemia:* Dyspnoea in association with pallor and fatigue can also be indicative of anaemia, which may be treated with a transfusion.
- *Bronchodilators:* Dilate the airways, loosen secretions, promote expectoration and maximise airway space that is not compromised by other sources.
- *Opioids:* Reduce the distress of respiratory exertion by reducing the perception of breathlessness and decreasing the ventilatory response to hypoxia and hypercapnia.
- *Benzodiazepines:* Relieve the anxiety of palliative dyspnoea.
- *Corticosteroids:* Reduce tumour bulk and oedema where these are related to infiltration of lung space by tumour.
- *Anticholinergics:* Assist to dry secretions.
- *Oxygen:* Oxygen is not routinely prescribed, as there is no benefit for a client who is not hypoxic and can therefore be contraindicated [26].

Nurses also need to initiate discussion with carers and formulate a plan regarding home management strategies in relation to medications for dyspnoea. The discussion should include:

- The availability and use of additional sedation for management of acute episodes.
- Whether the carer is willing or able to give a subcutaneous bolus of morphine.
- How much support is available and who is likely to be involved in future support for the client.
- Reassessment for continuing home care and resources that will be required.
- The use of home oxygen and the willingness of a carer to undertake the management of oxygen therapy.

A major role for the community nurse in the management of clients with dyspnoea is the identification of symptoms. Nurses should be aware of changes in the severity and onset of symptoms and should not assume that symptoms are related to the diagnosed disease.

Cough

Persistent cough is a distressing symptom for the client and carers. Support for the client with this symptom requires careful assessment, including assessment of the home environment. The nurse must determine triggers for the cough as well as provide information to the client and carer about the need for a well-filtered environment as possible prevention for this symptom. Causes include:

- Foreign matter in airways.
- Excessive bronchial secretions.
- Stimulation of receptors.
- Unrelated primary illness.
- Respiratory infection.
- Fatigue.
- Heart failure.
- Pulmonary fibrosis.
- Pulmonary effusion.

The mechanism of coughing is very important for the clearance of secretions from the airways; hence, intervention by way of prescribed cough suppressants may be contraindicated. For this reason all drug regimes must be dependent on the cause of the cough:

- *Bronchodilators and corticosteroids:* Reduce bronchospasm.
- *Mucolytic agents:* Thin airway secretions, which are easier to expectorate.
- *Nebulised saline and liquid opioids:* Moisten airways and reduce cough reflex.

Respiratory congestion or 'death rattle'

When death approaches, the client is not able to swallow saliva or cough up mucous from the trachea. Mucous pools in the trachea and larynx and breathing becomes laboured. This type of breathing is commonly known as a 'death rattle' and occurs in approximately 92% of people who are dying [13]. Family and carers may find this distressing. The community nurse plays an important role in management of death rattles in the following ways:

- Support and reassurance of carers is essential.
- Frequent repositioning of the client may also assist. Suctioning of the client has been found to have limited value as it causes mechanical trauma and is distressing to both client and carer.
- Anticholinergics, useful as a prophylactic at the first indication of secretions, when the client can no longer cough independently [21].

Hiccups

Hiccups are a spasmodic involuntary contraction of the diaphragm that results in uncontrolled inspiration of air [19]. Hiccups can disrupt client sleep for prolonged periods and the spasmodic action can bring on more pain. Causes of hiccups in a palliative care client are:

- Metabolic disturbances related to renal or hepatic failure, e.g. uraemia.
- Diseases which irritate the diaphragm, e.g. tumours of the stomach and abdomen.
- Intercranial pathology which disrupts the phrenic and vagal nerves.

The community nurse can encourage the client to attempt any number of simple non-pharmacologic measures to assist to eradicate the hiccups:

- Position the client in an upright position.
- Pharyngeal stimulation – frequent small drinks from the 'wrong' side of a cup, eating granulated sugar or placing pressure on the tongue by squeezing with a warmed flannel (held down by client fingers).
- Self-induced hypercapnia – holding breath or rebreathing into a paper bag.

If these measures fail or the client is too weak to attempt the measures, the following pharmacologic intervention may be required:

- Nebulised saline – pharyngeal stimulation.
- Sedatives or antispasmodics – relax the client and/or cause gastric relaxation.

However, there is little documented evidence of the success of these interventions and treatment should not be continued if the client does not respond [25].

Gastrointestinal symptoms

The client's inability or refusal to eat may be perceived by the carer as failing in their duty or that the client has 'given up'. There is often a strong belief in carers that if a good diet can be maintained, then death can be postponed [25].

Constipation

Constipation is a condition in which waste matter is hard to pass or in which bowel movements are infrequent [19]. It can be physically exhausting and often painful for the client. Constipation can cause the client pain, physical exhaustion when trying to defecate/evacuate and embarrassment. The nurse may consult with the client about how they self-manage constipation rather than only enquiring about bowel function [27]. Table 18.3 shows the causes of constipation [27].

Special issues in relation to management of constipation for a client receiving palliative care are:

Table 18.3 Causes of constipation [27].

Cause	Assessment	Management	Drug therapy
Opioids	History of altered bowel function	Review and monitor bowel habits daily	Oral laxative, wetting agent
Anticholinergics	History of aperient intake and response	Encourage carers to monitor daily	Oral laxative, stimulant
Antidepressants	Disease history	↑dietary fibre	**Fibre laxative not recommended**
Tumour obstruction	Dietary intake	↑oral fluids (if possible)	Osmotic agent softener
Stricture	Fluid intake	Massage	Enema
Dehydration	Analgesic history	Exercise	
↓bowel tone	Physical assessment		
Neurological disease			
Trauma – anal/rectal			
Haemorrhoids			Topical anaesthetic
Hypercalcaemia		Reverse hypercalcaemia	
Hypokalaemia		Reverse hypokalaemia	

- To promote dignity, a private, warm, comfortable environment for the client that is close to toilet facilities is paramount when supporting a client in their home.
- Diarrhoea may be overflow from impacted faeces. Consider concurrent rectal intervention when prescribing aperients to clients with faecal impaction.
- Anorexia, nausea and/or vomiting may be signs of impaction and/or obstruction.
- Constipation may precipitate urinary incontinence.
- The use of aperients in palliative care is extensive and is often influenced by the client's personal preference and habits. Failure to prevent constipation or manage it appropriately can lead to distress for clients and carers. Knowledge of the action and appropriate use of common aperients is basic to good palliative care.

For more information about the management of constipation, refer to the Chapter 11 of this book.

Anorexia

At any point on the alimentary tract – the mouth, throat, stomach, gut or bowel – a disturbance to normal function can affect the person's ability and desire to eat. Factors such as nausea and vomiting, dysphagia due to tumour obstruction, mucositis from chemotherapy or radiotherapy, constipation, altered taste and inadequately controlled pain should be discussed with the client, an assessment conducted and remedies or management options offered. Anorexia, a loss of appetite and reduced caloric intake affects between 80 and 85% of clients with cancer and is the second most frequently reported symptom [26, 28, p. 123]. Drug therapy is one option to encourage appetite:

- ETOH (alcohol) can stimulate appetite, increase calorie intake and provide subtle analgesia.

- Antiemetics can stimulate appetite.
- Corticosteroids can stimulate appetite.
- Progestational agents stimulate appetite and improve weight gain.
- Multivitamins can improve quality of calorie intake [21].

To support the client experiencing anorexia, careful explanation of the causes and choices to manage the symptoms and counselling of clients and carers need to occur. Clients often feel pressured to eat, thus causing stress, which can affect their quality of life. Carers should be praised for their good effort and reassured of the diminished importance of eating for the client, as the client deteriorates.

Nausea and vomiting

Nausea and, to a lesser extent, vomiting are very debilitating symptoms, which affect around 50% of people with cancer, and are frequently undertreated. The mechanisms producing nausea and vomiting are complex and may be multifactorial in a particular client. Nausea and vomiting are controlled by the midbrain vomiting centre that receives input from many neural pathways and neurotransmitters [26].

Communication with the client and conducting an accurate assessment ensures that treatment for nausea and vomiting specifically matches the cause, and is as prompt as possible for client comfort. Nausea and vomiting may be caused by:

- Stimulation of drugs, radiotherapy or chemotherapy.
- Gastric irritation due to drugs or by a distension of the stomach or peptic ulceration.
- Stimulation of the part of the brain (vestibular apparatus) which controls balance and motion, e.g. motion sickness and infection.
- Physical or psychological stimuli, such as anxiety and pain.
- Obstruction of any part of the bowel, e.g. constipation, faecal impaction or tumour mass.
- Oesophageal obstruction or irritation.
- Any type of compression on the stomach, e.g. enlarged liver, ascites or tumour.
- Elevated intracranial pressure.
- Metabolic disturbances, e.g. hypercalceamia, hyponatraemia and uraemia.

Communication with the client is needed to assess the likely aetiology of the nausea and vomiting. This should also include a combination of a client history, physical examination, diagnostic tests and prompt communication with the multidisciplinary team.

Medication management will be dependent on the aetiology of the nausea and/or vomiting. Drugs to control nausea and vomiting act either on the CNS or on the GI tract. If nausea and vomiting control is not acceptable to the client, combining medications (CNS and GI acting) may be successful [26].

Cachexia

Cachexia is a complex syndrome of progressive wasting seen in clients with advanced cancer, chronic heart failure and some dementia types. It is due to a combination of malnutrition and/or metabolic or nutritional requirements of a tumour. The role of nutrition is minor and cachexia cannot be prevented by enteral and parenteral nutrition [26].

Hypodermoclysis

Hypodermoclysis is the practice of administering up to 1.5 L of isotonic solution (normal saline) via a subcutaneous infusion to maintain hydration. The rate of infusion is not critical because subcutaneous fluids absorb at their own rate.

Weakness and fatigue

Weakness and fatigue are associated with a generalised feeling of exhaustion. These symptoms are most frequently associated with the progression of a life-limiting illness and do not respond to increased relaxation or rest by the client. Fatigue affects the physical, psychosocial and social well-being of the client and is known to be both multifactorial and multidimensional [29]. There are three types of fatigue:

- Generalised physical weakness – making it difficult to initiate activities
- Reduced physical stamina – producing early tiring
- Psychological fatigue – with loss of motivation, drive, memory and concentration

Often people experience all three types of fatigue, which may further complicate drowsiness, sleepiness and altered sleep behaviour. As weakness and fatigue are common and impact on many facets of the client's life, the nurse must assess the client for treatable causes, which may enhance the client's quality of life.

Pain management

Pain is what the client says it is [21]. Pain is the most common symptom for a client in the last days of life [30]. Pain in terminal conditions may be due to the disease process, treatment or unrelated causes, and many clients may have more than one pain. Physical pain is often compounded by psychological, emotional, social, cultural and spiritual factors, which must be understood if the community nurse is to be successful in managing pain [31].

Pain management principles

- Pain management must be approached in a holistic manner, considering the whole client and not just one aspect of his/her condition.
- Pain is a constantly changing phenomenon and distress related to pain symptoms has an impact on the client's well-being [32].
- Pain may be modified by psychological, cultural and spiritual factors and attention to these is essential to support the client and manage their pain.

Table 18.4 Pain management [21, 26].

Type of pain	Drug therapy	Non-drug options
Somatic	Non-opioid analgesic Weak opioid Strong opioid Non-steroidal anti-inflammatory drugs (NSAIDs) Steroids Antidepressants	Radiotherapy immobilisation heat/cold irrigation of mucosa
Visceral	Non-opioids analgesic Weak opioid Strong opioid NSAIDs Steroids Antispasmodics Antidepressants	Radiotherapy pressure/heat chemotherapy
Neuropathic	Opioids – often in other drug combinations Membrane stabilisers Steroids Epidural local anaesthetic neurolitic procedure	Radiotherapy transcutaneous electrical nerve stimulation
Psychogenic	Antidepressants anxiolytics	Counselling/support

- Establish the cause of the pain before commencing or changing any therapy.
- Communication with the client to ascertain aspects of pain assessment are crucial.
- Pain assessment must occur regularly, respecting the client's cultural and personal values, in order to plan care strategies to support the client in their home environment.

Pain involves physical and psychological factors which are shown in Tables 18.4 and 18.5 and Figure 18.1 [21, 26]. Pain from physical causes may be:

Nociceptive – The activation of normal pain fibres, causing impulses to be carried along peripheral nerves to the spinal cord. These impulses are carried up the spinal cord, through the brain stem to the thalamus, and delivered to various areas of the cerebral cortex, which allows the perception of, and reaction to, pain. This pain may be:

- Somatic, involving skin or superficial structures.
- Visceral, involving deeper structures (such as organs or muscle).

Neuropathic – Due to nerve damage or nerve compression occurring anywhere in the pain pathway. Such pain may be

- Peripheral (sciatica).
- Central (post-therapeutic neuralgia).

Table 18.5 Types of pain [21, 26].

SOMATIC – The stimulus for somatic pain may either be superficial or deep

Cancer-related cause	Non-cancer-related cause	Treatment-related cause

Superficial somatic
  Malignant ulcers
  Stomatitis
Deep somatic
  Related to tumour
  Bone metastases
  Liver capsule distension
  or inflammation
	Pre-existing conditions such as
	arthritis
	Pressure due to immobility
	Immobility itself
		Post-radiotherapy
		Mucositis

Description of pain: Superficial somatic is often described as burning or stinging, whilst deep somatic is reported as dull or aching

Localisation (to site of stimulus): In both superficial and deep somatic pain, localisation is well defined

VISCERAL – Poorly localised, diffuse and often aching in quality

Cancer-related cause	Non-cancer-related cause	Treatment-related cause

Capsular stretch
  Liver secondaries
  Primary kidney mass
  Colic spasms
  Any obstruction of the
  hollow viscera
	Bowel obstruction
	Constipation
	Cardiac pain
		Constipation due to
		medication regime

Description of pain: Visceral pain is often described as dull or aching in quality

Localisation (to site of stimulus): It is poorly defined

NEUROPATHIC – Neuropathic is described as either mixed or pure in aetiology

Cancer-related cause	Non-cancer-related cause	Treatment-related cause
Tumour invasion or compression of nerve pathway Oedema causing pressure on nerve	Post-surgical neuropathic pain Post-hepatic neuralgia Phantom pain	Nerve damage due to any cause, e.g. surgery Chemotherapy Radiotherapy

Description of pain: Neuropathic pain may present in many ways: abnormal sensation, pins and needles, tingling, burning, shooting and phantom

Localisation (to site of stimulus): Nerve or dermatome distribution

PSYCHOGENIC: Any type of cancer-related pain plus any psychogenic pathology, e.g. anxiety, or known psychiatric condition is considered psychogenic pain

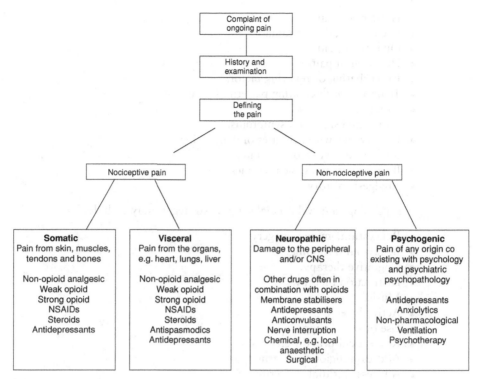

Figure 18.1 Pain management.

Radiotherapy and chemotherapy for pain management

Radiotherapy – Radiotherapy remains the most effective treatment of local metastatic bone pain with response rated consistently of the order of 80% within 48–72 h after initiation of therapy [33] and complete pain relief in a significant proportion of clients.

Chemotherapy – The use of chemotherapy in pain management has some benefits; however, it is dependent on the type of tumour, sites of spread and phase of illness.

Transcutaneous electrical nerve stimulation – Transcutaneous electrical nerve stimulation (TENS) can be offered to the client as an alternative or to complement drug pain management. This electrical device transmits electrical impulses and blocks pain impulses from the peripheries to the CNS and has been found useful for some clients with neuralgia and for a variety of aches of soft issue origin.

Clinical assessment of pain

Good pain management starts with accurate assessment of the cause, type and pathophysiology of the pain. Clinical assessment of pain requires a comprehensive review, including:

- Is there one pain.
- Site of pain, does it radiate.
- Quality of pain.
- Duration of pain.
- Exacerbating or relieving factors.
- Temporal or fluctuating pattern of pain.
- Exact onset.
- Associated signs and symptoms.
- Interference with activities of daily living.
- Impact on psychological state.
- Response to analgesic therapies.
- Analgesic history.

Psychological/psychosocial support strategies may include:

- Relaxation, guided imagery.
- Behavioural training.
- Cognitive therapy.
- Distraction therapy.
- Music.
- Active listening.
- Use of social support.
- Respect cultural differences.
- Address religious concerns.
- Address spiritual concerns.

Chronic pain

Chronic pain persisting after healing is expected to be complete or is caused by a chronic disease. It can be further categorised into cancer and non-cancer pain. Transdermal synthetic opioids (such as fentanyl patches) offer a non-invasive approach to pain management for clients with chronic cancer and non-cancer pain, whose compliance with oral medication (possibly due to nausea, dyspnoea or dysphagia) is poor [34].

Principles to manage chronic pain

- Analgesia – 24-h pain relief.
- Commence regular non-narcotic medication.
- Assess and identify characteristics of pain.
- Prophylactic antiemetic.
- Oral/parenteral/topical routes most common.
- Regular aperients essential.
- 2/24 breakthrough dose orders.
- With opioids use caution in renal impairment.
- When stable – consider converting to 12-hourly slow-release preparations.

Parenteral opioid

- If converting oral opioid doses to parenteral doses, remember to review current opioid conversion rates (e.g. 30-mg *oral* morphine = 10-mg IM/SC/IV morphine).
- For safety reasons, opioid infusions should be by subcutaneous route.
- For opioid naïve clients, SC prn orders may be more appropriate than a continuous infusion.
- Antiemetic may be mixed in the same syringe with opioid and administered by subcutaneous infusion if nausea and/or vomiting are prominent.

Mouth care

Regular and thorough assessment of the condition of the client's mouth should be a principal consideration in the nursing care of the palliative care client. Thorough inspection of all mucosal surfaces such as the tongue and throat should be undertaken if the client is agreeable or physically able to assist. Removal of dentures will aid the viewing of the entire oral mucosal membrane.

Importantly, the mouth is a vital organ and so poor mouth hygiene can affect many social interactions for the client, such as power of speech, ability to smile and the ability to eat and drink [21].

Management options

Encourage the client or carer to carry out the following mouth care 'as required' wherever possible:

- Inspect oral cavity regularly using torch and tongue depressor.
- Encourage frequent mouth rinses and regular mouth care.
- Brush teeth, gums and tongue.
- Use 'Jumbo' swabs for dependent or unconscious clients.
- Establish presence of dentures and ensure removal during oral hygiene regime – soak dentures overnight.
- Apply lubricant to lips frequently.
- Support the application and administration of medications, e.g. antifungal, local anaesthetic and analgesia.
- Promote the use of frozen fresh-fruit cubes, e.g. pineapple or melon.
- Promote the use of effervescent soft drinks, e.g. soda water, ginger ale and champagne.

Neurological/psychological symptoms

Anxiety/fear

Anxiety is a conscious feeling of fear and danger without the ability to identify immediate objective threats that could account for the feelings [13]. The symptoms of anxiety may occur in different situations in clients with cancer and should be regarded as a continuous clinical spectrum ranging from normal to psychiatric, mild and fleeting to severe and disabling [21].

Fear is a common experience in the face of death, not only for the client but also for their family, and is seldom expressed in words. The client may experience either fear of death, fear of the unknown, or feeling out of control in the process of dying. The client may experience emotional or spiritual fears, triggered by a sense of guilt or punishment for some hidden wrongdoing [35]. The physical or somatic manifestations of anxiety overshadow the psychological and are the symptoms the client most often reports. Anxiety occurs in response to the stress and crises associated with cancer and its treatment. It is a personal experience influenced by past feelings and situations.

Some anxiety can however be related back to physical causes and the nurse needs to assess for treatable causes of anxiety, through a thorough assessment and effective communication with the client or carer. Treatable causes of anxiety include pain, hypoxia, any uncontrolled or severe physical symptom, and drug withdrawal or drug reactions.

Strategies for management of anxiety include:

- See the client at regular intervals (where possible), as the development of trust and rapport with the client provides reassurance and facilitates ongoing expression of feelings.
- Work towards relieving physical discomfort wherever possible.
- Listen to what the client is saying and avoid premature reassurances.
- Correct the client's or carer's misconceptions about the disease, its treatment and pathophysiology. Information can reduce uncertainty and provide clients with a sense of control over their circumstances.
- Complementary therapies such as visualisation, meditation and massage may be useful.

Pharmacological treatment of anxiety involves the following classes of medication:

- Benzodiazepines – both short and long acting, as an antianxiety agent.
- Antihistamines – act as a sedative to reduce anxiety.
- Opioids – reduce respiratory drive (where anxiety is related to dyspnoea) [36].

Depression

The National Palliative Care Programme defines depression as 'a pervasive and sustained lowering of a person's mood and demeanour. A cluster of symptoms which include guilt, tearfulness, irritability, lethargy, poor concentration and poor sleep patterns' [37, p. 81]. Symptoms of depression are reported to occur in approximately 25% of clients with a terminal illness. Sadness and depressed mood can be an appropriate response in the terminally ill client; 50% of clients will experience a symptomatic adjustment reaction [21]. As a client approaches death, depression may be one of the stages which they experience.

Depression not only impacts on clients' and carers' quality of life but also on their acceptance of palliative treatments and therapies [37]. Furthermore, there is evidence of an association between difficult physical symptoms and depression.

Whilst pharmacological interventions are offered to the client for the management of depression, the client's prognosis and the time frame for treatment play an important role in determining the treatment selected. Optimal therapy is known to succeed only when other aggravating or causative factors, such as pain or anxiety relating to social, cultural or spiritual issues, are discussed and/or resolved with the client. Resolutions may take some time and much support, and some anxieties for the client may never be resolved. The role of the nurse here is to offer the client options such as counselling, pharmacological intervention or privacy/time.

The choice of antidepressants depends on the side-effect profile, existing medical conditions and drug interactions:

- *Tricyclic antidepressants:*
  - Improve sleep within days
  - Stimulate appetite and weight gain
  - Coanalgesic effect within 3–7 days
  - Antidepressant effect within 2–4 weeks
- *Selective serotonin reuptake inhibitors (SSRIs):*
  - Antidepressant effect within 4 weeks
- *Monoamine oxidase inhibitors (MAOI) – not recommended*
  - Antidepressant effect within 4 weeks (severe drug and food interactions) [22]

Confusion/delirium

Confusion/delirium is a common symptom that is distressing to the carer/family and can be a challenge to remedy. In more than half the cases, a definitive diagnosis of the cause(s) cannot be made. Investigation must be appropriate to the stage of the client's disease and the prognosis. Mild states of confusion or non-frightening hallucinations may not require intervention especially if the client does not show noticeable signs of distress. For moderate-to-severe states of confusion, antipsychotics or sedatives can be used with caution.

Caring for a client who is confused, delirious and agitated is extremely challenging for carers and families and is associated with feelings of helplessness. Carers need reassurance and education about their role in helping to support and calm the client. For the carer, feelings of helplessness and desperation are usually worse at night, and the provision of a night nurse to stay with the client may help to ease this duty, while the client is stabilised. This may take more planning if the client lives in a rural or remote area and care delivery is hard to access.

Terminal restlessness

As death approaches, between 40 and 80% of clients may experience motor restlessness (terminal restlessness), fear, anxiety, mental confusion with or without hallucinations, or a combination of these symptoms [21]. Communication with the client becomes progressively difficult and rapid deterioration usually occurs as the client progresses from being semiconscious to unconscious. Even if the client appears unconscious, he or she may respond to words spoken by a significant loved one. This may alleviate or help to reduce client and or carer/family distress.

The causes of restlessness may be physical, psychological, environmental, pharmacological, social and spiritual. Providing prompt and appropriate attention to the reversible physical causes (e.g. distended bladder or faecal impaction) will greatly aid in settling the client.

Other resources to assist with restlessness should be considered, including referral to social workers, counsellors and pastoral care workers. Effective communication between all members of the caring team and carers is essential to ensure that appropriate and supportive treatment strategies are initiated.

Complementary therapies such as music, touch or massage may assist. Frequent reassessment is essential and increased visits from community nursing services may be required in consultation with the carer.

Oncological emergencies

People with cancer or other life-limiting illnesses are at risk of life-threatening medical emergencies caused by complications of the disease itself or its treatments. Nurses who know which clients are at risk can promote early detection and treatment of oncological emergencies, many of which are completely reversible if treatment is administered promptly.

Superior vena cava obstruction

SVC obstruction, as shown in Table 18.6, is a disorder of venous congestion caused by obstruction of venous drainage in the upper thorax. The SVC is particularly vulnerable to obstruction because of its thin walls, low venous pressure and anatomic location.

Table 18.6 Superior vena cava obstruction [21].

Causes	Clinical features	General treatment	Drug therapy
Enlarged lymph nodes	Oedema, face, neck, upper limbs	Bed rest with head elevated	Oxygen administration
Thoracic tumour	Dyspnoea	↓fluids and NaCl	Chemotherapy
Thrombosis	Dilated hand veins Cough/hoarseness Chest pain Dysphagia Headache Blurred vision Vertigo, syncope	Aid airway patency Support client Educate carer/family	High-dose diuretic Radiotherapy Stat. corticosteroids Thrombolytics Anticoagulants

Table 18.7 Spinal cord compression [21].

Clinical features	General treatment	Drug therapy
Central back pain[a]	Surgery	Corticosteroids
Bladder distention	Rehabilitative, supportive care	Radiotherapy
Paraesthesia	Physiotherapy	Analgesia only (terminal)
Loss of anal tone	Carer education, support	
Faecal leakage		

[a]Back pain is the earliest sign of SCC and occurs in more than 95% of clients with this condition approximately 6–7 weeks prior to the onset of any clinical features [21]. Successful reversal requires very prompt treatment.

The onset of symptoms is often slow, and varies greatly between clients. Diagnosis of SVC obstruction is made on assessment of suspicious findings; chest X-rays or computed tomography scans will usually reveal a mediastinal tumour.

Spinal cord compression

SCC, as shown in Table 18.7, is a disorder caused by direct pressure on the spinal cord. A tumour (usually a bony metastasis in the vertebra) grows and causes compromised vascular supply to the area, resulting in spinal cord infarct or vertebral collapse. Approximately 5% of people with metastatic disease develop SCC [21, p. 157].

Hypercalcaemia

Hypercalcaemia is the most common life-threatening metabolic disorder associated with cancer, occurring in more than 10–20% of clients with cancer and as many as 20–40% of clients with cancer of the bronchus [38, p. 448], breast, kidney, lymphoma or multiple myeloma. Hypercalcaemia is defined as a serum calcium or corrected calcium, greater than 11 mg/dL. It usually occurs in the context of advanced disseminated malignancy and can produce a number of distressing symptoms for the client. Causes and general management are shown in Table 18.8.

Table 18.8 Hypercalcaemia [38].

Causes	Clinical features	General management	Drug therapy
Listed cancers	Pruritus	Rehydrate	IV hydration
Dehydration	Hypertension	Encourage mobility	Diuretics
Immobilisation	Cardiac arrhythmias	Weight bearing	Bisphosphonates
Fractures	Polyuria/dehydration		Corticosteroids
Renal insufficiency	Excessive thirst		
	Confusion		

Table 18.9 Catastrophic haemorrhage management [21].

Causes	General management	Drug therapy
Erosion, infection of vessels	Prevention – chemotherapy, radiotherapy, surgery	Sedation – to reduce awareness of fear
Malaena Heamaturia Malignant wounds Haemoptysis Thrombocytopenia Obstructive jaundice Haematemesis	Absorb blood in dark towels Discuss client fears Discuss carer fears	Opioids

The goal of medical management of hypercalcaemia is to *reduce* bone reabsorption of calcium and increase renal excretion of calcium. Repeated treatment for hypercalcaemia is usually offered to the client monthly, depending on the client's condition and prognosis.

Catastrophic haemorrhage

Major haemorrhage in palliative care is rare; however, the fear of haemorrhage is common, as shown in Table 18.9. There are a range of conditions that predispose people to a high risk of catastrophic haemorrhage. In these situations it is essential that preparation, education and support of the client and caregiver have been provided. Practical advice such as having easy access to dark-coloured towels, administration and access to subcutaneous medication (e.g. opioids and/or sedatives) and calling for assistance is fundamental. Careful consideration needs to be given to the appropriateness of teaching some caregivers in the management of medication administration in this situation, due to its stressful nature. Importantly, however, any caregiver who has had to manage a catastrophic haemorrhage at home will require prompt follow-up and support to assist them in the early bereavement period.

Complementary therapies

Many complementary therapies offer a holistic approach, which incorporates body, mind and spirit, similar to the fundamental philosophy of nurses. This closeness of complementary therapy to the concept of holism means that nurses must have an understanding of the basic concepts of complementary therapies, which in turn encourages them to think and work in new and modern ways [39, 40].

It is important that nurses have a general understanding of specific therapies that their clients are engaging in. Nurses should not sabotage the relationship and trust with the client through insensitive enquiry about why they are pursuing a particular therapy. In a sensitive manner, it is appropriate for the nurse to investigate:

- The understanding for the client of the potential benefits, side effects and costs of the treatment.
- The treating practitioner's qualifications and affiliations and their ease with working with other treating medical officers.
- Practicalities of alternative therapy commencement in the client's home (client privacy, space and comfort).
- An inadequate knowledge of either the nurse or the client about a particular therapy or a concern that the therapy may be harmful.

Some of the most popular complementary therapies are acupuncture, massage, meditation, aromatherapy, dietary manipulation, homeopathy, music therapy, lymphatic massage, faith and spiritual healing, hypnosis, visualisation therapy, herbal medicine and vitamin and mineral therapies.

Understanding and learning about the particular alternative therapy your client is engaged in will not only assist your ongoing symptom management assessment and care planning, but also provide a perspective and understanding of how the client prioritises their needs and treatment strategies in relation to their disease process.

Researching alternative therapies requires time and effort on behalf of the practitioner but has valuable outcomes for the client, their caregivers and the treating practitioners. Maintaining trust, professionalism and respect for people's choices in relation to their treatment preferences is always essential to care delivery; however, the planning and delivery of care must always be balanced with 'duty-of-care principles'. Requests by clients to receive treatments that are not approved by the Therapeutic Goods Association (TGA) require sensitive discussion with the client on boundaries of professional practice requirements. Seeking further guidance from the wider treating team can be useful if uncertainty exists on safe practice codes.

Carer support and assessment

A carer can be defined as a person who provides a substantial amount of care on a regular basis for which they are not paid in any form [41]. The majority of caring is provided to a dying client by the family or carers or close friends, 24 h a day.

To support informal carers the nurse needs to be acutely aware that the welfare of the client and carer are inextricably linked. Deterioration in the welfare of one will inevitably affect the other. Key aspects to carer support include:

- *Provide information and explanations:* For example keep carers informed of clinical changes and plans for the future needs of the client and involve caregivers in decision making if the client is agreeable.
- *Provide practical help and social support for caregivers:* For example ensure carer has 24-h phone support/advice phone numbers; prompt the carer to develop a roster system among friends and relatives to provide respite; recognise different coping styles of individual family members (social worker referral may assist); and suggest respite to ease the stress and burden of care. Remember that volunteers

are a valuable resource that can be accessed through palliative care services, local councils, church or community groups.

- *Provide caregiver with education:* Take time to explain and train caregivers in particular skills required for client care outside of nursing visits; provide clear written instructions for all procedures, where possible, to reduce carer feelings of frustration or inadequacy; and encourage written records of the client's progress and administered medications.
- *Provide emotional support:* Encourage carers to verbalise any difficulties they are experiencing; provide information about support groups for carers which are available in most areas, both during the terminal illness and in the bereavement period; and acknowledge the importance and involvement of carers in providing care.

Carer assessment

The carer's ability and willingness to continue to support a dying family member or friend at home may change with time, depending on numerous factors, including:

- The nature of the relationship between the client and the carer.
- The carer's physical health and strength.
- The carer's emotional state, which may fluctuate from day to day.
- The duration of care and the carer's expectations of the experience.
- The nature of the client's symptoms, and how well they can be managed.
- The level of support available from family, friends and the community.

These factors may change from day to day, and from hour to hour, and the nurse needs to assess the carer at each visit and provide the support that is likely to help the carer to cope with each factor. Effective communication with a carer will not only provide a forum to verbalise their concerns and fears but allow for reflection and the potential realisation that home-based palliative care can result in life-enriching experiences for the carer [42].

Psychospiritual issues in palliative care

Culture

Nursing philosophy embodies the belief that a high standard of care should be provided to individual clients regardless of their beliefs, practices, race, religion, colour or creed – otherwise known as 'culturally competent care'.

Particular issues for nurses related to culture include:

- Intergenerational conflict.
- Insensitivity of health professionals (i.e. lack of knowledge relating to cultural differences).
- Communication barriers (i.e. identify the decision maker within the cultural context).
- Issues of gender (i.e. women preferring female rather than male nurses attending personal care).

Strategies for upholding clients' cultural beliefs include:

- Show a genuine willingness to learn from and accept the guidance of carers.
- Arrange a family meeting – preferably early in the care process. A family meeting can serve to establish the ground rules for the nurse and the client/carer/family that will support a plan of care.
- Offer the use of an interpreter to enable the client to 'speak freely' in their own language.
- Access culturally appropriate community groups.
- Provide information about the community nursing service.
- Discuss the cultural aspects of death, dying and funeral procedures which are important to the client and the family [43].

Spiritual care

Spiritual care involves recognising the value of the individual and their personal beliefs and feelings, hopes and fears, and affirming who they are with unconditional acceptance. Spirituality encompasses the relationships and partnerships that can emerge among nurses, the client and family or carer [16], and has a central role to play in the provision of care for the terminally ill client [44]. Positive health outcomes for the client associated with spirituality include:

- Enhanced coping skills.
- Improved quality of life.
- Reduction in anxiety and depression [45].

Feeling comfortable with listening to a client's anguish in searching for answers to questions like 'why me?' and 'why now?' and the meaning of 'mental suffering' or their anticipation of whether there is life after death, or merely oblivion, requires mental energy rather than answers.

Death of a client and bereavement care

As the client's condition deteriorates and enters the terminal phase, the client and family may request support and assistance to prepare them for the death. Contacting a funeral director in advance to support and facilitate a client's involvement in the planning of their own funeral may be a request.

Anticipating and initiating discussion about management of the death at home can be difficult but is usually welcomed by the carers, who may have little or no experience in this area. It is important to remember that the way in which people die will remain in the memories of those who live on [46, p. 483].

Immediately following the death

Families deal with death in their own way. Some wish to keep their loved one's body at home for a longer time to say farewell, while some are quite distressed and want to have their loved one's body removed as soon as possible. There is no need to wash or lay out the body, but if the family wishes to be involved, they are often grateful for the opportunity to help the nurse wash and tidy the body before other family and friends arrive.

In Australia, certification of death is normally required from a medical officer prior to funeral directors collecting the body from the home. The death certificate (showing causes) can be written later. It is important that nurses are aware of the *requirements specific to their regional area of work* (e.g. who will certify death after hours in their region? Where is the best place to store the body until funeral directors can attend in remote and rural areas?) These are essential pre-planning requirements of any home death and it is important that the family and caregivers have a clear understanding of this process to minimise confusion and distress following the death of the client.

Bereavement support

Bereavement is a time for remembering and supporting the family/carer in the reality of loss or grief by way of active listening and acknowledging occasions for tears, and not discouraging expressions of grief [47]. It is important for the nurse to understand the following four phases of bereavement:

- Shock.
- Anger.
- Despair.
- Acceptance/adjustment.

and to reassure the bereaved that changed 'feelings' and state of mind after the loss of a loved one is normal and that support is available.

Grief follows a similar path to bereavement and it is important that loved ones are supported through this process, offered professional counselling if necessary and contacted again by the nurse up to 1 month after the death to offer continued support. Knowledge of local grief support groups and professional counsellors will assist prompt referral of carers to appropriate services if required.

Community and professionals' support networks

Working within the field of palliative nursing can provide many personal challenges and rewards in the daily work environment. In some situations, working effectively with those issues and challenges will require support and professional guidance from others. It is important for all personnel working in palliative care to know and understand their local and wider professional support networks to assist them in the provision of good service delivery. Some examples are palliative care nurse forums; regional palliative care and hospital services; regional hospice networks; and local counselling services.

Information and support is also available via the internet, and one of the most common palliative care websites is Palliative Drugs Ebulletin (www.palliativedrugs.org/), where exchange of ideas about medication use is utilised in a variety of settings.

Summary

This chapter has demonstrated the importance of nursing knowledge in palliative care, including client assessment, management of disease complications and support for family/carers, including bereavement support. As the population ages and more life-limiting disease conditions are managed within community settings, nurses will continue to need to strengthen their knowledge in the area of palliative care delivery.

Acknowledgement

The authors acknowledge that the contents of this chapter have been adapted from the RDNS' *Principles of Palliative Care: Clinical Practice Guidelines* (2006).

References

1. Doyle, D. (2003) Editorial. *Palliative Medicine*, 17, 9–10.
2. Palliative Care Australia (2005) *Standards for Providing Quality Palliative Care for All Australians*. Palliative Care Australia, Canberra.
3. Commonwealth Department of Health and Ageing (2003) *Evidenced Based Clinical Practice Guidelines in Palliative Care for the Multi-Disciplinary Team*. The National Palliative Care Program, Commonwealth Department of Health and Ageing, Canberra.
4. Van Kleffens, T., Van Baarsen, B., Hoekman, K. and van Leeuwen, E. (2004) Clarifying the term 'palliative' in clinical oncology. *European Journal of Cancer Care*, 13, 263–71.
5. Johnson, D., Kassner, C. and Kutner, J. (2004) Current use of guidelines, protocols, and care pathways for symptom management in hospice. *American Journal of Hospice and Palliative Care*, 21(1), 51–7, 80.
6. Tearfund, A., Mathew, A., Cowley, S. and Bliss, J. (2000) The development of palliative care in national government policy in England, 1986–2000. *Palliative Medicine*, 17, 270–82.
7. Goncalves, J. (2003) Palliative care and the principles of biomedical ethics. *European Journal of Palliative Care*, 10(4), 158–9.
8. Buckley, J. (2002) Holism and a health-promoting approach to palliative care. *International Journal of Palliative Nursing*, 8(10), 505–8.
9. McNeal, G.J. (2002) End of life issues in a palliative care framework for a critically ill adult African American with cystic fibrosis: A case study. *Journal of Cultural Diversity*, 9(4), 118–27.
10. Seymour, J.E. (2004) Negotiating natural death in intensive care. *Social Science and Medicine*, 51, 1241–52.
11. Bayliss, J. (2004) Counselling skills in palliative care, in B. Nyatanga (ed.) *Aspects of Social Work and Palliative Care*. Cromwell Press, Wiltshire, UK, p. 176.
12. Cannaerts, N., de Casterle, B. and Grypdonck, M. (2004) Palliative care, care for life: A study of the specificity of residential palliative care. *Qualitative Health Research*, 14(6), 816–35.
13. The National Palliative Care Program (2004) *Guidelines for a Palliative Approach in Residential Aged Care*. Edith Cowan University Publishing, Cowan, Western Australia.
14. Simpson, M. (2003) Principles and practice of palliative care. *Nursing Management*, 9(9), 9–12.
15. Goodwin, D, Douglas, H. and Normand, C. (2003) Effectiveness of palliative day care in improving pain, symptom control, and quality of life. *Journal of Pain and Symptom Management*, 5(3), 202–12.

16. Hudson, R. (2003) Aged care nursing, in S. Carmody and S. Forster (eds) *A Guide to Practice*. Ausmed Publications, Melbourne.

17. Venning, M. (ed.) (1996) Palliative nursing care: A community perspective. Care of the terminally ill client and their family. *1996 NRS018 Diploma of Nursing Course Booklet*. South Australian Health Commission Publishing, Adelaide, Australia.

18. National Consensus Project for Quality Palliative Care. (2004) *Clinical Practice Guidelines for Quality Palliative Care*. National Consensus Project, Pittsburgh.

19. Miller-Keane, B. (1992) *Encyclopedia and Dictionary of Medicine, Nursing and Allied Health*, 5th edition. W.B. Saunders Publishing, Sydney, Australia.

20. Hoskin, P. and Makin, W. (1998) *Oncology for Palliative Medicine*. Oxford University Press, New York.

21. Palmer, E. and Howarth, J. (2005) *Palliative Care for the Primary Care Team*. Issues for the Primary Care Team. Butler and Tanner Limited, Somerset, UK.

22. Commonwealth Department of Health and Aged Care (2000) *Australian Medicines Handbook*. Finsbury Press, Thebarton, South Australia.

23. Gray, M. (2005) Skin care of the incontinent patient. *Advances in Skin and Wound Care*, 18(3), 138–9.

24. Henoch, I. and Gustafsson, M. (2003) Pressure ulcers in palliative care: Development of a hospice pressure ulcer risk assessment scale. *International Journal of Palliative Nursing*, 9(11), 474–84.

25. Therapeutic guidelines (2001) *Palliative Care Version 1*. Therapeutic Guidelines Limited, Melbourne.

26. Whitecar, P, Maxwell, T. and Douglass, A. (2004) Principles of palliative care medicine. Part 2: Pain and symptom management. *Advanced Studies in Medicine*, 4(2), 88–100.

27. Cadd, A., Keatinge, D. and Hessen, M. (2000) Assessment and documentation of bowel care management in palliative care: Incorporating patient preferences into the care regimen. *Journal of Clinical Nursing*, 9(2), 228–35.

28. Waller, A. and Caroline, N. (1996) *Handbook of Palliative Care in Cancer*. Butterworth-Heinemann, Boston.

29. Coackley, A., Hutchinson, T. and Saltmarsh, P. (2002) Assessment and management of fatigue in patients with advanced cancer: Developing guidelines. *International Journal of Palliative Nursing*, 8(8), 381–8.

30. Bravemen, C. and Cohen, L. (2000) Dialysis discontinuation and palliative care. *American Journal of Kidney Diseases*, 36(1), 140–44.

31. Mitchell, G., Bowman, J. and McEniery, H. (February 2001) The blue book of palliative care: Evidence based clinical guidelines for primary practitioners. *Australian Journal of Rural Health*, 9(1), 53–4.

32. Volker, D.L. (2003) Assisted dying and end-of-life symptom management. *Cancer Nursing*, 26(5), 392–9.

33. Frassica, D.A. (2003) General principles of external beam radiation therapy for skeletal metastases. *Clinical Orthopaedics Related Research*, 41(5), 158–64.

34. Noyes, M. and Irving, H. (2001) The use of transdermal fentanyl in pediatric oncology palliative care. *The American Journal Hospice Palliative Care*, 18(6), 411–16.

35. Maddocks, I. (1994) Part 2: Patient assessment, in *Symptom Control (Education Package of GPs)*. Southern Hospice Foundation, Adelaide.

36. Lloyd-Williams, M. (1996) An audit of palliative care in dementia. *European Journal of Cancer Care*, 5(1), 53–5.

37. Hotopf, M., Chidgey, J., Lan, L. and Addington-Hall, J. (2002) Depression in advanced disease: A systematic review: Part 1, Prevalence and case finding. *Palliative Medicine*, 16(2), 81–97.

38. Doyle, D., Hanks, G. and MacDonald, N. (eds) (1996) *Oxford Textbook of Palliative Medicine*. Oxford University Press, New York.

39. Bennett, J. and Robinson, A. (2005) District nursing: Evolution or extinction. *Journal of Community Health Nursing*, 19(4), 26–8.

40. Bennett, J. and Robinson, A. (2005) District nursing: Opening the doors to reality. *Journal of Community Health Nursing*, 19(3), 26–7.

41. Hearn, F. (2004) Setting up a support group for carers in palliative care. *European Journal of Palliative Care*, 11(5), 204–6.

42. Stajduhar, K. (2003) Examining the perspectives of family members involved in the delivery of palliative care at home. *Journal of Palliative Care*, 19(1), 27–35.

43. Ahmed, N., Ahmedzai, S., Vora, V., Hillam, S. and Paz, S. (2005) *Supportive Care for Patients with Gastrointestinal Cancer* [Review]. The Cochrane Library, The Cochrane Collaboration. John Wiley & Sons, Ltd, UK.

44. Nyatanga, B. and Astley-Pepper, M. (eds) (2005) *Hidden Aspects of Palliative Care*. Tranbridge, Cranwell Press, Wiltshire.

45. Wasner, M., Longaker, C., Fegg, B. and Masio, G. (2005) Effects of spiritual care training for palliative care professionals. *Palliative Medicine*, 19(2), 99–104.

46. Rabow, M., Hauser, J. and Adams, J. (2004) Supporting family caregivers at the end of life: 'They don't know what they don't know'. *Journal of Advanced Medicine*, 291(4), 483–91.

47. Funnell, R., Katarkidis, G. and Lawrence, K. (2005) Loss, grief and death in nursing care, in E. Tabbner (ed.) *Theory and Practice*. Marrickville, Elsevier, NSW.

Further reading

Palmer, E. and Howarth, J. (2005) *Palliative Care for the Primary Care Team*. Quay Books, London.

Chapter 19

Personal care

Scott King and Elaine Tooke

Introduction

The purpose of this chapter is to examine those activities identified as personal care and to understand the community nurse's role in assisting people to perform personal care. Personal care activities are a fundamental part of everyday life. They are activities that most people do each day without thinking and are skills that everyone has learnt from a young age for maintaining cleanliness, social image and social acceptance. As we grow and develop, we learn to care for ourselves in a number of ways and develop routines and patterns for life. Community nurses may assist people in personal care when the person is unable to attend to these activities.

For many nurses, personal care conjures up images of showering and sponging, which are often seen as meaningless tasks that have a relatively low rating on the scale of importance. These tasks are not glamorous; they are not usually highly technical and may be considered by some to be arduous, but needing to be performed anyway. Known also as activities of daily living (ADLs), these include eating, bathing, dressing, toileting and transferring. Such tasks are engaged in by all in order to maintain health and social acceptability. Each individual has their own ideas on how they like to look (the way we dress, the way we do our hair). Often these preferences make us who we are; they are the image we present to the world and are intrinsic to how we perceive ourselves and can also be a mirror to how we feel.

The Northern Territory Home and Community Care Personal Care Standards (2004) consider personal care to be:

- Assistance with daily self-care tasks, such as:
  - Bathing, showering or sponging.
  - Dressing and undressing.
  - Shaving, hair care and grooming.
  - Toileting.
  - Limited nail care, only following appropriate professional assessment.
  - Mobility and transferring (getting in and out of bed and moving about).
  - Eating, drinking, cooking and food preparation.

– Monitoring with self-medication.
– Fitting and the use of appliances such as splints, hoists, hearing aids and communication devices [1].

When people are unable to perform these activities independently, due to frailty, illness or disability, there is a risk of loss of independence, loss of self-esteem, alterations to skin integrity, inadequate nutrition, constipation and urinary and faecal incontinence which may lead to their needing assistance and may require the person to move from their home into institutionalised care [2].

Feeling independent is essential to an individual's quality of life and well-being [3]. The term 'independence' attracts widespread emphasis and debate in policy and research. What is also important is the individual's perception of what constitutes independence. Perception is an essential component of nursing assessment which will be addressed later in detail in this chapter, as the person being assessed may perceive that they are managing well despite any contradictory evidence [3].

The scope of the issue

Although people across the lifespan may experience difficulties performing personal care, the prevalence of people requiring assistance is higher for older people. Within the older persons population, assistance with ADLs rises steeply with advancing age and is particularly high for persons aged 85 years and over [4]. This need may primarily arise as the persons functional ability, movement and dexterity are affected, which in turn readily turns into lethargy. Chronic diseases such as arthritis, dementia, heart disease and chronic obstructive airways disease are common diseases that affect older people's ability to adequately self-care. People with disabilities are living longer and have an increased need for care assistance. For people with a disability, recognising a deterioration in health and being able to access appropriate services may also be an issue.

In 2003 the Australian Bureau of Statistics conducted a survey titled 'Disability, Ageing and Carers in Australia'. The results showed that:

- One in five people in Australia (3 958 300 or 20.0%) had a reported disability. The rate was much the same for males (19.8%) and females (20.1%).
- Of those with a reported disability, 86% (3 387 900) were limited in the core activities of self-care, mobility or communication. Most people with a disability (76%) were limited in one or more core activities.
- There were 3.35 million people aged 60 years and over (17% of the population), compared with 3.0 million people (16%) in 1998. In 2003, just over half had a reported disability (51%) and 19% had a profound or severe core activity limitation.

Of people aged 60 years and over, 41% reported needing assistance because of disability or age-related decline, to manage health conditions or cope with everyday activities. However, people aged 85 years and over reported a much greater need for assistance than those aged 60–69 years (84% compared with 26%) [5].

With the Australian community comprising a large number of people who are ageing or who have a significant disability, or both, it is inevitable that community nurses will be engaged at some time to care for people requiring assistance with personal care. The community nursing role may incorporate assessment, liaison, referral and establishment of a system of personal care that is viable to meet the health needs of the person, whether in a support and maintenance capacity or a postacute capacity.

The intimacy of personal care

Nurses provide care to complete strangers that at times can be intimate and invasive, in an environment that stretches social boundaries and comfort zones. So unique is this work of nurses, it can entail managing, discussing and confronting issues and sensitive topics that society in general may consider taboo. Some of these sensitive topics may include, but not be limited to, issues of sexuality: a man performing work that has traditionally been seen as female orientated, performing work that is considered 'dirty' by definition of dealing with and managing body products and waste and functions and invading intimately the personal space of a person in the performance of body care. These issues are considered private and personal by society, but are primary tasks and functions that nurses undertake in dependent situations numerous times and in diverse environments.

The care and touch provided by nurses can also be very comforting to people who are suffering or who require help. Bottoroff [6, p. 303] states that 'the nurse patient touch, has frequently been linked to caring, and this is the connection that many nurses make initially when developing rapport and therapeutic relationships. The reverse of this is that a comforting touch can also be invasive and can reduce a person's sense of being – to feeling nothing more than an object or thing, not a person – particularly when they are feeling unwell or self-esteem is greatly compromised [7]. This is of particular importance when considering that the environment in which community nurses work is the person's own home, which is often where people feel most safe, secure and in control.

Nurses' perceptions

Nurses' attitude and the perception of how nurses show care for the person's body are important. Biases and opinions are critical points to consider when analysing attitude. Personal care can be categorised or prioritised by some nurses into degrees of importance, considering the impact on people's quality of life. Acknowledgement of our own biases, whether good or bad, is critical to avoid people being made to feel or being considered as objects of care. A way of illustrating this, and to assess clinicians' attitudes, is to reflect on two situations (Scenarios 19.1 and 19.2). Both these situations require tact, diplomacy and a great deal of empathy in management; however, traditionally they are managed quite differently. Consider the impact that you could have either positively or negatively on each scenario, with your current attitude and biases regarding personal care and how that may change when considering and acknowledging this attitude.

Scenario 19.1

Allesandra is a successful 32-year-old business woman. She has undergone a double mastectomy due to metastatic breast cancer. She requires palliative support as well as personal care daily. Allesandra is angry and scared and is struggling with her perceptions of no longer feeling or looking like a woman. Allesandra has not allowed her boyfriend of 7 years to see her naked since her operation.

Scenario 19.2

Reginald is an 85-year-old war veteran. He suffered a stroke 2 years ago and has substantial health issues including mobility and faecal incontinence. Reginald has offered you as the community nurse keys to his home. When being visited for personal care, Reginald is often incontinent of faeces and is embarrassed and depressed by his inability to control his bowels.

The community nurse would invest time into planning care which could include resourcing, case management, counselling and advocating when working with both clients. The nurses would be cognizant of working with Allesandra to increase her self-esteem. Rapport building and the development of a solid relationship between nurse and client would be critical to the success of any interventions with both of these clients. In each scenario, the nurse's attitude and awareness of their own biases are essential in the development of therapeutic and mutually respectful nurse/client relationships.

The development of interpersonal relationships can be a challenge for any community nurse. The community nurse is a visitor in home-based care and as such relies on their communication skills to quickly develop a rapport to facilitate cooperation with care. McCann and Baker [8, pp. 532–5] suggest some useful strategies that can easily and effectively enable the development of a rapport with clients in the community who are living with a mental illness. These strategies have a high degree of relevance to anybody suffering from a self-care deficit. The strategies include:

- Try to understand the client's experience of living with a dysfunction that affects the ability to self-care. Allow extra time to listen to their experiences and their perspectives on how well or how much difficulty they are experiencing.
- Be friendly. This is a critical strategy to attempting to enable a mutually respectful and cooperative relationship.
- Tune in. The key point of tuning in is to be ordinary. This requires nurses to give consideration to their own appearance and mannerisms when interacting with clients. It also requires taking into account and adjusting to the way the client dresses, communicates and the types of approaches that the client prefers, to gain cooperation and even influence health behaviours.
- Reveal yourself. When appropriate, be open with clients and talk about yourself. The process of self-disclosing is a useful strategy to help put both clients and the

nurse at ease. Although revealing could be perceived as dissolution of professional boundaries, it does not imply that nurses reveal private and personal information. In fact extreme care should be taken to avoid this. It is important to try and improve the client's perception of power, so they have the ability to make informed choices and influence their own care. This can be instrumental in achieving better health outcomes as well as improving emotional and general health, in comparison with clients who perceive themselves as not having a choice and hence lacking power [8]. Be present for the person. It is important to be reliable and accountable for the care that is provided to the client.

- Maintain confidentiality. It is the primary premise for a safe, professional relationship [9].

Culture, gender and other considerations

Community nurses working with people from diverse cultures must act with cultural sensitivity. To be culturally sensitive a model of person-centred care is critical. A person-centred care approach acknowledges the beliefs, values, wants, needs and desires of individuals. The approach also demands that professional relationships develop that enable and promote flexibility, mutuality, respect and care [10]. Within a person-centred care approach, culture is an essential component when assessing, planning, implementing and evaluating the personal care of individuals. Within Australian communities, there may be subcultures of people from diverse ethnic backgrounds. In order to make an accurate assessment of the person's needs there may be a need to modify an existing assessment tool to include some questions about culture. Spradley and Allender [11] suggest six factors to include when modifying an existing assessment tool for cultural assessment:

1. Ethnic or racial background.
2. Language and communication patterns.
3. Cultural values and norms: what are their values and standards regarding roles, education, family functioning, ageing, child-rearing, death and dying, and rites of passage?
4. Biocultural factors: are there any predispositions to disease or illness?
5. Religious beliefs and practices: how do they influence health and illness?
6. Health beliefs and practices: what are the beliefs regarding prevention, treatment and cause?

Personal culture

In addition to traditional culture, personal culture is a subissue that needs careful consideration in the assessment and planning phase of care. Individuals may not align themselves with a particular culture. However, they may appreciate and practice small components of many cultures and establish their own rules or morals to abide by, coined a 'personal culture' [12]. Without a thorough assessment of needs, personal cultural issues can easily be overlooked and this can be very detrimental to the relationship that needs to develop between the nurse and the person requiring care.

Rapport building is a critical skill in these circumstances and the demonstration of an attitude that is non-judgemental and non-biased. There are numerous issues that could develop from this oversight, including embarrassment, difficulties with language (written or verbal), comprehension and poor communication. For example an older woman may not want a male nurse to provide personal care. This may not be a direct link to a particular culture, but may be more of a personal cultural issue. Some may rightfully say that this is allowing for choice, but a critically thinking nurse will reflect on why the woman has chosen this stance? Perhaps one answer is that it is a direct reflection of the individual's personal culture, what they believe is right and morally acceptable for them. In turn, it may not be the person themselves; it may be advocates who are advocating a culture, whether that be personal or otherwise. Again, an issue could arise where parents of a daughter with a disability may not want a male carer to provide intimate and invasive personal care. These instances could pose significant resourcing problems for service agencies and require careful consideration.

Consent

Consent can be verbal or non-verbal, whether that is written, indicated by nodding or implied. It is critical that in a dependent situation, for example in the provision of personal care, the nurse cannot assume that it is reasonable and okay to touch a person without consent. For frail older people or people with a disability, relationships with health professionals can be threatening as they can involve an unequal power relationship and expose vulnerabilities [13]. In the work environment of community nurses, this may translate to a threatening situation where the perception is that the nurse is assessing the person to determine their capacity to cope at home or if higher level care is required. This 'threat' or perceived threat may translate to a person who desperately needs personal care or other nursing care to refuse entry into the home, which in turn could greatly jeopardise the longevity of the person staying at home. Adversely, community nurses have great potential for enabling people to cope, positively focusing on strengths and developing supports for their weaknesses. In regard to personal care practices, community nurses can make a critical difference in supporting or eroding people's sense of self, their sense of self-power and esteem and their identity [13].

Gender and culture

Gender issues are another consideration in the management and maintenance of the body. Particular issues that can be impacted on by gender are communication, self-expression and sexuality. In relation to communication, there are many cultures where men have limited communication and interaction with women. For Indigenous Australians, 'women's business' and 'men's business' are held separately and not discussed in front of the opposite sex [14]. This can pose a particular barrier and issue for clinicians in assessing an Indigenous person of the opposite gender. It may be considered more appropriate to talk to people other than the person when discussing particular issues or situations. It is important for community nurses to manage these situations with sensitivity, tact and diplomacy.

Sexuality

Self-expression, sexuality and body image during personal care may be challenging and confronting for community nurses. With touching, caressing and washing of body parts including genitals, physical reactions can occur in both men and women. In people who may have difficulty in differentiating reality, or who may be suffering from isolation, deprivation of human touch and depression, provision of personal and intimate care may be taken as a gesture of consent to reciprocate. It is critical in these situations that boundaries be established and that if such situations occur, the person is left alone in a safe and secure environment to deal with any issues that they need to attend to. Attitudes and the reaction of the nurse are important in not berating or marginalising the person. In the community setting it may be necessary that the nurse leaves the person's home. This highlights the uncontrolled work conditions of community nurses who are required to assess risk and employ strategies to promote safety for themselves and clients at all times.

Body image

Body image is another issue to consider in the overall managing of personal care. Body image can be seen as the person's concept of their physical appearance. This concept is fluid and changes as people grow, age and mature. It is body image that is responsible for a person's sense of identity [15]. The term 'alteration in body image' is one that appears frequently in care plans of clients who may have undergone radical surgery, trauma, medical treatment, processes of ageing or disabilities, whether physical, intellectual or both [16]. Community nurses can assist clients by affirming their feelings, fears, hopes and aspirations. It is this connection, contact and level of interaction that enables community nurses the privilege to assess and better address issues of body image disturbances [16].

The astute clinician with good observation skills would identify and make correlations between alterations in body image and appearance and the environment that the person is living in. This may be as simple as the client looking outwardly different, not washing or grooming and their house being dirtier or more unkept than usual. Correlations can be clearly made in this instance when the change in body image is seen with a changing environment, which is real, tangible, symbolic, internal and external to the physical body [16]. Observations such as this can be subtle but are critical in early detection and management of some complex issues such as depression and isolation. Often these noted changes can trigger further assessments by the community nurse and guide early intervention and management strategies to prevent them from becoming worse or critical. It may entail referral to other agencies for services, consultations with general practitioner (GP) and other specialists and perhaps even more intense family involvement.

Counselling is an important aspect of addressing body image change with clients, who may be going through a grieving process. Counselling may assist the client to see, address and accept the change and other complicated issues such as sexuality and their expression of themselves. Remember that body image is the outward expression of who we are, what has made and created us, and what we have to endure on a daily basis [16].

Specific roles of the community nurse and community programmes

With policy changes and reallocation of funds from acute care to community settings, trends are focused on supporting older people and those with disabilities to remain at home and receive care, instead of being relocated to hospitals or aged care facilities. Community programmes can be tailored to meet specific needs. Governments are supportive of this redirection of funds to meet the needs and preferences of people and to reduce the costs to the taxpayer [13]. In the 2007/2008, Australian budget funds of up to $411 million have been allocated to support older people to remain in their own homes. An increase in aged care packages supporting people with low- and high-level needs has occurred, from 5000 places in 1996 to 40 000 places in 2007/2008 [17]. These statistics have implications for the provision of nursing care in the community and the shift in the type of care to be provided.

Assessment

It is clearly evident that community nurses have a critical role to play in the assessment, planning, implementation and evaluation of personal care.

Enabling and capacity building to encourage people to stay at home for longer are critical components of a successful strategy to support this trend. Accurate, useful and timely assessment is crucial. The community nurse is in an excellent position to undertake an effective functional assessment to identify strengths, highlight weaknesses and enable effective planning to support and maintain current abilities.

The first step when receiving a referral for personal care support is to conduct a holistic assessment, using an appropriate and user-friendly assessment tool. With this, the community nurse can begin to identify areas where supports or aids are required and to develop a plan of care. Assessment can begin from the first contact a nurse has with the client. For example if the first contact is a telephone call to make a time for the community nurse to visit, a lot of information can be revealed. During the telephone call the nurse can assess how alert the person is, whether the client or family member is stressed and whether the client has a good understanding as to why a visit is being scheduled [18]. The initial assessment should also include a discussion with the client and family members about what they perceive the personal care needs to be [12].

Once face-to-face contact is made with the client, an accurate assessment can identify whether the client is able to manage independently, or whether assistance from devices or aids may help, or if another person is required to assist them [4]. Assessment involves seeing how much the person can do themselves – are there skills that they can be taught to promote and maintain independence?

Table 19.1 provides a list of considerations and observations to stimulate thought regarding what an assessment may entail for community nurses, particularly when

Table 19.1 Assessment considerations.

Observations of client

Normal physiologic ageing and/or current functional ability secondary to a disability	What is a 'normal' or acceptable level of functioning for the person? Would this be considered the 'norm' for another person with a similar ailment?
Overall well-being and perception of health including ability to cope independently	General appearance: Is the clothing and expression of self (e.g. hair, make-up, shaving) appropriate to the time of the day? How is the person presenting themselves?
Physical issues including mobility and transfers	Movement, breathing, ability to move around
Pain	Does the person experience any pain? Are they able to state where it is, what type and how severe it is? What impact does the pain have on their everyday life?
Skin	Look for breakdown, sores that are unhealed, reddened areas, dry and flaky skin; is their skin clean?
Psychological and emotional health	How interactive is the person and are they communicating well? Making eye contact? Emotional lability
Cognitive and behavioural considerations	Look for increased confusion, behaviour changes. Observe the client: Are they acting in a way that would normally be accepted of other individuals in a similar situation? Are there any signs of depression?
Nutrition	Note food in the fridge, monitor weight of person, look at their skin and lips. Do they look well hydrated? Do they access any community nutrition services? Do they prepare their own meals?
Medications	What medication is the person taking? What are the common side effects? Are there any medications that may interact with each other? Is the client safely taking their own medications? Do any of these medications greatly impact the person's ability to undertake personal care practices?
Communication	Are there language difficulties? Do they communicate verbally or by other means? Do they require additional time for the assessment? Do they require any aids to be turned on, put on, inserted, cleaned and maintained?
Social characteristics – including issues of gender and culture	Are you the best person to be assessing this client? Is your presence compromising the findings of the assessment?
Client perspective	What are the main issues for the client? Do they wish to remain in their current setting?

Observations of environment

Cleanliness	Is the environment clean and safe? Risk assessment is essential as personal bias can greatly affect this outcome. Given the environment, is there substantial risk to the client's health if they continue living here?
Lighting	Is there adequate lighting in rooms and passages? Does inadequate lighting pose a falls risk?

Table 19.1 (*continued*)

Safety	Are there grab rails in the bathroom and toilet and near steps? What other safety devices/aids might assist the client in remaining safely in their own home?
Other supports	
Family supports and services	What supports does the person have? Who does their shopping and cooking and cleaning? What are the issues for the family?
Current services utilised and impact on quality of life	Are current services effectively meeting the need? Are they being reviewed and by whom?
Recreation and leisure status	Is the person confined to home? Are they able to and are they maintaining social supports?
Domestic considerations	What is the person's ability to undertake other skills such as cooking, cleaning and laundry?
Client perspective	Does the client express any problems with personal care? If so, what are the issues for the client? They may not necessarily be the same issues that the nurse identifies

Adapted from [18].

undertaking functional assessments for personal care. The points are not a definitive list, simply a starting point. The nurse will need to adapt their assessment skills depending on the needs of the individual client.

Safety

Safety is critical and should form part of the overall assessment of functional capacity. Safety and risks should be formalised with a risk assessment to analyse aspects of frequency of exposure to the risk, likelihood of injury and the examination of any control measures to aid in minimising the risk. Some unique safety challenges facing community nurses include, but are not limited to:

- The client's desire to bathe in a bath with no lifting equipment.
- Shower lips (recesses), shower screens, no shower hose, restricted areas.
- Poor lighting and temperature control.
- Limited access to mechanical aids or other equipment such as mobile shower chairs.
- Narrow passageways and doorways that allow little manoeuvrability with equipment and positioning.
- Slippery floors
- The client's desire to use toiletries that pose a risk to the clinician (e.g. talcum powders on slippery floors).

In order for the community nurse to address some of these hazards, it is important that they have a sound knowledge of the hierarchy of control measures in order to creatively assist in resolving some of the challenges. The hierarchy of control includes the following steps:

- Eliminate the hazard.
- Substitute the hazard with a lesser risk.
- Isolate the hazard.
- Use engineering controls.
- Use administrative controls and use personal protective clothing [19].

Safety assessments can be instrumental in assisting the client to make safe care choices regarding methods of care. The most common forms of care include showering, sponging, bathing, face/hands/back, hot towel bath and head and tail (face washing and genital washing). These choices should actively engage the client to facilitate and encourage self-care and to promote control, self-esteem and participation in care. One approach to maintaining self-care skills involves maximising continuity between an individual's past and present routines. This involves promoting what is familiar to the client. Continuing with routines learnt through long-term practice can help prevent premature decline in normal ageing and can slow the decline in independence that frequently occurs with conditions such as dementia [20]. In some instances the client might desire a particular practice that cannot be safely executed. Consider the following example and the application of the hierarchy of control in managing the choice.

The client wishes to bathe in a low bath with limited space. The client requires assistance to stand and significant assistance to move to a standing position from a sitting position as in the bath. A risk assessment would determine that this occurs on a regular basis (exposure to the risk occurs daily) and there is high risk of injury to the community nurse and the client. The hierarchy of control will be applied to determine alternatives:

- Eliminate the hazard – do not bathe the client at all due to the high risk.
- Substitute the hazard for a lesser risk – will the client accept showering as an alternative or another care option?
- Isolate the hazard – establish a contract of care highlighting the safety concerns of this practice and place effective bans on this practice.
- Use engineering controls – determine the possibility of using mechanical lifting aids, with appropriate slings and that there is enough room to manoeuvre the aid safely. Can the client stand up independently with the use of rails appropriately placed?
- Use administrative aids – use safe workplace practices, effective manual handling practices with appropriate training to facilitate the choice.
- Use of personal protective clothing – there is no personal protective equipment (PPE) that would protect from injury in this circumstance [19].

It is important to practice person-centred and individual care; however, it is just as important to work in a safe and secure environment. There is a very fine balance between the two, between clinicians working in a safe environment and minimizing risk of injury and harm and meeting the unique needs of the client empowering them to make choices regarding their care arrangement. The community nurse needs to engage advanced communication and negotiation skills to achieve the best possible outcomes for the client as well as for the clinician.

Other key points that need to be addressed as part of a thorough safety assessment are:

- Can the person perform this task with teaching or modifying a skill? It is important for the nurse and client to jointly determine the learning plan [12].
- Are there some environmental factors that have to be changed so that the person can perform the task independently and safely (e.g. rails in the bathroom, shower stool)?

Caregiver

Further questions to ask in an assessment include:

- Does the person have a caregiver?
- Can the person's caregiver provide this task – do they need teaching/coaching or support to do this?
- What training or resources does the caregiver require in order for them to provide the care?
- Is the provision of this care appropriate for a family caregiver to provide? For example is it appropriate for a grandson to administer vaginal medication to his grandmother?
- What is the impact on the caregiver?
- Is providing the care for the person putting a strain on the caregiver?

Many people who are caregivers are older or unwell themselves. A survey conducted by the Australian Bureau of Statistics in 2003 showed that there were 2.6 million carers who provided some assistance to people who had a health need secondary to disability or age. About one-fifth of these (19%) were primary carers, that is, people who provided the majority of the informal help needed by a person with a disability. Just over half (54%) of all carers were women. Of those providing care, 1.0 million (39%) were in the 35- to 54-year age range. This age group's caring responsibilities involved children, partners and/or ageing parents [5].

A study by Smith [21, p. 338] found that there were key factors that contributed to stress in people who were caregivers to family members needing high-technology care in the home. The key factors were:

- Length of time that care is provided.
- Amount of preparation that has been provided to the caregiver.
- Motivation of the caregiver to care and provide services.
- The amount of mutual assistance that may be required from other family members.
- Financial considerations.
- Coping mechanisms within the family.
- Periodic or situational depression within the caregiver role.

Another issue to consider is the length of time it takes to provide the care. Are there other family members who also need support from the caregiver? Caring is often a role performed around the clock and so the community nurse may need to determine if assistance is provided by other members of the family or community groups. Often people give up their ability to earn an income to become a caregiver and so financial issues also need to be discussed.

The coping ability of the caregiver needs to be assessed – does he/she have supports within their family or community? In some situations, support may be provided to the caregiver from a registered nurse or careworker as part of a community package. There are numerous local government supports and state- and federal-funded programmes that can provide in and out of home respite, care support, domestic and garden support through either government or non-government agencies to prevent carer burn out and specialised support. Carer support networks are also useful outlets for carers who can benefit greatly from discussing issues and talking with other carers to find that their challenges are not unique and that help is always available.

Careworkers

When assessing clients' needs, the community nurse may ask if the care can be provided by a careworker. One issue that has been debated in recent times is when it may be appropriate that someone provides the care other than a registered nurse. It is widely thought that it is not the care activity that determines the distinction; it is the person offering the care [4, 22]. So whatever caring activity or task is being undertaken, it is the knowledge, skills and experience of individual staff that will determine the outcomes of care. Although an untrained carer will bring individual experience and skills, the registered nurse has an assessed level of skill and knowledge and works to a prescribed standard of care. The key to this decision is assessment [4]. Decisions about whether a nurse or another level of worker should provide personal care can only be based on the characteristics of the person requiring the care as well as the activities to be performed.

Deciding to delegate the care raises delegation issues: Each nurse should be aware of the delegation issues in his/her own state or territory. Delegation has been defined as:

> the conferring (often referred to as transferring or assigning) of authority to perform specific functions or tasks in a specific situation, to a person whose role and function allows them to perform them but does not have the authority to perform the function or task autonomously without supervision of an appropriately qualified health professional [23, p. 14].

Table 19.2 outlines some of the questions that need to be considered before deciding that care can be provided by another level of carer.

Table 19.2 Assessment of client needs.

Client	• Is the client's health stable?
	• What are the acuity and complexity of client's health needs?
	• Is there a health plan in place?
Careworker	• What is the level of competency of the individual careworker?
	• Is the procedure within the careworker's scope of practice?
	• What supports are available for the careworker?
Enrolled (Division II) nurse	• Is the procedure within the nurses's scope of practice?
Environment	• Has an assessment of environment where care is to occur been undertaken?
	• Are there available resources?
Procedure	• What is the suitability and complexity of the task?
	• Is there a predictable outcome?

Adapted from [22, p. 14].

Perception and self-neglect

Perception is the key to understanding individuals, their patterns and coping mechanisms. Some clients may perceive themselves to be coping when their environment reveals they are not. There are a number of cues that the community nurse can draw on in their assessment of the client and their environment to determine gaps in perception and reality as described above. Discretion is essential in this process, because when confronted clients may not cooperate effectively in the assessment, jeopardising any benefits and influences that the clinician can provide to the client.

In 2004, Wang *et al.* [3] undertook research to examine the relationship between activity limitations and independence and whether these factors are mediated by an individual's coping capacity. They used four domains to collect data for this study. Manipulation of the principles of these measures provides the community nurse with a base from which to assess personal care practices. The first domain is self-perceived independence. This domain is important in all assessment activities, as it aids the clinician to determine to what extent any problems or issues the client is experiencing impact on their independence. An example of a relevant question could be, 'How much does your back pain affect your independence?'

The second domain is the activity variable. This can involve asking the client about the level of ease or difficulty they have in achieving activities. The list can include personal care activities such as bathing, showering and grooming; household tasks such as dusting, vacuuming and doing the laundry; community ability such as getting in and out of taxis or on-and-off public transport; and in-home mobility such as getting in and out of bed or climbing stairs. There are a number of assessment tools that aid in gathering information. Two of the most commonly used tools are the Barthel index and the functional assessment measure [24, 25]. The tools use rating scales to measure dependency such as from 1 to 5 or 10, with 1 being no problem at all and 5 or 10 being a lot of difficulty. Tools can add a degree of objectivity to the assessment process and help to develop consistency between assessments by different caregivers. In addition, assessment tools identify areas of need in a systematic approach to assist in care planning.

The third domain is the sociodemographic variable. This domain addresses issues such as age, education and income. The rationale behind assessing this domain is to address questions such as do differing levels of education affect the ability of individuals to access and better comprehend health promotion activities or initiatives? Does income positively or negatively impact on the individual's ability to purchase or hire equipment to aid and promote independence?

The fourth domain is coping efficacy. This domain addresses the client's confidence in undertaking different aspects or components of their own care. In practice, these domains could be used in a scenario where the community nurse is assessing a client's postcerebral vascular accident (CVA) as in Table 19.3.

Client perception can be skewed at times and contradict the evidence that lies before the community nurse. This contradictory evidence can reveal signs of self-neglect. Self-neglect can be defined as 'the failure to engage in those self-care actions necessary to maintain a socially acceptable standard of personal and household hygiene and/or a failure to adequately care for one's own health' [26, p. 14]. The issue of who has the problem in relation to self-neglecting behaviours can appear to be absurdly obvious

Table 19.3 Assessment domains for a client following cerebral vascular accident.

Self-perceived independence	Activity variables	Sociodemographic variables	Coping efficacy
Do you feel that your stroke has affected your independence? How dependent do you feel on other people?	What activities do you find the easiest and hardest to undertake since you have suffered from your stroke?	*This domain is an indicator of the client's ability/capacity to understand how to and where to access community services (i.e. local council services, GP, community health centres, pharmacy). A critical association to this is the person's ability to understand the importance of blood pressure monitoring, although this may not be directly associated with a sociodemographic variable*	How confident would you feel in showering yourself since you suffered from your stroke without any help from another person or aid?
This provides the clinician crucial information that could include needs such as grief counselling and carer respite and provides a profile of the client's self-esteem and psychological health			*This provides critical information on potential ongoing care or community service requirements*

that it is the client. However, this may not always be the case. Reports of self-neglect can be made by people who appear to be affected by the self-neglecter, such as family, friends or neighbours who make a complaint to health agencies to aid in 'fixing' the problem of issues such as incontinence, poor appearance and body odour. Some may argue that this is a lifestyle choice that the client wishes to engage in and hence the 'problem' of self-neglect is not the client's, but that of the people around the client [26].

Theories exist regarding self-neglect, such as the personal construct theory [27] where a client makes a deliberate decision to live in conditions that others would find incomprehensible, but which the client perceives to be a lifestyle preference. The structuralist–functionalist theory [28] is based on the principle that the self-neglecter is not fulfilling a role that enables a smooth function in society. Hence, the person's behaviour is open to judgement by health professionals as abnormal and they have a medical diagnosis placed on them as a measure of social validation and legitimacy. Almost a diagnostic excuse if you will. Other theories exist such as the attribution theory, which are based on a medical diagnosis, often a mental health disorder, which overemphasise mental health dysfunction to the exclusion of other equally important factors or considerations [29]. Self-neglect is also at times referred to as a health behaviour [30]. This term is more of a trigger for clinicians to recognise that extensive work from a multidisciplinary team is required to achieve positive outcomes. Coping mechanisms and determining the cause is critical in addressing this 'behaviour'.

The ability to self-care may be limited in a number of situations and as a result of a number of factors, often outside the control of the client. Orem's theory of self-care suggests that a client's behaviour is normally rational and open to appropriate choice except in situations where the ability to reason is compromised [20]. There can be numerous causes or impetuses for clients to self-neglect. Some of these include:

- Capgras' syndrome.
- Loss of control.
- Cognitive impairments and intellectual disabilities.
- Advanced age.
- Social isolation and poor social support.
- Depression.
- Learning disability.
- Poor role modelling.
- Chronic medical conditions.
- Fear of institutionalisation.
- Frontal-lobe dysfunction.
- Functional impairment.
- Lifestyle choice.
- Malingering.
- Schizotypal and paranoid personality disorders.
- Substance misuse.
- Major life stressors [29–31].

Some manifestations and signs of these causes to be observant of and that could require further investigation include, but are not limited to:

- Poor personal hygiene and appearance.
- Smelling of urine or faeces.

- Unclothed or dressed in inappropriate clothing for the weather.
- Skin rashes and deterioration.
- Dehydration, malnourishment or weight loss.
- Absence of needed aids such as dentures, glasses, hearing aids and walkers.
- Increased confusion and disorientation.
- Unexpected or unexplained worsening of health or living conditions.
- Isolation.
- Lack of interest or concern about life.
- Untreated medical conditions.
- Self-destructive behaviours.
- Hallucinations and/or delusions.
- Drug and alcohol abuse.
- Treasured animals looking unkempt and uncared for [26, 29–31].

Nursing intervention in these instances requires careful assessment, diplomacy, negotiation, mediation and communication skills. One of the most important strategies is to reduce the impact of isolation on the client. Case conferencing may be an appropriate tool here; however, it is important not to draw conclusions without a thorough and holistic assessment. Enabling the client to accept help is critical to any case-conferencing process. If they are unwilling to accept help, considerable effort may need to be employed into encouraging uptake of services. This can be very difficult, particularly if the client perceives that they do not need assistance. Client-orientated goal setting is required here, again to determine what some of the issues are and who determines that a problem exists. The final and perhaps sometimes the hardest intervention is the acknowledgement that a vulnerable person chooses to neglect and this should be respected as a choice, with the community nurse helping the best they can. In instances of self-neglect the critical factor is that of the risk of deterioration to health due to the living conditions. Personal bias and values cannot enter into the assessment, as they will skew objective findings into subjective and liable conclusions.

Health promotion

Health promotion is a fundamental principle that drives many clinical challenges in community health care, including personal care. In the context of personal care, health promotion includes strategies to promote healthy lifestyles and to adopt appropriate health behaviours. Many Australians attribute a healthy lifestyle to diet and exercise, psychological well-being, relaxation and maintaining quality relationships [32].

Self-care choices and acceptance of assistance to promote good hygiene can be seen as a positive step and an appropriate health behaviour. There is an expanding awareness that clients are becoming more accountable for their own health and choices related to their health, including self-care, and are contributing more to the principles of self-care [30]. Community nurses have a pivotal role in encouraging self-care practices, not only with everyday practices such as personal care, but also with the management and promotion of self-care of chronic conditions. The enabling and promoting of good self-care practices, numerous benefits for the client and the health system include:

- Increase in life expectancy.
- Better control over symptoms.
- Reduction in pain, anxiety and depression levels.
- Improvement in quality of life with greater independence (for example it may enable the client to stay in their own home longer before moving to an institution).
- Improved quality of consultations.
- Visits to GPs can reduce by 40–69%.
- Hospital admissions can reduce by up to 50%.
- Number of days in hospital may decrease by up to 80%.
- Outpatient visits can reduce by 17–77%.
- Accident and emergency visits can reduce significantly.
- Medication intake reduced, e.g. steroids.
- Medicine utilisation is improved by 30% [33].

Positive health behaviours which influence health promotion vary significantly amongst client populations. Some influences that affect client motivation include loss of health and control, self-discipline, social support, value orientation, income, education, employment, self-esteem, attractiveness and health [30]. Within communities and cultures, there may be a focus on health promotion and screening campaigns. People with disabilities or the elderly may be less likely to take up screening if they do not understand the benefits, have poor access to services, are reliant on carers who are less health aware or cannot afford the service.

Many health promotion opportunities exist such as free breast screening for people aged over 50 years; however, these government-funded services are not equipped to screen people with multiple and severe disabilities, as mammograms can often not be performed with clients in wheelchairs. One way to ensure that the client receives the appropriate screening is to have an ultrasound, which is not a free service and leaves the client with significant out-of-pocket expenses. Thus health promotion resources may not always be accessible to people with a disability, the aged or people with language difficulties. However, consumers are becoming aware that it is better to take care of themselves when possible and remain healthy than to neglect their health and have to treat an illness or injury [12].

Nurses who practice community-based nursing need to understand the community within which they practice. Knowledge of the community helps the nurse maintain quality of care and provide safety features for themselves and their clients. The nurse is responsible for identifying available resources and identifying constraints or limitations of care that exist in the community [12].

Summary

Just as communities vary widely, the health and personal supports available in each community also vary. The challenge for community nurses is to promote independence, empower the client and caregiver with an agreed plan of action, promote positive health behaviours, engage in health promotion activities and promote self-care. Providing personal care is an integral part of the total care of the person. The basis is assessment of the person and the supports around them. It is essential not to assess the task or person in isolation, but to look at the complete picture, including the psychological and emotional impacts on care provision, while keeping account of the unique challenges that face community nurses in the provision of personal care.

References

1. Department of Health and Community Care, Northern Territory Home and Community Care (HACC) (2004) *Personal Care Guidelines.* Department of Health and Community Care, Northern Territory.
2. Dill Linton, A. and Lach, H. (2007) *Matteson and McConnell's Gerontological Nursing – Concepts and Practice,* 3rd edition. Elsevier/Mosby, New York.
3. Wang, P., Badley, E. and Gignac, M. (2004) Activity limitation, coping efficacy and self-perceived physical independence in people with a disability. *Disability and Rehabilitation,* 26(3), 785–93.
4. Heath, H. and Phair, L. (2000) Defining nursing and personal care. *Elderly Care,* 12(2), 26–7.
5. Australian Bureau of Statistics (2003) *Disability, Ageing and Carers, Australia: Summary of Findings.* Available at http://www.abs.gov.au/AUSSTATS/abs@.nsf/Lookup/ 4430.0Main+Features12003?OpenDocument (viewed 6 December 2007).
6. Bottoroff, J.L. (1991) A methodological review and evaluation of research on nurse patient touch, in P. Chinn (ed.) *Anthology of Caring.* National League for Nursing Press, New York, pp. 303–44.
7. Parker, J. (1997) The body as text and the body as living flesh; metaphors of the body and nursing in post modernity, in J. Lawler (ed.) *The Body in Nursing.* Churchill Livingstone, Melbourne, pp. 11–29.
8. McCann, T. and Baker, H. (2001) Mutual relating: Developing interpersonal relationships in the community. *Journal of Advanced Nursing,* 34(4), 530–37.
9. Australian Nursing and Midwifery Council (2006) *National Competency Standards for the Registered Nurse,* 4th edition. Australian Nursing and Midwifery Council, Dickson ACT.
10. McCormack, B. (2004) Person-centredness in gerontological nursing: An overview of the literature. *Journal of the Clinical Nursing,* 13(3a, Suppl 1), 31–8.
11. Spradley, B.W. and Allender, J.A. (1997) Cultural considerations, in R. Hunt and E.L. Zurek (eds) *Introduction to Community Based Nursing.* Lippincott-Raven, Philadelphia, p. 103.
12. Hunt, R. and Zurek E.L. (1997) *Introduction to Community Based Nursing.* Lippincott-Raven, Philadelphia.
13. Kendig, H. and Brooke, L. (1999) The social context/experience of ageing: Issues for geriatric nursing, in R. Nay and S. Garratt (eds) *Nursing Older People: Issues and Innovations.* Maclennan & Petty, Sydney, pp. 135–50.
14. Wenitong, M. (2003) Cultural issues in health delivery. *Royal Australasian College of Physicians News,* 22, 6–8.
15. Leksell, J., Johansson, I., Wibell, L. and Wikblad, K. (2001) Power and self-perceived health in blind diabetic and nondiabetic individuals. *Journal of Advanced Nursing,* 34(4), 511–19.
16. Burch, J. (2006) Psychological problems and stomas: A rough guide for community nurses. *British Journal Community Nursing,* 10(5), 224–7.
17. Pyne, C. (8 May 2007) *Budget Secures the Future for Aged Care* [Press release]. Australian Government, Canberra.
18. Lemone, P. and Burke, R. (2000) *Medical Surgical Nursing,* 2nd edition. Prentice Hall Health, New Jersey.
19. Safework, S.A. (2007) *The Hierarchy of Control.* Available at http://www.safework. sa.gov.au/contentPages/EducationAndTraining/HazardManagement/Electricity/ TheAnswer/elecAnswerHierarchy.htm (viewed 11 August 2007).

20. Cohen-Mansfield, J. and Jensen, B. (2007) Dressing and grooming preferences of community dwelling older adults. *Journal of Gerontological Nursing*, 33(2), 31–9.
21. Smith, C. (1997) Home healthcare nursing, in R. Hunt and E.L. Zurek (eds) *Introduction to Community Based Nursing*. Lippincott-Raven, Philadelphia, p. 338.
22. Nurses Board of South Australia (2005) *Delegation by a Registered Nurse or Midwife to an Unlicensed Healthcare Worker*. Adelaide, South Australia.
23. Australian Nurses' Federation (2005) *Role Boundaries in the Provision of Personal Care Policy*. Available at www.anf.org.au (viewed 2 April 2007).
24. Collin, C., Wade, D.T., Davies, S. and Horne, V. (1988) The Barthel ADL Index: A reliability study. *International Disability Study*, 10, 61–3.
25. Wright, J. (2000) *The Functional Assessment Measure*. The Center for Outcome Measurement in Brain Injury. Available at http://www.birf.info/home/bi-tools/tests/fam.html (viewed 9 December 2007).
26. Gibbons, S. and Launder, W. (2006) Self neglect: A proposed new NANDA diagnosis. *International Journal of Nursing Terminology Classification*, 17(1), 10–19.
27. Kelly, G.A., cited in Launder, W., Anderson, I. and Barclay, A. (2002) Sociological and psychological theories of self neglect. *Journal of Advanced Nursing*, 40(3), 334.
28. Wolinksy, F.D., cited in Launder, W., Anderson, I. and Barclay, A. (2002) Sociological and psychological theories of self neglect. *Journal of Advanced Nursing*, 40(3), 334.
29. Launder, W., Anderson, I. and Barclay, A. (2002) Sociological and psychological theories of self neglect. *Journal Advanced Nursing*, 40(3), 331–8.
30. Carter, K. and Kulbok, P. (2002) Motivation for health behaviours: A systematic review of the nursing literature. *Journal of Advanced Nursing*, 40(3), 316–30.
31. Launder, W. (2001) The utility of self care theory as a theoretical basis for self neglect. *Journal of Advanced Nursing*, 34(4), 545–51.
32. Jackiewicz, J., James, R. and Campbell, C. (2006) Is the term 'lifestyle' appropriate to use in health promotion today? *Health Promotion Journal Australia*, 16(3), 179–83.
33. Department of Health, UK (2007) *Self Care Support – The Evidence* [Summary pack]. Department of Health, United Kingdom.

Chapter 20

Stoma care

Carmen George

Introduction

This purpose of this chapter is to examine the principles of stoma management and consider the community nursing role when caring for people with a stoma. Stoma surgery may have life-changing impact on a person and hence this chapter offers some practical ways to ensure that life for people at home with stomas is as good as it can be. The community nurse can play a vital role in assisting the client to adjust to an altered body image and waste elimination process. In this chapter, we also consider the products available to manage stoma output and the rationales for choosing one product over another in the management of an individual's stoma.

Types of stomas

A stoma is an artificial, surgically made opening into a body part [1]. Stomas may be found in the gastrointestinal (GI) tract, the genitourinary (GU) tract and the respiratory tract (see Table 20.1). For the purpose of this chapter, tracheostomy care is excluded; however, attention will be given to fistula management. A fistula is an unnatural opening between one organ and another and for the purposes of this chapter between the GI or GU tracts and the skin [1].

A *stoma* usually takes on the name of the body part it is made in. Hence, a gastrostomy is an opening into the stomach; a jejunostomy is where a portion of the jejunum has been exteriorised; an ileostomy is where a portion of the ileum has been exteriorised; and a colostomy is where a portion of the colon has been exteriorised. These openings may be feeding, draining or decompressing (venting): the main reason a gastrostomy is made is for feeding purposes; a jejunostomy may be feeding or draining; ileostomies are generally draining as are colostomies. Decompressing (venting) stomas may be in any part of the GI tract and are made to decompress the gut proximal to an occlusion or blockage.

A *mucous fistula* is the name given to an end stoma that may be draining, but is not functional in the same way as an ileostomy or colostomy. Stomas made in the GU tract

Table 20.1 Types of stomas.

Type of stoma[1]	Anatomy	Output	pH	Usual status
Gastrostomy	Below diaphragm	Nil	1.0–3.5	Feeding
Jejunostomy	Left epigastric region	High liquid	7.5–8.9	Draining
Ileostomy	Right iliac fossa	Moderate- to high-thick faecal fluid	7.5–8.9	Draining
Transverse colostomy	Right epigastric	Paste consistency	7.8	Draining
Sigmoid end colostomy	Left iliac fossa	Formed stool	7.8	Draining
Mucous fistula	Above symphasis pubis or elsewhere	Pus/blood mucous		Venting
Urostomy	Right iliac fossa	Urine	4.5–8.0	Draining

are draining. The output one should expect from the stoma is dependent on where in the GI/GU tract it is.

It is important to understand the surgery the person with a stoma has had and why they have had it so that when problems arise it is easier to understand the mechanism behind the problem and how to tackle it [2]. Consider the following clinical scenario:

> Two people, both with end colostomies, shortly after discharge home report experiencing brown staining on their underpants and sore bottoms, but one has had an abdominoperineal excision of their rectum (APR) and the other has had a Hartmann's procedure. The person who has had the APR will quite likely have an old blood or haemoserous discharge from their perineal excision and may need some wound care. The person who has had the Hartmann's procedure may have retained faeces in their rectal stump and require an enema.

Surgical interventions

Cancer of the rectum, anus, bladder, penis, diverticular disease, inflammatory bowel disease, trauma, ischaemic bowel and disorders of defaecation are just some of the health disorders that may lead to surgical intervention inclusive of stoma formation [1]. These stomas may be temporary or permanent; they may be end, loop or abcarian stomas (see Figures 20.1 and 20.2).

- An *end stoma* is where the segment of bowel ends at the stoma, the bowel is inverted and the inner mucosal lining of the bowel is what is seen.
- A *loop stoma* is where the exteriorised segment of bowel is only partially divided (cut through) and inverted so that there is a proximal evacuating end and a distal defunctioned end.

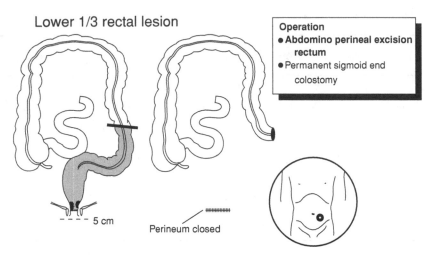

Figure 20.1 End colostomy.

- An *abcarian stoma* is where the functioning end is exteriorised and the divided distal end is sewn under the skin adjacent to the stoma. This facilitates easy access by the surgeon when reversal of the stoma is to take place [1].

An *ileal conduit* is when a length of ileum with its blood supply has been isolated from the faecal stream and converted into a conduit. The ureters are implanted into one end and the other end is exteriorised and inverted to form a stoma. This is generally called a urostomy or an ileal conduit, to avoid confusion with ileostomies that put out faecal fluid.

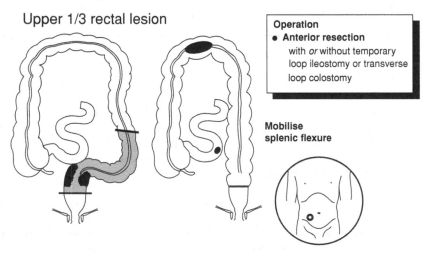

Figure 20.2 Loop stomas.

Planning for discharge into the community

Discharge planning begins with hospital admission. In the case of the person who has stoma surgery, the stomal therapy nurse (STN) in the hospital starts planning for life after the stoma as soon as they meet the person [3]. The initial assessment of the person preoperatively, in addition to informing the STN about the type of surgery being planned and why, will also give the STN information about the person's attitude to having the surgery, their general health, their support systems, their physical abilities, their living arrangements and their coping mechanisms. During hospitalisation, the STN develops a therapeutic relationship with the client and utilises this client information to guide the person to the most appropriate product to use for the management of their stoma. This client information also informs the STN about how the person may cope once at home. This includes determining what community resources are available for the client to access, ensuring that the community nurse is aware of the pending discharge from hospital and that the client is discharged home with sufficient supplies and information regarding the management of their stoma and the availability of ongoing support.

The product chosen for the client's use is determined by its availability and its manageability by the client at that point in time. Frequently, while the client is in hospital, the abdomen is distended, the stoma is oedematous, the output is variable and the client is not in the best learning situation. This may mean that what was working in hospital might not be totally suitable at home. Further, as the stoma shrinks, the opening on the appliance needs to be modified. Stoma shrinkage may take up to 4 weeks after surgery [4]. With shortened hospital stay and the trend to send frail clients home via a rehabilitation centre, errors of judgement in the choice of an appliance may be made. This would evidence itself by either the client experiencing persistent leakage problems or their inability to manage the chosen system. In these instances the community nurse may need to contact the hospital STN for advice and to reassess the client.

Living with a stoma

Whatever their age, gender, social status, living conditions or mental ability, every person with a stoma should be confident that they can live, knowing they have a reliable, leak-proof and easy-to-manage appliance. It is the experience of some people however that they struggle for many years having an unsatisfactory stoma appliance. This may impact on the individual's ability to participate in their community and live a normal life and to engage in activities that they enjoy (see Case study 20.1). The International Charter of Rights for people experiencing ostomy surgery advocates that people should [5]:

- Receive preoperative counselling to ensure that they are fully aware of the benefits of the operation and the essential facts about living with a stoma
- Have a well-constructed stoma placed in an appropriate site and with full and proper consideration of the comfort of the client

Case study 20.1

The son of an older woman, Mrs C, asked the community nurse if anything could be done about her 'smell'. He said that his children did not want to be in the car or same room as their grandmother as she smelt so bad. Further, his mother kept running out of bags and the colostomy association would not give her any more without a certificate from an STN. After meeting Mrs C and examining her stoma and the appliance she was using, the community nurse saw that the large woman was trying to manage her end colostomy using a one-piece paediatric drainable appliance with no filter. It transpired that she had had a Hartman's procedure for a bowel obstruction caused by a diverticular mass. The surgery had been performed in a small suburban hospital. No STN had been involved in her care either preoperatively or postoperatively. The ward staff had put her on the small drainable bag as that was all that they had in the cupboard. (This bag had in fact been donated to the hospital by the company representative for use on draining wounds.) They had shown her how to cut a hole in it and ordered more of these same bags from the colostomy association.

Challenges identified:
- Actual bag was too small – a large person does not get large by eating a small amount. This lady had to change the bag minimum of two to three times a day as the bag filled up.
- No filter – with no mechanism for getting rid of flatus, the little bag would fill up with flatus and dislodge.
- Cutting surface of skin barrier was too small – the stoma measured 35 mm, which was the outer area of the bag, so there was no margin for error when Mrs C applied it.
- Mrs C had difficulty seeing her stoma as it was out of her normal range of vision. She had to stand in front of a mirror to apply the bag.
- When Mrs C went out she could not stand in front of a mirror or change the appliance herself which is why she smelt because the bag would often fill up and start coming off whilst she was out.
- Mrs C could not empty the faeces out of the drainable opening of the bag because the faeces were too firm.
- The skin around Mrs C's stoma was red and sore from frequent exposure to faeces and frequent removing of bags.
- Mrs C had no knowledge about her stoma or the resources available to her or any problem-solving ability.
- Mrs C was becoming socially withdrawn and isolated. She was aware of the faecal odour and thus was avoiding contact with other people.

Solutions and strategies:
- Mrs C's stoma was measured, her dexterity was assessed and a pre-cut two-piece clip on closed appliance with a filter was chosen.
- Mrs C was shown that if she *sat down* whilst changing the base plate, she could actually see her stoma.
- Mrs C was taught how to *adequately clean the peristomal skin* and apply the correctly fitting base plate. This required changing only twice a week. She soon learnt how to change the clip on bag when it was one-third full and also how to use deodorising drops in the bag.
- Mrs C's skin readily improved as it was protected from both faeces and constant removal. She was taught how to *dispose of the bag and its contents when out*.
- She was given *simple explanations and written information* about her stoma and provided with available resources.

- Receive experienced and professional medical support and stoma nursing care in the preoperative/postoperative period both in hospital and in their community
- Receive full and impartial information about all relevant supplies and products available in their country
- Have the opportunity to choose from the available variety of ostomy management products without prejudice or constraint
- Be given information about their national ostomy association and the services and support which can be provided
- Receive support and information for the benefit of the family, personal carers and friends to increase their understanding of the condition and adjustments which are necessary for achieving a satisfactory standard of life with a stoma

The community nurse may play an important support role as a person learns to adapt to living with a stoma in their home environment.

Rehabilitative process

Shortened hospital stays mean that a person with a newly created stoma is unlikely to achieve the goal of independence in all aspects of their own stoma care whilst in hospital. They certainly are unlikely to retain information about potential problems and how to solve them. The need for appropriate ongoing support and education at home becomes paramount [6] and may be an area where the community nurse has significant impact.

> The feeling of lack of preparedness for discharge was a recurring theme. The shorter hospital length of stays obviously impacting on both the stomal therapy nurse and the client [7, p. 24].

Communication between the hospital STN and the community STN or registered nurse needs to be appropriate and support the transition of the client from the hospital to the community. There is a tool available for use by hospital STNs to communicate with the community nurse. A copy of this is available in the *Journal of Stomal Therapy Nursing* [8]. This tool is useful in ensuring that all relevant clinical information is forwarded to the community nurse. The provision of ongoing education, support and anticipatory guidance enables the planning of realistic strategies so that clients and carers are able to manage in the event of a crisis [9].

The community nurse will need to assess not only what the client or carer can actually do with regard to stoma care but also how confident and effective they are in managing the stoma. From this, the community nurse will be able to determine what the client's specific learning needs are and the client's readiness and willingness to learn.

Although most hospital STNs would have discussed changes to body image and sexuality with the client and included counselling into their care, it 'is unlikely that clients will successfully adapt psychologically and emotionally to the body image changes related to stoma formation if they have not achieved confidence and competence in practical stoma care' [3]. Adaptation takes time and the community nurse may be an excellent source of support for the client.

Rural and remote clients

With access to the internet, email and telemedicine, people with stomas and those who care for them are often no more isolated than others in the community. Website addresses are included at the end of this chapter, which may be of use to community nurses and people learning to live with a stoma. All major hospitals have 'telehealth' centres and, if necessary, a consultation with a qualified STN can be arranged through this system.

People being discharged home to rural or remote communities should have written care plans, sufficient equipment and the name of a health professional to contact in their region, as well as the name and contact details of their discharging STN. These can also be an important source of information for the community nurse.

A stoma care manual can be ordered through the post [10]. This is designed for people with stomas, so some hospitals may give one to the client on discharge. All people with stomas need to be joined to their local stoma association as this organisation distributes their stoma supplies. Once a member of an ostomy association, they should automatically receive the latest copy of the ostomy magazine. This magazine is a very useful tool as it not only has current information and stories from other ostomates but all the product advertisements have website addresses and free call numbers.

Cultural differences

Clients from non-English-speaking backgrounds ideally should have had access to an interpreter during their hospitalisation and decision making regarding the management of their illness. Many hospitals that have large numbers of clients from specific ethnic backgrounds have literature translated into appropriate languages. Attitudes to illness in some cultures may be different from what we would consider usual. 'In Muslim, Jewish, Hindu and certain orthodox Christian religions, cleanliness and an intact body are prerequisite to performance of obligatory religious rituals. Although dispensations have been made by these religions' for bodily changes that promote health and prolong life it is not uncommon for people from these backgrounds to initially refuse ostomy surgery' [1].

Muslim clients

The International Ostomy Association (IOA) sought clarification from the Fatwa Commission regarding the concerns of Muslims with stomas and the need for ritual cleanliness prior to praying five times a day. Muslim clients will be reassured by being given a copy of this Fatwa which gives them absolution from this requirement and is available on the IOA website www.ostomyinternational.org.

Stoma Appliance Scheme

Most stoma appliances are manufactured overseas from where they are imported into Australia. The Pharmaceutical Benefits Scheme has a stoma appliance division called the Stoma Appliance Scheme (SAS) [11]. The government sets the price for equipment and the volume of products available each month for each person. In this country people with a stoma currently pay nothing for their products. They may however have to pay a membership fee to belong to a stoma association which distributes the appliances on the behalf of the government and may have to pay postage if they require their supplies to be posted rather than picked up.

Department of Veterans Affairs (DVA) gold-card holders do not have to pay membership fees or postage; the DVA pays for these but the ostomate still has to become a member of their local association. The SAS is available to all Australians with a Medicare card. The predetermined allocation of supplies by the SAS is generous; the associations are unable to distribute more than the monthly allocation without an authority signed by an STN or general practitioner (GP). Other ancillary products are available through the scheme, such as urinary drainage bags, catheter straps and adhesive remover wipes. For a full list of stoma products available on the SAS, go to www.health.gov.au, search for Stoma Appliance Scheme and then click on schedule. This will give the current listings and the volume people may order each month.

Types of appliances

All products that adhere to the skin or contain the stoma output or are used as accessory products are called appliances [1]. Terms such as bag, appliance or pouch can be used to describe the actual containing device. The flat base that adheres to the skin in two-piece appliances is called a base plate. Other terms that may be used to describe the skin-adhesive part of the two-piece system are flanges, wafers and skin barriers. Technically, 'flange' refers to the part of the base plate that a bag clips on to; however, as some of the newer two-piece systems do not have flanges, this term is defunct; wafer describes the square of 'hydrocolloid' as does 'skin barrier'. The correct comprehensive term is base plate.

Stoma appliances can be one piece or two pieces, opaque or clear, and are either closed, drainable or have a tap. The skin barrier may be either soft and mouldable or rigid and convex. The appliance may be designed to last a week or may be designed for more frequent removal. The companies that manufacture these products invest enormous amounts of money into research and development to find new and more effective products that will ultimately enhance outcomes for people with stomas. For example filter technology, integrated closure mechanisms and adhesive low-profile two-piece appliances are three technological advances that have impacted on the quality of the available products.

Accessory products and when and how to use them

The following products are available [12]:

- *Adhesive remover wipes*
  - May be helpful to remove well-adhered appliances from sensitive or hairy skin.
  - Caution must be taken to ensure that all residual substance has been thoroughly washed off skin prior to applying the next bag or base plate.

- As with all chemicals, in some individuals they may cause a skin reaction or irritant dermatitis.
- *Skin-protective barrier wipes*
  - May be useful in applying a protective layer between the skin and the product adhesive. This chemical barrier is not an adhesive, but may enhance the effect of the adhesive on the stoma appliance.
  - Caution should be taken when using on broken or eroded skin as most contain alcohol.
  - Alcohol-free barrier wipes are available.
  - As with all chemicals, in some individuals they may cause a skin reaction or irritant dermatitis.
- *Deodorants*
  - These are liquids that are inserted into the bag/pouch to reduce the odour when the appliance is being changed, emptied or removed.
  - Generally used with colostomies.
  - Most ileostomy output is inoffensive smelling; therefore, deodorants are rarely needed for this.
  - Not designed for use in urostomy appliances.
- *Lubricants*
  - Lubricating deodorants are available to assist with the dropping of faeces into the bag.
  - Need to be smeared around the inside of the bag to be effective.
  - Generally useful with colostomies when 'pancaking' of the faeces over the stoma occurs; however, increasing fluid intake and modifying diet to ensure less solid faeces should be considered or faecal softeners such as coloxyl.
- *Tablets for controlling wind*
  - These tablets are generally designed to be used with liquid faeces, i.e. ileostomy output. Fermentation of the faecal fluid continues in the bag; these tablets are designed to mix with the liquid faeces and chemically prevent the fermentation from occurring.
  - Generally, half a tablet is sufficient. May be useful at night.
- *Gelling agents*
  - A product designed for ileostomies to thicken output in the bag making it easier to empty.
  - May be useful at night in bed when gravity is not available and pooling of faecal fluid over the stoma may result in leakage.
- *Pastes*
  - These hydrocolloid pastes have alcohol in them and are used to fill dips and gullies in the peristomal skin to facilitate the adherence and performance of the stoma appliance.
  - Not glue. Designed to be used as a filler or 'no more gaps'.
  - Caution should be used if applied to broken or eroded skin.
- *Seals*
  - Seals are used to lengthen wear time of an appliance, mould into creases or crevices or provide convexity around the stoma.
  - Seals may be made from hydrocolloid-type substances or karaya.
  - May be flat or convex.
  - May be thin or thick.

- *Powders*
  - A hydrocolloid powder designed to adhere to moist surfaces.
  - Useful on lesions on the actual stoma.
  - May be useful to adhere onto moist denuded skin prior to applying a bag or base plate.
- *Cleansing wipes*
  - These are individually wrapped 'wet ones'.
  - May be useful when water and a soft lint-free cloth are not available for cleansing around the stoma.
  - May be useful when going out.
- *Catheter straps*
  - Designed to secure the tubing from the overnight bag to the thigh to avoid kinking of the tubing when the person with a urostomy moves in bed.
- *Overnight drainage bags*
  - Used to connect to urostomy bag at night.
  - Enables free drainage from the stoma appliance to a larger container.
  - Prevents the need for the person with a urostomy to get up at night to empty the bag.
- *Stoma belts*
  - Designed to fit onto some bags or base plates.
  - Useful to ensure pressure around the stoma which may facilitate the stoma protruding more and the output from the stoma draining into the bag more readily.
  - Needs to be firmly applied to be of any use.
  - Only four per year per person available from SAS and therefore should not be discarded thoughtlessly.
- *Stoma support belts/garments*
  - Designed to reduce the risk of parastomal herniation or to support reduction of an established parastomal hernia.
  - Needs to be accurately fitted and ostomate needs to be taught how to apply properly and when to use.
  - Only three available per year per person on SAS and are very expensive and so should be judiciously prescribed by a STN.

Changing an appliance, basic hygiene and application of a new appliance

When working with people to help them adjust to life with a stoma the community nurse can offer the following advice and hints [13]:

- The person can bathe or shower with the pouch (bag) *on* or *off*. There is no guarantee that the stoma will not function while bathing, but once a pattern is established, people may find a satisfactory time of day or evening when it will be safe to bathe with the pouch off.
- If the person chooses to bathe/shower with a two-piece appliance on, show them how to remove the pouch only and clean around the site with water and a clean soft washcloth. If they shower with a one-piece appliance on, check if the filter needs to be covered.

- Avoid the use of bath oils or creams as they may interfere with the adhesion of the pouch. Some premoistened wipes may contain lanolin.
- Encourage the person to establish a regular routine for changing the appliance. This is best done when the bowel is least active, e.g. prior to breakfast. Never wait for leakage to occur before changing the appliance.
- The person may find it easier to fit their new appliance if they view it by changing the appliance using.
- A stoma is not sterile. Wash the stoma and surrounding skin with warm water and then pat dry.
- Allow plenty of time to change the appliance. Talk to the person about reducing the possibility of interruptions by taking the phone off the hook or turning the answering machine on while changing the appliance.
- Advise the person to not let the pouch become too full before emptying it. One-third to half-full is a good guide.
- Remember that the opening on the wafer or pouch should expose no more than 2 mm of skin around the stoma. Too large an opening can cause skin excoriation and leakage under the wafer/pouch. Too small an opening may cause the stoma to become swollen or ulcerated.
- Plain warm water is the best cleanser for around the stoma.
- People may notice a trace of blood when cleaning the stoma – this is usual.
- Keep hairs around the stoma trimmed or shaved. Hold tissue, toilet paper or a soft, clean cloth over the stoma to protect it whilst shaving.
- Clothes pegs are ideal for holding clothes away from the appliance when necessary.

Special note. Never mend a leaking pouch or appliance. The whole appliance needs to be changed.

Common stoma complications

- *Ischaemic stoma*
  - Although this is an immediate postoperative complication, the long-term consequence may be that the stoma never protrudes as much as one would like and may even become stenosed or retracted.
  - This has implications for management and will contribute to the choice of appliance needed to remedy these problems.
- *Mucocutaneous separation*
  - This is a postoperative complication that may become manifest immediately postoperatively or within the first 10 days after surgery as the abdominal distension and stoma oedema diminish (see Figure 20.3).
  - Mucocutaneous separation may be circumferential or partial.
  - This wound needs to be dressed and isolated from the faecal or urinary output of the stoma.
  - The presence of a mucocutaneous separation may delay client independence, as they may not be able to dress the wound themselves prior to applying the skin barrier.
  - This may have long-term management implications as the healed wound may cause stenosis.

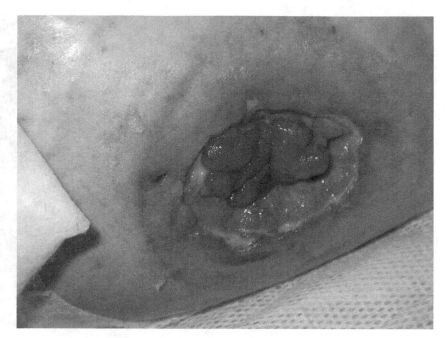

Figure 20.3 Mucocutaneous separation.

- This should not prevent discharge from hospital back into the community.
- This can be easily managed by a community nurse with stoma therapy skills [14].
- *Leakage*
  - May cause both physical and psychosocial problems for the client [15].
  - Most leakage problems are solvable.
  - Cause of leakage needs to be established.
  - Prevention of leakage should be paramount when choosing an appliance.
- *Granulomas and mucosal implants*
  - Mucosal implants are 'bubbles of bowel mucosa [which] proliferate when epithelial cells are inadvertently transplanted from bowel mucosa into the epidermis during maturation of the stoma'[1, p. 203] (see Figures 20.4 and 20.5).
  - Mucosal implants are seen on the skin around a stoma.
  - Granulomas are 'heaped up granular bodies' [16, p. 20].
  - May be seen on the actual stoma or on the mucocutaneous junction.
  - Both will respond to silver nitrate treatment, which is discussed later in this chapter [17, p. 283].
- *Retraction*
  - Retraction is the term given to a stoma that has pulled back below the level of the skin (see Figure 20.6).
  - In the immediate postoperative phase, this is closely monitored to ensure that the stoma does not completely retract into the abdominal cavity.
  - By the time the person is discharged from hospital, any retraction of the stoma simply becomes a management challenge.

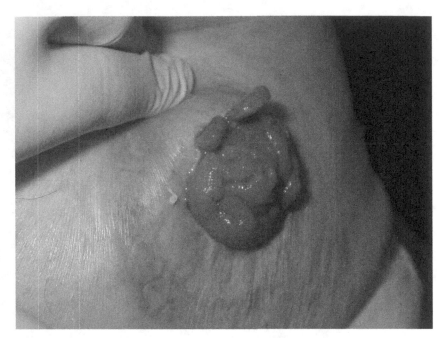

Figure 20.4 Granulomas on the mucocutaneous junction before treatment.

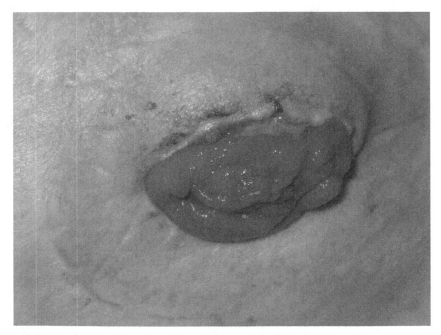

Figure 20.5 Same stoma after treatment of granulomas with silver nitrate.

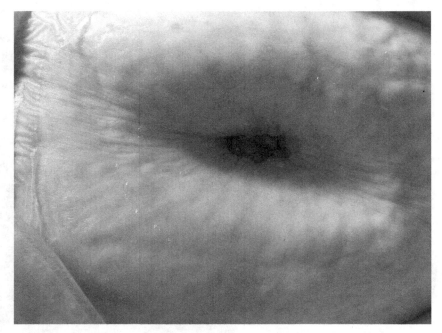

Figure 20.6 Retracted stoma – needs convex appliance.

- As the stoma retracts below the level of the skin, a 'moat' will develop around the stoma.
- Unless correctly pouched, the stoma output will seep into this 'moat' and cause leakage.
- *Stenosis*
  - The stoma opening is narrowed and may even appear closed over.
  - May restrict drainage.
  - May cause pain when formed faeces try to get through narrowed opening.
  - May cause loin pain in urostomates [1].
  - May need surgical revision.
  - May benefit from digital dilatation.
  - Faecal output should be kept loose, and dietary modification and aperients may be required.
- *Oedema*
  - Generally, this is an immediate postoperative complication; however, it may occur in severe electrolyte imbalance or following injury to the stoma or if the stoma prolapses.
  - Openings in stoma appliances will need to be modified to accommodate the enlarged stoma.
- *Prolapse*
  - Generally prolapse occurs in the distal loop of a transverse colostomy; however, any stoma may prolapse out (see Figures 20.7 and 20.8).
  - Prolapse can be unsightly and frightening for the person.

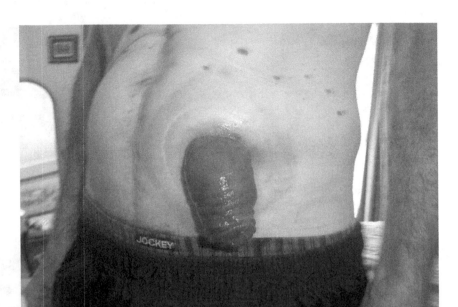

Figure 20.7 Prolapsed colostomy.

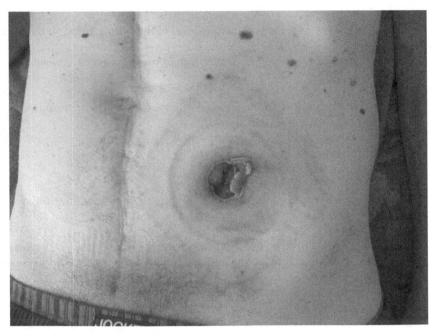

Figure 20.8 Manually reduced prolapsed colostomy – note the granulomas.

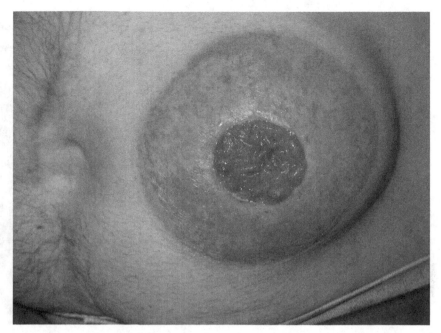

Figure 20.9 Contact dermatitis and parastomal hernia.

   – May be manipulated back in.
   – May need appliance modification or change of size to accommodate the stoma.
   – Should be reviewed by an STN.
   – May require referral for surgical revision.
- *Parastomal hernia*
   – Incisional hernia around the stoma resulting in a parastomal bulge.
   – Stretching of the stoma causes alteration in stoma size, i.e. larger, flatter stoma.
   – Potential for strangulation of bowel (surgical emergency).
   – Corrective surgery is not always successful.
   – Use of an abdominal support garment may reduce risk of occurrence and may reduce potential for further enlargement.
- *Dermatitis*
   – May be irritant, allergic or contact (see Figure 20.9).
   – Usually caused by contact of the skin with stoma output.
   – Usually will heal when the causative substance is removed.

Management principles

Skin protection and containment of output are the two practical principles of stoma management (see Figure 20.10). If the peristomal skin is protected from irritants such as stomal output and the stomal output is contained within the appliance, then these principles have been implemented. The other important principle is independence.

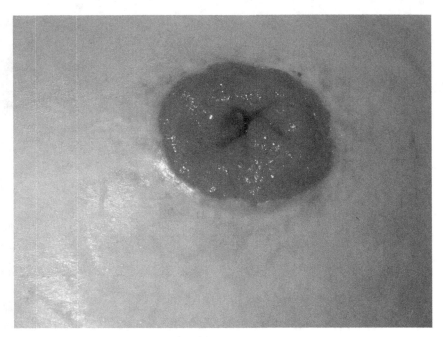

Figure 20.10 Perfect peristomal skin and end stoma.

- *Correct fit*
  - There should be the minimal amount of skin showing around the stoma. Any skin that is not protected by the skin barrier will be exposed to the stoma output with potential for irritation and denudation of the skin.
  - Using the measuring guides provided, cut appliances to fit, ensuring that the correct size is cut or if using a pre-cut appliance ensure that it is the correct size.
- *Convexity*
  - Is an in-built outward curving on a base plate which begins at the opening of the base plate extending outwards.
  - Advised when the stoma is in a 'moat' or the stoma opening is below skin level or for flush urostomies or ileostomies (see Figure 20.11).

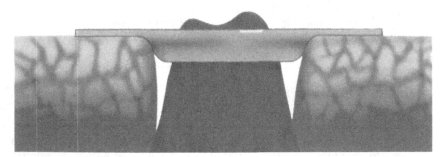

Figure 20.11 Convex appliance.

- Useful to use in an emergency situation such as persistent leakage as by applying firm pressure immediately around the stoma, this may have the twofold effect of preventing stoma output from leaking underneath the appliance and may also result in the stoma protruding more.
- *Changing appliances whilst out*
  - Advise the person to carry a spare appliance with some individually wrapped wet ones and some toilet paper. These can be put into a small zip-lock bag inside a brown sandwich bag.
  - The appliance can be removed in a public toilet and placed in the zip-lock bag and then inside brown paper bag for disposal in garbage.
  - If the client is concerned about odour when changing the appliance when out, advise them to carry a small deodorant aerosol spray to use.
  - If the client is planning to travel overseas, advise that they may not have access to similar appliances or products. Advise the client to pack adequate supplies in their luggage and hand luggage so that if luggage is misplaced they will still have access to some supplies.
- *Disposal*
  Encourage the person to dispose of used stoma appliances thoughtfully:
  - Appliances should be emptied of content prior to disposal.
  - For closed bags this can easily be achieved by having a dedicated pair of scissors, cutting two-third of the bottom of the bag open and holding into the flush of the toilet so that the content empties out and the bag is cleaned at the same time.
  - Wrapping used appliances in newspaper and then tied up in a plastic bag will prevent odour in the garbage.
  - Some people use commercially available nappy sacks for disposal.
  - Sanitary disposal units in female toilets can be used for one off disposals, but if being used every day, such as in a workplace, then the disposal unit company should be informed to change the unit more frequently.

Use of silver nitrate

The following factors need to be taken into account when using silver nitrate ($AgNO_3$) for management of granulomas on or around stomas [16, p. 25]:

- Diagnose and describe the condition $AgNO_3$ is to be used on.
- Identify causative factors for this condition and attempt to eliminate them.
- Inform the client about the rationale for using $AgNO_3$ and its mode of action and side effects.
- Obtain client consent for use of this product.
- Protect your own hands from staining by wearing gloves.
- Avoid run off of $AgNO_3$ onto tissue not to be treated by protecting non-treated areas of the client from staining.
- Moisten tip of $AgNO_3$ stick with water or with moisture obtained from the lesion.
- If using tap water, place water in a container prior to moistening tip to ensure that staining of enamel sink does not occur.
- When using on hypergranulation in a wound, clean area afterwards with normal saline.

- Document use of AgNO$_3$ as well as other interventions.
- Review treated area at a designated time.
- Evaluate treatments.

Conclusion

This chapter has described surgical interventions leading to formation of a stoma and has addressed the challenges that both clients and community nurses face when managing a stoma in the home environment. Many things can go wrong for these people, from surgery to the day-to-day living with a stoma.

All people with stomas have the right to expect a leak-proof appliance that will enable them to live without the burden of feeling insecure about leakage and odour. There are many resources available to people with stomas and the health professionals working with them. If the client or carer is not able to maintain intact skin and contained stoma output, it is important that help is obtained from a credentialed STN, or for those clients living in remote areas, a nurse with stomal care knowledge.

Useful resources

Ostomy Magazine: Distributed to all members of registered ostomy support groups and distribution centres

Stoma associations: All associations listed at the back of *Ostomy Magazine* or on their website www.australianstoma.com.au

Australian Association of Stomal Therapy Nurses (standards for stomal therapy nursing practice available on website): www.stomaltherapy.com

World Council of Enterostomal Therapy Nurses: www.wcetn.org

Wound Ostomy Continence Association: www.wocn.org

International Ostomy Association: www.ostomyinternatinal.org

Stoma appliance company websites and their representatives within Australia:

- Hollister   www.hollister.com.au
- Convatec   www.convatec.com.au
- Coloplast   www.coloplast.com.au
- Eakin   www.eakin.co.uk
- Dansac   www.dansac.com
- BBraunn   www.bbraun.com.au

References

1. Blackley, P. (2004) *Practical Stoma Wound and Continence Management*, 2nd edition. Research Publications, Victoria, Australia, p. 95.
2. Cox, C. and McVey, M. (1996) Models of care, in C. Myers (ed.) *Stoma Care Nursing – A Client Centred Approach*. Arnold Press, London, pp. 220–35.
3. Allison, M. (1996) Discharge planning for the person with a stoma, in C. Myers (ed.) *Stoma Care Nursing – A Client Centred Approach*. Arnold Press, London, pp. 267–81.

4. Borwell, B. and Breckman, B. (2005) Types of bowel stoma and why they are created, in B. Breckman (ed.) *Stoma Care and Rehabilitation*. Elsevier, Churchill Livingstone, London, pp. 70–80.

5. AL-AZHAR (2007) *Complex of Islamic Research Fatwa Commission*. Available at www.ostomyinternational.org (viewed 18 December 2007).

6. Breckman, B. (2005) Towards rehabilitation, in B. Breckman (ed.) *Stoma Care and Rehabilitation*. Elsevier, Churchill Livingstone, London, pp. 133–42.

7. George, C. and Charles-Barks, C. (2005) Patients' perception of their involvement in the choice of their appliance. *The Journal of Stomal Therapy Australia JSTA*, 25(3), 24.

8. White, C. (2005) Calvary health care adelaide inc stomal therapy discharge summary. *The Journal of Stomal Therapy Australia JSTA*, 25(2), 28.

9. Forsyth, J. (2005) Some thoughts about discharging people with new stomas back into the community. *The Journal of Stomal Therapy Australia JSTA*, 25(2), 24.

10. Hayes, D. (2007) The stoma care manual. *Ostomy Australia*, 16(1), 8.

11. Commonwealth Department of Health and Ageing (2008) *Stoma Appliance Scheme*. Available at www.health.gov.au.

12. Erwin-Toth, P. and Doughty, D. (1992) Principles and procedures of stomal management, in B.G. Hampton and R.A. Bryant (eds) *Ostomies and Continent Diversions*. Mosby Year Book, St Louis, USA, p. 41.

13. Australian Association of Stomal Therapy Nurses (AASTN) Education and Professional Development Subcommittee (2007) *Handy Hints for Stoma Clients. Stomal Therapy Client Information Pamphlets*. Available at www.stomaltherapy.com (Updated 2007).

14. George, C. (2003) Wounds adjacent to stomas: Mucocutaneous separation. *The Journal of Stomal Therapy Australia JSTA*, 23(1), 14–15.

15. Bourke, R. and Davis, E. (2003) Is convex the preferred appliance for pouching loop ileostomies? *The Journal of Stomal Therapy Australia JSTA*, 23(1), 7–12.

16. George, C. (2003) Use of silver nitrate in clinical practice. *The Journal of Stomal Therapy Australia JSTA*, 23(3), 20.

17. Hampton, B. (1992) Peristomal and stomal complications, in B.G. Hampton and R.A. Bryant (eds) *Ostomies and Continent Diversions*. Mosby Year Book, St Louis, USA, pp. 105–25.

18. Breckman, B. (2005) Problems in stomal management, in B. Breckman (ed.) *Stoma Care and Rehabilitation*. Elsevier, Churchill Livingstone, London, pp. 277–96.

Chapter 21

Wound management

Sue Templeton

Introduction

Within Australia, the majority of wounds are managed by nurses in community settings [1]. Whilst chronic and enduring wounds are predominant, all types of wounds are managed by community nurses. The community setting provides unique opportunities and challenges for wound management. The nurse provides wound management in collaboration with the client and other health care professionals.

This chapter addresses the role of the community nurse in wound management and discusses clinical competency standards, assessment and documentation requirements and legal responsibilities related to this type of care. The principles of wound management, including assessment, wound classification, pain management, dressing choice and factors that impede healing, are also presented.

Background

Wounding is an interruption to the integumentary system resulting in tissue damage. Causes of wounds include disease processes, trauma, toxic substances, thermal or chemical exposure and surgery. The majority of wounds will heal in a timely and uncomplicated manner. For some persons, however, wound healing can become lengthy, requiring complex interventions and specialised skills. For a small number of clients, healing might not be a realistic outcome and the community nurse works with the client to manage their wound over a prolonged period. Working with clients to assist them to participate in and contribute to their care is vital to ensure that optimal outcomes are obtained.

The role of the community nurse in wound management

Community nurses are pivotal in wound management for many clients. The nurse's care has the potential to facilitate or delay healing [2]. Many community clients receive multidisciplinary wound management (e.g. regularly attend a hospital outpatient department, general practitioner, medical specialist or allied health professional). Often it is the community nurse, however, who sees the person and the wound on a day-to-day basis and is able to best understand the client's response to interventions, their home environment and psychosocial factors. Community nurses may not appreciate their pivotal role in wound management.

> It is not well understood by the community, nor perhaps by medical doctors and healthcare managers that nurses and midwives are not passive implementers of medical practitioners' orders, and do not work under medical supervision. Nurses and midwives hold direct legal and ethical accountability for their clinical practices and that of their colleagues. Thus, all Registered Nurses (RN)s and Registered Midwives (RM)s are regarded legally as autonomous health professionals [3, p. 8].

The community nurse therefore is both responsible and accountable to ensure wound management is based on contemporary evidence and is appropriate for the individual client. Professional autonomy and accountability bring with them expectations. For example it is the nurse's responsibility to communicate information to other members of the health care team in a timely, accurate and professional manner. If another health practitioner recommends a particular treatment and this is deemed by the clinical evidence to not be appropriate for the client, the community nurse can, with the client's consent, alter the treatment to better suit the client's needs. For example another practitioner requests that community nurses apply calcium alginate dressings to a wound with low exudate and the dressings become adhered to the wound, causing pain and trauma on removal. The community nurse does not continue this management, but applies a different dressing, more appropriate to the exudate level. However, care must be based on thorough assessment and a sound, documented, defensible rationale. Where appropriate, the nurse should inform the practitioner who recommended the care of the change and the reasons for this.

Evidence-based wound management

Wherever possible, sound, contemporary evidence should be used in the planning and implementation of wound management. Contemporary evidence and information to support wound management practice can be derived from a number of sources such as recent textbooks, journal articles in peer-reviewed journals, Cochrane reviews and publications of the Joanna Briggs Institute. Evidence-based standards and clinical practice guidelines can also be useful to guide and underpin practice. The Australian Wound Management Association (AWMA) has published standards for wound management [4]. These standards are reflective of best practice and are intended to guide practitioners, educators and researchers to achieve optimal outcomes for persons with a wound. The broad nature of the standards allows for flexible application in a variety of settings [4]. Other resources include clinical practice guidelines, systematic reviews, meta-analyses, websites, company-produced publications, newsletters, short articles, presentations and expert opinion.

Organisations might have policies, guidelines and work instructions to guide and regulate wound management practice within a particular setting. Policies can range from broad documents to those focused on a specific practice issue. Specific policies relevant to community nursing settings might include application of compression bandaging, undertaking and ankle brachial pressure index (ABPI), performing conservative sharp wound debridement or taking a wound swab. Policies help protect community nurses and their employers by guiding interventions and setting practice expectations [5].

When assessing what information to use in practice the community nurse must consider whether it is contemporary and based on sound methods and evidence and is applicable to the client and the practice setting. It is the integration of information from many sources with personal experience and skills that informs practice. Specific procedures or protocols (such as algorithms) must be based on evidence where it exists and should allow some flexibility for individual client circumstances and preference. The community nurse has a responsibility to themselves, their employers, clients and colleagues to ensure wound management knowledge and skills meet expected standards and reflect best practice. The nurse needs to understand and document the reasons for interventions and be able to identify expected outcomes. The nurse's role is also to evaluate whether interventions are achieving the expected outcomes and adjust care, when necessary, in consultation with the client. Organisations have a responsibility to develop policies, procedures and guidelines that are based on evidence. The community nurse can be placed in a difficult position when a particular wound management intervention (e.g. which dressing product to use) is insisted on by a practitioner in another organisation, but does not meet contemporary best practice or suit the client or the community nursing context. For example in some private community nursing settings, the nurse is employed by another practitioner (e.g. medical officer), or continuing referrals are reliant on following another practitioner's instructions. As autonomous practitioners with a duty of care to clients, nurses are encouraged to communicate and negotiate with practitioners to achieve best practice.

Clinical competencies

There are several ways to evaluate performance, knowledge, skills, attitudes and beliefs relevant to the nurse's scope of practice. One method of setting a standard for and evaluating knowledge and skills is the development of competencies. In wound management, a competency can be developed to evaluate a specific task, such as applying a compression bandage or performing an ABPI measurement using hand-held Doppler ultrasound. This can take the form of a checklist that might require completion under supervision prior to that skill being performed alone. Competencies can also be used to determine the nurse's clinical application of their knowledge base and attitudes. These aspects can be assessed through scenario-based competencies, where the nurse is given a set of questions based around a particular clinical situation. Competencies can be developed using existing frameworks such as the Australian Nursing and Midwifery Council (ANMC) competency framework. One way of achieving this is to develop specific wound-related competency elements and cues. The community nurse then provides a scenario from their clinical practice that demonstrates competency. Exercises involving short answer and multiple-choice questions may also be useful. Different methods or a combination of methods for confirming competence are useful for different aspects of wound management. As an example, Table 21.1 outlines

Table 21.1 Programme to achieve competence in ABPI measurement using hand-held Doppler ultrasound.

- Attend a 2-h training session with theoretical and practical components
- Complete a self-directed study guide on leg ulcer management and ABPI
- Perform at least two ABPI measurements under the supervision of another accredited registered nurse in the clinical setting
- Complete a set of questions related to clinical aspects of ABPI measurement. This includes scenario-based questions and multiple-choice questions
- Complete an ABPI competency checklist under the supervision of a nurse specifically trained to evaluate ABPI performance

the programme used to develop competence in ABPI measurement using hand-held Doppler ultrasound for the Royal District Nursing Service, South Australia. This programme integrates several methods of competency assessment.

In the community setting, evaluating competence requires innovation to manage the issues of home-based care, including independent nursing practice and limited access to resources. Technological advances such as intranets, videoconferencing, email and other opportunities must be maximised to develop, maintain and confirm the community nurse's competence in wound management.

Classification of wounds

There are several ways to classify wounds. The most commonly used classification definitions are:

Duration

- Acute – a wound that heals in a timely, predictable manner (often quoted in literature as within 6 weeks) [1].
- Enduring – a wound that heals over a prolonged time frame (greater than 6 weeks). An enduring wound is often a large wound healing by secondary intention (e.g. venous leg ulcer, pressure ulcer). Enduring wounds can be chronic wounds where the factors impairing healing have been overcome, leading to healing progressing in a measurable, observable manner.
- Chronic – a wound that has evolved into a non-healing state [6]. Chronic wounds result from cellular and/or physical and/or chemical imbalances that impair or stop the normal healing processes.

Depth

- Partial thickness – a wound that penetrates through the epidermis and possibly into the dermis. The wound does not extend into the subcutaneous tissue.
- Full thickness – a wound that extends into the subcutaneous tissue and possibly deeper.

Type of healing

- Primary intention – a wound that heals via sutures, staples or closure devices that completely approximate the wound edges.
    - Delayed primary closure is undertaken when a wound is contaminated or requires removal of foreign bodies. Primary intention is delayed by several days to allow intensive cleansing or debridement [7].
- Secondary intention – a wound that heals via granulation and contraction.

There are several specific wound classification systems. These include staging/classification systems for pressure ulcers, skin tears and foot ulceration in people with diabetes.

Stages of wound healing

Table 21.2 describes the stages of wound healing.

Table 21.2 Stages of wound healing.

Stage and duration	Processes
Haemostasis (immediate)	Haemostasis (coagulation) initiates the healing process [33]. Reduced oxygen tension at the wound site leads to vasoconstriction, formation of a platelet plug, and formation and degradation of a blood clot [7]
Following haemostasis, tissue repair occurs in three distinct but overlapping phases:	
Inflammation (0–3 days)	Vasodilation occurs in the tissues around the area of injury. Polymorphs and macrophages protect the area from bacteria and prepare for tissue repair by digesting dead bacteria and debris. Clinically, the chemical and cellular processes result in the normal manifestation of redness, heat, swelling and pain [1]
Reconstruction (2–24 days)	In the destructive phase, devitalised tissue is removed from the injured area. In the proliferative phase, fibroblasts proliferate to synthesise collagen, elastin and fibronectin. New capillaries are formed. This forms the framework of granulation tissue that fills the wound space [1]. Granulation tissue appears as pink-red, firm, vascular and bumpy. During this phase, contraction of the wound occurs simultaneously. This powerful force, mediated by myofibroblasts, speeds the healing process by pulling the wound edges towards each other, thus reducing the amount of granulation tissue required for tissue repair [2]. Finally, re-epithelialisation occurs, resurfacing the defect and restoring skin integrity
Maturation (24 days–1 year)	Once the wound has resurfaced, the new scar is remodelled. Collagen is simultaneously broken down and synthesised. New collagen fibres are oriented along the lines of mechanical stress to maximise tensile strength. However, the maximal tensile strength of a scar will only be 80% of unscarred skin. During this process, the scar becomes flatter and less vascular [7]

Anatomy and physiology of the integumentary system

A basic understanding of the anatomy and physiology of the integumentary system is assumed; hence, this will not be explored in depth within this chapter. As most wounds involve injury to the skin and associated structures, it is important for nurses to have a sound understanding of the normal structure and function of the skin. The skin is one component of the integumentary system that also includes the hair and nails. The skin is the largest organ of the human body and therefore intact skin is the first and best defence against injury [8]. The skin has several functions and these include:

- Production of vitamin D
- Excretion
- Physical and chemical barrier
- Thermal regulation

The skin is composed of two main layers: the outermost epidermis and the underlying dermis. The epidermis has four or five layers (depending on anatomical location). Epidermal cells originate in the innermost layer. As new epidermal cells arise, the older cells move towards the surface and mature, to finally be shed.

Normal wound healing

Normal wound healing follows a timely and orderly process to restore the skin's integrity. The process of repair varies, depending on the depth of wounding [2].

Partial-thickness wound healing

If only the epidermis is injured, healing proceeds as regeneration through epithelial proliferation and migration. If dermal injury also occurs, collagen formation occurs simultaneously with epithelial repair to close the wound. Partial-thickness wound healing results in re-establishment of the normal skin layers and function [2].

Full-thickness wound healing

Full-thickness wound healing results in scar formation. This is a complex process. 'Injury sets into motion a series of physiologic responses that are coordinated and sequenced and, in the healthy host invariably result in healing' [2].

Principles of wound management

There are a number of discrete principles that should be followed in wound management for every client with a wound. These principles are [9]:

1. Define wound aetiology.
2. Determine and where possible control factors impairing healing.
3. Determine long- and short-term objectives.

4. Implement local wound management.
5. Reassess and evaluate progress towards identified objectives.
6. Achieve identified objective/optimal outcome.

Each of these will now be considered in detail.

Define wound aetiology

The underlying cause of a wound must be determined to ensure appropriate management. Common aetiologies of wounds in the community include (but are not limited to):

- Venous leg ulcers
- Arterial leg ulcers
- Mixed leg ulcers (where there is coexisting venous and arterial disease)
- Pressure ulcers
- Neuropathic ulcers
- Surgical wound breakdown
- Skin cancers
- Traumatic wounds (including skin tears)

Sometimes clients are referred for community nursing care for wound management with a wound that does not have a determined aetiology. If the aetiology of a wound is unsure or cannot be determined by the community nurse, it might be necessary to liaise with other health practitioners so that further investigations can be undertaken. At any time during a client's treatment it may become evident that the original diagnosis was not correct. Reassessment might be needed to determine the correct diagnosis. Case study 21.1 provides an example of the importance of determining correct wound aetiology

---

Case study 21.1

A client is referred to a community nursing organisation for 'leg ulcer management'. In the first instance the nurse undertakes an assessment and determines that the cause of the leg ulcer is most likely venous disease. The nurse institutes compression therapy. During the course of treatment (which is successfully healing the original wound), another wound develops on the other leg. The clinical picture is also consistent with venous disease; therefore, compression is commenced. However, the second wound does not respond and slowly increases in size. As the wound is not responding, the community nurse liaises with the client's general practitioner regarding further investigations. The client is referred to the local hospital, where tests reveal the second wound to be a squamous cell carcinoma (SCC). The SCC is excised and a skin graft applied. The original wound heals with compression therapy.

Determine and where possible control factors impairing healing

The systemic factors impairing healing are covered within this chapter in the section titled, 'Physiological factors impairing healing'. The community nurse undertaking a systemic assessment process identifies these factors and takes steps to minimise their impact on healing. For example a client with diabetes can be offered education and encouraged to achieve improved blood glucose control through diet, lifestyle and adherence to medication regimens. One of the benefits of blood glucose control is improved wound-healing capacity.

Achieving and maintaining a healthy nutritional status for clients with wounds can be challenging for the community nurse. Environmental and psychosocial factors influencing healing must also be considered. These can include, but are not limited to:

- The client's willingness and ability to participate in their care (physical and psychological)
- The client's financial situation
- Involvement of carers and significant others
- The care setting (home, clinic, rural, remote)
- Resources available (nursing expertise, dressing products, equipment, e.g. pressure redistributing surfaces such as pressure mattresses)

Determine long- and short-term objectives

Following a structured and systematic assessment of the client, their environment and their wound, the community nurse can, in consultation with the client, determine objectives. Whilst these objectives might change over time, they should be identified using the best available information at that time. Objectives should be measurable, achievable and realistic.

Long-term objectives

The long-term objective is the expected final outcome for the client and their wound. The community nurse is often in the unique position of being able to follow a client through their care over a long period or until healing. To avoid frustration for both nurse and client, it is important that the long-term objective is realistic. For some clients healing might not be a realistic objective, as the factors impairing healing are unable to be controlled to an extent that will allow healing to occur. For example it might be unrealistic to expect a client with arterial ulcers due to severe, inoperable peripheral vascular disease to heal in a timely manner. Other examples of wounds unlikely to heal include malignant wounds and neuroischaemic wounds associated with Charcot foot. It is very important that the community nurse supports clients with such wounds to maximise their quality of life whilst living with their wound. The following time frames may be used to articulate the long-term objective, based on assessment of clients and their wound(s):

- Timely healing   Healing expected in 3 months or less   Acute wound
- Slow healing   Healing expected in 3–6 months   Enduring wound
- Prolonged healing Healing expected in 6–12 months   Enduring wound
- Unlikely healing   Healing doubtful or not likely to occur Chronic wound

Short-term objectives

Short-term objectives are generally related to wound-specific interventions identified following a systematic, structured assessment of wound characteristics. Short-term objectives might include (but not be limited to) one or more of the following:

- Remove non-viable tissue (slough, necrosis)
- Prevent or reduce the clinical signs of infection
- Control exudate
- Resolve maceration
- Reduce pain during dressing changes

Short-term objectives also must be realistic, measurable and achievable. Regular assessment should be undertaken to determine if the objectives have been met and new objectives set based on wound and client reassessment. For example if a client has recently sustained a skin tear to their forearm, the initial short-term objectives might be to (1) optimise viability of the skin flap, (2) protect fragile periwound skin and (3) prevent infection.

Implement local wound management

Ideal conditions at the local wound environment will facilitate optimal outcomes. The term 'wound bed preparation' is often used to describe the processes used to achieve this [10]. The mnemonic TIME has become synonymous with the components of wound bed preparation [10]:

*T*issue management
*I*nfection and inflammation control
*M*oisture control
*E*dge of wound advancement

Tissue management is the elimination of non-viable tissue from the wound [11]. This can be achieved through one or more of the following debridement techniques:

- *Autolytic.* Using moist wound management, through dressings, to enhance the body's natural processes. Autolytic debridement is the easiest debridement method to use but the process can be prolonged [12].
- *Mechanical.* Using external force, e.g. wet-to-dry saline-soaked gauze, high-pressure irrigation, forceful cleansing with gauze or scraping the wound with a blunt instrument such as forceps. Can be useful but should be used with caution as some techniques can damage healthy tissue or cause pain and/or trauma.
- *Conservative sharp.* Using sterile, sharp metal instruments (scissors and scalpels). This can be a rapid, cost-effective, efficacious method of debridement. However, the community nurse must possess the necessary skills and knowledge to perform this.

- *Biological.* Also referred to as maggot therapy or larval therapy. Larval therapy using specifically bred sterile maggots is used in some community settings. If the community nurse is required to undertake this procedure, they should check with the supplier of the maggots regarding appropriate protocols for use. In the community setting, accidental larval infestation is not uncommon. If this has occurred, the maggots should be removed from the wound and disposed of appropriately.
- *Surgical.* Debridement generally performed under general anaesthesia by a surgeon. More extensive than conservative sharp debridement. Usually involves excision of all non-viable tissue down to a healthy, bleeding base.
- *Chemical.* Using chemicals to break down non-viable tissue, e.g. sodium hypochlorite. Generally not used in modern wound management due to the possible deleterious effects on healthy tissue.
- *Enzymatic.* Using enzymes. There are currently no enzymatic wound debridement agents available in Australia. However, overseas this is a commonly used technique.

In chronic wounds, repeated sharp debridement might be necessary to remove the physical and cellular burden impairing healing. In the community setting, autolytic, mechanical and conservative sharp wound debridement are the most commonly used techniques.

Reassess and evaluate progress towards identified objectives

Regular assessment of client and wound progress is used to guide management. An informal assessment is undertaken every dressing change. During this assessment the community nurse evaluates whether or not the dressing is meeting the needs of the client and the wound. It is important that the community nurse has an understanding of what the wound appearance was previously in order to make a sound judgement as to whether the wound is static, improving or deteriorating. It may not always be possible for the same community nurse to undertake consecutive dressing changes as many nurses work part-time or on a casual basis. Therefore, good documentation is relied on by all health professionals involved in the client's care to provide information for comparison. A formal, systematic, documented reassessment of wound characteristics should be undertaken every 1–4 weeks, based on clinical judgement, or at any time there is a significant change in the wound [13]. When determining the optimal frequency for formal assessment, the following factors are considered:

- The type of wound
- The expected duration of the wound
- The care setting (e.g. clinic, remote, residential, domiciliary)

A well-designed wound assessment chart that is quick and easy to complete can guide a systematic assessment by prompting the necessary parameters and allowing easy comparison of wound characteristics over time.

The community nurse undertaking reassessment must consider whether the client and the wound are moving towards the identified long-term objective. For example, if timely healing is the long-term objective and the wound dimensions have not changed in 2 weeks, a reassessment should be undertaken that considers the local wound environment and client factors influencing healing. For example, it might be that the wound has developed a mild infection that requires treatment or the client with diabetes has poorly controlled blood glucose levels.

Achieve optimal outcome

Optimal outcome will vary. For the majority of clients healing will be the expected outcome. For a minority of clients healing might not be realistic, as the factors impairing healing cannot be adequately overcome. Whilst it is the community nurse's role to work with the client to achieve the highest quality of life while living with a wound, it becomes even more important when healing is unlikely. This might occur in persons with malignant wounds or ischaemic wounds.

A wound that has epithelialised is viewed as healed. However, as new scar tissue is yet to reach its maximal tensile strength, care of the new scar is important to prevent breakdown. Regular moisturising helps keep tissue supple. Regular massage of the scar and/or some topical applications (e.g. stretch adhesive tape or silicone sheets/gel) might have some benefit in reducing the appearance of scar tissue.

Factors impairing wound healing

There are many factors that can impair the wound-healing process and outcomes. It is important that the community nurse undertakes a systematic, comprehensive assessment of the client with a wound to determine any such factors. A well-constructed wound assessment chart provides a framework to record these factors. Information gained from the client, other practitioners, written records, significant others such as parents or guardians in the circumstance of a child client and the community nurse's own observations are used to assist in determining the objectives for the client with a wound.

Community nurse influence on wound healing

Lifestyle changes and optimal control of comorbidities can positively affect wound outcomes and should be encouraged by the community nurse. A combination of verbal and written information with encouragement for the client can be useful. Delivering care in someone's own home is quite different to delivering care in a hospital setting. If a client perceives the community nurse as too forceful or directive, they might decide not to heed the advice given or even refuse to have a particular community nurse attend their care. Therefore, developing a trusting professional relationship and good rapport with the client and/or carers is essential. The community nurse often finds that they are also responsible for explaining medical terminology, disease processes, test results and other health-related issues whilst providing direct clinical wound care for the client.

Physiological factors impairing healing

Table 21.3 outlines some of the most common physiological factors that may impair healing and their mechanism of action.

Table 21.3 Physiological factors impairing healing [1, 2, 7, 18, 33–35].

Factor impairing healing	Mechanism of action
Systemic/general	Factors relevant to the general health status of a client that can impair healing
Increasing age	Multiple influences on healing. Slows down metabolic processes. Decreased skin thickness. Decrease in collagen content of skin. Impaired inflammation and tissue repair
Poor nutritional state	Inadequate nutrients will reduce the formation and strength of vital wound-healing components
Poor vascularity	Inadequate blood supply results in inadequate delivery of oxygen and nutrients to the wound. Reduced transport of waste products
Smoking	Can lead to hypoxia, impaired epithelialisation, vasoconstriction, enzymatic system toxicity, poor tissue perfusion, reduction in collagen synthesis and reduction in cutaneous blood flow
Diabetes	Effects of raised blood glucose levels can include compromised vascular supply, aberrant metabolic pathophysiology and impaired leukocyte function
Malignancy	Can result in locally compromised blood supply and decay of tissues, increased risk of infection. Poor nutritional state is common. Chemotherapy and radiotherapy can impair healing
Corticosteroid medications	Inhibits epithelial proliferation. The powerful anti-inflammatory effects impair wound healing
Rheumatoid arthritis	A chronic inflammatory process. Anti-inflammatory drugs given to control the condition can suppress wound inflammation and predispose to infection
Inflammatory bowel disease	Associated with malabsorption and poor nutrition. There is increased risk of infection and reduced energy available for tissue repair
Renal disease	A raised blood urea impairs granulation tissue formation. Can lead to anaemia, fluid and electrolyte imbalance, and increased risk of infection
Hepatic failure	Lowers the level of circulating haemoglobin. Increases the risk of wound dehiscence
Stress, anxiety, depression	Reduces immune system efficiency
Local	Factors at the local wound environment that can impair healing
High bacterial load/infection	Prolongs inflammatory phase. Can cause additional tissue destruction, delayed collagen synthesis and epithelialisation, endotoxins and metalloproteinase production. Biofilm might form
Non-viable tissue	Increases the risk of infection and prolongs the inflammatory response. Can mechanically obstruct contraction
Foreign bodies	Lead to increased risk of infection or chronic inflammation
Trauma, pressure, shear	Can compromise or occlude local blood flow. Can damage local circulation and tissues. Ischaemia with subsequent tissue necrosis can occur
Poor wound management practices	Includes poor dressing technique, inappropriate dressing product selection, inappropriate use of antiseptics, failure to act on factors impairing healing, failure to correctly identify aetiology and treat appropriately

Psychological and social factors impacting on wound healing

Psychological and social factors can also contribute significantly to wound outcomes. Managing the social and/or psychological factors impacting on healing often requires innovation, flexibility and compromise with the client. If the client cannot understand the reasons for the recommended treatment, due to poor explanation, communication or language difficulties, cognitive impairment or mental illness, it can make concordance difficult. Behaviours such as constantly disturbing or removing dressings, getting dressings wet, regularly missing appointments for care or refusing contemporary wound treatments may produce challenges for the nurse and lack of wound progress for the client. Issues such as alcoholism, substance abuse, homelessness, self-neglect and aggression can impact significantly on the ability to deliver nursing care safely in the community. It is important for health professionals across care settings to communicate potential social or behavioural challenges in order to maintain a safe working environment. Working with clients in the community can require negotiation and compromise to deliver the best possible care that is acceptable to both the client and the community nurse.

Nutrition

Improving nutritional intake is a major challenge for some community clients. Protein and vitamins are vital for wound healing [14]. The community nurse should not presume adequate nutritional intake of the client. If the client consents, the community nurse could check the amount and quality of food in cupboards or the refrigerator. If possible, it is helpful to weigh the client regularly as unintentional weight loss can signify inadequate diet or underlying disease (e.g. malignancy). Even if meals are delivered through a community organisation (such as Meals on Wheels), the nurse will need to ascertain how much the client is eating. For example some clients will feed their delivered meals to the pet or will make the one meal last an entire day. Offer education to clients regarding eating a balanced diet. In particular, reinforce the importance of protein as essential for wound healing [14]. For example suggest good-quality protein sources such as lean meat, fish, eggs, nuts, legumes and dairy products, and strategies such as fortifying milk with skim milk powder can increase protein intake. Some clients might benefit from a vitamin and mineral supplement if it is suspected that dietary intake is inadequate. Commercially prepared nutritional supplements are available. Some of these, such as preparations containing the essential amino acid arginine, claim to assist wound healing [15, 16]. Occasionally, specific vitamin supplements are required under the direction of a medical officer. For example vitamin D deficiency is not uncommon in clients who rarely venture outdoors.

Infection and inflammation control

Infection and inflammation control is the management of wound bacterial load and the chronic, inflammatory process often associated with chronic, non-healing wounds. No wound is sterile and wounds will heal with a level of bacteria [17]. However, a high level of bacteria or the presence of multiple species of bacteria can overwhelm the body's defence mechanisms resulting in impaired healing and local and systemic effects [18]. It is now also recognised that bacteria can form organised communities comprising various species that secrete an exopolymeric substance referred to as biofilm [19]. This biofilm coats the bacterial colonies and makes them resistant to antibiotics and topical preparations. Management of infection and chronic inflammation of wounds in the community setting usually involves topical antimicrobials or systemic treatment (antibiotics).

Topical antimicrobials such as silver-containing dressings and cadexomer iodine are widely used in community settings to prevent and treat high bacterial load in wounds. There are several points to consider in relation to using topical antimicrobials:

- Undertake a comprehensive and systematic assessment prior to commencement of the therapy. These products are used when it is believed that the wound healing is or has a high potential of being impaired by bacteria. Certain types of silver-containing dressings might also be useful in reducing chronic wound inflammation [18]. Antimicrobial dressings can be used as a primary treatment for superficial infections or as an adjunct to systemic antibiotics in the treatment of local or spreading infection.
- Ensure control of other underlying client factors prior to commencement of therapy, e.g. good compression therapy for venous disease and adequate pressure redistribution for pressure ulcers.
- Generally these products will not penetrate thick slough or eschar; therefore, this needs to be removed prior to dressing application.
- Choose a product with proven efficacy as the composition of silver-containing dressings varies considerably [20]. Look for supporting studies or literature.
- Choose a product appropriate for the wound characteristics and apply it according to the manufacturer's recommendations. There are several presentations of cadexomer iodine and many variations of silver-containing dressings. Choose a product appropriate for the wound exudate level, the client and the type of wound (see 'Dressing procedure and cleansing techniques' section in this chapter).
- Set a defined period for evaluation of the effect. If it is expected that the wound will improve with use of a topical antimicrobial, measurable progress should occur within 2–4 weeks [21]. If the wound has not demonstrated improvement (e.g. reduction in size, improvement in tissue quality, reduction in exudate and reduction in pain) in 4 weeks, consideration should be given to systemic antibiotic therapy or other factors that might be the cause of the impaired healing.

Pain in wound management

Pain is commonly associated with wounding and can be associated with the physiological effects of impaired healing (see Table 21.3). Pain is described as 'an unpleasant sensory and emotional experience associated with actual or potential tissue damage, or described in terms of such damage' [22, p. xx]. It should be assumed all wounds are painful unless proved otherwise [23]. In wound management pain is often poorly assessed and managed. Clients sometimes endure severe pain in the misguided belief that it is a necessary and normal part of healing. A holistic wound management model must include pain management.

Types of pain

Nociceptive pain

Normal, nociceptive pain is typically localised, constant and often with an aching or throbbing quality. It is an appropriate, physiological response [23] that alerts the body to actual harm and forces the person to rest the part, facilitating healing. Nociceptive pain is usually associated with acute wounds and is self-limiting [24].

Neuropathic pain

Neuropathic pain is an inappropriate physiological response that is usually associated with nerve damage [22]. The pain frequently has burning qualities. Neuropathic pain is the main cause of chronic pain [22]. In chronic wounds, the prolonged inflammatory response can result in hypersensitivity and increased pain that is seemingly more severe than expected for the stimulus. This can manifest as [22]:

- Primary hyperalgesia: severe pain occurring in the wound itself
- Secondary hyperalgesia: severe pain occurring in the skin surrounding the wound
- Allodynia: intense pain brought on by minimal stimuli (such as movement of air over the wound)

Chronic, neuropathic pain usually requires specialised assessment and management by a medical pain management specialist. In wound management, neuropathic pain is often underestimated and clients might not receive adequate pain control. Chronic pain can lead to impaired wound healing and significant psychological, social and financial harm [13].

The individual interpretation of pain and the meaning each of these types of pain has for a client is dependent on:

- Psychosocial influences, e.g. pain threshold and tolerance, age, culture, gender, education, anxiety and fear
- Environmental influences, e.g. timing of the procedure, setting, techniques used, positioning and tools used

In wound management, common causes of pain include:

- Inappropriate dressing choice (e.g. dressings that become adhered to the wound or slip or pain due to the qualities of the product itself)
- Aggressive cleansing or debridement techniques (e.g. wet-to-dry saline-soaked gauze, which is likely to cause pain on removal).
- Application of hot or cold topical preparations
- Prolonged exposure of wounds to the air
- Frequent dressing changes

Pain assessment

Systematic, comprehensive, regular assessment is used to understand the client's experience of pain. It is important for the community nurse to respect and believe the client's description of their pain and to use open, non-judgemental questions. Assess the cause(s) of pain, location, duration, quality, triggers and relievers. It is recommended that a validated pain assessment scale (of which there are several) is used to assess pain [13]. Special consideration should be given to persons who cannot articulate their pain, such as the very young, intellectually disabled, clients with a neurological impairment or clients who cannot speak fluent English. Pain assessment should occur at regular intervals, in particular following interventions aimed at reducing pain (e.g. administration of analgesia) to determine their effectiveness. In wound management it is also important to consider the particular challenges associated with clients who do not experience pain. Clients with paraesthesia due to neuropathy or spinal cord injury are at high risk of wounding, as they do not feel a normal pain response when tissue damage occurs.

Management of pain

Pain management should be individualised for each client. If possible, the community nurse should implement strategies to remove the cause of the pain. For example wound infection or cellulitis should be managed with appropriate antibiotic therapy; ischaemia should be assessed and managed by a vascular surgeon. For pain which is assessed as 'complex', the community nurse might need to facilitate referral to an appropriate practitioner.

Pharmacological management

Pharmacological agents can be used when other strategies are not possible or are ineffective. A combination of pharmacological and non-pharmacological agents is usually the most effective in managing chronic pain. The choice of agent is based on a comprehensive assessment of the client. Ensure:

- The choice of agent is appropriate for the pain and the client
- The client receives adequate educational information related to the agent, dose, administration, expected effects and possible adverse effects
- There is adequate assessment of effect
- Adverse effects are monitored and reported to the prescribing medical office or nurse practitioner if they occur

Acute pain often responds well to regular doses of traditional analgesia [13]. Treatment with some antidepressants and anticonvulsants has been demonstrated to reduce chronic pain associated with wounds [13]. Other strategies such as local anaesthetic infusions and transcutaneous electrical nerve stimulation can also be offered to the client to assist in the control of neuropathic pain.

The community nurse should advocate for the client to ensure that a comprehensive, appropriate and effective pain management plan is implemented that reflects the client's wishes, if the client is unable to do so.

Dressing procedure and cleansing techniques

Wound cleansing is the removal of excess exudate, wound debris and old dressing product, with the aim of achieving an optimal wound environment for healing to proceed [25]. The procedures and techniques associated with wound cleansing and application of dressings are performed routinely by nurses in the community. However, many techniques are embedded in tradition and folklore rather than evidence [26]. There is an urgent need for rigorous research related to wound-cleansing techniques and solutions [27]. There are three main wound-cleansing techniques:

- *Sterile*. Using sterile equipment, sterile solutions, sterile gloves and multiple sterile fields. Usually performed in the operating theatre.
- *Aseptic*. Using sterile equipment, sterile solutions and a 'non-touch' technique. A commercially prepared dressing pack is usually used and forceps are used to handle any dressing products. Gloves are not required to be worn unless there is a risk of contamination with blood or body fluids.
- *Clean*. Using non-sterile equipment, non-sterile solutions and limited handling of dressing products using clean, non-sterile gloves.

In the community most wounds can be cleansed using a clean technique, with some requiring aseptic technique [4]. The AWMA's wound management standards related to wound-cleansing and -dressing techniques are described as follows:

An aseptic wound technique will be used when: the client is immunosuppressed, the wound enters a sterile body cavity (i.e. nephrostomy or central venous line), during the peri-operative period, or the wound healing environment is compromised. A clean wound management technique, i.e. washing or showering of wounds, may be implemented when the criterion [for an aseptic technique] is not demonstrated or when policies and procedures dictate [4, p. 9].

In the community setting the client's floor or a table is often used as a dressing preparation area. Whatever the setting, the community nurse must undertake procedures in a manner that minimises the risk of introducing new bacteria to the wound environment. The principles of wound field concept should apply no matter what technique is used. The 'wound field' consists of the wound and the dressing preparation area, whether that is the upper surface of the sheet in a dressing pack or a clean dressing towel [26].

The main solutions used to clean wounds in the community are sterile saline and tap water of drinking quality. 'Antiseptics are not justified in the majority of cases, but they may have some benefit on heavily colonised or infected wounds' [25, p. 157]. The community nurse is also required to manage availability of dressing products. Individual organisations should consider implementing guidelines for the use, storage and transfer of dressing products. These can include:

- Whether an unused portion of a dressing product can be used at a later date on the same client; e.g. if the wound requires a clean technique for cleansing, a clean dressing should suffice. However, if the wound requires aseptic technique, a sterile dressing is generally used.
- Whether it is acceptable to save and use partially used products. If so, storage techniques should minimise the risk of contamination or soiling; e.g. a plastic zip-lock bag is useful for this.

- Transfer of excess stock-out of the client's home for use on others. If undertaking this, only sealed, clean packets that can be wiped with detergent or disinfectant should be transferred out of clients' homes. Transfer of excess stock is generally not appropriate for clients with multiresistant organisms or an infectious disease.

Assessment and documentation

Structured, systematic and comprehensive assessment is vital. The AWMA's standards for wound management state that 'clinical decision making includes evidence of a comprehensive assessment of the individual, their wound, their risk of wounding and healing environment' [4, p. 7].

Wound assessment has two main components:

1. Collection of baseline information. This might include:
   - Location of wound(s)
   - Date of wounding
   - Mechanism of injury
   - A brief history of any previous wounds
   - A list of other health care practitioners involved in the client's care
   - Factors impairing healing
   - Client's understanding of their wound and their expected outcome
   - Biochemical data, e.g. blood tests and radiology results

Baseline information is used for professional communication and to assist in determining the client's long-term outcome.

2. Collection of information regarding wound characteristics includes:
   - Wound dimensions
   - Tissue types
   - Exudate amount and quality
   - Odour
   - Surrounding skin
   - Pain level
   - Possibly specific factors such as a wound swab or biopsy

Documentation forms part of the enduring legal nursing record. It is important that documentation is timely, accurate, complete, comprehensive, objective, relevant and concise. It is important that organisations have policies regarding expected documentation and that nurses understand those expectations.

Tools of documentation

There are many tools of documentation available. These range from the very simple to the more complex. A brief overview of the most commonly used tools to assist in wound documentation follows:

Ruler

Many of the dressing product manufacturers supply disposable rulers to assist with measurement of wound dimensions. These should be used once and then discarded. Rulers allow measurement of maximum wound length, width and, possibly, depth. Length and width must be measured perpendicular to each other [28]. Unless the wound is round or square in shape, multiplying the length and width does not provide an accurate surface area or volume. However, simple measurements can assist the community nurse to determine whether or not contraction (and therefore healing) is occurring. Some companies manufacture wound probes with centimetre/millimetre graduations printed on them. These can be very useful for measuring wound depth (including undermining and sinuses).

Tracing

Tracing of wound size onto clear plastic is a simple, yet very useful, way of determining wound progress. Some dressing product manufacturers can supply tracing grids. These often have room for client details and have a 0.5-cm or 1.0-cm grid marked on them. Some are multilayered, enabling the surface that contacts the wound during the tracing process to be discarded. However, a clean piece of thick plastic or acetate can be used if other grids are not available. If serial tracings are kept, they can be compared over time to assist in determining wound progress. Tracing is a skill that requires some expertise. When a plastic grid is placed over a wound, condensation can form, obscuring the wound edges and making tracing difficult. Sometimes it is necessary to hold the grid down and gently lift edge sections as they are traced to ensure that the marker is in the correct position. Client positioning, body curvature, tapering of limbs and the thickness of the marker can also affect tracing accuracy [29].

A more sophisticated tracing method is available with the Visitrak™ from Smith & Nephew®. This is a battery-powered, portable, digital device. The Visitrak™ can calculate wound length and width, surface area and surface area of a secondary area (e.g. undermining or necrosis). If previous data is available, the Vistrak™ can calculate a change in wound surface area over time. A computer program to enter client and wound details and track changes over time is available with the Visitrak™.

Photography: The rapid evolution of digital cameras has provided community nurses with an affordable, easy method to accurately record wound appearance. Digital images can also be shared across electronic networks between community nurses and other health practitioners. This is particularly helpful to those community nurses working in remote areas who have limited contact with wound specialists (both nursing and medical). In utilising digital photography for wound documentation there are several issues to consider. These include:

- Ensure that the camera battery is adequately charged and the nurse is familiar with how to use the camera.
- It is recommended that written consent is obtained from clients [30]. This is particularly important where images might be used for education or publication.
- Wherever possible, avoid including identifying features in images.
- Take a minimum of two images. One image should be from enough distance to allow overall perspective of the area. For example if the photograph is of a leg

ulcer, one photo should include the whole lower leg. Another photo taken closer should identify detail. Holding a disposable ruler adjacent to the wound within the photograph can assist with identification of wound dimensions.

- Avoid busy or glossy backgrounds (such as floral prints or plastic). If possible, use a dark, matt background such as a clean towel or sheet.
- Hold the camera at 90° to the wound to avoid skewed perspective.
- Always check the quality of the images before dressing the wound. Blurry images are not useful.
- Ensure there is a process for saving and printing photographs. Higher resolution cameras will give very sharp images but these use considerable storage space on a computer. The process for saving photographs should allow easy retrieval at a later date if required.

Photographs do not replace the need for written wound documentation. Recording of exudate level and type, odour, the appearance of surrounding skin and pain level remains necessary because these elements are not captured by a photograph.

Computer programs

Sophisticated computer programs such as the Alfred Medseed Wound Imaging System (AMWIS™) allow the user to obtain considerable information from a digital photograph. This can include surface area, types of tissues in the wound and a detailed client history. Programs such as this offer significant benefits for community, rural and remote nurses as images and information, with the client's consent, can be shared across electronic networks. This concept of 'telehealth' means nurses can communicate with other health practitioners in major health centres and receive advice. Clients benefit from not having to travel to the city for a consultation and have the opportunity to receive expert input from a distance.

Sinuses and undermining

Obtaining an accurate description and/or diagrammatic representation of sinuses and undermining can be difficult. One method of describing these is to use a clock-face analogy [31]. This is achieved by using grid lines or imagining a clock face over the wound. The centre of the 'clock face' should be the centre of the wound. Twelve o'clock is always towards the head. In this way, descriptions can be used such as '2 cm deep undermining from one o'clock to five o'clock'. The same method can be used for sinuses. For example '4-cm-deep sinus at seven o'clock'. Figure 21.1 illustrates this technique.

To assist in tracing undermining accurately, place a soft-tipped probe gently in the undermining until resistance is felt. Feel for the end of the probe with a finger on the skin above (like feeling for a toe through a shoe). Use a marker to place a small mark on the client's skin where the end of the probe can be felt. Move the probe a few centimetres, following the undermining, and repeat the process. Once the extent of the undermining has been marked out, a tracing grid can be used to record the wound and undermine by tracing over the marks made on the client's skin.

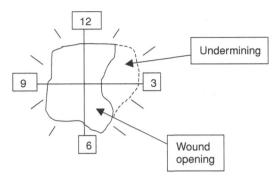

Figure 21.1 Using a clock-face analogy to describe undermining and sinuses.

Moisture control (dressings)

Dressings are applied to the wound primarily to regulate moisture, thereby achieving and maintaining optimal moisture balance at the wound to facilitate the ideal healing environment. Maintaining a moist wound environment can accelerate healing up to 50% over dry wound healing [17]. The ideal dressing is one optimised for each individual according to the wound characteristics, client factors and the care setting. The ideal dressing fulfils all the following criteria [17, 32]:

- Regulates wound moisture effectively, avoiding desiccation or maceration of the wound and periwound area
- Provides thermal insulation, maintaining an appropriate wound temperature
- Maintains an effective barrier against bacterial penetration
- Does not adhere to the wound, nor allow leakage of exudate
- Does not contain any toxic, irritant or pain-causing components
- Does not cause damage to the wound or periwound area
- Is able to be applied and removed without causing pain and/or trauma
- Is acceptable to the client (including appearance) and their social and economic circumstances

As dressings are primarily moisture regulators, it is useful to classify them according to their functionality. Table 21.4 outlines the main categories of basic moist wound-healing dressing products.

In addition to moisture regulation, the nurse should consider the following when choosing the most appropriate dressing to use:

- The location and dimensions of the wound
- The types of tissue present in the wound
- The long-term objective

Whilst the majority of wounds can be managed using the basic products outlined in Table 21.4, there will be circumstances when a specialty dressing or therapy will be required. There are a burgeoning number of specialised dressings available. Characteristics of specialty dressings include:

- A particular dressing suitable for a range of wound exudate levels (e.g. rapid capillary action dressing)
- A dressing with an active component (e.g. silver) in different presentations for various exudate levels
- Additional functions, including (but not limited to) dressings designed to reduce odour through the addition of carbon, dressings that claim to reduce bacterial load through the addition of silver or iodine, dressings that offer wound cleansing or debridement (e.g. foam with additives, wet therapy or high-sodium dressings) and dressings that minimise trauma to the wound and periwound area (e.g. silicone-coated dressings)

The community nurse must sometimes consider other factors that influence what dressing is used in the community. These can include:

- Client acceptability – the dressing needs to suit the client's lifestyle. The ability and willingness of the client to accept and participate in their care must be considered.
- Availability – in some areas, there might be very limited resources or the dressing product range might be restricted.
- Cost – in areas where the client or family is required to meet the costs of dressings this can influence dressing choice. Even where dressing products might be provided at no direct cost to the client, a limited or inadequate organisational budget line can limit the availability and use of dressing products. A cost–benefit analysis based on outcome is recommended, rather than focusing on cost per dressing. For example a more expensive dressing product might heal a wound in a shorter period, thereby saving considerable money for a nursing organisation.

Table 21.4 Basic dressing products according to functionality.

Exudate level	Dressing functionality	Generic products	Notes
None. Dry wound	Hydration	Hydrogel High-sodium gel	Occlusion of dressing will ensure optimal product performance. Prior to rehydration of dry eschar on extremities ensure the client has adequate arterial blood supply to support healing
Low	Moisture retention	Hydrogel Hydrocolloid Thin foam	Usually an occlusive dressing is required to ensure moisture is retained at the wound surface
Moderate	Exudate management	Regular foam Calcium alginate	Absorbency characteristics should help retain exudate in the dressing, thereby preventing maceration or leakage
High	Exudate management	Thick foam Expanding foam Hydrofiber Specialty absorbent dressings	

In choosing which dressing product to use, the nurse assesses the client and their wound and collaborates with the client and other health practitioners involved in the client's care. Dressing choice is influenced by the community nurse's knowledge and confidence, past experience, available products and the recommendations of other health practitioners. Some guiding principles to assist in optimising dressing performance include:

- Understand the dressing product being used. Source information from companies, colleagues, journals and other publications and internet sites. The community nurse needs to understand how the dressing functions, the main components and structure of the dressing, how to apply the dressing correctly and expected wear time.
- Assess the old dressing. This will provide information on dressing performance, including durability, exudate quality and quantity, and moisture regulation.
- Avoid frequently changing the types of products used. The following list notes some of the bona fide reasons to change the type of dressing product being used:
  - The dressing is inappropriate for the wound exudate level or the exudate-level changes. This might result in the dressing being adhered to the wound bed. Dressings should not need to be soaked off. Alternatively, the dressing might leak. An inappropriately applied dressing may affect dressing performance. In a community setting, some strike through of wound exudate to the outside of the dressing might be determined to be acceptable, depending on the wound, the client and the care setting.
  - The client has developed sensitivity to the product. This often manifests as a rash where the dressing was contacting the skin.
  - The dressing causes prolonged pain or irritation.
  - The wound becomes or ceases to be infected.
  - The wound has not met expected short-term objectives in a 4-week period.

If the community nurse ceases using a dressing product, the rationale for this must be clearly stated in the client's notes. The reasons/rationale for choosing an alternative product should also be described.

Edge of wound advancement

Wound contraction (reduction in wound dimensions) is an indicator of wound healing. Healthy wound edges are pink, flat and somewhat indistinct. Raised, rolled, indurated (hard), overhanging, distinct wound edges might indicate impaired or stalled wound healing. 'A wound that is not 30% smaller between weeks 0 and 4 is unlikely to heal by week 12' [17, p. 32]. Therefore, accurate, regular, comparative recording of wound dimensions and margin appearance is vital. The rate of wound-edge advancement can help guide wound treatment choices. If dressings fail to improve the wound, consideration should be given to further investigations or more advanced therapies.

Wound bed preparation aims to remove the physical, cellular and chemical burdens that can impair healing. Wound bed preparation presumes that other factors impairing healing are identified and controlled and therefore this concept should not be viewed in isolation from the whole client and their circumstances.

Conclusion

This chapter has addressed the issues and challenges faced by community nurses when caring for a client with a wound. Guiding principles have been linked to competency standards to offer the reader an understanding of the standard of care required to not only manage a wound from a clinical perspective but also offer the client a service which is informative and inclusive of their needs.

Wound management in a community nursing setting can be challenging, rewarding and interesting. New developments in wound management mean the community nurse needs to keep abreast of changes to ensure practice is contemporary and evidence based. This will assist to ensure that clients are involved in their care choices and will achieve the optimal outcome.

References

1. Myles, J. (2006) Woundcare: Assessment and principles of healing. *Practice Nurse*, 32(8). Accessed online 29 March 2007.
2. Bryant, R.A. (1992) *Acute and Chronic Wounds: Nursing Management*. Mosby Year Book, Missouri, USA.
3. Nurses Board of South Australia (2006) *Nursing and Midwifery Career Structure Discussion Paper, Nursing Office*. Department of Health, South Australia.
4. Australian Wound Management Association (2002) *Standards for Wound Management*. Australian Wound Management Association, ACT.
5. Crofton, C. and Witney, G. (2004) Understanding nursing documentation, in C. Crofton and G. Witney (eds) *Nursing Documentation in Aged Care: A Guide to Practice*. Ausmed Publications, Melbourne, Australia.
6. Moore, K. (2003) *Wound Physiology: From Healing to Chronicity, Emap Healthcare*. London, England.
7. Carville, K. (2005) *Wound Care Manual, Silver Chain Nursing Association*. Osborne Park, Western Australia.
8. Sibbald, R.G., Campbell, K., Coutts, P. and Queen, D. (2003) Intact skin – an integrity not to be lost. *Ostomy/Wound Management*, 49(6), 27–41.
9. Templeton, S. (2005a) Assessment and documentation, in S. Templeton (ed.) *Wound Care Nursing: A Guide to Practice*. Ausmed Publications, Melbourne, Australia.
10. Falanga, V. (2004) *Wound Bed Preparation: Science Applied to Practice*. European Wound Management Association, Position document: Wound Bed Preparation in Practice. MEP, London, England.
11. Swanson, T. (2005) Wound bed preparation, in S. Templeton (ed.) *Wound Care Nursing: A Guide to Practice*. Ausmed Publications, Melbourne, Australia.
12. Enoch, S. and Harding, K. (2003) Wound bed preparation: The science behind the removal of barriers to healing. *WOUNDS: A Compendium of Clinical Research and Practice*, 15(7), 213–29.
13. Keast, D.H., Bowering, K., Evans, A.W., Mackean, G.L., Burrows, C. and D'Souza, L. (2004), MEASURE: A proposed assessment framework for developing best practice recommendations for wound assessment. *Wound Repair and Regeneration*, 12(3 Suppl), S1–17.
14. Hess, C.T. (1999) *Clinical Guide: Wound Care*. Springhouse Corporation, Pennsylvania.
15. Waitzberg, D.L., Saito, H., Plank, L.D., Jamieson, G.G., Jagannath, P., Hwang, T.-L., Mijares, J.M. and Bihari, D. (2006) Postsurgical infections are reduced with specialized nutritional support. *World Journal of Surgery*, 30, 1–13.

16. Desneves, K.J., Todorovic, B.E., Cassar, A. and Crowe, T.C. (2005) Treatment with supplementary arginine, vitamin C and zinc in patients with pressure ulcers: A randomised controlled trial. *Clinical Nutrition*, 24, 979–87.
17. Sibbald, R.G., Williamson, D., Orsted, H.L., Campbell, K., Keast, D., Krasner, D. and Sibbald, D. (2000) Preparing the wound bed – debridement, bacterial balance and moisture balance., *Ostomy/Wound Management*, 46(11), 14–35.
18. Warriner, R. and Burrell, R. (2005) Infection and the chronic wound: A focus on silver. *Advances in Skin and Wound Care*, 18(Suppl 1), 2–12.
19. Percival, S. (July 2004) *Understanding the Effects of Bacterial Communities and Biofilms on Wound Healing*. World Wide Wounds. Available at www.worldwidewounds.com (viewed 9 November 2007).
20. Thomas, S. and McCubbin, P. (2003) An in-vitro analysis of the antimicrobial properties of 10 silver-containing dressings. *Journal of Wound Care*, 12(8), 305–8.
21. Templeton, S. (2005b) Management of chronic wounds: The role of silver-containing dressings. *Primary Intention*, 13(4), 170–79.
22. World Union of Wound Healing Societies (WUWHS) (2004) *Minimising Pain at Wound Dressing-Related Procedures*. A consensus document. MEP, London.
23. Hollinworth, H. (2005) *Pain at Wound Dressing-Related Procedures; a Template for Assessment*. World Wide Wounds. Available at www.worldwidewounds.com (viewed 29 October 2005).
24. Templeton, S. (2006) *Minimisation of Pain and/or Trauma During Wound Management, the Pursuit of Excellence*, 41, 1–5. Available at www.rdns.org.au
25. Carr, M. (2006) Wound cleansing: Sorely neglected? *Primary Intention*, 14(4), 150–61.
26. Ellis, T. and Beckmann, A. (1997) The wound field concept: A new approach to teaching and conceptualising wound dressing. *Primary Intention*, 5(2), 28–34.
27. Joanna Briggs Institute (2006) Solutions, techniques and pressure in wound cleansing: Best practice evidence based information sheet for health professionals. 10(2), 1–4.
28. Pudner, R. (2002) Measuring wounds. *Journal of community Nursing*, 16(9), 36–42.
29. Flanagan, M. (2003) Wound measurement: Can it help us to monitor progression to healing? *Journal of Wound Care*, 12(5), 189–94.
30. Swann, G. (2000) Photography in wound care. *Nursing Times Plus*, 96(45), 9–12.
31. McConnell, E.A. (2000) Measuring a wound. *Nursing*, 30(12), 17.
32. Pudner, R. (1997) Choosing an appropriate wound dressing. *Journal of Community Nursing*, 11(9), 34–9.
33. Smith and Nephew (2001) Science of wound management: Wound bed preparation.
34. Fergusson, J.A.E. and MacLellan, D.G. (1997) Wound management in older people. *The Australian Journal of Hospital Pharmacy*, 27(6), 461–67.
35. Rayner, R. (2006) Effects of cigarette smoking on cutaneous wound healing. *Primary Intention*, 14(3), 100–104.

Chapter 22

Systemic reactions and anaphylaxis

Deryn Thompson, Kate Visentin and Colleen Smith

Introduction

The focus of this chapter is systemic reaction and anaphylaxis in community nursing settings. The historical perspective of nursing management in emergency situations related to allergic reactions is explored followed by identification of the important elements of relevant drug therapy, risk assessment and problem solving. This chapter aims to establish the foundations for safe community practice at a time when the prevalence of allergic reactions is increasing [1], and hence the emergency management of anaphylaxis is detailed. Whilst the focus is on community nursing, the information provided is applicable to any situation in which anaphylaxis may occur including urban, rural or remote practice settings.

We discuss nursing response and intervention to allergic reactions defined as 'immediate' or 'delayed', as these are the most common reactions that community nurses will encounter. Knowledge of key elements of a risk assessment and effective nursing intervention will minimise risk to the client should an allergic reaction occur. Information about other types of allergic reactions is available from the 'Useful resources' section at the end of the chapter.

Defining the terms

The key terms discussed throughout this chapter are defined as follows.

Anaphylaxis

Anaphylaxis is a rapidly evolving, generalised, multisystem allergic reaction characterised by one or more signs of respiratory and/or cardiovascular involvement *and* involvement of other systems such as the skin and/or gastrointestinal tract [2, 3].

It is important to be able to distinguish anaphylaxis from a generalised allergic reaction.

Generalised allergic reaction

'A generalised allergic reaction is characterised by one or more symptoms or signs of skin and/or gastrointestinal symptoms *without* respiratory and/or cardiovascular involvement' [4, p. 2].

Allergy

Allergy (also known as hypersensitivity) occurs when a person's immune system reacts abnormally to substances (called allergens) that the body would usually find harmless. Reactions can be either immediate or delayed [5].

Immediate allergic reaction

Immediate reactions (called type 1 hypersensitivity) are mediated by antibody (immunoglobulin E, IgE), whereas delayed reactions (type 4 hypersensitivity) are mediated by immune cells called T cells [6, 7]. Immediate reactions are those such as asthma, allergic rhinitis or anaphylaxis. Immediate reactions can be in two phases:

- The early phase reaction is termed 'immediate hypersensitivity', occurring from a few seconds, a few minutes and up to 2 h after exposure to the allergen [8].
- The late phase reaction occurs 4–6 h after the first phase symptoms appear to have gone [3, 9].

Background

'Allergic diseases have increased dramatically throughout the 20th century, a change that has been described as an epidemic' [1, p. 226]. Australia has one of the highest incidences of allergic diseases in the world [1]. While asthma prevalence has plateaued after rising for many years, eczema rates have dramatically increased between 1993 and 2002 [1]. Food allergy and anaphylaxis are also on the rise [10, 11]. There are a number of hypotheses for this increasing prevalence, which are the focus of research being conducted in Australia and other countries. Some hypotheses are:

- The 'hygiene hypothesis' where a reduced or lack of exposure to infections, parasites and endotoxins may induce allergic responses to allergens [1]
- More comfortable, sealed homes, perhaps favouring increase in conditions in which house dust mites breed [8]
- Gut microflora in infants that plays a role in the newborn's immune system development [8]

The tendency to develop allergies and allergic diseases is called atopy and is known to have a genetic link [8, 9]. Allergic diseases include allergic rhinitis (hayfever), eczema, asthma and food allergy and can cause reactions ranging from urticaria (skin rashes) to anaphylaxis. Atopic individuals are at increased risk of developing an allergic reaction to latex, but the risk of developing allergy to medications or insect venoms is similar in atopic and non-atopic individuals [12].

After initial exposure to an allergen, the body produces sensitising antibodies that are specific to that allergen only. These sensitising antibodies are known as immunoglobulin E (IgE) and bind to specific receptor sites on mast cells [13, 14]. Mast cells are found just under the skin and near blood vessels of connective tissue and mucosal tissue of the gastrointestinal and respiratory tract. They are in largest concentrations in areas that are in contact with the external environment and they have a role in the inflammatory response of the body [5].

Mast cells can survive for years and cause no symptoms if no further exposure to the allergen occurs. This is known as 'sensitisation', a type of 'allergy memory' [5, p. 11]. On further exposure to the allergen, the mast cells are activated through the allergen-specific IgE on their surface, which sends signals into the cell to activate it [13, 14]. Activated mast cells release chemical mediators and enzymes (such as histamine, cytokines, prostaglandins, tryptase and leukotrienes) in an allergic reaction [5, 7], which results in:

- Leakage and dilation of blood vessels – causing oedema, skin redness (flushing), excess mucous production, sneezing, urticaria and angioedema
- Stimulation of sensory nerve endings – itchiness and stinging sensations
- Contraction of smooth muscle – bronchospasm, wheezing, coughing, uterine or abdominal cramps [15]

Delayed allergic reaction

Delayed reactions (type 4 hypersensitivity) are mediated by immune cells called T cells and termed 'cell mediated' [6, 7]. In a cell-mediated reaction, sensitised lymphocytes (T cells) are activated and produce symptoms, such as rashes, urticaria or eczema, that can occur hours or days after the exposure [8, 9]. Nurses working within community health care settings need to be aware of these reactions, because while often not the cause of anaphylaxis, this type of reaction may occur in clients that have been exposed to oral or topical medication and other substances, such as disinfectant washes, used within the community setting. Clients may experience a range of different manifestations, including:

- Gastrointestinal reactions to foods or medications
- Skin reactions to certain medications
- Contact allergy on the skin to things such as latex, glove powder, topical creams, disinfectants, nickel or plants [8, 9]

If delayed-type sensitivity is suspected, consultation with a general practitioner is necessary. Referral of the client to the appropriate specialist (usually an allergist or a dermatologist) for expert diagnosis and testing is recommended.

Anaphylaxis

Anaphylaxis is characterised by life-threatening upper airway obstruction, bronchospasm and/or hypotension [16]. Unfortunately, there is no universal agreement on the 'definition of anaphylaxis' [8, 14]. The lack of universal agreement on the

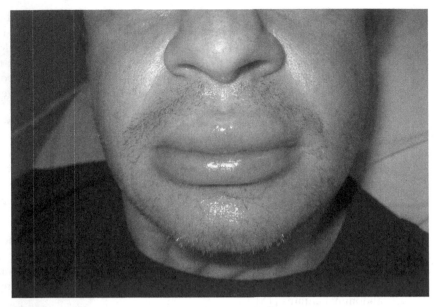

Figure 22.1 Angioedema.

'definition of anaphylaxis' is thought to have contributed to some incidences of ana-phylaxis not being diagnosed nor being correctly treated [16, 17]. The Australasian Society of Clinical Immunology and Allergy (ASCIA) specialists state that although anaphylaxis is not rare, deaths from anaphylaxis are rare [18]. It is estimated that there are ten deaths each year in Australia caused usually by medication or blood transfusion [18]. There have been claims that adverse outcomes of an allergic reaction, including death, appear to be increasing, with two deaths during a 6-month period reported in Sydney [19].

Anaphylaxis should be considered in any episode of severe, acute-onset respiratory distress, bronchospasm or cardiovascular collapse even if skin features are absent [16]. (These features can be absent in up to 20% of cases.) Sometimes the rapid onset of hypotension masks the skin rash, which becomes visible only after the adrenaline has been administered [20]. Figure 22.1 shows an example of angioedema (swelling of soft tissue) caused by oral ingestion of an angiotensin-converting enzyme (ACE) inhibitor, while Figure 22.2 shows how skin urticaria (hives) may present. Both these symptoms can be associated with anaphylaxis.

Possible causes

The majority of anaphylactic reactions are caused by:

- Foods
- Medications
- Insect venom [16]

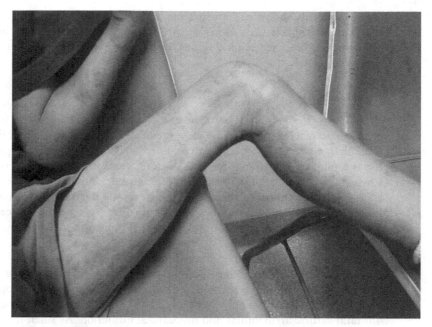

Figure 22.2 Skin urticaria (hives).

It is also recognised that a *combination of factors*, such as allergen exposure, *and*

- physical exercise,
- concomitant medication such as non-steroidal anti-inflammatory drugs (NSAIDs),
- recurrent infection may provoke an anaphylactic reaction [16].

If the cause of anaphylaxis is not able to be determined, it is termed 'idiopathic anaphylaxis' [2, 16]. The most likely time community nurses would be involved in the treatment of anaphylaxis would be following administration of medications, either oral or parenteral.

Acute management of anaphylaxis

Anaphylaxis and allergic reactions can occur in a variety of settings. Community nurses are most concerned with pre-hospital management of anaphylaxis and as such, availability of emergency equipment will vary.

The acute management of anaphylaxis involves the following:

- If another person is present, have them call an ambulance immediately.
- Place the person in the supine position or left lateral if vomiting.
- Administer intramuscular (IM) adrenaline.
- Resuscitate with intravenous (IV) saline (may not be easily available in a community setting).
- Begin oxygen therapy (if available).
- Maintain airway, breathing and circulation.
- Call the ambulance at this point, if only nurse and client are present [16, 17].

Adrenaline, also known as epinephrine, is generally the only drug available for use by community nurses [21]. Other medications will be administered by paramedics and medical officers when an ambulance arrives and the person is transferred to an emergency service.

Adrenaline

Adrenaline is the first-line treatment and the most important drug for any severe anaphylactic reaction, as it is the only medication proved to reverse the symptoms of anaphylaxis [10, 17, 18, 21]. Adrenaline, 0.01 mg/kg of body weight (maximum dose 0.5 mg), can be administered IM in the anterior lateral thigh every 5–15 min as necessary [17]. More frequent injections can be administered as necessary by the expert emergency clinician. The evidence suggests administration of adrenaline at 3- to 5-min intervals [15]; however, most community nurses will not have access to multiple doses of adrenaline and so prompt transfer of the client to an emergency department is paramount.

Two doses of self-injectable adrenaline are available in Australia – EpiPen Jr® (0.15 mg) and EpiPen® (0.3 mg). Administration of adrenaline via the subcutaneous route delays absorption when compared with the IM route and therefore is less effective in the treatment of anaphylaxis [21–23]. IV administration has been associated with fatal cardiac arrhythmias and myocardial infarction. As such, it is reserved only for those clients with unresponsive anaphylaxis and should only be administered by medical officers with appropriate training and experience [16, 21, 22].

Drug legislation controls the use of adrenaline and there is some variance across the states. There is also specific legislation related to a health care profession's practice, including nurses and medical practitioners, that impacts on drug practices. It is the responsibility of the community nurse to ascertain their responsibility and accountability under their state/territory/country's legislation governing nursing practice.

Antihistamines, corticosteroids and salbutamol

Adrenaline is the most important treatment and must not be delayed by the administration of antihistamines, corticosteroids or asthma medications, as these have been shown to have little impact on the immediate and dangerous effects of anaphylaxis [17, 18, 21]. Antihistamines are useful for the symptomatic treatment of urticaria/angioedema and itching [17]. Corticosteroids are sometimes administered in anaphylaxis, but there is no evidence proving they are effective [17]. The use of beta 2 agonists (such as salbutamol) may be effective for bronchospasm, but must not be used instead of adrenaline [18, 21].

Observation post-anaphylaxis

Anaphylaxis usually responds rapidly to treatment and does not usually relapse, but sometimes symptoms may:

- Fail to improve
- Worsen (termed protracted)
- Return after early resolution (termed biphasic) [16]

Clinicians are not able to distinguish which people are most at risk for a biphasic reaction, so it is recommended that there is a 4- to 6-h observation period, post-anaphylaxis, within an acute hospital setting or rural/remote clinical centre [24]. For some people, more prolonged observation is required, e.g. those with severe or refractory symptoms and those with reactive airway disease [16, 17].

A version of the new wall chart on emergency management of anaphylaxis in the community setting is available from the Australian Prescriber website http://www.australianprescriber.com/upload/pdf/articles/913.pdf. This document has been designed to help health professionals working within community settings. It is endorsed by several major Australasian professional bodies associated with management of allergic disease and anaphylaxis [24].

Treatment of anaphylaxis will be the same regardless of the cause [16]. Allergic reactions to latex, antiseptics or disinfectants, gelatin and medications may also be encountered by the community nurse. These reactions may or may not progress to anaphylaxis. From an ethical and legal stance, community organisations have a responsibility to ensure that policies, procedures and training are in place to ensure nurses and clients are informed about the risks of allergic reactions.

Latex allergy

Nurses and clients in the community setting may be exposed to latex through a variety of products such as gloves, urinary catheters, tourniquets, resuscitation equipment, IV equipment, parenteral feeding tubes, adhesive tapes and dressings, to list a few. Non-medical product examples are balloons, condoms and hair extensions. Most of these products do have non-latex substitutes. Health workers regularly using gloves and clients regularly needing procedures involving products that are made from latex are at higher risk of latex allergy, as are people having an atopy tendency (such as allergic rhinitis or asthma) [12, 25].

Presentation

Latex allergy can present as either immediate (IgE) or delayed allergic reactions. Allergy to latex can be caused by proteins contained within the latex of a glove or to the chemical compounds used in the actual production of latex and manufacture of the gloves [12]. In powdered gloves, latex protein can be carried on the powder, which becomes airborne when gloves are put on or removed. Only 1% of the population show clinical signs of latex allergy and those exposed to latex within the course of their work (for example medical personnel, food preparation staff), those with spina bifida and those who undergo multiple surgical procedures are at the greatest risk of developing sensitivity reactions [25, 26].

Symptoms

Symptoms of latex allergy depend on the route of exposure such as mucous membranes, respiratory tract or skin [12]. Skin contact with latex gloves may commonly cause itching or a mild rash (irritant dermatitis), which is not true latex allergy. Urticaria (hives) at areas of contact is a symptom of true type 1 latex allergy [27]. Delayed skin reactions can also occur due to hypersensitivity to the chemical compounds used in the manufacture of latex [27].

Delayed sensitivities involving the skin are uncomfortable but are not anaphylaxis. These will not be dealt with in the scope of this chapter, but referral to a dermatologist for patch testing is recommended if this type of sensitivity is suspected. Nurses need to be aware that clients and other nurses may not associate the delayed symptoms with latex exposure and thus awareness about the potential sensitisation of latex is important.

If the latex protein is airborne, such as when glove powder is released on removal of gloves, respiratory symptoms such as rhinoconjunctivitis (hayfever) and asthma may occur. Anaphylaxis can also occur from airborne particles and may be life threatening. The greatest likelihood of anaphylaxis occurs when the latex is in contact with the mucous membranes as with surgical, gynaecological and dental procedures [12].

Risk management

Education of health care employees and clients about latex allergy is important to raise awareness of this potential problem. Instigating measures for employees to have reduced exposure to latex by providing latex alternatives can reduce exposure and reduce the risk of sensitisation [28]. The employing organisation has a responsibility to provide a safe working environment for its employees and this should include providing latex-free equipment. Legal cases have reflected the need for employers to take appropriate precautions for workers [25].

Community nurses and clients can undertake the following measures to reduce the chances of developing latex sensitivity [25]:

- Use vinyl gloves or if this is not possible, insist on provision of non-powdered gloves.
- All resuscitation equipment should be latex free.
- Equipment required by the nurse to carry out his/her duties and treatments should be latex free.
- When obtaining a client history, questions about allergy to any substance, medications or foods should be included. Ascertain if the client has or does suffer from allergic rhinitis, eczema and/or asthma.
- Use appropriate signage alerting other health personnel to the client's allergy(ies).
- If it is suspected that a client or nurse has latex allergy, an appointment with an appropriately trained allergy specialist is essential as soon as possible, to develop a latex allergy health plan.

Antiseptics and disinfectants

Reactions to disinfectants and antiseptics may present as either anaphylaxis, generalised allergic reactions, such as rash, flushing and redness, or as allergic contact dermatitis. There are many different preparations used in wound care and infection control and these preparations will vary between organisations. Community nurses need to be aware of the possibility of sensitisation to these products by clients, or indeed themselves, and must apply the appropriate risk management strategies. Referral to an allergist or dermatologist may also be appropriate if an allergy is suspected. Anaphylaxis to chlorhexidine, a skin disinfectant commonly used in wound management, and to povidone/iodine is reported in the literature [29, 30].

Medication administration: reducing the risks

It is difficult to ascertain from the literature the frequency of anaphylaxis caused by medication. In one study, 28% of all cases of anaphylaxis seen in an Australian emergency department ($n = 164$) were caused by medication. Antibiotics (cephalosporins, penicillin and trimethoprin) were the most common, followed by NSAIDS and ACE inhibitors [20]. Blood products such as plasma, red blood cells and platelets can all trigger anaphylaxis [31, 32]. There have also been reported cases of anaphylaxis to gelatin [33, 34]. Gelatin is found in products such as vaccines, plasma expander infusions and medication such as suppositories [35].

Anaphylaxis to medications is characterised by a high frequency of cardiovascular collapse that has a rapid onset (within minutes). Older people are especially at risk [36]. Hypotension is usually associated with drug-related anaphylaxis, with other symptoms being confusion, collapse, unconsciousness, nausea, vomiting, abdominal pain and incontinence [16]. The route of administration of the medication can be an important factor in the severity and speed of an allergic reaction; for example oral administration is generally safer than parenteral administration. However, oral medications can also be the cause of fatal anaphylaxis [37–39].

Clients receiving home-based community care may be on multiple medications. Allergic adverse reactions to medications (anaphylaxis and rashes) should be distinguished from pharmacological effects. Assessment by an appropriately trained medical practitioner or accredited pharmacist for diagnosis, dose modification and altered management options is essential [26]. Pharmacological reactions are often dose dependent and may be predictable.

Medication by parenteral routes

The administration of medications by parenteral routes (injection or infusion) is common practice in community settings. Blood products are also sometimes administered in community settings. Community nursing organisations providing medication administration services must consider the potential for allergic reaction. As previously mentioned, *anaphylaxis is life threatening, progresses rapidly and requires urgent treatment.*

An Australian study in 2001 reported that only one-third of individuals admitted to the emergency department with medication-induced anaphylaxis had a previous history of allergy to that medication [20]. This has implications for community nurses administering medications in the client's home, as it means that all medications' doses are a potential risk for inducing anaphylaxis. The key to successful management of each client with severe anaphylaxis is the education of nurses to ensure [40]:

- Comprehensive assessment
- Early identification of anaphylaxis
- Prompt initiation of treatment

Risk management

The community nurse avoids exposing clients to unnecessary risks. Procedures such as the administration of medications and transfusions do pose risks to clients, particularly if they are performed without due care [41]. All community nurses need to have the knowledge and skills to competently assess clients, be alert for a history of past reactions, know the types of procedures that put a client at risk of anaphylaxis, know protocols for managing a reaction when it occurs and document any events. If any of these factors are absent, there is potentially a breach of duty of care.

Conducting a risk assessment

It is important to assess the risk for a client receiving nursing care in a non-clinical setting, such as a home or community-nurse-led clinic/centre. Questions to ask include:

1. Does the client have a history of any adverse drug reactions or anaphylaxis?
   - It is essential that nurses accurately assess past reactions as a history of anaphylaxis to one drug increases the risk even when drugs are unrelated [37].
   - If a client reports a history of any allergic-type adverse reactions, consultation with an allergy specialist may be required prior to commencing therapy.
2. Is the client currently taking beta blockers, tricyclic antidepressants or monamine oxidase inhibitors?
   - These drugs can have an effect on the way in which the person responds to adrenaline [22].
3. Does the client have fast access to a telephone? Do caregivers know which number to ring in an emergency?
   - In case of emergency all clients need access to a working phone. As some allergic reactions are delayed, the nurse may no longer be with the client.
4. Can the client understand the signs and symptoms of an allergic reaction? Are they able to communicate this to the community nurse?
   - Consider people from culturally and linguistically diverse backgrounds.
   - Consider people with limited cognitive ability.
5. Does the person have access to a capable support person who can stay with the client during and after the procedure?
   - It is important that another person is available in case there is an emergency.
6. Does the person have poorly controlled asthma?
   - Asthma is associated with an increased risk for fatal anaphylaxis especially in children [16, 17, 22]. Medical consultation may be necessary to ensure optimal control of asthma *before* commencement of treatments.

The onset of anaphylaxis post-medication administration varies, although it is usually rapid. American guidelines for allergen immunotherapy suggest that individuals are observed for at least 20–30 min post-administration so that reactions can be recognised and treated promptly [42]. The Australian Immunisation Guidelines recommend at least 15 min of observation [43]. Vaccination, immunotherapy and intravenous medication can all trigger anaphylaxis and so similarities can be drawn. Medication-induced anaphylaxis can occur at any stage during treatment, not only on the first dose [37, 44]. Organisations may need to seek advice about implementing processes for risk reduction and to determine the possible resource implications of managing risk.

Many community nursing services, such as hospital at home, immunisation nurses and some district nursing services are now routinely carrying emergency kits for the treatment of anaphylaxis. Each of these services differs in terms of what the kit contains, as each organisation develops its own risk analysis in terms of client profile and medical supports. It is essential that community nurses are aware of the symptoms of anaphylaxis and respond to the situation appropriately. Diagnosis and effective management of anaphylaxis involves cooperation and collaboration between the client, community nurse and an interdisciplinary team of health care professionals using up-to-date, evidence-based information. Community nurses can help educate clients to distinguish between mild allergy symptoms and those requiring immediate medical attention.

To summarise, we suggest that organisations consider the following:

- Provide clear guidelines that outline prevention and management of allergic reactions and anaphylaxis.
- Provide a competency-based staff education programme that includes allergy history assessment, recognising and managing anaphylaxis and preventative measures.
- Develop consent forms, client and health professional information sheets and adverse reaction recording sheets for use in the community setting.

Assessment and care planning for allergy

In addition to planning for safe administration of medications, the community nurse should ensure that any past history of allergy or any current symptoms are discussed and documented as part of routine assessment and history processes. Discussion with the client may reveal known allergies, allergic reactions or anaphylaxis. Allergies may have been unaddressed for a number of years. Discussion should include questions such as:

- Have you ever been told that you have anaphylaxis? If yes:
  - Do you have an anaphylaxis action plan?
  - Were you ever prescribed an EpiPen®? If so, is it within the expiry date?
  - Do you feel confident in recognising the signs of anaphylaxis?
  - Do you feel confident about using your EpiPen®?
  - How long ago did you discuss your allergy with an allergy specialist?

If anaphylaxis has previously occurred, self-injectable adrenaline should be carried (EpiPen® for people over 20 kg or EpiPen Junior® for those under 20 kg. Can it be made consistent, or do these forms) [4]. This must be prescribed by an allergist or a medical professional who has discussed the particular client situation with an allergist [4].

There has been an increase in the number of EpiPens® being prescribed for individuals believed to be at risk of anaphylaxis [1]. The literature, both nationally and internationally, highlights some problems with EpiPen® use in the community, including underuse by those prescribed EpiPen® [45]. Research has shown that, even when individuals have access to an EpiPen®, it is frequently not used in an emergency [46]. Education about diagnosis and management of anaphylaxis is recommended to increase confidence in using the EpiPen® [45].

If a client requires more information and assessment of their allergy status, it may be necessary to discuss referral to a specialist. If they have seen a specialist, it may be an opportunity to revise their action plan or check that the client understands EpiPen® administration technique. Other allergy reactions such as hives, allergic rhinitis, intolerance to foods or asthma may be raised by the client and the nurse should recommend to the client that they seek the advice of a medical practitioner.

For clients with a history of allergy, community nurses should emphasise the importance of consistency of consulting the same general practitioner and pharmacist. Seeing the same doctor and pharmacist can be useful for ongoing monitoring and education.

What is an anaphylaxis action plan?

People who have had anaphylaxis should have a medical plan termed an 'anaphylaxis action plan' completed by the specialist diagnosing the allergy. There is one version for adults and one for children [47]. These are available at http://www.allergy.org.au/aer/infobulletins/index.htm#anaph.

The plans contain patient's name and carer contact details together with instructions and diagrams on how and when to administer the Epipen® [4].

Note that EpiPens are manufactured in the United States of America and the product information insert differs from the Australian Guidelines for prescribing EpiPen Jnr®, in particular [47] (see 'Useful resources' section). To avoid confusion nurses offer clients and health personnel education about this important fact, which could result in an Epipen® not being administered when needed.

Correct technique for using EpiPen®

Nurses should not assume that clients have received education about the correct way to administer an EpiPen®. If a client is known to have been prescribed the device, the nurse needs to check the client has received correct instruction on how to use it. If not, or if the client seems unsure, the community nurse must demonstrate how to use the device. If an 'EpiPen trainer' is not available, care must be taken whilst demonstrating, not to activate the EpiPen®. Using a 'trainer' EpiPen® is advisable. Trainers can be obtained from Anaphylaxis Australia (see 'Useful resources' section).

To correctly use an EpiPen:

- Remove it from packaging and remove from the covering tube with the coloured end.
- Place in palm of the hand, with the end with the grey cap pointing towards the thumb.
- Clasp the fingers around the pen to form a fist around the pen.
- Remove the grey safety cap with the other hand.
- *Do not* place thumb over the end from which you have just removed the safety cap.
- Place black end of the EpiPen® on the anterior, lateral aspect of the thigh. (If the leg, from knee to thigh, is divided into three, the site of administration would be in the middle section.)
- Press the device very firmly against the skin until a loud 'clicking' noise is heard.
- Hold the EpiPen® on the area for 10 s to allow administration of the contents.
- Lift the EpiPen® from the leg, taking care with the black end, as a needle will now be protruding.
- Rub the area where the EpiPen® was administered for 10 s to aid distribution of the adrenaline.
- Replace the EpiPen® into the tube cover, taking care not to be injured by the needle.

The client must be transferred to hospital immediately via an ambulance.

Storage and expiry of EpiPens®

- EpiPens® should be stored between 15°C and 30°C.
- They should be stored in their protective containers and inside the packaging box to protect them from light.
- They must *not* be stored in the refrigerator nor left in a vehicle for any part of the day.
- The date of expiry must be checked regularly and contact made with a medical practitioner to obtain a repeat prescription, *before* the expiry date has passed.

People can purchase an EpiPen® without a prescription.

Medical alert jewellery

The wearing of medical alert jewellery is recommended, by allergy specialists, for the client at risk of anaphylaxis [16]. Medical alert jewellery is important when the trigger for the anaphylaxis was a medication which may be administered in an emergency (for example penicillin) or if the client has an impairment that might prevent them from being able to communicate information about the allergy. Medical alert jewellery can be authorised by the client's doctor or a specialist. Nurses can check that the information on a client's medical alert jewellery is up to date. If 5–10 years have elapsed since it was updated, the community nurse should ensure that the client has the situation reviewed by an allergist or appropriate medical practitioner. Nurses can obtain further information from the Medic Alert Foundation website [48].

Ambulance plan

For clients known to be at risk of anaphylaxis, nurses should check if the client has appropriate health insurance cover in the event of an ambulance being required. If the client does not have cover, this needs to be discussed, explaining both the health and financial risks of not having any cover and the need for the client to discuss it further with their medical practitioner. Nurses should also document clearly that such a discussion has taken place. The responsibility does rest with the client but nurses do have a duty of care to explain the issues to the client. The lack of health insurance cover, however, should not be a factor that delays the community nurse calling an ambulance in a health emergency.

Considerations in rural and remote areas

Clients in rural and remote areas may need to have additional adrenalin prescribed if there is extensive distance to medical help [15]. This needs to be discussed with the client's medical practitioner/specialist and the closest ambulance and hospital facility.

Documentation

Documentation is an important and integral part of community nursing work. It provides an ongoing account of a client's progress and may be required as evidence in court. Documentation should be accurate, legible and of a high standard in order to meet legislative requirements [49]. Accuracy may become an important factor should the records become important in the defence of the community nurse or medical practitioner treating the client. Accurate documentation may also provide information that can assist the medical practitioner subsequently assessing the allergic reaction. Documentation should occur as near as possible to the event if it is to be considered reliable evidence [49].

The need for accurate documentation cannot be stressed enough. A risk assessment should be completed and documented and any matters causing the community nurse concern must be followed up as soon as possible and *before* any treatment or medication is given [49].

Consent

All registered health professionals are subject to mandatory consent standards. Community nurses have a responsibility to ensure informed consent has been obtained before implementing treatment interventions. Different states of Australia have different legislation related to consent. Nurses need to be aware of the consent legislation in the state/territory/country in which they are practising and practise within that legislation.

Clients have the right to determine the treatments or tests they receive; thus, obtaining a client's informed consent for any procedure is mandatory. Failure to inform clients about the risk of anaphylaxis, when consenting to treatments such as blood transfusion or intravenous medications, may be considered a breach of duty of care.

Oral, written and implied consent are different ways in which valid consent can be obtained. When a person is unable to consent, such as in an emergency situation where the client is suffering from anaphylaxis, a community nurse can proceed with measures to save a life and prevent severe injury [49].

When obtaining informed consent, open-ended questions are the best format to allow parents, guardians or clients to discuss their concerns before the treatment is given or the test performed. Information should be available which describes the intervention, what they can expect and the risks, however rare, of the treatment or test compared with the risks, however rare, from not having it performed or given. If the person to give consent has English as a second language or is illiterate, the information must be translated or interpreted. This is best done by a trained interpreter. Careful consideration of these issues may reduce the risk of harm to clients. This process must be accurately documented by the community nurse at the time of gaining consent.

It is up to the client to decide when he/she has received enough information to make an informed decision about whether or not to consent to treatment. Nurses must provide the available information that the client needs to make an informed decision. People require different information and different amounts of information.

Summary

It is imperative that nurses can recognise the potential significance of allergic reactions and their responsibilities in risk assessment, recognition and management of these reactions. This requires an understanding of the allergic response and manifestations of 'immediate' and 'delayed' allergic reactions. Assessment of the client and interventions to reduce risk has been highlighted. Through this knowledge nurses can inform and work with clients to prevent and manage allergic reactions more effectively.

Acknowledgement

Thank you to Dr William Smith, Clinical Immunologist and Allergist, for critiquing this chapter.

Useful resources

Various websites are available to clients and nurses who wish to access more information about education and support in managing systemic reactions and anaphylaxis:

1. Australasian Society of Clinical Immunology and Allergy (ASCIA)
   at http://www.allergy.org.au
   - Anaphylaxis resources (including action plans and EpiPen® information)
   - ASCIA educational resources
   - Clinical immunologists and allergists
   - Position papers and guidelines

- Website links
  Australian Prescriber-Emergency Management of Anaphylaxis in the Community, 2007, 30(5). Available at
  http://www.australianprescriber.com/magazine/30/5/artid/913/
2. Anaphylaxis Australia at http://www.allergyfacts.org.au
   - Local support groups exist in some states with further information available on the website.
3. Health Insite: An Australian Government Initiative at
   http://www.healthinsite.gov.au/content/internal/page.cfm?ObjID=000940B6-510F-100C-B65883032BFA006D
   - Anaphylaxis, community nursing
4. HealthySA Your gateway to healthy living at
   http://www.healthysa.sa.gov.au/results-az.asp?action=load&keyword=Anaphylaxis
5. Medic Alert Foundation at http://www.medicalert.com.au/
6. Nurses' acts for each state or territory are available from the nurses board in each state/territory.
7. Royal Prince Alfred Allergy Unit Resources at
   http://www.cs.nsw.gov.au/rpa/allergy/resources/allergy/default.cfm
8. Child Health and Education Support Services (CHESS) at
   http://www.decs.sa.gov.au/speced2/pages/health
9. World Allergy Organisation (WAO) at http://www.world allergy.org

References

1. Kemp, A., Mullins, R. and Weiner J. (2006) The allergy epidemic: What is the Australian response? *Medical Journal of Australia*, 185(4), 226–7.
2. Australasian Society of Clinical Immunology and Allergy (ASCIA) (2005) *What Is Anaphylaxis? Educational Resources*. Available at www.allergyfacts.org.au/whatis.html (viewed January 2006).
3. Anaphylaxis Australia (2007) *What Is Anaphylaxis?*. Available at http://www.allergyfacts.org.au/whatis.html (viewed March 2007).
4. ASCIA (2004) *Guidelines for Epipen Prescription*. Available at http://www.allergy.org.au/anaphylaxis/ASCIA_EpiPen_prescription_guidelines.pdf (viewed 20 March 2007).
5. Mygind, N., Dahl, R., Pedersen, S. and Thestrup-Pedersen, K. (1996) *Essential Allergy*, 2nd edition. Blackwell Science, Oxford.
6. World Allergy Organisation (2007) *IgE in Clinical Allergy and Allergy Diagnosis*. Available at http://www.worldallergy.org/professional/allergic_diseases_center/ige/index.shtml (viewed March 2007).
7. Jevon, P. and Dimond, B. (2004) *Anaphylaxis a Practical Guide*. Butterworth Heinmann, Edinburgh.
8. Smith, H. and Frew, A. (2004) *Your Questions Answered: Allergy*. Livingstone, Edinburgh.
9. Walls, R. (1997) *Allergies and Their Management*. Maclennan and Petty Ltd, Sydney.
10. Allen, K., Hill, D. and Heine, R. (2006) Anaphylaxis: Risk factors for recurrence. *Medical Journal of Australia*, 185(7), 394–400.
11. Mullins, R. (2003) Anaphylaxis: Risk factors for recurrence. *Clinical & Experimental Allergy*, 33(8), 1033–40.
12. Katalaris, C. (2006) Latex allergy. *Medical Journal of Australia*, 185(6), 339.
13. Lydyard, P., Whelan, A. and Fanger, M. (2000) *Instant Notes in Immunology*. Springer, New York.
14. Hannigan, B. (2000) *Biomedical Sciences Explained: Immunology*. Arnold, London.
15. Brown, S. (2006) Clinical concepts and research priorities. *Emergency Medicine Australasia*, 18(2), 155–69.

16. Brown, S., Mullins, R. and Gold, M. (2006) Anaphylaxis: Diagnosis and management. *Medical Journal Australia*, 185(5), 283–9.

17. Sampson, H.A., Muñoz-Furlong, A., Campbell, R.L., Adkinson, N.F., Jr, Bock, A., Branum, A., *et al.* (2006) Second symposium on the definition and management of anaphylaxis: Summary report – Second National Institute of Allergy and Infectious Disease/Food Allergy and Anaphylaxis Network symposium. *Journal Allergy Clinical Immunology*, 117(2), 391–7.

18. ASCIA (November 2005) *Anaphylaxis Training Resources: For Educators and Allied Health Professionals*. Australasian Society of Clinical Immunology and Allergy, Balgowlah, NSW, Australia.

19. Tong, W. and Anderson, E. (2007) Cross-reactivity of penicillins and cephalosporins. *Australian Prescriber*, 30(1), 25–6.

20. Brown, A., McKinnon, D. and Chu, K. (2001) Emergency department anaphylaxis: A review of 142 patients in a single year. *Journal of Allergy and Clinical Immunology*, 108(5), 861–6.

21. Resuscitation Council (UK) (2005) *The Emergency Medical Treatment of Anaphylactic Reactions for First Medical Responders and for Community Nurses*. Resuscitation Council, UK.

22. McLean-Tooke, A.P.C., Bethune, C.A., Fay, A.C. and Spickett, G.P. (2003) Adrenaline in the treatment of anaphylaxis: What is the evidence? *British Medical Journal*, 327(7427), 1332–5.

23. Sampson, H.A., Munoz-Furlong, A., Bock, A., Schmitt, C., Bass, R., Chowdhury, B.A., *et al.* (2005) Symposium on the definition and management of anaphylaxis: Summary report. *Journal Allergy Clinical Immunology*, 115(3), 584–91.

24. Australian Prescriber (2007) Emergency management of anaphylaxis in the community. *Australian Prescriber*.

25. Noonan, A. and Moyle, M. (2004) Latex glove allergy in health care. *Australian Nursing Journal*, 12(3), 1–3.

26. Thein, C. (2006) Drug hypersensitivity. *Medical Journal of Australia*, 185(6), 333–8.

27. Yip, E. and Roman, M. (2003) Latex Protein Allergy and our choice of gloves: A balanced consideration. *Medical Surgical Nursing*, 12(1), 20–26.

28. Tarlo, S., Easty, A., Eubanks, K., Parsons, C., Min, F., Juvet, S., *et al.* (2001) Outcomes of a natural latex control program in an Ontario teaching hospital. *Journal Allergy Clinical Immunology*, 108(4), 628–33.

29. Aalto-Korte, K. and Makinen-Kiljunen, S. (2006) Symptoms of immediate chlorhexidine hypersensitivity in patients with a positive prick test. *Contact Dermatitis*, 55(3), 17307.

30. Beaudouin, E., Kanny, G., Morisset, M., Renaudin, J., Mertes, M., Lexenaire, M., *et al.* (2004) Immediate sensitivity to chlorhexidine: Literature review. *Allergy Immunology*, 36(4), 123–6.

31. The International Collaborative Study of Severe Anaphylaxis (2003) Risk of anaphylaxis in a hospital population in relation to the use of various drugs: An international study. *Pharmacoepidemiology and Drug Safety*, 12(3), 195–202.

32. Gilstad, C. (2003) Anaphylactic transfusion reactions. *Current Opinion in Hematology*, 10(6), 419–23.

33. Sakaguchi, M. and Inouye, S. (2001) Anaphylaxis to gelatin-containing suppositories. *Journal Allergy Clinical Immunology*, 108(6), 1033–4.

34. Apostolou, E., Deckert, K., Puy, R., Sandrini, A., de Leon, M., Douglass, J., *et al.* Anaphylaxis to gelofusine confirmed by in vitro basophil activation test: A case series. *Anaesthesia*, 61(3), 264–8.

35. Nockleby, H. (2006) Vaccination and anaphylaxis. *Current Allergy Asthma Reports*, 6(1), 9–13.

36. Moneret-Vautrin, D., Morisset, M., Flabbee, J., Beaudouin, E. and Kanny, G. (2005) Epidemiology of life-threatening and lethal anaphylaxis: A review. *Allergy*, 60(4), 443–51.

37. Thong, B., Motala, C. and Vervloet, D. (2007) *Drug Allergies. Allergic Diseases Resource Center* (sic). Available at www.worldallergy.org/professional/allergic_diseases_center/drugallergy/index.shtml (viewed 8 May 2007).

38. Pumphrey, R. and Gowland, M. (August 2007) Further fatal allergic reactions to food in the United Kingdom, 1999–2006. *Journal of Allergy and Clinical Immunology*, 119(4), 1018–19.

39. Pumphrey, R.S.H. (August 2000) Lessons for management of anaphylaxis from a study of fatal reactions. *Clinical & Experimental Allergy*, 30(8), 1144–50.

40. Ferns, T. and Chojnacka, I. (2003) The causes of anaphylaxis and its management in adults. *British Journal of Nursing*, 12(17), 1006–12.

41. Staunton, P. and Chiarella, M. (2005) *Nursing & the Law*, 5th edition. Elsevier, Marrickville, NSW.

42. Joint Task Force on Practice Parameters (2003) Allergen immunotherapy: A practice parameter. *Annals of Allergy, Asthma, & Immunology*, 90(1, Suppl 1), 1–40.

43. National Health and Medical Research Council (2003) *The Australian Immunisation Handbook*. Australian Government Department of Health and Ageing, Canberra.

44. Langran, M. and Laird, C. (2004) 8 Management of allergy, rashes, and itching. *Emergency Medical Journal*, 21(6), 728–41.

45. Sicherer, S. and Leung, D. (2006) Advances in allergic skin disease, anaphylaxis, and hypersensitivity reactions to foods, drugs, and insects. *Journal of Allergy and Clinical Immunology*, 118(1), 170–77.

46. Kim, J., Sinacore, J. and Pongracic J. (2005) Parental use of EpiPen for children with food allergies. *Journal of Allergy & Clinical Immunology*, 116(1), 164–8.

47. ASCIA (2003) *Anaphylaxis Action Plans*. Available at http://www.allergy.org.au/aer/ infobulletins/index.htm#anaph (viewed 20 March 2007).

48. Medic Alert Foundation (2007) Website. Available at http://www.medicalert.com.au (viewed 31 March 2007).

49. Mair, J. (2000) Chapter 2 in *An Introduction to Legal Aspects of Nursing Practice*. MacLennan & Petty Pty Ltd, Sydney.

Chapter 23

New and emerging technologies

Moya Conrick

Introduction

The aim of this chapter is to define and discuss the new and emerging technologies that are available to support community nursing practice and health care. It offers the community nurse an insight into these technologies and examines best practice related to them.

Information technology (IT) is a powerful tool that supports clinicians because it can deliver clinical information quickly, consistently and in a form that can be read and understood. IT can contribute to improve health outcomes, provide seamless on-line communication across the health system and organise client-specific information from diverse, linkable databases. IT supports health service delivery across the spectrum, from clinician and consumer education to the collection of information used in planning services.

The exponential rise in health costs, particularly those associated with hospital admissions, means that an increasing range of health problems are treated in the community. Patterns of care are changing in response to the increase in chronic health problems associated with changes in population demographics, the expansion of public health interventions, technology and changing diagnostic tools and therapies. Governments are implementing strategies to reduce demand on hospitals by providing health care for frail older people and those with chronic conditions where they reside. Telehealth is seen as an integral part of this strategy and 'smart home' technology is being promoted to reduce hospital admissions for frail older people [1, 2].

The health system is made up of many disparate groups with multiple perspectives and subcultures. Each group sees things slightly differently, but they must all capture, communicate, reliably retrieve and reuse information between each other and across multiple settings [3]. These differences affect the introduction of widespread health-sector computing and although health care informatics has been undergoing rapid change and development funding has begun to flow, research funding has not kept pace.

In this chapter, every attempt has been made to include published guidelines on each topic. However, accessibility to many guidelines is restricted, and in fact some of the literature suggests that they may not be required [4, 5]. This chapter supplements guidelines that are accessible with a compilation of reported best practice based on the limited available research, integrated with well-considered concept papers. Most of these have not undergone the extensive evaluation required by validated guidelines.

Definitions

Hand-held technologies are a category of pocket-sized computing devices that integrate miniaturised computer technology. They include smart phones,[1] wearable computers, high-end personal digital assistants (Pads) or small tablet computers. Most can connect to other computers via the internet, using wireless technology (Bluetooth) or infrared interfaces.

Laptop or *notebook computers* are small mobile computers with their weight and cost depending on their size, incorporated hardware, materials used and other factors. Most now perform the same functions as desktop computers. They are miniaturised and optimised for mobile use and efficient power consumption. Laptops have a touch pad or a pointing stick in addition to a built-in keyboard for input. There are several variants but the most common are:

- *Tablet* computers are a variation of the laptop. They have touch-screen interfaces and writing and sometimes voice recognition software. Data are collected by means of a stylus/digital pen or fingertip rather than a keyboard or mouse.
- *Convertible* notebooks are perhaps the most popular form of tablet computers. They look like a laptop and are usually heavier and larger than a tablet. The display is attached by a swivel hinge joint to the base, which enables 180° rotation. The display folds on top of the keyboard providing a flat writing surface. There is a sliding design that locks into place to provide the laptop mode.

Telehealth is the use of telecommunications to provide health information and services, that is, a health-related activity carried out at a distance [6]. *Telenursing* is a subdiscipline of telehealth.

Videophones are telephones that communicate in both audio and video between individuals. Although of some use in health care, they are generally expensive and disappointing. Web-cam conferencing has the principles of videophone and is much more cost effective.

Wireless (WiFi): There are several types of wireless connectivity that can be used: Infrared and Bluetooth[2] offer short-range or local-area communication, while CDPD- and CDMA-type standards enable long-range or wide-area communication.

---

[1] *Smartphones* are full-featured mobile phone and personal organiser with added personal computer (PC)-like functionality. Most smartphones have an in-built camera, support email and some can install applications for enhanced data processing and connectivity.

[2] *Bluetooth* is an industrial specification for wireless personal area networks (PANs). Bluetooth provides a way to connect and exchange information between devices such as mobile phones, laptops, PCs, printers and digital cameras over globally unlicensed short-range radiofrequency.

Mobile computing

One of the biggest challenges for consumers and health care providers at the point of care is the limited flow of essential health information associated with paper-based health records and office processes. Community nurses are constantly challenged in their need for current, reliable and accurate information at the point of care and often have to make decisions based on incomplete patient data. They have little access to current guidelines or evidence-based resources and the body of health care literature changes so quickly that it is impossible to keep abreast of the changes [1]. The potential consequence of this is that nurses make decisions based on incomplete client data and without access to current guidelines or evidence-based resources.

Mobile computing incorporates wireless connectivity and can deliver timely and complete information from centrally located clinical systems. It can also provide timely access to decision support systems, clinical guidelines and evidence-based resources at the point of care. RSS (really simple syndication) feeds that make it possible for nurses to keep up with the latest literature in an automated manner are also available.

General guidelines for purchasing mobile devices

- Understand your need.
- Know and understand what is on the market.
- Evaluate your business and clinical processes.
- Look for opportunities to streamline those processes.
- Map/measure/understand your current workflow and workflow issues.

General guidelines for evaluating mobile products

- Know the features but do not be blinded by them – not all 'bells and whistles' are always necessary or useful.
- More expensive is not necessarily better.
- Check how much the software will assist with replicating your workflow processes.
- Check whether the software does things you do not expect/want and whether you are paying for this.
- Check how much tailoring is required.
- Check how staff will react and whether they will see technology as a threat or an opportunity.
- Consider the occupational health and safety issues associated with any devices. A mobile product may be considered lightweight until a nurse needs to carry it for long periods of time.
- Consider storage options, particularly when a community nurse is working from diverse settings such as a car.

Hand-held computing guide

Hand-held devices have long been promoted as enabling devices for clinicians and as the 'Holy Grail' of point-of-care data entry. Many organisations promote these technologies as part of their clinical IT strategy because they enable timely access to clinical information and facilitate communication across healthcare.

PDAs, Pocket PCs and Smartphones are the major classes of hand-held computers but these are rapidly evolving and their functions are converging. The major difference between the three classes is the operating system (OS) used and the focus: PDAs use the Palm OS, while the Pocket PC uses a Windows environment. Both of these are data centric; that is, they are centred on the manipulation of data.

Mobile phone technology has gradually changed and with added functionality has moved into the hand-held space. It is voice centric and uses the Symbian or Lynux OS. It has phone, personal computer and data-processing capabilities. Microsoft now incorporates Smartphone technology into its Pocket PC OS and the boundaries between these devices have become very blurred.

There are numerous programs written specifically for health clinicians and others have been modified to suit these 'miniature' environments. The Palm OS probably has more of these at this time. Programs such as MIMS for PDA and various drug programmes have been modified as have literature databases. The National Library of Medicine for instance offers its abstract database PubMed for this environment.

Functionality

Hand-held computers are small and easy to carry [7] and now perform similar functions which are summarised in Table 23.1. Most clinicians use the basic PDA functions (marked with '*' in Table 23.1). Most community nurses access clinical software including drug databases, medical reference, client care and client tracking [8, 9].

Several models incorporate global positioning systems (GPS) with street maps, verbal directions and trip-and-time meters, which are all very useful and time-saving functions for community health workers. GPS can also be used as a safety device for tracking nurses' whereabouts when mobile in cars. All are battery powered and easily

Table 23.1 Functions of hand-held computers.

Calculator*	Spreadsheet
Calendar*	Web browsing
Address book*	Global positioning system
Notes*	Email
Reminder lists*	Internet access
Address book*	Video recording
Clock*	Portable media player, e.g. MP3
Word processing	Bar coding
Some models video capable	Radiofrequency identification (RFID) readers
Phone	Camera

transported. Data can be uploaded through a docking station or via a wireless link or modem to the host computer.

Performance issues

- Most have wireless limitations specifically related to rural and remote areas [10].
- Small display size: some say they are difficult to read [11, 12] particularly for an ageing workforce [13, 14]; others report them as clear and easy to read [7].
- Input mechanisms difficult/limited [13, 14] and slow [9].
- Insufficient processing power [14].
- Insufficient storage requiring frequent synchronisation [11–13] especially in the community [13].
- Easily dropped, lost or stolen [14].
- Screen damage – as this is also the input device.
- Ease of navigation [13, 14].
- The screen's pixels affect how much text can be read at one time [4].
- Most internet browsers have limitations although Internet Explorer for Pocket PC is fairly functional.
- The OS determines what software can be used and thus its usefulness [15].

Data input

Hand-held computers have touch screens, with pen-based data entry and/or small built-in keyboards for input, although portable external keyboards, both virtual and real, are available. Some keyboards are small and are not fully functional; others fold to the same size as the hand-held computer but unfold into a full-size keyboard [15]. The virtual laser keyboard is a useful technology but is in its infancy and at this time tends to be error prone.

The more sophisticated (and more expensive) Pocket PCs have writing recognition and intelligence. (They learn over time.) The inbuilt keyboard is small and not generally comfortable and it requires a stylus to point to the letters on the board – fingertips are generally too big. Using systems in this way can be laborious, error-prone and sometimes slow. Handwriting recognition is improving but remains somewhat hit and miss. Generally, community nurses find that using the pen is easier when entering data into structured fields, rather than handwriting [16]. An evaluation of the use of hand-held computers in bedside nursing care found that community nurses:

- Were frustrated at having to learn how to write for the handwriting recognition software
- Regarded data accuracy as poor
- Complained that handwriting was not always recognised by the software
- Could not write continuously as on paper
- Found that the pause for each letter to be recognised interrupted the flow of documentation
- Felt the process would be too slow for them to use an interface that used a pen for textual data entry [16]

Download and synchronisation

Pocket PCs exchange data via download on demand, where data are obtained in real time using wireless connectivity or downloaded periodically by synchronisation [2]. Data synchronisation ensures that the user has accessed the same information as is on the host computer. Synchronisation by short-range wireless communication or 'beaming' is also possible. This process required users to be in close proximity (2–3 m) and because of this is being surpassed by wireless. Download on demand enables members of the care team to share data with each other at any time and then pass on the most current data to the next shift quickly, accurately and comprehensively.

Security issues

Hand-held computers store large amounts of data; they are portable, concealable and easily stolen [17]. They have basic access security, but this is usually not sufficient because many publicly available programs can bypass it. Some vendors provide enhanced password protection and cryptographic standards such as Blowfish, IDEA, SAFER-SK and 3DES [18].

All hand-held computers are susceptible to the introduction of viruses, but to date the Palm OS with its multiple-level protections has been relatively safe. However, Windows-CE-based hand-held computers are vulnerable to the thousands of viruses that target the Windows environment and Microsoft products in general.

User satisfaction

Nurses' perceptions of and satisfaction with hand-held computers seems to vary depending on their exposure to the technology. Nurses who are not familiar with such technology regard their introduction quite differently from nurses who are regular computer users [14]. However, hand-held computers are seen to enhance productivity and the quality of client care and service [14]. In addition:

- PDAs are not good for writing a lengthy client history – a full keyboard is faster [11, 14].
- Writing observations on PDAs is faster than finding the paper charts or an available PC [14].
- Displays are clear and easier to read if they have good resolution and colour [7].
- Built-in cameras and phones are useful [15]. For example photos of wounds can be compared daily to judge the rate of healing and the client can send vital signs measurements via email to their clinician [16].
- Resolution is not high enough for reading some diagnostic images.

Portable computer guide

Laptops, notebooks and tablets are often used by community nurses and as point-of-care devices in institutions. Their relevant features have been described in the definitions presented earlier.

Functionality

Laptops and notebooks have many of the features of a PC. They are portable, have an integrated liquid crystal display (LCD), full-sized keyboard, a pointing device(s), WiFI (wireless), infrared ports, modem and network cards. Feature to feature they are more expensive than PCs. Notebooks are larger and heavier than laptops, mostly because of additional features. However, they are becoming smaller and lighter and the boundaries between the two have blurred.

Tablets may or may not have all of the features of laptops and notebooks. However, the measures of advantages and disadvantages of Tablet PCs are subjective because what appeals to one user may frustrate another. Generally tablets cost more and may have less power than conventional laptops. They may not have in-built compact disc (CD) drives or the larger applications found on more powerful machines; while this reduces costs it may be problematic for the user because of the ubiquitous nature of the CD and functionality of the larger programs. Again this is changing as the technology advances and large memory sticks become the portable data transport device of choice.

Although not as easily transported as hand-held computers, mobile computers are still very portable. They are made even more convenient by mounting them on specially designed trolleys for point-of-care access in community nursing centres/rooms.

Performance issues

Historically, mobile computers have been less powerful than desktop PCs because they prioritise energy efficiency, portability and compactness over absolute performance, whereas it is the converse for desktops. Tablets have some specific characteristics such as:

- More natural input by handwriting. However, handwriting may be slower than typing.
- Gesture (moving the stylus in special patterns over the screen) recognition which increases efficiency. Many applications can be programmed to respond specifically to certain gestures.
- Note taking or drawing diagrams increase productivity. Notes can be automatically searched if handwriting recognition is implemented.
- Because the screen is the input device, Tablet PCs are at higher risk of screen damage. They are handled more than conventional laptops, yet are built on conventional notebook frames.
- Some tablet digitisers cannot keep up if the user writes too quickly, reducing the fluidity of the lines the computer captures.
- The signal from the pen may become distorted near the edges of the screen [19].

Security issues

Mobile computers are portable, store large amounts of information [17] and may be easily stolen. Therefore, the security issues discussed for hand-held computers are applicable here. However along with encryption, passwords and biometric scanning, laptops can use virtual private network (VPN) technology to protect information being transmitted over the internet. This allows users to securely access the resources on their office network through the internet from geographically dispersed areas [20]. Public key infrastructure (PKI) provides encryption and digital signing of messages, enabling the secure transfer of emails.

User satisfaction with mobile computing

In most studies, mobile computers have been well received [7, 8, 14, 21]. Overall user satisfaction has been similar for PDAs and laptops except for the writing of client notes [22]. Some of the reasons for this may be that:

- Responsiveness of hand-held computers is better than laptops or tablets and more suited to the continuous interruptions and lengthy shifts of clinical practice [14].
- Using a PDA takes nurses significantly less time to look for vital signs measurements, enter fluid balance measurements and enter a daily assessment than on a laptop [22]. However, it takes significantly less time to read a paragraph, enter a set of vital signs and write on a laptop [22].
- The horizontal orientation of Tablet PCs and the small size of PDAs do not interrupt line of sight, which is important in therapeutic relationships.

Guidelines for safe use of IT

- Keep computers protected from malicious attack and vulnerabilities. Routinely scan them with up-to-date virus and spyware detection programs (such as AVG) and install a strong firewall.
- Watch for changes in the computer's OS.
- Always scan for viruses after installation of new programs.
- Before backing up hard drives use a virus scan to check the system for viruses.
- Treat public domain and freeware software with caution.
- Use volume labels on all discs and be aware if changes are made.
- Authenticate source when swapping files.
- Institute frequent backup procedures.

Guidelines for exchanging health data

Electronic health data exchange must adhere to security and confidentiality standards that include:

- Data encryption or the translation of data into a secret code. (An encrypted file can only be read if you have access to a secret key or password that enables you to decrypt it.)
- User authentication or identifying an individual, usually based on a username and password. In other words, it ensures that the individual is who he or she claims to be, but says nothing about the access rights of the individual.

- User authorisation. Gives an individual access rights to various system objects or information based on their identity.
- Audit logs. Audit logs or audit trails records who did what to what, when, the duration and on which area of the system. In principle it is possible to detect and record every keystroke of any user at any workstation or device.

All electronic health information on mobile devices should be encrypted and access password protected to prevent access from unauthorised people. During any synchronisation or wireless data transfer, suitable user/device authentication should be required before transmitting data and be encrypted during transmission. An audit trail is essential. Beaming is relatively safe as it requires close physical proximity (2 m or less) to the beaming device and the recipient must accept incoming beams. There can be no unsolicited beam; that is, a device cannot access another device without the recipient granting permission.

Guidelines for using passwords

Passwords should be a word or phrase with meaning for the user but mixed up by adding symbols or numbers to increase its security. A password should:

- Be changed regularly
- Combine mixed-case alphabetic characters, numbers and symbols – for example a strong password would be M3ht?rt6, while a weak password would be Ann25
- Be easy to remember – so you do not have to write it down
- *Never* be shared
- Have at least eight characters

Guidelines for email communications between clinicians and clients

Email communication should be treated the same as any other correspondence with clients. The majority of the following guidelines are taken from the General Practice Computing Group Australia [23] and the American Medical Informatics Association guidelines [24].

- Reduce risk by establishing clear policies and procedures before undertaking any online communication [25].
- Provide an information sheet on how you use email.
- Set up password and encryption on all desktops that receive emails from clients.
- Treat all emails as official correspondence.
- Add all emails to the client record – the client should also keep a copy [24].
- Establish turnaround time for messages – consider whether to use email for urgent matters.
- Inform clients about privacy issues and that messages will be included in their record.
- Establish types of transactions and sensitivity of the subject matter permitted over email.
- Check for accuracy and appropriateness of language before sending.

- Include the full text of previous emails with your reply to ensure that you and your client are in accord.
- Follow up with the client to clarify details.
- Ask the client to put their full name in the body of the email.
- Ask clients to state the nature of the transaction in the subject line of the message so that it can be filtered (for example 'Friday visit' or 'leg ulcer').
- Ask the client to notify a change to their email address.
- Ensure that the community nurse and client use the 'read receipt' and 'automatic reply' functions of the email system.
- Establish a system for checking the inboxes of absent staff, or set the system to automatically forward their incoming messages. Request and document client consent.

Computing best practice

Best practice for computing use is to:

- *Never* share passwords – you are responsible for any data written in your name.
- Read and comply with the institution's policies.
- Know your IT support and their role in information security.
- Report information security incidents.
- Recognise when your computer may be compromised.
- Implement security recommendations.
- Avoid activities that may compromise security, like replying to unsolicited email.
- Log out of accounts when you are finished.
- Remain updated with computer user technology by completing IT education.

Telehealth and telenursing

Nurses have been using the telephone to communicate with colleagues and clients for years, so telenursing is nothing new. What has changed is access to more sophisticated technologies that enable different models of care and services. Telehealth is beneficial where distance and a lack of health practitioners dictate the type of service delivered [6.] The exchange of information may be local, national or international or:

- Client with practitioner
- Practitioner with practitioner
- Client with client (for mutual support)
- Practitioner or client accessing sources of health information [6]

Telehealth interactions require equipment to capture, transmit and display the information. However, the quality of communication is largely dependent on how comfortable the practitioner is with the technology, their communication skills and the appropriateness of the clinical application to the telehealth setting [26].

Functionality

Determining the suitability of systems is dependent on need, which varies from one application to another:

Audio

The most common audio is the transmission of speech, for example in the use of teletriage or electronic stethoscopes to transmit heart or breathing sounds [6, 7].

Text

Analog messages can be transmitted via fax but digital transmission produces better-quality data. Computer files are already digital. Printed documents can be digitised using a scanner or a digital camera and then transmitted as still images [6].

Still images

Transmitted for diagnosis, management and education. Low-cost digital cameras can capture good-quality images. Flatbed scanners can produce digital images of charts, ECG (electrocardiographic) traces, wounds [27] or X-rays. However, for high-quality diagnostic images the equipment can be costly [5].

Videoconference

Groups or individuals interact during real-time clinical consultations. Can include centres such as nursing homes or assisted living facilities [28]. Minimum equipment specifications, etiquette and the room set-up are important [25].

Remote monitoring

Sensors capture and transmit biometric data. They can be used for remote intensive care units, pacemakers and monitoring and can enable clients to maintain independent lifestyles [21, 28]. For client self-monitoring, the technology must be easy to learn and use with well-structured graphical design, have intuitive navigation, be low cost and error resistant [29].

Networked programs

Link tertiary care hospitals and clinics with outlying clinics and community health centres in rural or suburban areas [28].

Point to point

Private networks are used by hospitals and clinics that deliver services to independent medical service providers at ambulatory care sites and within the community nursing setting [28, 30].

Web-based ehealth client service sites

Provide direct consumer outreach and services over the internet [28, 30].

Guidelines for infrastructure

- Record or log start time, end time, technical problems, user problems and problem resolution [27].
- The quality of communications must be sufficiently high. Inadequate infrastructure hampers many telehealth projects, especially in rural areas [6, 27].
- Regular preventative maintenance may include equipment checks, software updates, spare parts on hand, interoperability checks and pre-session tests.
- Equipment should be interoperable; in other words, it should have the ability to exchange information and to use the information that has been exchanged. It should adhere to standards for data exchange, remote management, audio quality and video streaming [2]. Such standards make it possible to:
  - Easily exchange information
  - Adapt new applications to existing systems without undue effort and expense
  - Ensure availability, integrity and confidentiality of information
  - Accommodate the wide variety of technological infrastructure in different clinical settings

Performance

Reliable technology that delivers many years of failure-free operation is critical. Analogue telephone transmission is inappropriate for many telehealth purposes because noise on the lines and low bandwidth may degrade the signal [6]. Digital signal transmission on the other hand can be transmitted for long distances without degradation. Bandwidths need to be much higher and satellite delivery of the signal is available [6].

Legal and security issues

Telenursing presents regulatory challenges and possible legal issues that have yet to be fully addressed [31]. There is the potential for a nurse or midwife to participate in cross-border nursing or midwifery practice and, in some cases, provide services in a state/territory/country where they are not registered to practise [30, 31].

User issues in telenursing

- Policies with respect to legal coverage and payment for telenursing services must be addressed.
- Education that specifically addresses communicative behaviours in telehealth must be provided [26].

- Although the literature is varied on their value [4, 5], specific practice guidelines in telemedicine triage should be discussed [26] and developed by the service organisation.

Guidelines for telenursing

It is essential that clients cannot be viewed or heard without their permission and that photography is not used without informed consent. The following excerpt from Australian Nursing and Midwifery Council (2007) targets clinicians. (The full document is available at http://www.anmc.org.au/.) These guidelines say that nurses and midwives practising telehealth:

- Have a duty to provide their full name, qualification and registration status, including the state/territory in which they are registered, to consumers of telehealth services. They should also supply the name(s) of the regulatory authority(s) with which they are registered.
- Should obtain informed consent to the telehealth process before proceeding and inform consumers of the process, including other persons/professionals who may be participating or present in the telehealth consultation, the use of telehealth technology and the purpose and use for which the information is destined.
- Must comply with government and institutional policies relating to privacy, confidentiality, informed consent, information security and documentation during the provision of telehealth care.
- Are required to document all interactions during the telehealth consultation, including the caller and for whom the advice is being sought (child, self or other), the details of the caller, the time of the call, the reason for the advice being sought (as described by the caller), the advice given and details of any referrals for further care. Consent must be sought from the caller should there be a need to transmit information to another health professional. Any information transmitted to another health professional should be followed up to ensure that it is received in an appropriate time frame either at the intended destination or by the intended recipient.
- Advice given should be based on evidence-based guidelines, developed, where possible, utilising the National Health and Medical Research Council guidelines process for the development of clinical practice guidelines.

Inclusion and exclusion guidelines must describe clients who are eligible and ineligible for the service and be made available to community nurses [27, 32]. Significant factors determining the possible use of telenursing include primary diagnosis, number of interventions, patient age and type of intervention [33]. Among the conditions most amenable to telenursing care are management of patients with acute exacerbation of chronic conditions, at-risk elderly people living alone at home and care interventions such as those required for support, education or review [34]. Other considerations for inclusion and exclusion criteria may be as follows:

Client enrolment and consent [32] should be written and provided to nurses.

- Written consent should be obtained from the client and placed in the client record.
- Clients should be screened for eligibility during a face-to-face encounter. A comprehensive client and caregiver assessment must be conducted [32].

Client/caregiver education [32]. Both the client and caregiver should be provided with written and verbal instruction on using the technology. They should practice and demonstrate competence in using the technology.

- Education should also include proper handling, storage and operation of the technology.
- Clients require instruction on managing emergency situations, if they have the capacity to do so.

Performance improvement must include client satisfaction [33]. This can be determined via verbal or written feedback and should relate to:

- Type of services (e.g. bathing, medication, physical therapy and consultation)
- System characteristics (e.g. set-up time, quality of image and quality of vocal communication)
- Changes in service use (e.g. the number of visits before and after using telemedicine)
- How satisfied the client was with the service (perhaps using a 1–5 Likert scale)

Further considerations

The type of technology should be based on the client's clinical needs, their functional ability to use it and the availability and cost-effectiveness of the technology to meet their needs. A plan of action for equipment failure must be instituted and communicated to clients.

Policies and procedures should be developed regarding equipment quality control standards, storage, cleaning and maintenance.

Ageing in place technology

Ageing in place technology is a relatively new concept that will impact on nursing in the community [1]. The issues already discussed cover individual device but IT also needs to be considered as a whole package to be implemented in a client's home. This will require nurses to adjust to different modes of service delivery driven by the need for further cost containment and patient demands for a greater role in shared decision making [34].

Electronic enhanced assistive technologies or 'smart' technologies are embedded with IT/intelligence; they are interactive and adaptive [34]. They adjust to the user or learn about them and communicate with humans and other technologies [35, 36]. They provide the user with control of furniture, the bed and the ambient environment and facilitate the operation of entertainment and communication equipment. Telehealth supplements these technologies, connecting the household to external parties, such as remote caregivers, community nurses or alarm centres. Telecare in smart homes monitors crucial health parameters to provide 'early warnings' of health problems and enhances the capacity of care providers to respond to emergency situations occurring in the home environment [37, 38].

Wireless sensor networks consist of spatially distributed autonomous devices using sensors to cooperatively monitor physical or environmental conditions such as temperature, sound or, more importantly, for a community practitioner, motion [39]. These can alert for falls or when a person is mobilising, going out the door, when a bed is wet, lights and stoves are left on and so forth.

Summary

The implementation of IT and other emerging nursing technologies will continue to change the way health care workers deliver client care [40] particularly as the population ages. IT is the tool of a modern health system but nursing must be cognizant of the issues associated with its use. The guidelines in this chapter are eclectic and have been complied using evidence derived from a variety of disciplines. They should provide the reader with a sound basis for procuring and using new and emerging technologies in their practice.

Useful resources

The American Telemedicine Association. *Telemedicine, Telehealth, and Health Information Technology*. The American Telemedicine Association, Washington, 2006.
A comprehensive report found at www.americantelemed.org/news/policy_issues/HIT_Paper.pdf
Journal of Mobile Informatics. Available at http://www.pdacortex.com
Online journal offering medical PDA product reviews, discussion forums, documents and software
MD on TAP Medline for hand-held devices available at http://archive.nlm.nih.gov/proj/pmot/pmot.php
PDA cortex available at http://www.rnpalm.com/software_palm.htm
A large collection of medical and nursing software for Palm
Vertical PDA network available at http://www.pdamd.com
Resources dedicated to the promotion and education of health care professionals on the use of mobile and wireless technology

References

1. Essen, A. and Conrick, M. (2007) Visions and realities: Developing smart homes for seniors in Sweden. *Electronic Journal of Health Informatics*, 2(1).
2. Soar, J., Yuginovich, T. and Whittaker, F. (2007) Reducing avoidable hospital admissions of the frail elderly using intelligent referrals. *Electronic Journal of Health Informatics*, 2(1).
3. Conrick, M., Walker, S., Scott, P. and Frean, I. (2006) Health information interchange, in M. Conrick (ed.) *Health Informatics: Transforming Healthcare with Technology*. Thompson/Social Science, Melbourne, pp. 20–38.
4. Rutenberg, C.D. (2000) What do we really know about telephone triage? *Journal of Emergency Nursing*, 26(1), 76–8.
5. Simonsen-Anderson, S. (2002) Safe and sound. *Nursing Management*, 33(6), 41–3.
6. Edirippulige, S. and Wootton, R. (2006) Telehealth and communication, in M. Conrick (ed.) *Health Informatics: Transforming Healthcare with Technology*. Thompson/Social Science Press, Melbourne, pp. 406–16.

7. Lapinsky, S.E., Weshler, J., Mehta, S., Varkul, M., Hallett, D. and Stewart, T.E. (2004) Handheld computers in critical care. *Journal of the American Medical Informatics Association*, 10, 139–49.

8. De Groote, S. and Doranski, M. (2004) The use of personal digital assistants in the health sciences: Results of a survey. *Journal Medical Library Association*, 92(3), 341–9.

9. Lewis, J. (March–April 2003) Personal data assistants: Using new technology to enhance nursing practice. *American Journal Maternal Child Nursing*, 28(2), 6–71.

10. Afrin, L. and Daniels, M. (2001) Palm OS-based access to the enterprise clinical data repository and clinical documentation assistant. *Proceedings/Amia Symposium ... Annual Symposium*, 848.

11. Embi, P.J. (2001) Information at hand: Using handheld computers in medicine. *Cleveland Clinic Journal of Medicine*, 68(10), 840–42.

12. Ebell, M. and Rovner, D. (2000) Information in the palm of your hand. *Journal of Family Practice*, 49(3), 243–51.

13. McManus, B. (2000) Mobile computers in a community NHS Trust: Is this a relevant context and environment for their use? *Personal Technologies*, 4(2), 96–101.

14. McAlearney, A.S., Schweikhart, S.B. and Medow, M.A. (15 May 2004) Doctors' experience with handheld computers in clinical practice: Qualitative study. *British Medical Association*, 328(7449), 1162.

15. Al-Ubaydli, M. (15 May 2004) Handheld computers. *British Medical Association*, 328(7449), 1181–4.

16. Young, P., Leung, R., Ho, L. and McGhee, S. (2001) An evaluation of the use of hand-held computers for bedside nursing care. *International Journal Medical Informatics*, 62(2–3), 189–93.

17. Carroll, A.E., Saluja, S. and Tarczy-Hornoch, P. (2002) The implementation of a personal digital assistant (PDA) based patient record and charting system: Lessons learned. *Proceedings/Amia Symposium ... Annual Symposium*, 111(5).

18. Yale University IT Department (2007) *Mobile Technology and Security*. Available at http://www.yale.edu/its/security (viewed 21 February 2007).

19. Tablet Computer (2006). Available at http://en.wikipedia.org/wiki/Tablet_computer (viewed 14 December 2006).

20. VPNS (2004) *Virtual Private Network Security*. Available at www.infosec.gov.hk (viewed 30 November 2007).

21. Schreier, G., Kollmann, A., Kramer, M., Messmer, J., Hochgatterer, A. and Kastner, P. (2004) Mobile phone based user interface concept for health data acquisition at home, in *Computers Helping People with Special Needs*. Springer, Berlin, pp. 29–36.

22. Rodriguez, N.J., Borges, J.A., Soler, Y., Murillo, V., Colon-Rivera, C.R., Sands, D.Z., *et al.* (2003) PDA vs. laptop: A comparison of two versions of a nursing documentation application, in Organizing and Program Committee (eds) *Computer-Based Medical Systems, 2003 Proceedings 16th IEEE Symposium*. New York, pp. 201–6.

23. General Practice Computing Group (2005) *Emails Between You and Your Patients*. Available at www.gpcg.org.au/ (viewed 24 April 2007).

24. Kane, M., Daniel, Z. and Sands, M. (1998) Guidelines for the clinical use of electronic mail with patients. *Journal of the American Medical Informatics Association*, 5(1), 104–11.

25. Loane, M. and Wootton, R. (2002) A review of guidelines and standards for telemedicine. *Journal of Telemedicine and Telecare*, 8(2), 63–71.

26. Hogenbirk, J.C., Brockway, P.D., Finley, J., Jennett, P., Yeo, M., Parker-Taillon D, *et al.* (2006) Framework for Canadian telehealth guidelines: Summary of the environmental scan. *Journal of Telemedicine and Telecare*, 12(2), 64.

27. Kinsella, A. (2000) Learning home telehealth: New opportunities. *Home Healthcare Nurse*, 18(8), 507–11.

28. The American Telemedicine Association (2006) *Telemedicine, Telehealth and Health. Information Technology*. The American Telemedicine Association, Washington.

29. Schreier, G., Kollmann, A., Kramer, M., Messmer, J., Hochgatterer, A. and Kastner, P. (2004) Mobile phone based user interface concept for health data acquisition at home, in *Lecture Notes in Computer Science, ICCHP Wien*. Springer, New York, pp. 29–36.

30. Dillon, E., Loermans, J., Davis, D. and Xu, C. (2005) Evaluation of the western Australian Department of Health telehealth project. *Journal of Telemedicine and Telecare*, 11(Suppl 2), 19.

31. Australian Nursing and Midwifery Council (2007) *Guidelines for Nurses and Midwives on Telehealth Practice*. Available at http://www.anmc.org.au/position_statements_ guidelines/guidelines.php (viewed 6 November 2007).

32. Britton, B. (2003) Telehealth clinical guidelines: Developed by the American telemedicine association. *Home Healthcare Nurse*, 21(10), 703–6.

33. Allen, A., Doolittle, G.C., Boysen, C.D., Komoroski, K., Wolf, M., Collins. B., *et al.* (1999) An analysis of the suitability of home health visits for telemedicine. *Journal of Telemedicine and Telecare*, 5(2), 90–96.

34. Black, S., Andersen, K., Loane, M.A. and Wootton, R. (2001) The potential of telemedicine for home nursing in Queensland. *Journal of Telemedicine and Telecare*, 7(4), 199–205.

35. Junestrand, S. (1998) *IT och bostaden, ett arkiterktoniskt perspektiv*. Available at http://www.arch.kth.se/'junestrand/licrapport/tekniklicrapport.pdf (viewed 2 April 2007).

36. Peterson, F. (2000) Smarta hem och smarta ting. Hur datorerna tar plats I världen och förändrar vårt vardagliga liv. CID rapport.

37. Barlow, J. and Venables, T. (2004) Will technological innovation create the true lifetime home? *Housing Studies*, 19(5), 795–810.

38. Hagberg, J.-E. (2004) Old people, new and old artefacts: Technology for later life, in B.-M. Öberg (ed.) *Changing Worlds and the Ageing Subject*. Ashgate, Aldershot.

39. Hong, D. and Woo, W. (2005) Wear-UCAM: A toolkit for wearable computing, in S. Eea (ed.) *The First Korea/Japan Joint Workshop on Ubiquitous Computing & Networking Systems*. Korea, pp. 1047–57.

40. Conrick, M. (2005) Nursing informatics, in R. Funnell, G. Koutoukidis and K. Lawrence (eds) *Tabbner's Nursing Care: Theory and Practice*, 4th edition. Churchill Livingstone, Melbourne, pp. 248–52.

Index

Printed in the United States
By Bookmasters